AF556747

Instructional Course Lectures Hip Volume 2

Edited by
Craig J. Della Valle, MD
Associate Professor of Orthopaedic Surgery
Director, Adult Reconstructive Fellowship
Rush University Medical Center
Chicago, Illinois

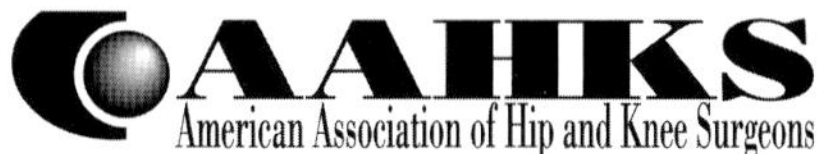

Developed with support from
American Association of Hip and Knee Surgeons

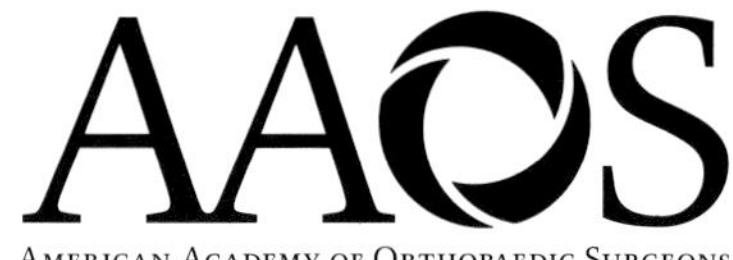

Published by the
American Academy
of Orthopaedic Surgeons
6300 North River Road
Rosemont, IL 60018

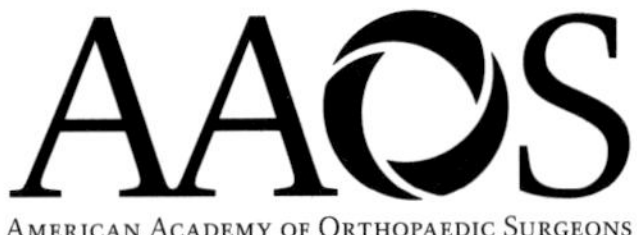

First Edition

6300 North River Road
Rosemont, IL 60018

ISBN 978-1-62552-099-9
Printed in the USA

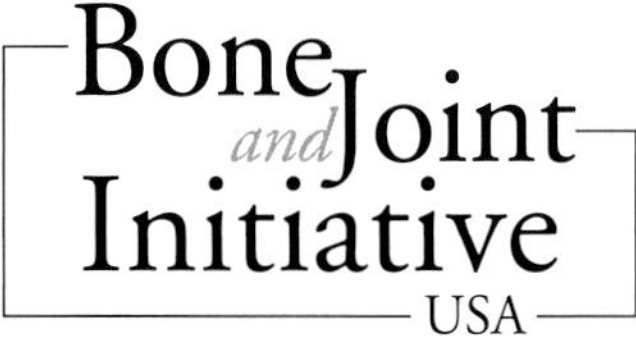

Editorial Board

---

*Dr. Della Valle or an immediate family member serves as a paid consultant to Biomet, Convatec, and Smith & Nephew; has stock or stock options held in CD Diagnostics; has received research or institutional support from Smith & Nephew and Stryker; and serves as a board member, owner, officer, or committee member of the American Association of Hip and Knee Surgeons, the Arthritis Foundation, and The Knee Society.

Contributors*

David J. Allen, MBChB, FRCSEd, MSc
Department of Orthopaedics
Ottawa General
Ontario, Canada

Jeffrey O. Anglen, MD, FACS
Professor and Chairman
Department of Orthopaedics
Indiana University
Indianapolis, Indiana

David D. Aronsson, MD
Professor
Department of Orthopaedics and Rehabilitation
University of Vermont College of Medicine
Burlington, Vermont

Robert L. Barrack, MD
Charles and Joanne Knight Distinguished Professor of Orthopaedic Surgery
Washington University School of Medicine
St. Louis, Missouri

Michael R. Baumgaertner, MD
Professor
Chief, Orthopaedic Trauma Service
Orthopaedic Department
Yale University School of Medicine
New Haven, Connecticut

Paul E. Beaulé, MD, FRCSC
Associate Professor
Head, Adult Reconstruction
Department of Orthopaedic Surgery
University of Ottawa
Ottawa, Ontario, Canada

Keith R. Berend, MD
Associate, Joint Implant Surgeons
Clinical Associate Professor
Department of Orthopedics
The Ohio State University
New Albany, Ohio

Gert J. Breur, DVM, PhD, DACVS
Professor of Small Animal Orthopaedics and Neurosurgery
Department of Veterinary Clinical Services
Purdue University
West Lafayette, Indiana

John J. Callaghan, MD
Lawrence and Marilyn Dorr Chair
Department of Orthopaedics and Rehabilitation
University of Iowa
Iowa City, Iowa

Ryan Carr, MD
Resident, Department of Orthopaedics
University of Illinois
Chicago, Illinois

Isabelle Catelas, PhD
Associate Professor and Canada Research Chair (Tier II)
Mechanical Engineering
Department of Surgery
University of Ottawa
Ottawa, Ontario, Canada

Charles R. Clark, MD
Michael Bonfiglio Professor of Orthopaedics and Rehabilitation
Department of Orthopaedics and Rehabilitation
University of Iowa
Iowa City, Iowa

John C. Clohisy, MD
Associate Professor, Co-Chief
Adult Reconstructive Surgery
Barnes-Jewish Hospital at Washington University School of Medicine
St. Louis, Missouri

Craig J. Della Valle, MD
Associate Professor of Orthopaedic Surgery
Director, Adult Reconstructive Fellowship
Rush University Medical Center
Chicago, Illinois

**The information listed for each contributor is his or her affiliation at the time of publication of the most recent chapter or commentary in this volume.*

Douglas A. Dennis, MD
Assistant Clinical Professor
University of Colorado Health Sciences Center
Colorado Joint Replacement
Denver, Colorado

Kyle F. Dickson, MD, MBA
Professor, Department of Orthopaedic Surgery
University of Texas Medical School
Chief of Trauma, Memorial Hermann Hospital
Houston, Texas

Clive P. Duncan, MD, MSc, FRCSC
Professor, Division of Lower Limb Reconstruction and Oncology
Department of Orthopaedics
University of British Columbia
Vancouver, British Columbia, Canada

Andrew Dutton, MD, FRCS
Clinical Fellow
Department of Orthopaedic Surgery
Massachusetts General Hospital
Boston, Massachusetts

Kenneth A. Egol, MD
Vice Chairman, Associate Professor
New York University Hospital for Joint Diseases
New York, New York

Jill A. Erickson, PA-C
Physician Assistant
Department of Orthopaedics
University of Utah
Salt Lake City, Utah

Richard J. Friedman, MD, FRCSC
Clinical Professor of Orthopaedic Surgery
Medical University of South Carolina
Charleston, South Carolina

Kishor Gandhi, MD, MPH
Senior Resident
Department of Anesthesiology
Thomas Jefferson University Hospital
Philadelphia, Pennsylvania

Reinhold Ganz, MD
Professor and Chair Emeritus
Orthopaedics Department
Inselspital, University of Bern
Bern, Switzerland

Donald S. Garbuz, MD, MHSc, FRCSC
Associate Professor, Division of Lower Limb Reconstruction and Oncology
Department of Orthopaedics
University of British Columbia
Vancouver, British Columbia, Canada

Kevin L. Garvin, MD
Professor and Chairman
Department of Orthopaedic Surgery and Rehabilitation
University of Nebraska Medical Center
Omaha, Nebraska

Andrew H. Glassman, MD
Staff Surgeon
Department of Orthopaedic Surgery
Grant Medical Center
Columbus, Ohio

Mark H. Gonzalez, MD, MEng
Professor and Head, Department of Orthopedic Surgery
University of Illinois at Chicago
Chicago, Illinois

Steven B. Haas, MD, MPH
Chief, Knee Service
Department of Orthopaedic Surgery
Hospital for Special Surgery
New York, New York

George J. Haidukewych, MD
Academic Chairman
Chief of Orthopedic Trauma and Adult Reconstruction
Level One Orthopedics
Florida Orthopaedic Institute
University of Central Florida
Orlando, Florida

Curtis W. Hartman, MD
Assistant Professor
Department of Orthopaedic Surgery and Rehabilitation
University of Nebraska Medical Center
Omaha, Nebraska

Thomas W. Huff, MD
European Travelling Hip Society Fellow
Department of Orthopaedic Surgery
Maurice E. Müller Foundation of North America
London, Ontario, Canada

Joshua J. Jacobs, MD
Professor and Chairman
Department of Orthopaedic Surgery
Rush University Medical Center
Chicago, Illinois

William A. Jiranek, MD, FACS
Chief, Adult Reconstruction Section
Department of Orthopaedics
Virginia Commonwealth University
Richmond, Virginia

Madhav Karunakar, MD
Orthopaedic Traumatologist
Department of Orthopaedic Surgery
Carolinas Medical Center
Charlotte, North Carolina

Raymond H. Kim, MD
Orthopaedic Surgeon
Colorado Joint Replacement
Denver, Colorado

Philip J. Kregor, MD
Jeffrey W. Mast Chair in Orthopaedic Trauma and Hip Surgery
Associate Professor and Director
Vanderbilt Orthopaedic Institute
Nashville, Tennessee

Christopher M. Larson, MD
Director of Arthroscopic Hip Joint Preservation
Minnesota Orthopedic Sports Medicine Institute
Twin Cities Orthopedics
Edina, Minnesota

Michael Leunig, MD
Department of Orthopaedic Surgery
Schulthess Clinic
Zurich, Switzerland

Randall T. Loder, MD
Garceau Professor of Orthopaedic Surgery
Director of Pediatric Orthopaedics
James Whitcomb Riley Children's Hospital
Indianapolis, Indiana

Bassam A. Masri, MD, FRCSC
Professor and Chairman
Department of Orthopaedics
University of British Columbia
Vancouver, British Columbia, Canada

Toni M. McLaurin, MD
Assistant Professor
Department of Orthopaedic Surgery
New York University Hospital for Joint Diseases
New York, New York

John B. Medley, PhD, PEng
Professor, Department of Mechanical and Mechatronics Engineering
University of Waterloo
Waterloo, Ontario, Canada

William M. Mihalko, MD, PhD
Associate Professor
Campbell Clinic
Department of Orthopaedics
Chief Science Officer, InMotion Orthopaedic Research Center
Memphis, Tennessee

Berton R. Moed, MD
Professor and Chairman
Department of Orthopaedic Surgery
Saint Louis University School of Medicine
St. Louis, Missouri

Steven J. Morgan, MD
Associate Professor
University of Colorado
Department of Orthopaedics
Denver Health Medical Center
Denver, Colorado

Michael J. Morris, MD
Joint Implant Surgeons
New Albany, Ohio

Steven A. Mussett, MBChB, FRCSC
Fellow, Arthroplasty and Reconstructive Surgery
Department of Orthopaedics
The Ottawa Hospital
Ottawa, Ontario, Canada

Shahryar Noordin, MBBS, FCPS
Clinical Fellow, Division of Lower Limb Reconstruction and Oncology
Department of Orthopaedics
University of British Columbia
Vancouver, British Columbia, Canada

Javad Parvizi, MD, FRCS
Professor, Department of Orthopaedic Surgery
Thomas Jefferson University
Rothman Institute
Philadelphia, Pennsylvania

Deepan Patel, MD
Orthopaedic Surgery Resident
Department of Orthopaedic Surgery
New York University Hospital for Joint Diseases
New York, New York

Christopher E. Pelt, MD
Visiting Instructor
Department of Orthopaedics
University of Utah
Salt Lake City, Utah

Christopher L. Peters, MD
Professor and Medical Director of Adult Reconstruction and Hip Preservation
Department of Orthopaedics
University of Utah
Salt Lake City, Utah

Elizabeth Picinic, BS
Rothman Institute of Orthopaedics
Thomas Jefferson University
Philadelphia, Pennsylvania

Manny Porat, MD
Orthopaedic Resident
Department of Orthopaedics
Thomas Jefferson University Hospital
Philadelphia, Pennsylvania

Mark C. Reilly, MD
Associate Professor and Co-Chief of Orthopaedic Trauma Service
Department of Orthopaedics
New Jersey Medical School
Newark, New Jersey

Corey J. Richards, MD, MASc, FRCSC
Orthopaedic Reconstruction Fellow
Department of Orthopaedics
University of British Columbia
Vancouver, British Columbia, Canada

Richard H. Rothman, MD, PhD
Chair Emeritus
Department of Orthopaedic Surgery
Rothman Institute
Philadelphia, Pennsylvania

Harry E. Rubash, MD
Chief of Orthopaedic Surgery
Massachusetts General Hospital
Edith M. Ashley Professor
Harvard Medical School
Boston, Massachusetts

Perry L. Schoenecker, MD
Professor
Department of Orthopaedic Surgery
Washington University School of Medicine
St. Louis, Missouri

Peter F. Sharkey, MD
Professor of Orthopaedic Surgery
Jefferson Medical College
Rothman Institute
Philadelphia, Pennsylvania

Klaus A. Siebenrock, MD
Professor and Chairman
Department of Orthopaedic Surgery
University of Bern
Bern, Switzerland

Rafael J. Sierra, MD
Assistant Professor and Consultant
Department of Orthopedic Surgery
Mayo Clinic
Rochester, Minnesota

Wade R. Smith, MD
Director of Orthopaedic Surgery
Denver Health Medical Center
University of Colorado
Denver, Colorado

Scott M. Sporer, MD
Assistant Professor
Department of Orthopaedic Surgery
Rush University Medical Center
Chicago, Illinois

Benjamin M. Stronach, MD
Visiting Instructor
Department of Orthopaedics
University of Utah
Salt Lake City, Utah

Moritz Tannast, MD
Resident in Orthopaedic Surgery
Department of Orthopaedic Surgery
University of Bern
Bern, Switzerland

Thomas S. Thornhill, MD
John B. and Buckminster Brown Professor of Orthopaedics
Harvard Medical School
Chairman, Department of Orthopaedics
Brigham and Women's Hospital
Boston, Massachusetts

Paul Tornetta III, MD
Professor and Vice Chairman
Program Director, Department of Orthopaedic Surgery
Boston University and Boston Medical Center
Boston, Massachusetts

Robert T. Trousdale, MD
Professor of Orthopedics
Mayo Clinic
Rochester, Minnesota

Eugene R. Viscusi, MD
Director, Acute Pain Management
Department of Anesthesiology
Thomas Jefferson University
Philadelphia, Pennsylvania

Mark S. Vrahas, MD
Partners Chief of Orthopaedic Trauma Services
Department of Orthopaedic Surgery
Brigham and Women's Hospital
Massachusetts General Hospital
Boston, Massachusetts

Sharon Walton, MD
Orthopedic Resident
Department of Orthopedic Surgery
University of Illinois at Chicago
Chicago, Illinois

Stuart L. Weinstein, MD
Ignacio V. Ponseti Chair and Professor
Department of Orthopaedic Surgery
University of Iowa
Iowa City, Iowa

Geoffrey Westrich, MD
Associate Attending Orthopaedic Surgeon
Hip and Knee Service
Department of Orthopaedic Surgery
Hospital for Special Surgery
New York, New York

Bruce H. Ziran, MD
Director Orthopaedic Trauma
Associate Professor of Orthopaedics
Neoucom
St. Elizabeth Health Center
Youngstown, Ohio

Preface

There is probably no joint in orthopaedics with more literature devoted to its study than the hip. The orthopaedic surgeon's fascination with the hip joint is likely related to the devastating effects that occur on a patient's quality of life when the hip does not work properly and the vast improvements seen when function is restored. As the US population becomes both more athletic and older, hip disorders and problems are being seen more often in orthopaedic practices.

As knowledge of the hip joint continues to expand, so does the literature on the topic. Keeping current on the most recent advances is challenging for the practicing orthopaedic surgeon who must balance direct patient care and responsibilities to family and friends with the need to maintain up-to-date knowledge on orthopaedic developments and research. The instructional course lectures are one of the most popular activities at the Annual Meeting of the American Academy of Orthopaedic Surgeons (AAOS) because they allow members who are specialists in the field to share their knowledge and experience with other AAOS members. From the breadth of outstanding instructional courses presented over the past 5 years, I have selected some of the best lectures to provide the practicing surgeon with an up-to-date overview of a range of topics related to surgery of the hip. It would be difficult to imagine finding a more concise collection of literature in any form at any one location.

The section editors, who are all leaders in the field of hip surgery, have exercised their practical knowledge and expertise in working with me to select chapters that cover six different areas of hip surgery: the young adult hip, trauma, bearing surfaces, managing complications, and primary and revision total hip arthroplasty. Each section editor has written a commentary to tie together the individual chapters within his section and has provided updated information to augment the content of those chapters.

The AAOS and the American Association of Hip and Knee Surgeons view education as a major mission of their organizations; this volume represents the best of those efforts. It has been an honor to work on behalf of both organizations as the editor of *Instructional Course Lectures Hip 2*. It is hoped that this specialty volume will assist orthopaedic surgeons in providing their patients with optimal quality care. Many thanks go to the authors of the individual chapters, the section editors, and the AAOS staff, most notably Kathleen Anderson, for assisting me in compiling this volume.

Craig J. Della Valle, MD

Table of Contents

Section 1 The Young Adult Hip

Section 2 Fracture Care of the Hip

Section 3 Bearing Surfaces in Total Hip Arthroplasty

Section 4 Primary Total Hip Arthroplasty

Section 5 Managing Complications

Section 6 Revision Total Hip Arthroplasty

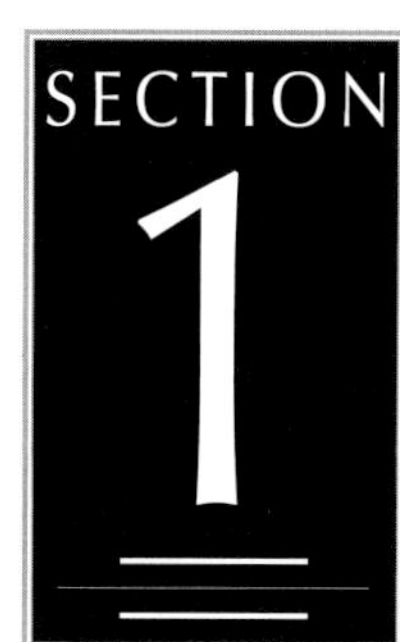

The Young Adult Hip

The Young Adult Hip

A virtual explosion in the diagnosis, management, and understanding of the painful hip in the young adult has occurred over the past 20 years. Although a painful hip in a young patient is not a new diagnosis, the ability of orthopaedic surgeons to properly diagnose and possibly offer early intervention to avoid or delay the progression of osteoarthritis has greatly expanded. This section presents chapters that cover the topic of femoral acetabular impingement (FAI), starting with a sound foundation in understanding hip pathoanatomy using conventional radiographs and transitioning into how to decide on the optimal treatment for affected patients. Arthroscopic, limited open, and open techniques are reviewed.

The first chapter, by Tannast and Siebenrock, reviews a comprehensive approach to the evaluation of the prearthritic hip using conventional radiographs. The key message is that an isolated AP pelvic radiograph may often be interpreted as normal in a prearthritic, young adult patient presenting with hip pain. If there is suspicion that the pain is related to the hip, additional imaging studies, including the cross-table lateral, Dunn-Rippstein, frog-leg lateral, and/or false profile views, can be helpful in distinguishing subtle anatomic variations that may be contributing to labral impingement and/or articular cartilage damage.

This chapter presents a comprehensive overview of the descriptions and characteristics of the two types of FAI and a detailed description of the various conventional radiographic studies, including proper techniques, the most common measurements, and common pitfalls in evaluating conventional radiographs in this patient population. Conventional radiographs performed in more than one plane are mandatory for a proper diagnosis and are imperative prior to ordering advanced imaging studies such as CT or MRI. Detailed figures of the proper radiographic studies are included to augment the text and help the reader understand various subtle radiographic findings.

The second chapter in this section, by Beaulé and associates, focuses on deciding on the optimal intervention for treating the young adult patient with hip impingement. After the correct diagnosis has been determined based on a comprehensive history, focused physical examination, and appropriate radiographic studies, the challenging question is how to best treat the patient. In most patients, the appropriate first step is a trial of nonsurgical management, including activity modification, anti-inflammatory medications, and range-of-motion exercises. Evidence is not clear that patients benefit substantially from these nonsurgical options. The authors offer a detailed description of the three categories of surgical techniques for treating FAI: (1) fully open surgical procedures (the femoral head is dislocated), (2) arthroscopic procedures that are sometimes augmented by a limited open arthrotomy (the femoral head is not dislocated), and (3) reorientation pelvic periacetabular osteotomy (limited to certain types of pincer impingement). The indications and clinical advantages and disadvantages of each surgical technique are discussed in detail. Beaulé and associates conclude that optimal treatment strategies are determined by careful evaluation of the patient (history, physical examination, and imaging studies) and tailoring treatment to the individual patient to adequately address the major underlying impingement deformities.

In the third chapter in this section, Larson discusses the arthroscopic management of hip pathology for both cam- and pincer-type FAI. The author emphasizes the importance of proper patient selection, the long learning curve for managing FAI arthroscopically, and the continuing evolution of specific techniques and indications for arthroscopic treatment. The chapter includes a comprehensive table that summarizes relevant clinical outcomes after arthroscopic treatment of FAI. Because of the variable patterns of FAI, Larson acknowledges the need for further long-term studies to better define the most appropriate surgical approach to treat this disorder.

In the fourth chapter in this section, Peters and associates discuss open surgical dislocation for managing cam- and pincer-type FAI. The authors describe the steps in a surgical technique that can safely dislocate the femoral head using a lateral approach to the hip with a trochanteric flip osteotomy. This approach allows for circumferential exposure of the acetabulum and the femoral head/neck and facilitates a more comprehensive surgical correction for patients with severe deformities. A table is included that summarizes clinical outcomes from studies using open surgical dislocation for FAI. A simple and effective treatment algorithm for the young patient with hip pain also is included in the chapter.

In the fifth and final chapter in this section, Leunig and associates describe

FAI treatments on the acetabular side (pincer impingement). The most common scenarios of pincer impingement are reviewed, including limited anterior overcoverage, acetabular retroversion, coxa profunda, and acetabular protrusio. Various surgical techniques (anteverting periacetabular osteotomy and surgical dislocation) and reported clinical outcomes are reviewed. The authors discuss the complexity of correcting acetabular-sided impingement deformity and the need for more comprehensive management with open procedures over arthroscopic management, which may not allow for global correction.

The chapters in this section address the entire spectrum of FAI with indications, radiographic assessment, proper diagnosis of the structural deformity, various surgical techniques, and clinical outcomes. The authors are international leaders in the field of the young adult hip and have provided an excellent and comprehensive overview of the topic. The authors stress the importance of proper patient selection, individualizing the treatment to the hip deformity, adequately correcting structural deformities, the continuing evolution of treatment techniques, and the importance of continued long-term research in this field. These chapters are a must-read for any orthopaedic surgeon who is considering treating patients with FAI.

Ryan M. Nunley, MD
Assistant Professor of Orthopaedic Surgery
Department of Orthopaedic Surgery
Washington University School of Medicine
St. Louis, Missouri

Dr. Nunley or an immediate family member serves as a paid consultant to Smith & Nephew, Wright Medical Technology, Medtronic, CardioMEMS, and Integra Sciences; has received research or institutional support from Biomet, Wright Medical Technology, Stryker, Smith & Nephew, EOS Imaging, and Medical Compression Systems; and serves as a board member, owner, officer, or committee member of the Missouri State Orthopaedic Association and the Southern Orthopaedic Association.

1

Conventional Radiographs to Assess Femoroacetabular Impingement

Moritz Tannast, MD
Klaus A. Siebenrock, MD

Abstract

Femoroacetabular impingement (FAI) is a pathologic condition of the hip joint in young adults that, if untreated, leads to end-stage osteoarthritis. It is characterized by early pathologic contact between primary osseous prominences of the acetabular rim (so-called pincer FAI) and/or the femoral head-neck junction (cam FAI). Conventional radiographs are often considered normal because classic radiographic signs of osteoarthritis are not present initially. The physician should be aware of the radiographic features for both types of impingement to recognize subtle pathologies.

Femoroacetabular impingement (FAI) is a purely mechanical hip disorder defined as abnormal contact between skeletal prominences of the acetabular rim or the proximal femur that leads to painful, prearthritic joint damage.[1] The estimated prevalence is 10% to 15%.[2] If untreated, FAI can lead to end-stage osteoarthrosis of the hip joint and may be one of the main causes of so-called primary osteoarthritis of the hip. Generally, FAI occurs as an isolated entity but can also present in combination with various hip disorders, such as developmental dysplasia or Legg-Calvé-Perthes disease (Table 1). The diagnosis of FAI is based on a positive correlation among symptoms, physical findings on clinical examination, suggestive conventional radiographs, and signs of chondrolabral degeneration on radial magnetic resonance arthrography. In the early stage of the disease, no classic signs of osteoarthritis (such as joint space narrowing, subchondral sclerosis, or bone cysts) are obvious on conventional radiography, although cartilage degeneration is already advanced.

Clinical Signs of Impingement

FAI often presents in active, young adults as groin pain of slow onset, usually noticed after an episode of minor trauma. The pain is intermittent and may be exacerbated by excessive physical demands on the hip, such as athletic activities or a normal activity of daily living such as walking. The pain also may occur after a prolonged period of sitting. Based on normal-appearing radiographs of the hip, patients with FAI sometimes are subjected to an extensive diagnostic work-up and even inappropriate surgical procedures.[1] Examination of the hip often reveals limited motion, particularly internal rotation and adduction in flexion.[3] A positive impingement sign is seen for anterior FAI if the forced internal rotation or adduction in 90° of flexion is reproducibly painful and for posterior FAI if forced external rotation in full extension is painful. The Drehmann sign is positive if hip flexion produces unavoidable passive external rotation of the hip. A positive impingement test has been closely correlated with labral lesions, as seen on specific radial magnetic resonance arthrograms of the hip.[4]

Radiographic Technique

Standard conventional radiographs for FAI include an AP pelvis radiograph and an axial cross-table view of the proximal femur.[5,6] The AP pelvis radiograph is taken with the patient supine and the legs internally rotated (to adjust for femoral antetorsion), with a film focus distance of 1.2 m. Obtaining a radiograph with the patient supine allows direct comparison with intraoperative and immediate postoperative radiographs during general anesthesia. The central beam should be directed to the midpoint between the superior border of the symphysis and a line connecting both the anterior and superior iliac spines, landmarks that can be easily and reproducibly palpated by the radiology technician. Centering of the beam is crucial and

Table 1
Description and Characteristics of the Two Types of Femoroacetabular Impingement

Criteria	Pincer Impingement	Cam Impingement
Main cause	Focal or general overcoverage	Aspherical head
Mechanism	Linear contact between overcovering rim and head-neck junction	Jamming of the aspherical head portion into the acetabulum
Gender distribution (M:F)	1:3	14:1
Average age (range)	40 years (40-57)	32 years (21-51)
Typical location of cartilage damage	Circumferential with contre-coup lesion	11 o'clock-3 o'clock
Average depth of cartilage damage	4 mm	11 mm
Associated pathologies	• Bladder extrophy • Proximal femoral focal deficiency • Posttraumatic dysplasia • Chronic residual dysplasia of the acetabulum • Legg-Calvé-Perthes disease • Slipped capital femoral epiphysis • After acetabular reorientation procedures • Idiopathic retroversion	• Slipped capital femoral epiphysis • Legg-Calvé-Perthes disease • Posttraumatic retrotorsion of the femoral head • Coxa vara • Pistol grip deformity • Head tilt deformity • Postslip deformity • Femoral retroversion • Growth abnormality of the femoral epiphysis
Radiographic signs on AP radiograph	• Coxa profunda • Protrusio acetabuli • Focal acetabular retroversion (figure-of-8 sign) • Lateral center edge (LCE) angle > 39° • Reduced extrusion index • Acetabular index ≤ 0° • Posterior wall sign • Ischial spine sign	• Pistol grip deformity • Triangular index R ≥ r + 2 mm* • Alpha angle > 68° (men) • Alpha angle > 50° (women) • Caput-collum-diaphyseal (CCD) angle < 125° • Horizontal growth plate sign
Radiographic signs on cross-table radiograph	• Linear indentation sign	• Alpha angle > 50° • Femoral offset < 8 mm • Offset ratio < 0.18 • Femoral retrotorsion
Secondary changes	• Herniation pits • Ossification of labrum • Appositional bone sign • Os acetabuli (acetabular rim fracture) • Posterior inferior joint space loss (on false profile view in pincer hips) • Late: classic signs of osteoarthritis	

*See text for explanation.

is different from preoperative planning for a total hip arthroplasty, where it is directed more caudally. The axial cross-table femoral view is also taken with the leg internally rotated, with a film-focus distance of 1.2 m and with the central beam directed toward the inguinal fold.[5] These technical prerequisites are mandatory for correct interpretation.

A false profile view[7] is rarely used for diagnosis because it does not show the relationship between the anterior and posterior acetabular walls. Rather, it can be used for the diagnosis of early joint degeneration in the posteroinferior part of the acetabulum, which is a relative contraindication for joint-preserving surgery described later in this chapter. As an alternative to the cross-table lateral view, a Dunn-Rippstein view[8] or a frog-leg lateral view[9] can be obtained for visualizing a cam deformity. To accurately measure a patient's pelvic tilt, a true lateral radiograph of the pelvis can be taken.[5] Knowledge of pelvic tilt is crucial for correct interpretation of the radiographic hip parameters. Gonadal shielding is not recommended because it can potentially hide important anatomic landmarks needed to quantify pelvic tilt and rotation.

Types of Impingement

Depending on the pathomechanism, two types of FAI, pincer and cam, can be distinguished (Figures 1 and 2). Isolated cam or pincer deformities are rare; in 86% of all affected patients a combined deformity is present.[10]

Pincer Impingement

In pincer impingement, a linear contact occurs between the acetabular rim and the femoral head-neck junction, with the maximal impact force tangential to the joint surface (Figure 2). The labrum (which acts like a bumper) is compressed between the two impinging bones and tears off its acetabular origin. The force is then further transmitted to the acetabular cartilage. In this type of impingement, the transmission of force to the cartilage is restricted to a narrow band of the acetabular rim. Therefore, these lesions are typically more benign in terms of visible cartilage damage than those seen in cam impingement. Generally, pincer impingement is caused by a focal or general acetabular overcoverage with a relatively normal femur, or rarely a large deformation of the femoral head. Repeated microtrauma induces cystic deformations of the labrum and bone growth at its base that subsequently ossifies. This rim ossification is responsible for additional deepening of the acetabulum and worsening impingement. Pincer impingement is more common in middle-aged women. The condition can occur as an isolated entity, in combination with various hip disorders, or iatrogenically (for example, after overcorrection in acetabular reorientation procedures [Table 1]).

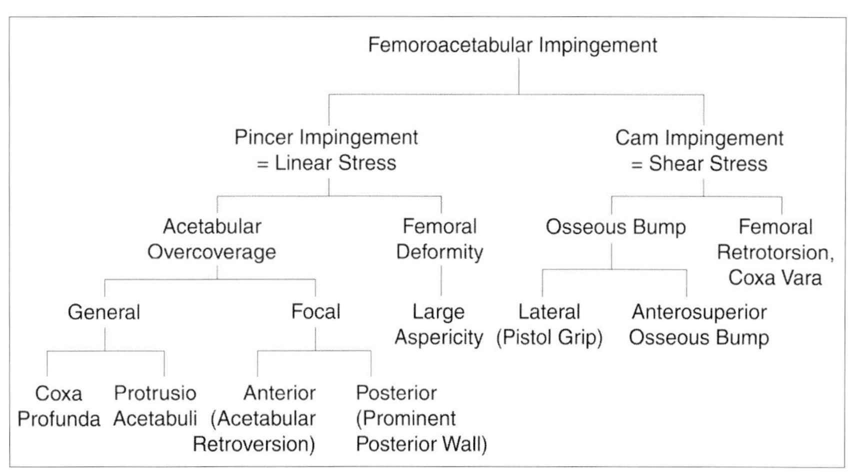

Figure 1 Overview of the different types of impingement.

General Acetabular Overcoverage

General acetabular overcoverage can be judged by the depth of the acetabular fossa. With normal depth, the acetabular fossa is lateral to the ilioischial line (Figure 3, *A*); with coxa profunda the acetabular fossa is touching or crossing the ilioischial line (Figure 3, *B*). With protrusio acetabuli, which represents the worst type of general overcoverage, the femoral head is crossing the ilioischial line (Figure 3, *C*). These joint configurations are primary pathologies and cannot be compared with secondary acetabular protrusion in end-stage osteoarthritis.

Coxometric measurements to quantify acetabular depth include the lateral center edge (LCE) angle of Wiberg, the acetabular index, and the femoral head extrusion index (Figure 3). The LCE angle is defined by a vertical line starting from the center of the femoral head and parallel to the longitudinal body axis and a line connecting the femoral head center with the lateral edge of the acetabular roof. Normally, this angle varies between 25° (defining a deficient acetabular coverage) and 39° (defining excessive coverage, Figure 3, *A*). The acetabular index (also called acetabular roof angle) is formed by a horizontal line and a line through the medial edge of the sclerotic zone and the lateral edge of the acetabulum. In hips with coxa profunda or protrusio acetabuli, the acetabular index typically is 0° or even negative (Figure 3, *B* and *C*). The femoral head extrusion index is defined as the horizontal portion of the femoral head that is uncovered by the acetabulum. Although there is a maximal extrusion of 25% (indicating dysplasia), no study has defined a minimal extrusion index.

It is assumed that the abrupt stop in pincer FAI leads to a slight joint subluxation with resulting joint damage in the opposite part of the joint (Figure 2). It can be seen in approximately one third of all patients with pincer impingement.[10] This posteroinferior joint damage can be seen as a subtle joint space narrowing on the false profile view, indicating an already advanced stage of joint degeneration with a limited prognosis (Figure 4). Therefore, this condition is a relative contraindication for joint-preserving surgery.

Hip radiographs made with the beam centered over the hip can show false depth of the acetabulum and are therefore not useful for interpreting radiographic signs of FAI (Figure 5). In addition, hip radiographs do not show the entire pelvis. This finding is important because anatomical reference lines (for example, the interteardrop line) cannot be determined.

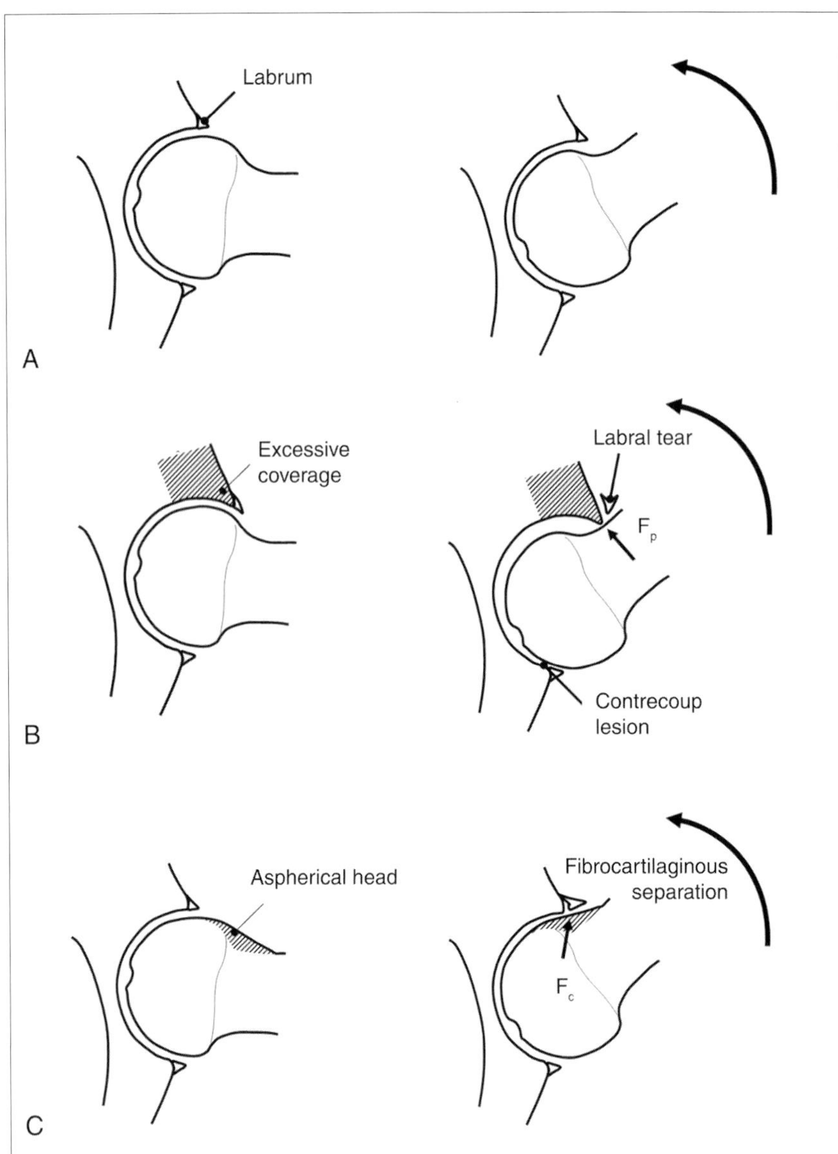

Figure 2 A normal hip **(A)** has an impingement-free range of motion within the physiologic amplitudes of joint motion. In pincer impingement **(B)**, the main impact force F_P is directed tangential to the joint surface, leading to a full tear of the labrum (mainly resulting from to acetabular overcoverage). In cam impingement **(C)**, the aspherical portion of the femoral head-neck junction is jammed into the acetabulum. The main impact force F_C is perpendicular to the joint surface, leading to a fibrocartilaginous separation (undersurface tear of the labrum).

Focal Acetabular Overcoverage

Focal acetabular overcoverage can occur in the anterior or posterior portion of the acetabulum. It can be assessed by carefully tracing the anterior and posterior acetabular walls on an AP radiograph. In a normal hip, the acetabulum is anteverted; the anterior wall runs medial to the posterior rim without crossing it (Figure 3, *A*). In relative anterior overcoverage, the anterior rim is projected more lateral than the posterior rim in the cranial part of the acetabulum. It crosses the posterior line caudally, which gives the appearance of a figure-of-8 sign (Figure 6). Often with this so-called acetabular retroversion, the ischial spine crosses the true pelvis medially (Figure 6, *A*).

Posterior acetabular coverage can be evaluated by determining the position of the posterior acetabular rim relative to the femoral head center. In a normal hip, the posterior border runs approximately through the femoral head center (Figure 3, *A*). With a too-prominent posterior wall, the projected line runs lateral to the femoral head center, indicating posterior FAI in extension and external rotation (Figure 6, *B*).

Differentiation of the anterior and posterior acetabular walls is sometimes difficult. As a helpful hint in clinical practice, the posterior wall can easily be identified when starting from the inferior edge of the acetabulum.

A positive crossover sign has to be assessed with caution if the technical radiographic prerequisites are not fulfilled. A crossover sign can be missed if the center of the beam is directed over the hip (Figure 7). Because of the conical geometry of the beams, the crossover sign can be increased if the film-focus distance is decreased (Figure 8).

In addition, acetabular retroversion can be created by an increased pelvic tilt or rotation to the ipsilateral side of the patient (Figure 9). Neutral pelvic rotation around the longitudinal axis is obtained when the tip of the coccyx points toward the middle of the symphysis. In men and women, neutral pelvic tilt around the horizontal axis can be roughly defined by a distance of 3.2 cm or 4.7 cm, respectively, between the upper border of the symphysis and the middle of the sacrococcygeal joint. To accurately determine individual pelvic

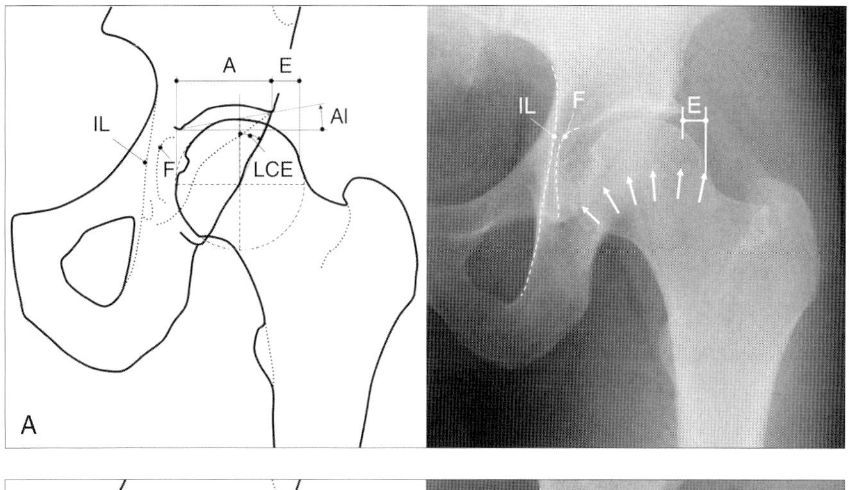

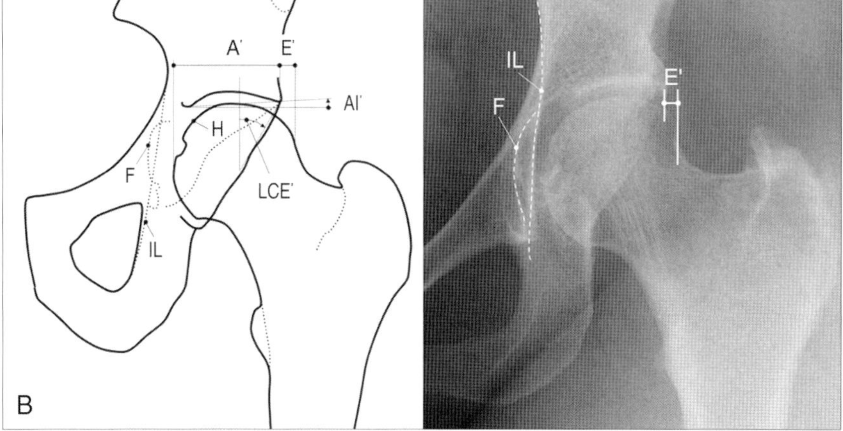

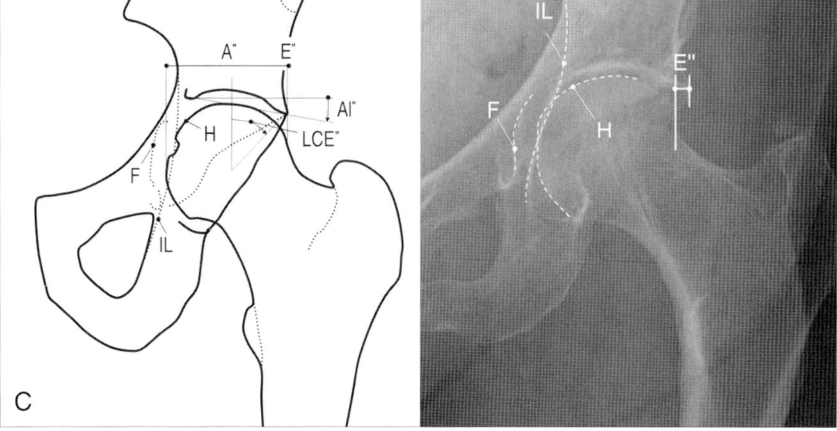

Figure 3 **A,** A normal hip with normal depth in a 35-year-old man. The acetabular fossa (F) lies lateral to the ilioischial line (IL). The lateral center edge (LCE) angle is between 25° and 39°. The extrusion index (E/[A + E]) is approximately 25%. The epiphyseal scar (arrows) lies within the femoral head circle. The acetabular index (AI) is slightly positive. The posterior wall goes through the femoral head center. See text for additional discussion. **B,** Coxa profunda in a 29-year-old woman is shown. The condition is defined by an overcrossing of the acetabular fossa with the IL. The AI and the femoral head extrusion are decreasing, the LCE angle is increasing. **C,** In protrusio acetabuli in a 42-year-old woman, even the femoral head line is crossing the IL.

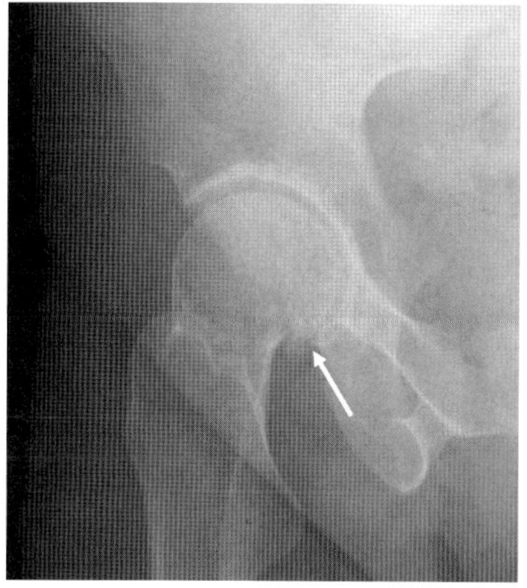

Figure 4 Because of the contrecoup lesion in the hip of a 36-year-old woman with pincer impingement, joint-space narrowing of the posteroinferior articular portion is visible on a false profile view (*arrow*).

tilt, a true lateral pelvic radiograph can be obtained.[3] A neutral pelvic tilt is indicated by 60° of pelvic inclination, which is defined by a horizontal line and a line connecting the symphysis with the sacral promontory. Modern software is available to correct the individual acetabular morphology to a standardized neutral orientation;[11] however, it still has to be shown if such an anatomically based standardization corresponds to the clinical symptoms.

Pincer impingement can lead to an indentation sign on the femoral side with compensatory cortical thickening (Figure 10). Pincer impingement also can occur without specific pathomorphology in patients with excessive hip motion, typically young hypermobile women (for example, ballet dancers).

Large Deformation of the Femoral Head

In rare instances, pincer impingement is caused by a large, deformed femoral head, typically in hips with

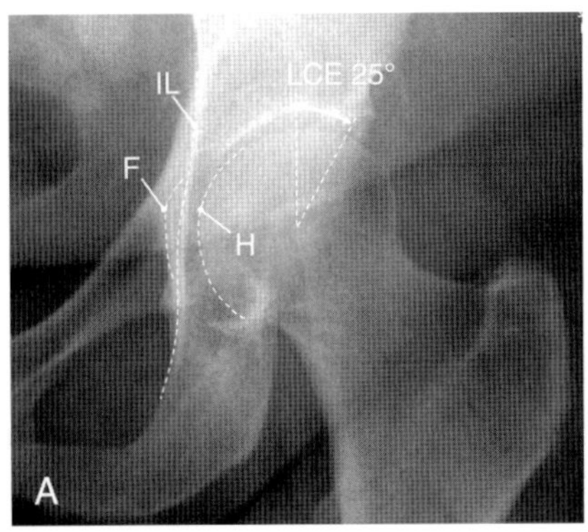

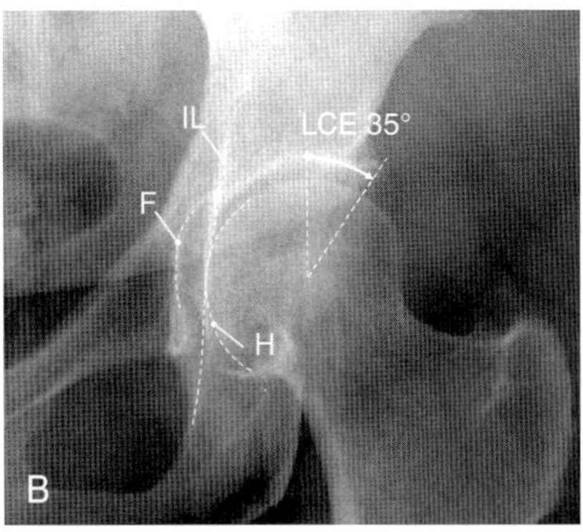

Figure 5 **A,** Radiograph of the hip of a 35-year-old woman shows a coxa profunda with an LCE angle of 25° if the beam is correctly centered over the pelvis. **B,** If the beam is directed over the hip, protrusio acetabuli is visible with a substantially increased LCE angle of 35°.

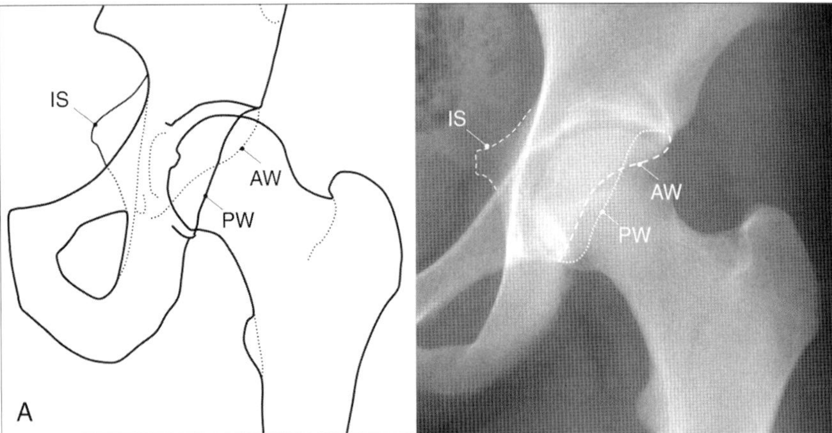

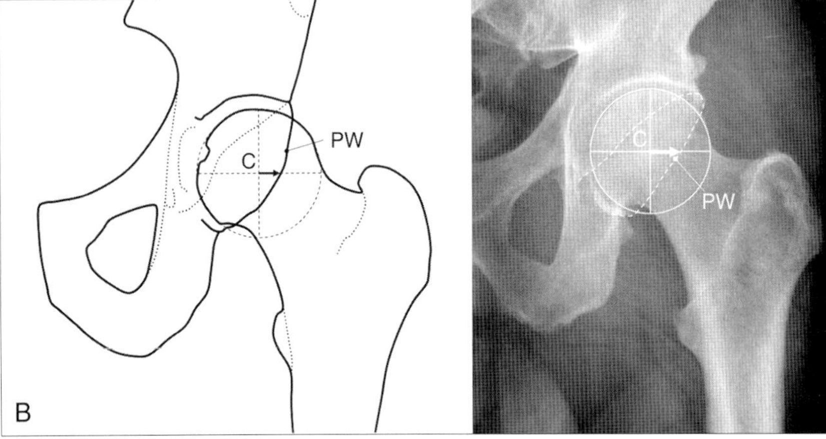

Figure 6 **A**, Drawing and radiograph of the hip of a 24-year-old patient show an acetabular retroversion with relative anterior overcoverage where the anterior wall (AW) crosses the posterior wall (PW), causing a figure-of-8 sign. As an indirect indicator, the ischial spine (IS) protrudes into the true pelvis. **B,** Drawing and radiograph of the hip of a 32-year-old man show posterior overcoverage, which is defined with the PW running lateral to the femoral head center (C). In normal hips, it runs approximately through the center (see Figure 3, *A*).

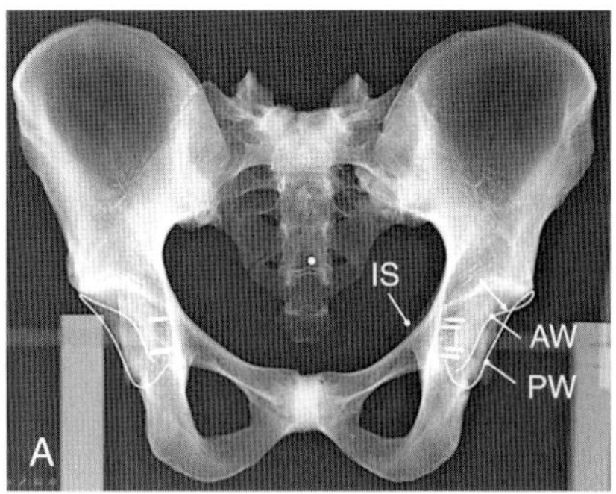

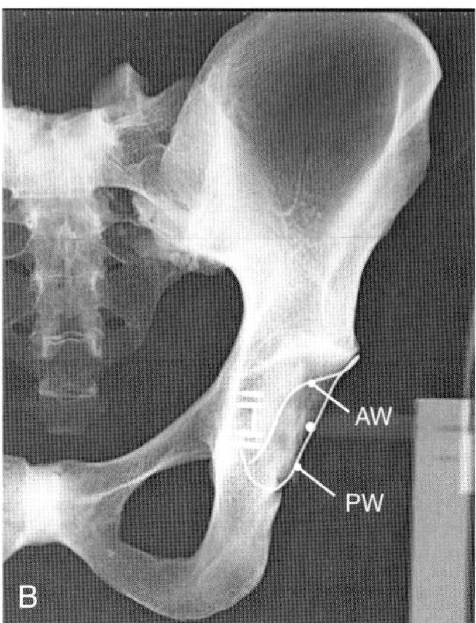

Figure 7 **A,** The correctly centered AP pelvic radiograph shows a cranial retroversion of the left acetabulum in a female cadaver pelvis. The center of the x-ray beam is marked with a radiodense ball. The ischial spine (IS) sign is positive. **B,** If the x-ray beam is centered over the hip, the crossover and the IS sign disappear.

Legg-Calvé-Perthes disease. Because the femoral head is too large to enter the joint, this leads to an abrupt stop at the final range of motion. These hips often show a femoral indentation corresponding to the early pathologic contact of the acetabular rim (Figure 11).

Secondary Changes in Pincer Impingement

Recurrent irritation in unrecognized pincer FAI leads to reactive ossification of the labrum (Figure 12). This also can be seen as a double contour of one of the projected acetabular rims. In an advanced stage, further deepening of the acetabulum is caused by additional reactive bone apposition at the osseous acetabular rim, thereby increasing impingement. Although there is significant and irreversible prearthritic damage of the cartilage, there is no joint space narrowing because only the quality of the cartilage and not its diameter is impaired in the early stage of the disease. Classic radiographic signs of osteoarthritis occur late and indicate advanced joint degeneration, a relative contraindication for joint-preserving surgery.

Cam Impingement

In cam impingement, the predominant abnormality is the contour of the anterosuperior femoral head-neck junction (Figure 2). The shearing stress between the femoral head-neck junction and the acetabulum is caused either by an irregularity of the femoral head-neck junction or by angular deformities of the proximal femur[12] (Figure 2; Table 1). Normally, the anterosuperior femoral head-neck junction has a concave, spherical configuration that is either flattened or convex in hips with cam impingement. This eccentric part slides into the acetabulum and induces compression and shear stress at the junction between the labrum and the cartilage and at the subchondral landmark. In contrast to pincer impingement, the maximal impact force is perpendicular to the joint surface (Figure 2). Therefore, the labrum is stretched and pushed outward, and the cartilage is compressed and pushed centrally, causing a separation between the labrum and the cartilage. The labrum with this undersurface lesion of its matrix remains partially attached on the acetabular rim.

The osseous irregularity can occur in the lateral (so-called pistol-grip deformity) or in the anterosuperior part of the femoral head-neck junction. Angular deformities include femoral retrotorsion and coxa vara. Cam impingement is most common in young athletic males.

Pistol-Grip Deformity

A pistol-grip deformity occurs in approximately 6% of men and 2% of women.[13] It is characterized on AP radiographs by flattening of the usually concave surface of the lateral aspect of the femoral head caused by an abnormal extension of the more horizontally oriented femoral epiphysis. It can be quantified by the α angle and the triangular index.[13]

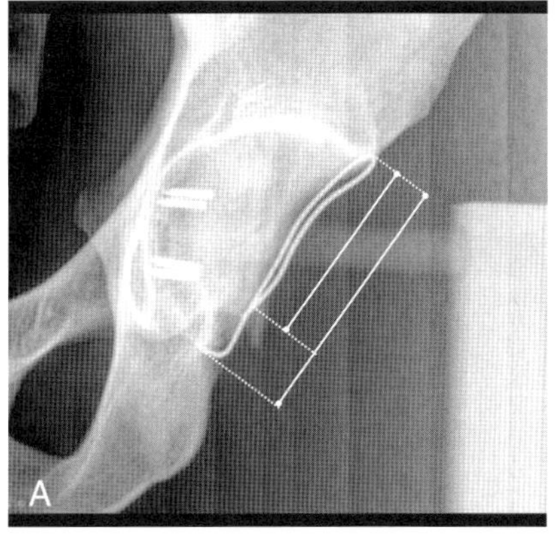

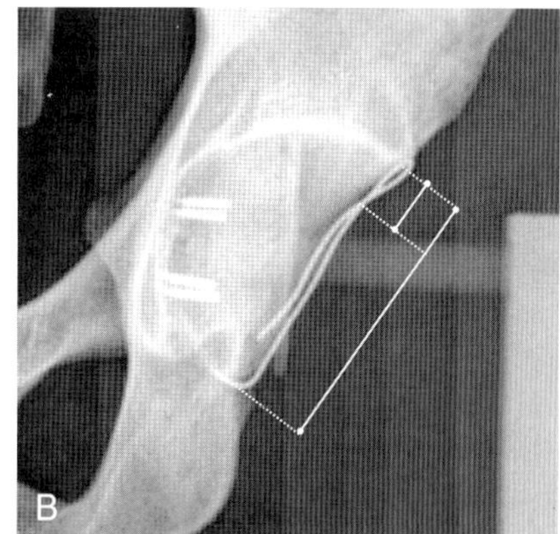

Figure 8 By changing the source-to-film distance, different projections of the acetabular morphology for this cadaver pelvis can be obtained. **A,** Radiograph showing a source-to-film distance of 0.8 m with large acetabular retroversion. **B,** Radiograph showing a source-to-film distance of 1.4 m; the retroversion index is reduced.

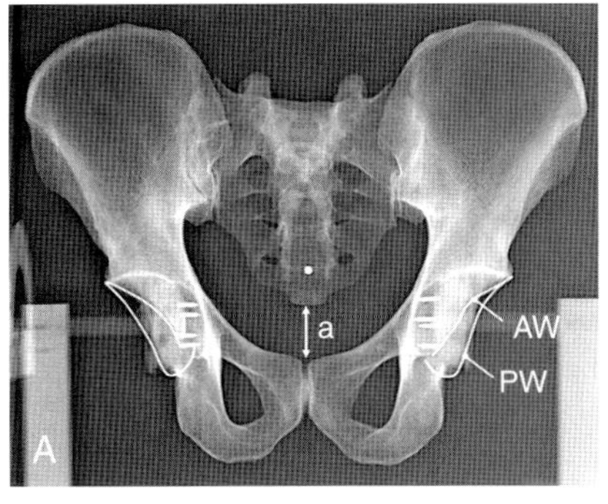

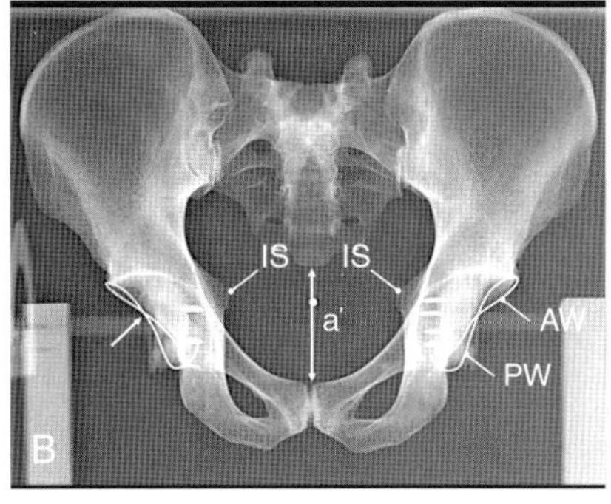

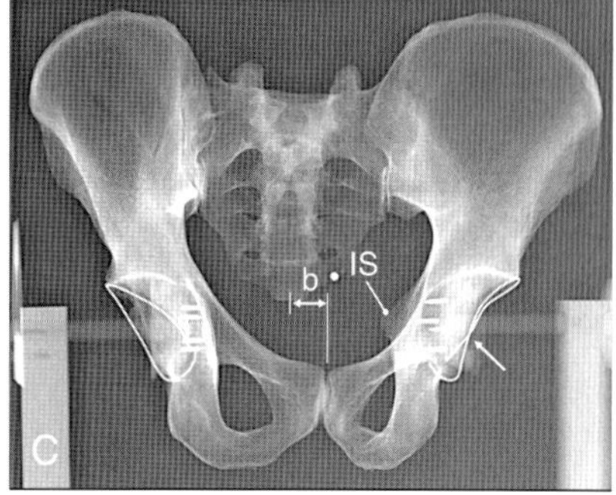

Figure 9 **A,** Radiograph showing normal acetabular version on both sides of a cadaver pelvis. **B,** By increasing pelvic tilt, an acetabular retroversion is visible on both sides. In addition, the ischial spine (IS) sign is positive. **C,** By rotating the pelvis to the left side, a crossover and IS sign can be created at the ipsilateral side.

The α angle is formed by the femoral neck axis and a line connecting the femoral head center with the point of beginning asphericity of the superior femoral head contour (Figure 13). This point can be determined with the Mose template method of concentric circles. The α angle can be underestimated if the femoral rotation is not controlled. The maximal normal α angle on the AP pelvic radiograph is 68° in men and 50° in women.[13]

The triangular index (Figure 13) is constructed as follows: on the femoral neck axis, half of the radius of the femoral head is measured. Then, a perpendicular line is drawn. The new radius is defined as the distance between the femoral head center and the intersection point of the perpendicular line with the superior femoral head-neck contour. The triangular index has better reproducibility than the α angle because it is constructed by clear geometric landmarks, whereas the α angle sometimes can be difficult to pinpoint. In addition, the triangular index is more independent from femoral rotation.[13]

Anterosuperior Osseous Bump

The anterosuperior osseous bump at the femoral head-neck junction cannot be seen on the AP pelvis radiograph, but it can be seen on additional radiographic views of the proximal femur such as the cross-table lateral view. It can be a primary osseous variant of the femoral head-neck junction or the result of subclinical slipped capital femoral epiphysis or Legg-Calvé-Perthes disease (Table 1). In addition, the anterosuperior osseous bump is seen in malunited femoral neck fractures.

As on the AP view, the amount of asphericity can be quantified on the lateral view by the α angle (Figure 14). The anterior femoral offset and the offset ratio also are used for description. An α angle larger than 50° is an indicator of an abnormally shaped femoral head-neck contour. The anterior offset is defined as the difference in radius between the anterior femoral head and the anterior femoral neck. In asymptomatic hips, the anterior offset is 11.6 ± 0.7 mm; hips with cam impingement have a decreased anterior offset of 7.2 ± 0.7 mm.[6] As a general rule for clinical practice, an anterior offset less than 10 mm is a strong indicator of cam impingement. The offset ratio is defined as the ratio between the anterior offset and the diameter of the head. It is 0.21 ± 0.03 in asymptomatic patients and 0.13 ± 0.05 in hips with cam impingement.[6]

It is important to recognize that these deformities are primary deformities, not osteophytes.

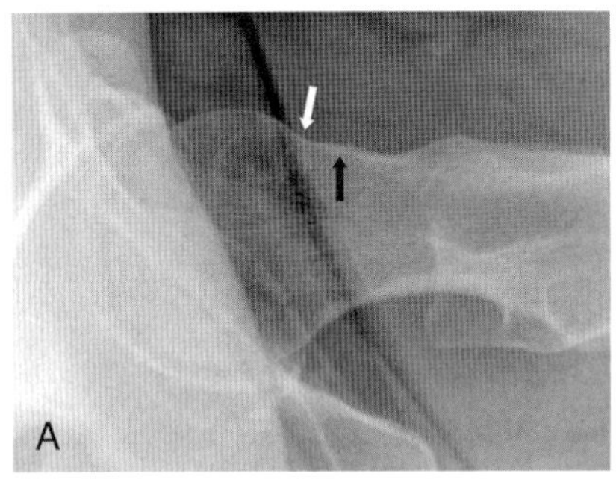

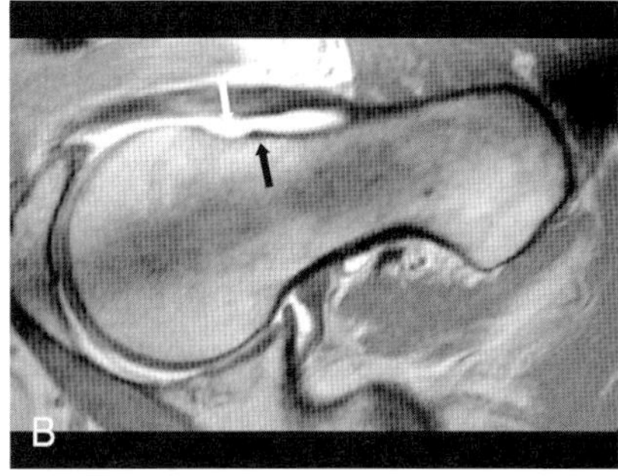

Figure 10 Cross-table lateral view **(A)** and corresponding magnetic resonance arthrogram **(B)** showing an indentation sign (*arrows*) on the femoral head-neck junction in a 38-year-old woman with pincer impingement.

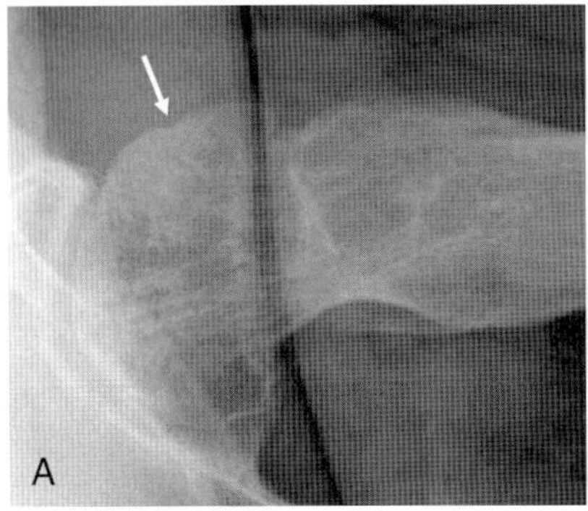

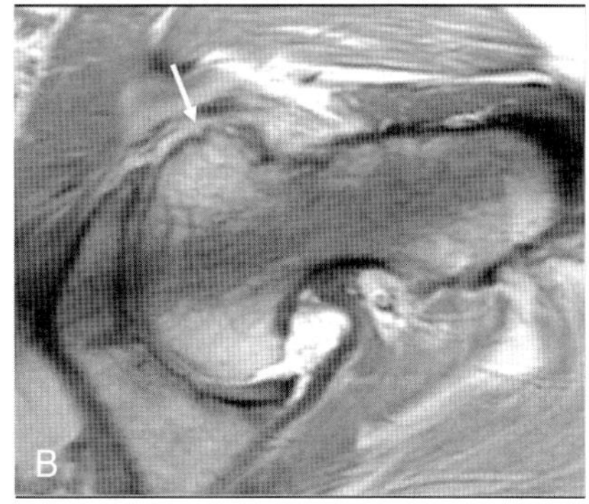

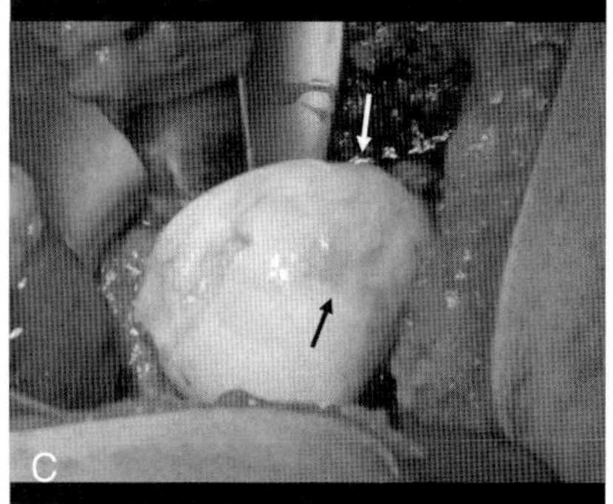

Figure 11 Pincer impingement caused by an extremely large femoral head that cannot enter the joint in a 28-year-old patient with Legg-Calvé-Perthes disease. Note the indentation (*arrows*) on the cross-table lateral view **(A)** the corresponding magnetic resonance arthrogram **(B)** and on an intraoperative view **(C)**.

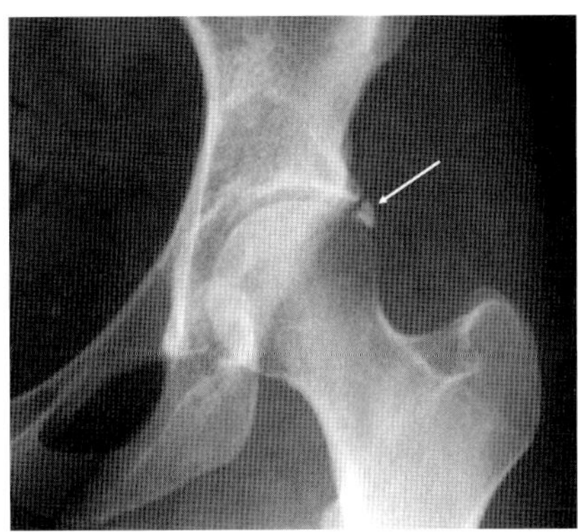

Figure 12 Radiograph showing secondary signs of FAI in the hip of a 34-year-old woman with coxa profunda: labral ossification (*arrow*).

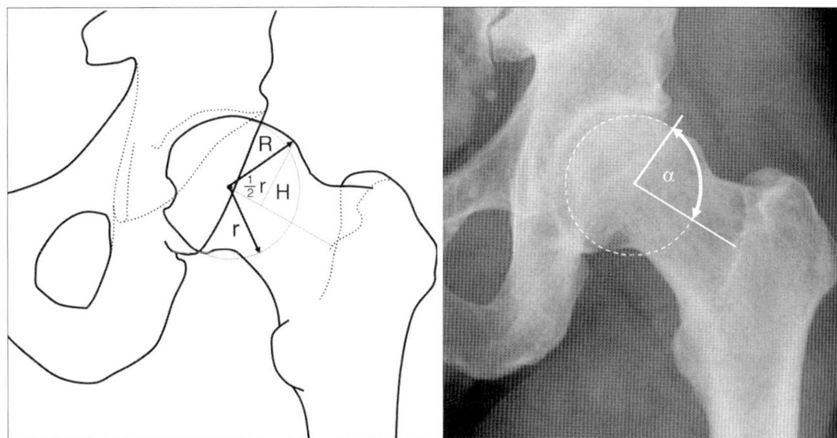

Figure 13 Drawing and radiograph from a 25-year-old patient with pistol-grip deformity. The triangular index R, or new radius, is pathologic if R ≥ r + 2 mm (estimated magnification, 1.2). An additional parameter for quantification of the femoral head-neck junction is the α angle. R = radius of the femoral head; H = perpendicular line; r = radius of the spherical portion of the femoral head.

Angular Deformities of the Proximal Femur

Other causes of cam impingement are femoral retrotorsion and coxa vara. Femoral retrotorsion can occur as primary pathology or in association with malunited femoral neck fractures. To accurately determine torsion of the femur, CT imaging studies are recommended. Coxa vara (defined by a caput collum diaphyseal angle of less than 125°) also can cause impingement. Although in these two pathologies the femoral offset might be normal, the femoral head-neck junction is closer to the acetabular rim during normal activities of daily living, leading to cam impingement.

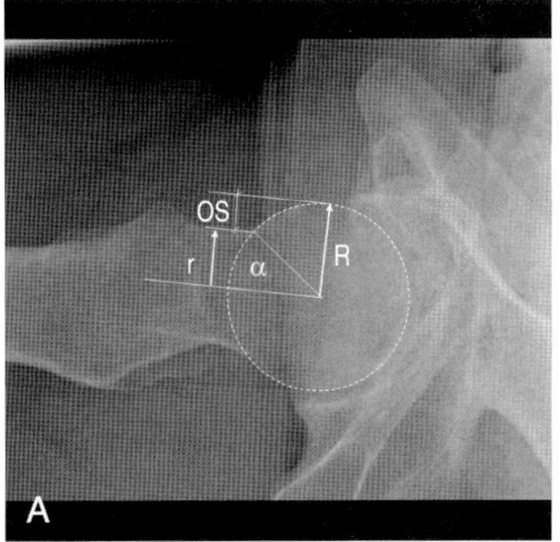

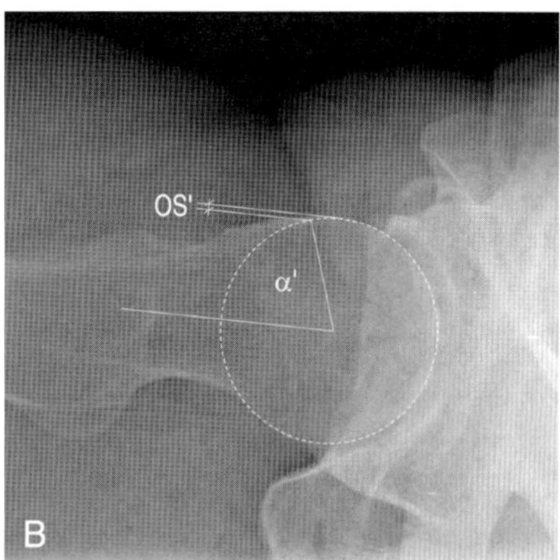

Figure 14 On a cross-table lateral radiograph, the asphericity can be quantified by the α angle, the femoral offset (OS), and the offset ratio. r = radius of the spherical portion of the femoral head; R = increased radius of the femoral head in the aspherical portion. **A,** Normal hip. **B,** Hip with cam impingement.

Secondary Changes in Cam Impingement

As with pincer impingement, labral ossifications can occur in cam impingment. The differential diagnosis of this ossification is hydroxyapatite deposition in the labrum. This calcification is usually resolved on follow-up radiographs at 6 weeks; with FAI (caused by the recurrent contact between the acetabular rim and femoral head-neck junction), labral radiodensity continues.

The recurrent irritation of the acetabular rim by the aspherical portion of the femoral head can cause stress fractures of the acetabulum (Figure 15, *A*). Because the initial appearance of the hip may be normal on an AP pelvis radiograph, these two damage patterns can be misinterpreted as incidental os acetabuli. However, the presence of a radiodense structure at the edge of the acetabular roof should raise suspicion of FAI.

Hips with FAI have a higher prevalence of herniation pits (Figure 15, *B*), which are believed to be benign.[14] They are radiolucencies surrounded by a sclerotic margin and typically located in the anterosuperior quadrant of the femoral neck. They are thought to be intraosseous ganglia at the femoral zone of FAI. Therefore, hips with these juxta-articular cysts should be considered a joint at risk for FAI rather than one with a benign lesion, but herniation

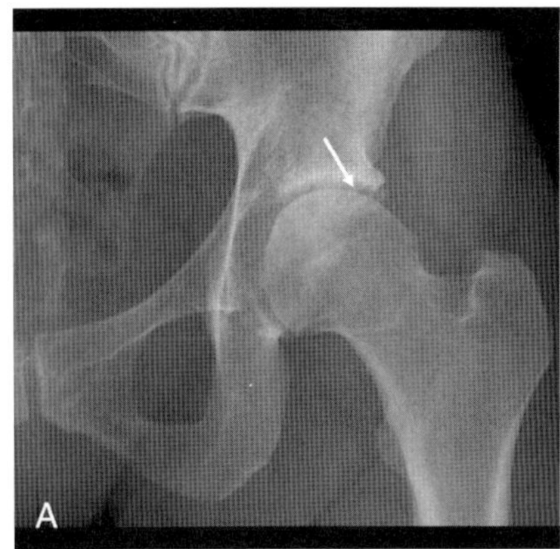

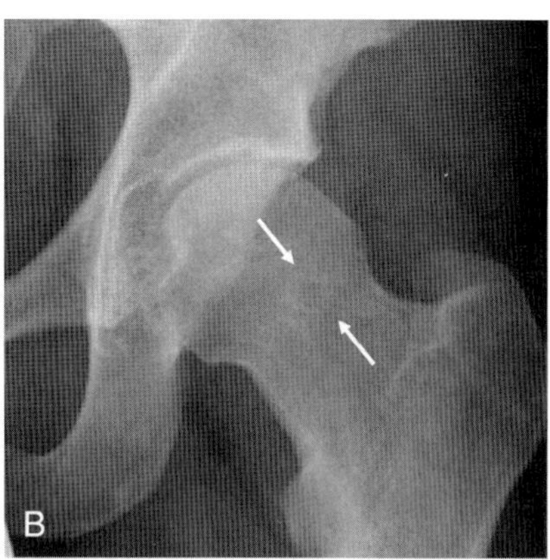

Figure 15 Secondary changes in cam impingement. **A,** Acetabular rim fatigue fractures can occur because of recurrent irritation by the aspherical portion. **B,** Herniation pits can occur in both forms of FAI and are located in the anterosuperior portion of the femoral head.

pits are not always associated with symptomatic impingement. They are usually present long before bone cysts occur in end grade osteoarthritis caused by FAI.

Summary

FAI is a condition of the hip joint that leads to osteoarthritis. Both the pincer and cam types have typical morphologic features on an AP pelvic radiograph and on a mandatory second view of the proximal femur. Despite significant intra-articular damage, classic radiographic signs of osteoarthritis are not present initially. Magnetic resonance arthrography is important for further evaluation of the disease.

References

1. Ganz R, Parvizi J, Beck M, Leunig M, Nötzli H, Siebenrock KA: Femoroacetabular impingement: A cause for osteoarthritis of the hip. *Clin Orthop Relat Res* 2003;417:112 -120.
2. Leunig M, Ganz R: Femoroacetabular impingement: A common cause of hip complaints leading to arthrosis. *Unfallchirurg* 2005;108:9-17.
3. Kubiak-Langer M, Tannast M, Murphy SB, Siebenrock KA, Langlotz F: Range of motion in anterior femoroacetabular impingement. *Clin Orthop Relat Res* 2007;458:117-124.
4. Nötzli HP, Wyss TF, Stöcklin CH, Schmid MR, Treiber K, Hodler J: The contour of the femoral head-neck: Junction as a predictor for the risk of anterior impingement. *J Bone Joint Surg Br* 2002;84:556-560.
5. Tannast M, Siebenrock KA, Anderson SE: Femoroacetabular impingement: Radiographic diagnosis. What the radiologist should know. *AJR Am J Roentgenol* 2007;188:1540-1552.
6. Eijer H, Leunig M, Mahomed MN, Ganz R: Crosstable lateral radiograph for screening of anterior femoral head-neck offset in patients with femoro-acetabular impingement. *Hip International* 2001;11:37-41.
7. Lequesne M, De Sèze S: False profile of the pelvis: A new radiographic incidence for the study of the hip. Its use in dysplasias and different coxopathies. *Rev Rhum Mal Osteoartic* 1961; 12:643-651.
8. Meyer DC, Beck M, Ellis T, Ganz R, Leunig M: Comparison of six radiographic projections to assess femoral head/neck asphericity. *Clin Orthop Relat Res* 2006;445:181-185.
9. Clohisy JC, Nunley RM, Otto RJ, Schoenecker PL: The frog-leg lateral radiograph accurately visualized hip cam impingement abnormalities. *Clin Orthop Relat Res* 2007;462:115-121.
10. Beck M, Kalhor M, Leunig M, Ganz R: Hip morphology influences the pattern of damage to the acetabular cartilage: Femoroacetabular impingement as a cause of early osteoarthritis of the hip. *J Bone Joint Surg Br* 2005;87:1012-1018.
11. Tannast M, Zheng G, Anderegg C, et al: Tilt and rotation correction of acetabular version on pelvic radiographs. *Clin Orthop Relat Res* 2005; 438:182-190.
12. Ito K, Minka MA II, Leunig M, Werlen S, Ganz R: Femoroacetabular impingement and the cam-effect: A MRI based quantitative study of the femoral head-neck offset. *J Bone Joint Surg Br* 2001;83:171-176.
13. Gosvig KK, Jacobsen S, Palm H, Sonne-Holm S, Magnusson E: A new radiological index for assessing asphericity of the femoral head in cam impingement. *J Bone Joint Surg Br* 2007; 89:1309-1316.
14. Leunig M, Beck M, Kalhor M, Kim YJ, Werlen S, Ganz R: Fibrocystic changes at anterosuperior femoral neck: Prevalence in hips with femoroacetabular impingement. *Radiology* 2005;236:237-246.

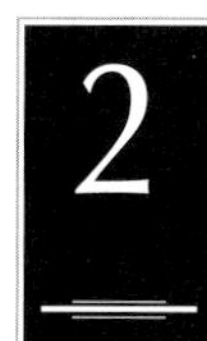

The Young Adult With Hip Impingement: Deciding on the Optimal Intervention

*Paul E. Beaulé, MD, FRCSC
David J. Allen, MBChB, FRCSEd, MSc
*John C. Clohisy, MD
Perry L. Schoenecker, MD
Michael Leunig, MD

Abstract

Femoroacetabular impingement is a recognized cause of hip pain and osteoarthritis in young adults. The clinical presentation of this pathology is quite varied in terms of the underlying deformity, patient age, and the degree of cartilage damage. Open hip surgery with surgical dislocation is the gold standard for treating femoral deformities and the damaged acetabular labral complex; however, less invasive techniques such as hip arthroscopy and arthroscopy combined with limited anterior hip arthrotomy may provide comparable outcomes with less surgical morbidity. Unresolved issues include the indications for acetabular rim trimming with labral refixation in the presence of acetabular retroversion and/or delaminated acetabular cartilage. Other issues involve the use of arthroplasty in older patients and/or in those with significant cartilage damage.

Femoroacetabular impingement is a relatively recently described condition in which an abnormally shaped proximal part of the femur causes interference between the femoral head-neck junction and the acetabular rim.[1,2] Although this can occur in normal hips with an increased range of movement, the condition is usually caused by abnormal morphology of the hip. Two mechanisms have been described.[1]

Cam-type impingement is caused by insufficient concavity of the femoral head-neck junction anterolaterally. This has been referred to as a pistol grip deformity or a head tilt deformity.[3,4] As a consequence, this region of the femoral head has an increased radius of curvature that is too large for the tightly congruent acetabulum. The repeated movement of the deformed femoral head in and out of the acetabulum produces shearing of the labrum and the adjacent acetabular cartilage. This can cause the labrum and articular cartilage to delaminate from the subchondral bone.[5,6] This damage is consistently seen at the anterosuperior aspect of the acetabular rim. The deformity may be secondary to Legg-Calvé-Perthes disease or slipped capital femoral epiphysis; however, most patients do not have a history of childhood hip disorders.[7-10]

Pincer-type impingement is caused by overcoverage of the femoral head by the acetabulum. This leads to contact of the labrum against the femoral neck during physiologic hip motion.[11,12] The labrum eventually fails, but damage to the articular cartilage is initially limited to the acetabular rim.[2] Heterotopic bone growth can occur at the base of the

**Paul E. Beaulé, MD or the department with which he is affiliated has received research or institutional support from Zimmer, Stryker, and Wright Medical Technology; has received miscellaneous nonincome support, commercially derived honoraria, or other nonresearch-related funding from Wright Medical Technology; and is a consultant for or an employee of Wright Medical Technology, BrainLab, and Maquet. John C. Clohisy, MD or the department with which he is affiliated has received research or institutional support from Zimmer and is a consultant for or an employee of Zimmer.*

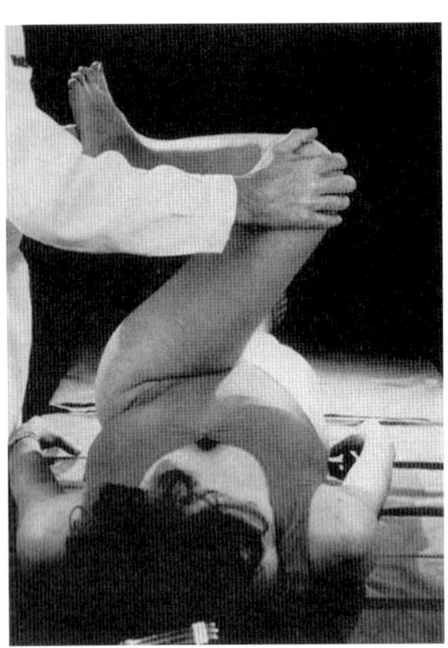

Figure 1 Impingement sign of the hip elicited by forced flexion, adduction, and internal rotation. (Reproduced with permission from Klaue K, Durnin CW, Ganz R: The acetabular rim syndrome: A clinical presentation of dysplasia of the hip. *J Bone Joint Surg Br* 1991;73:423-429.)

labrum in response to the repeated microtrauma. Pincer-type impingement may be associated with hip dysplasia or may be created by overcorrection after periacetabular osteotomy; more commonly, however, it is caused by a retroverted acetabulum producing impingement anteriorly or coxa profunda producing global impingement.[13,14] These two classic forms of impingement (cam and pincer) were shown by Beck and associates[2] to coexist in a large percentage of cases. In their study, 27 of 57 hips (47%) with cam impingement had an associated acetabular deformity, and 34 of 54 (63%) of hips with pincer impingement had an abnormally shaped femoral head. However, to what degree each coexisting deformity contributes to the intra-articular cartilage damage has yet to be clearly defined.

Diagnosis

Patients typically present with groin pain, which is usually of insidious onset and sometimes exacerbated by activity. The pain may be felt as the patient starts to walk after rising from a sitting position, or it may be a dull groin ache while the patient has the hip in a flexed position. The latter type can cause difficulty with sitting at a desk for a prolonged period or with traveling a long distance by automobile or airplane.[1,2,15] Patients with cam-type impingement most often have the onset of symptoms between ages 30 and 39 years, although the symptoms may occur earlier. Men are more commonly affected. Although the deformity is often bilateral, patients usually have symptoms on only one side. Pincer-type impingement is more common in women and often presents as groin pain after activity in patients between ages 40 and 49 years.[16]

The results of the physical examination may be normal, but most patients have a slightly antalgic gait. Typically, the patient has less than 20° of internal rotation with the hip in 90° of flexion and a positive impingement sign, which is groin pain with internal rotation combined with adduction of the lower limb with the hip in 90° of flexion[17] (Figure 1). Wyss and associates[18] found a strong correlation between a lack of internal rotation of the flexed hip and a lack of space between the acetabular rim and the femoral head-neck junction on MRI. The abdomen and low back should be examined to exclude referred pain, and an injection of bupivacaine into the hip joint may help to establish that the pain is from the joint.

Investigations

Cam-type impingement is characterized by asphericity of the femoral head. As the abnormality is typically in the anterolateral portion of the head-neck junction, it may not be seen on an AP pelvic radiograph or a simple lateral radiograph of the hip.[19,20] A cross-table lateral view (with the hip in 10° of internal rotation) or a Dunn view is required[21] (Figure 2). The authors of most studies have used an α angle (the angle between the axis of the neck and the point where the bone of the head-neck junction crosses outside the radius of curvature of the head) of greater than 50.5° to diagnose the abnormality.[20,22,23] In addition, a head-neck offset ratio[21] of 0.15 or less on the cross-table lateral radiograph has been reported to have a sensitivity and specificity of 68% and 82%, respectively, for diagnosing cam impingement.[19,21] The offset ratio is measured by dividing the anterior offset by the femoral head diameter. The anterior offset is the distance between two parallel lines, one adjacent to the anterior aspect of the neck and the other touching the most anterior part of the femoral head, with both parallel to the femoral neck axis. In a comparison of four different lateral radiographic views used to detect femoral head asphericity, Meyer and associates[20] found that the modified Dunn view (an AP radiograph of the hip in neutral rotation, 20° of abduction, and 45° of flexion) was the most sensitive, and the cross-table lateral view (with the hip in 10° of internal rotation) and the standard Dunn view (an AP radiograph of the hip in neutral rotation, 20° of abduction, and 90° of flexion) were quite satisfactory.

The AP pelvic radiograph is the most valuable study for confirming retroversion or coxa profunda in a patient suspected of having pincer-type impingement.[2,11] Pelvic posi-

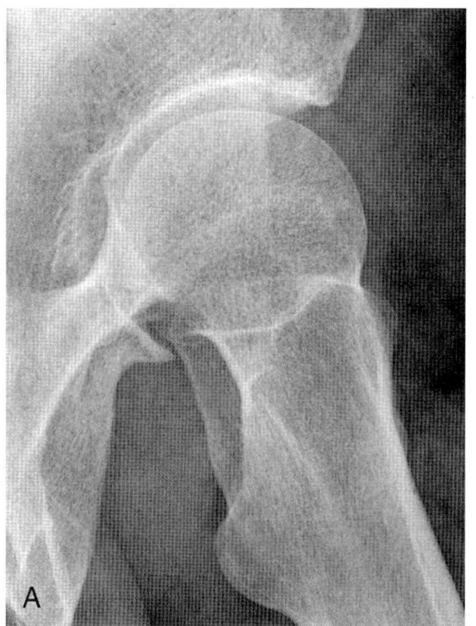

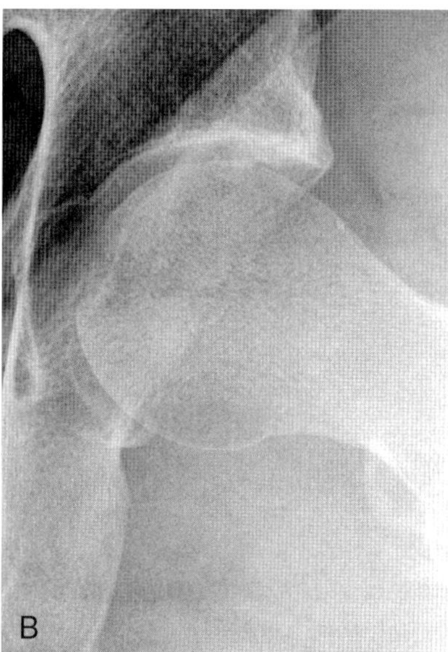

Figure 2 **A,** The impinging lesion can be underestimated on the basis of a standard lateral radiograph. **B,** The Dunn radiograph is more accurate for the assessment of the abnormality.

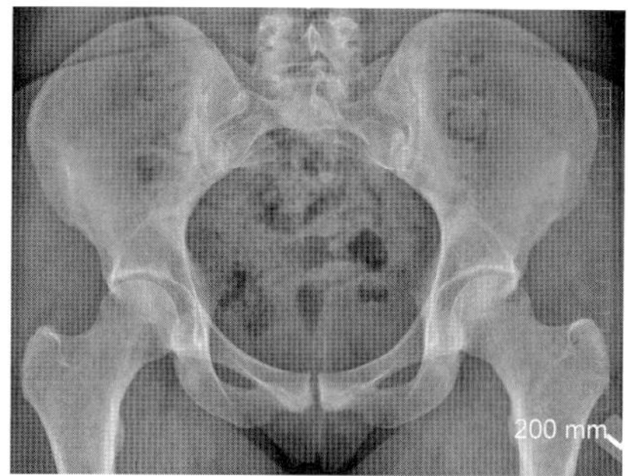

Figure 3 AP pelvic radiograph of a 24-year-old woman with evidence of acetabular retroversion. The crossover sign can be seen on both sides (where the anterior wall of the acetabulum crosses the posterior wall) and the ischial sign is present on both sides (as the ischial spine is visible).

tioning must be considered when interpreting the radiographic signs associated with pincer impingement. With the coccyx and symphysis pubis aligned, the pelvis should be in neutral flexion-extension, which means that the distance between the top of the pubic symphysis and the sacrococcygeal junction should be 32 mm for men and 47 mm for women.[24] The retroverted acetabulum is recognized on the basis of one of three findings: the anterior wall of the acetabulum crossing the posterior wall (the so-called crossover sign), the center of the femoral head lying lateral to the posterior wall (the so-called posterior wall sign), or the ischial spine projecting into the pelvic cavity on the AP pelvic radiograph (the so-called ischial sign)[11,12,25] (Figure 3). Coxa profunda is recognized on the AP pelvic radiograph when the medial wall of the acetabulum lies on or medial to the ilioischial line. Protrusio, which represents the more severe form of coxa profunda, is diagnosed when the femoral head crosses the ilioischial line.[2]

CT and MRI with gadolinium arthrography are useful as additional studies to confirm the impingement deformity, identify associated pathologic changes, and facilitate surgical planning.[23,26] CT scans provide three-dimensional surface renderings of the impingement deformity and aid in determining the area of resection to correct femoral head asphericity.[23] MRI with gadolinium arthrography can demonstrate abnormalities of the acetabular rim, such as labral tears, paralabral cysts, and cartilage delamination.[6,27] It has been demonstrated that MRI is useful for distinguishing dysplasia from impingement.[28] When there is impingement, the labrum may be normal in size or small, in contrast to the hypertrophied labrum associated with a dysplastic acetabulum.[28] Fibrocystic changes at the femoral head-neck junction (also known as Pitt's pit), which are often visible on plain radiographs but are more easily seen on CT or MRI studies, have been reported to be 91% specific and to have a positive predictive value of 71% for the diagnosis of femoroacetabular impingement.[26] When the plain radiographic examination is inconclusive, both MRI and CT scans provide radial images of the anatomy of the femoral head-neck junction that are more sensitive in detecting abnormal α angles as well as acetabular version.[19]

Management

Although we are not aware of any longitudinal studies on the issue, there is evidence that femoroacetabular impingement is a leading cause of so-called primary osteoarthritis of the hip.[1,2,16] Therefore, early intervention is aimed not only at providing pain relief and improving function but also at delaying and/or preventing subsequent osteoarthritis. Although we are not aware of any long-term follow-up studies demonstrating that the onset of osteoarthritis can be prevented and/or delayed with surgery, Beck and associates[5] reported no progression of joint-space narrowing in 19 hips at

4.7 years after surgical treatment of femoroacetabular impingement. However, it is becoming more apparent that one of the greatest challenges in treating femoroacetabular impingement is dealing with the associated damage to the acetabular labral chondral complex, which can range from fraying or irritation of the labral tip to large delaminated flaps of cartilage and/or chondral defects of the acetabulum.[2,29,30] In addition, the treatment of delamination of acetabular cartilage is still evolving. Localized débridement may be sufficient for small acetabular cartilage flaps, whereas larger lesions may require rim trimming to restore a stable cartilage edge.[30] Consideration is needed for the underlying morphologic abnormality causing the impingement (cam or pincer, or both); the presence or absence of deformity of the proximal part of the femur; and the physiologic age of the patient, especially one with early arthritic changes (1 to 2 mm of joint space narrowing), in whom a joint arthroplasty may offer a more predictable outcome. In contrast to a patient with advanced hip arthritis, joint-preserving surgeries may be inappropriate for a patient with relatively mild symptoms and/or advanced age. For young patients, joint preservation to delay and/or prevent arthritis may make even an open approach and femoral head dislocation appropriate. The following clinical factors should most strongly influence the treatment of a patient with femoroacetabular impingement: (1) the physiologic age of the patient; (2) joint space narrowing of 1 to 2 mm; (3) the extent of damage to the acetabular labral chondral complex; (4) in patients with pincer-type impingement, the severity of acetabular retroversion with or without the presence of cam-type impingement; and (5) in those with cam-type impingement, the absence or presence of proximal femoral deformity (for example, a high-riding greater trochanter) and the extent of head asphericity.

The best time for surgery is unknown. Symptoms are usually not as severe as those in patients requiring a joint arthroplasty, and delaying surgery may lead to irreversible cartilage damage. Nevertheless, a course of nonsurgical management, consisting of activity modification, anti-inflammatory medication, and range-of-motion exercises, is advisable for most patients. It is not clear that patients benefit substantially from such a regimen, however.[31]

There are three categories of surgical techniques for the treatment of femoroacetabular impingement: (1) a fully open surgical procedure in which the femoral head is dislocated, providing full access for the correction of cam impingement and trimming the acetabular rim as needed; (2) an arthroscopic technique, wherein the correction is done either arthroscopically only or combined with an arthrotomy (but the femoral head is not dislocated); and (3) a periacetabular osteotomy performed for certain forms of pincer-type impingement. Most patients with femoroacetabular impingement have a mixed type of impingement, and as yet there is no clear information about how to establish the predominant impingement type or if treatment of the cam or pincer-type deformity in isolation is sufficient.

Open Hip Surgery With Dislocation of the Femoral Head

The indications for this approach include (1) cam-type impingement with or without proximal femoral deformity, (2) pincer-type impingement associated with cam-type deformity, and (3) cam-type impingement with 1 mm of joint-space narrowing because this approach would allow possible conversion to arthroplasty.

Dislocation of the femoral head allows complete access to both the femoral head-neck junction and the acetabular rim.[32] The recommended technique for surgical dislocation was developed by Ganz and associates[33] for the treatment of intra-articular hip pathology. With this technique, the femoral head vascularity is protected, and osteonecrosis is avoided. In brief, the patient is placed in the lateral decubitus position, and the incision is centered over the greater trochanter and angulated slightly posteriorly. After the iliotibial band is released, the posterior border of the gluteus medius and minimus is marked. A trochanteric slide osteotomy is performed with a small sleeve of the gluteus medius left attached and with the vastus lateralis left attached to the trochanteric fragment. The osteotomy must be extracapsular and lateral to the piriformis fossa to avoid damage to the blood supply.[34] The trochanteric slide osteotomy is mobilized anteriorly, and the femoral head is dislocated anteriorly. This allows a complete view of the femoral head.

Both Beck and associates[5] and Murphy and associates[32] reported that, in their early experience with the treatment of femoroacetabular impingement with the surgical dislocation technique of Ganz and associates,[33] the results were good to excellent in more than 65% of patients. In a subsequent study, Espinosa and associates[35] reported significantly better outcomes (a 94%

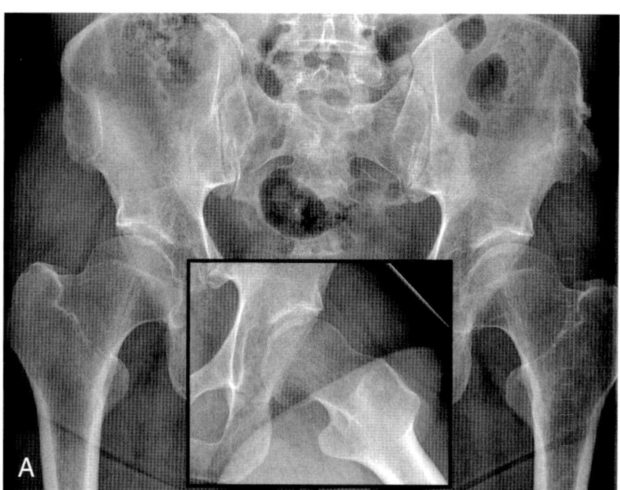

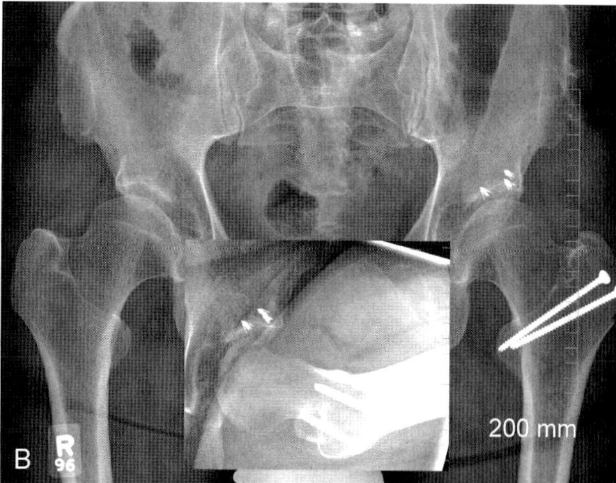

Figure 4 **A,** A 51-year-old man presented with bilateral hip and groin pain, which was worse on the left. The left hip had caused him discomfort for approximately 20 years, affecting his activities of daily living and limiting the distance that he was able to walk. The asphericity of the femoral heads and the short acetabular roofs are seen on the AP radiograph. The diminished anterior concavity of the femoral head is seen on the Dunn radiograph (inset). **B,** The patient was treated with surgical dislocation with osteochondroplasty of the femoral head-neck junction. Labral refixation was performed after the rim was trimmed to remove exposed subchondral bone and perform microfracture of the damaged articular surface. The restored head-neck offset is seen on the Dunn radiograph (inset).

rate of good to excellent results) when the labrum had been preserved as compared with when it had been resected ($P = 0.01$ Figure 4). After following the principles of labral preservation through partial débridement or refixation, Peters and Erickson[29] and Beaulé and associates[30] reported good to excellent clinical scores in more than 80% of patients, which was an improvement compared with the results in the initial series reported by Beck and assoicates[5] and Murphy and associates.[32] On the basis of these results, surgical dislocation appears to be a safe and effective technique for joint preservation that does not lead to osteonecrosis.[8] However, this technique has risks. Ganz and associates[33] reported 2 cases of sciatic neurapraxia, 3 trochanteric nonunions, and 11 cases of clinically relevant heterotopic ossification in a series of 213 hips. In addition, Beaulé and associates[30] reported 10 revisions directly related to the approach (such as screw removal or trochanteric nonunion).

Periacetabular Osteotomy

The indication for periacetabular osteotomy is acetabular retroversion with an associated posterior wall sign. A retroverted acetabulum is caused by external rotation of the entire acetabulum.[36] This produces overcoverage of the anterior aspect of the femoral head and less-than-normal coverage of the posterior part of the femoral head. This altered relationship between the anterior and posterior aspects of the hip leads to the posterior wall sign. This abnormality can be corrected with a periacetabular osteotomy (Figure 5), which also can be used to correct a retroverted acetabulum associated with a dysplastic hip.[37] The cartilage in the anterosuperior aspect of the acetabulum must be intact for a periacetabular osteotomy to be recommended; if it is not intact, acetabular reorientation will place poor cartilage in the main weight-bearing area. Siebenrock and associates[12] reported the results of periacetabular osteotomy in the treatment of femoroacetabular impingement secondary to a retroverted acetabulum in 29 hips in 22 patients. In conjunction with the periacetabular osteotomy, an anterior hip arthrotomy was performed in 26 hips to reshape the femoral head-neck junction. The result was good or excellent for 26 hips, and the average Merle d'Aubigné score improved from 14.0 points preoperatively to 16.9 postoperatively. Three patients required a revision, one each because of loss of correction, posteroinferior impingement, and recurrent signs of anterior impingement (caused by insufficient correction and lack of a head-neck offset). Pincer impingement caused by the relative prominence of the anterior

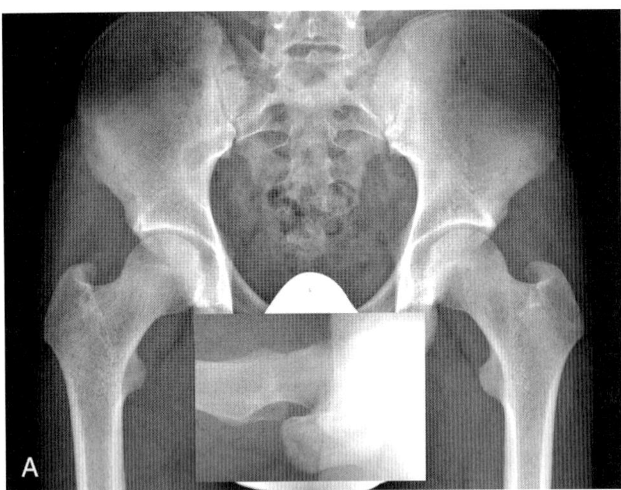

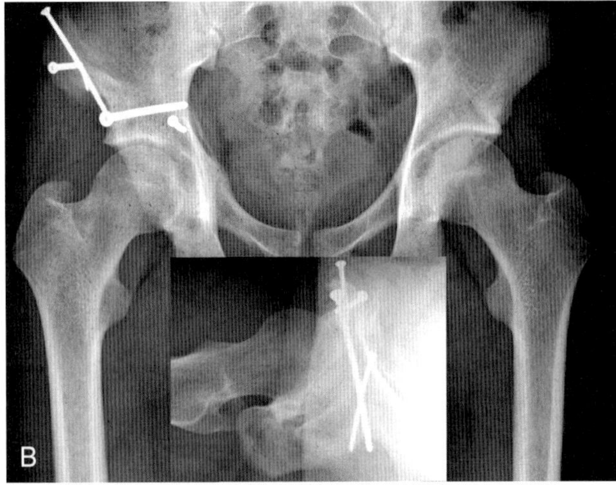

Figure 5 **A,** An 18-year-old male professional ice hockey player reported persistent pain in the right hip. Retroversion of the acetabulum with deficiency of the posterior acetabular wall (the lateral edge of the posterior wall lying medial to the femoral head center) is seen on the AP radiograph. Diminished anterior concavity of the femoral neck is seen on the cross-table lateral radiograph (inset). **B,** One year after a periacetabular osteotomy, the AP radiograph showed that the crossover sign has been corrected. The anterior concavity of the femoral neck has been restored (inset).

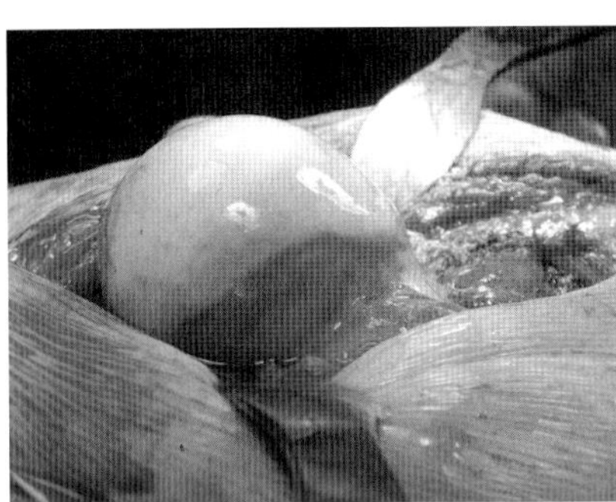

Figure 6 The extent of the deformity of a cam-type impingement is seen on this intraoperative photograph of a dislocated femoral head.

wall (the crossover sign) with an absent posterior wall sign (for example, with the lateral aspect of the posterior wall lateral to the center of the femoral head) is best treated with localized trimming of the rim, whereas coxa profunda requires global rim trimming; both procedures are best done with open surgery by means of surgical dislocation.

Hip Arthroscopy Combined With a Miniopen Anterior (Hueter) Hip Arthrotomy

Hip arthroscopy can be combined with a miniopen anterior (Hueter) arthrotomy as described by Frederic Laude (personal communication, 1999). The arthroscopy is performed first to inspect the joint as well as to treat labral and chondral pathology. Then the anterior hip arthrotomy is performed to correct a cam deformity, which is most commonly located on the anterior aspect of the femoral head-neck junction. In addition, it is possible to detach the labrum anteriorly to trim the acetabular rim. The direct anterior approach involves a dissection within the fascial sheath of the tensor fasciae latae to minimize the risk of damage to the lateral femoral cutaneous nerve. The fascia over the rectus femoris is then released, the rectus femoris is retracted medially, and a T-shaped capsulotomy is performed. Clohisy and McClure[37] argued that performance of the anterior hip arthrotomy allows a better exposure of the femoral head-neck junction than is possible with arthroscopy alone and that there is less potential for osseous debris to become trapped in the joint. Furthermore, the risk of an inadequate osseous correction is minimized. However, Ganz and associates[33] argued that the open technique with femoral head dislocation offers better inspection of the acetabulum than is possible with an anterior Smith-Petersen approach unless the tensor fasciae latae and gluteus medius are extensively detached from the pelvic brim. Clearly, the mini-anterior approach is not suitable for circumferential lesions of the femoral head or acetabulum (Figure 6). However, it may be appropriate for most patients in whom preoperative evaluation has demonstrated that the lesion is localized mainly anteriorly. Patients should be warned that there is a risk of injury to the lateral femoral cutaneous nerve with this approach. In addition, because the

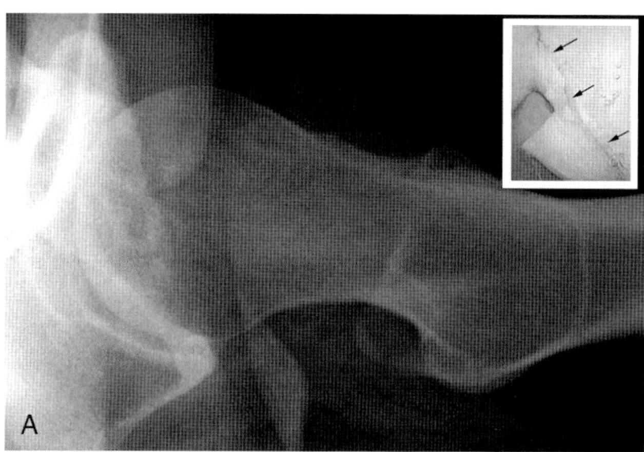

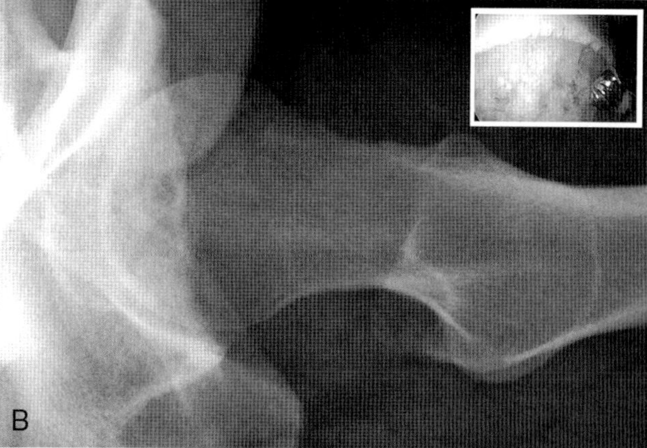

Figure 7 **A,** A cross-table lateral radiograph showing an insufficient anterior head-neck concavity. The inset shows the associated damage to the acetabular labral chondral complex (*arrows*). **B,** The concavity of the femoral head-neck junction has been restored by means of hip arthroscopy as seen on the postoperative radiograph. The resected head-neck area can be seen on the arthroscopic photograph (inset).

incision is not parallel to the tension lines of the skin, a hypertrophic scar may develop in some patients.

Hip Arthroscopy

The indications for hip arthroscopy include (1) cam-type impingement without proximal femoral deformity and (2) isolated acetabular retroversion with or without cam-type deformity. Arthroscopy is clearly an attractive alternative for patients because it involves smaller incisions, a shorter recovery time, and a lower morbidity rate. Today, the technique of arthroscopy of the hip can be divided into two approaches: one into the central compartment and one into the peripheral compartment. The central compartment includes the labrum and all parts medial to it. The peripheral compartment comprises everything lateral to the labrum within the capsule and includes the head-neck junction. Arthroscopy of the central compartment is typically performed with traction. The labrum can be inspected for tears that can be débrided or, in some cases, treated with refixation. Delaminated articular cartilage can be excised, and exposed acetabular subchondral bone can be treated with microfracture. With the traction released, the peripheral compartment can be entered through an anterolateral portal. A partial capsulectomy is then performed to facilitate instrument placement for reshaping of the femoral head-neck junction (Figure 7). In more advanced cases of osteoarthritis, peripheral osteophytes which can be removed. Incomplete visualization may lead to undertreatment, can lead to errors with defining the extent of rim trimming that is required, or can lead to excessive removal of bone at the femoral head-neck junction and subsequent fracture.[38] Neurovascular injury is rare but possible; it can be related either to the portals (the superior gluteal nerve can be damaged with creation of the anterolateral portal, and the lateral femoral cutaneous and femoral nerves can be damaged with creation of the anterior portal) or to the traction, which can especially affect the sciatic and pudendal nerves.

As with any new surgical technique, there is a risk of suboptimal results when arthroscopy is used for the treatment of femoroacetabular impingement.[39] With increasing clinical experience and training, arthroscopic treatment of femoroacetabular impingement will continue to expand. Ilizaliturri and associates[40] recently reported on 19 patients with pure cam impingement treated arthroscopically. Sixteen patients had significant improvement in their Western Ontario and McMaster Universities Osteoarthritis Index scores ($P = 0.001$), 2 had progression of arthritis, and 1 was advised to undergo total hip replacement. There were no major complications associated with this procedure. Other surgeons have reported on larger studies, but the duration of follow-up was short, and no validated scoring was provided.[38] More importantly, because the indications for and techniques of arthroscopic treatment of pincer-type impingement are still evolving, great caution should be exercised when considering trimming the acetabular rim, which is technically demanding and can create a dysplastic acetabulum if there is overcorrection.[41]

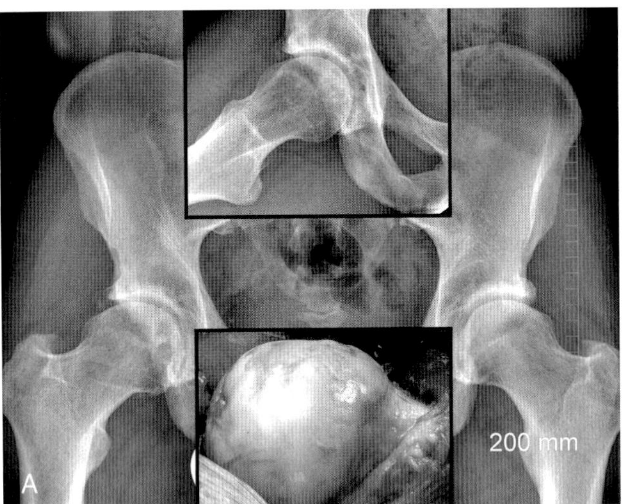

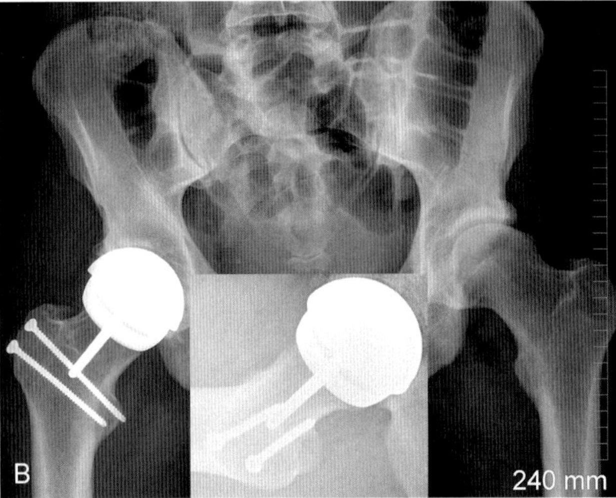

Figure 8 **A,** A 37-year-old man with pain in the right hip had cam-type impingement and joint-space narrowing. The Dunn radiograph (top inset) shows an insufficient head-neck concavity, and the intraoperative photograph (bottom inset) shows gross cartilage loss from the femoral head. **B,** Radiograph made following metal-on-metal hip resurfacing done through a surgical dislocation approach. The inset shows optimization of the femoral head-neck concavity.

Hip Arthroplasty

The presence of substantial cartilage damage at the time of surgery for the treatment of impingement has been associated with a poor outcome, with patients treated with joint arthroplasty in the short-term follow-up period.[5,40,42] However, it is often unclear whether joint preservation is still indicated or if arthroplasty is preferable to provide a more predictable outcome. One of the factors that has discouraged surgeons from proceeding with a total hip replacement is the large leap between joint preservation and resection of the femoral head-neck area to treat patients' symptoms. Hip resurfacing represents an attractive alternative bone-preserving option for a young patient with an arthritic hip.[43] When hip resurfacing is performed in a patient with osteoarthritis caused by femoroacetabular impingement, care must be taken to restore the femoral head-neck offset; otherwise, impingement can still occur.[19] In addition, restoration of the femoral head-neck offset allows optimization of the sizes of the femoral and acetabular components because the femoral head diameter drives the acetabular size.[44] It is recommended that anterior osteophytes be removed from the head-neck junction before the guide pin is placed.[44] One of the authors (P.E.B.) performed resurfacing arthroplasty in six patients, with a mean age of 42.4 years (range, 34 to 48 years), who had initially undergone surgery to treat impingement. All six patients had consented to both procedures because preoperative radiographs had demonstrated joint-space narrowing (Figure 8, *A*). All patients underwent hybrid metal-on-metal hip resurfacing with the Conserve Plus (Wright Medical Technology, Arlington, TN), and one patient also underwent a trochanteric advancement. All had substantial pain relief and improvement in function (Figure 8, *B*). Although there were no complications, two of the six patients required removal of the screws because of persistent bursitis.

Summary

Femoroacetabular impingement is a cause of hip pain in young adults, and there is evidence that it is a major cause of osteoarthritis. Treatment of femoroacetabular impingement has been reported to relieve symptoms and perhaps retard the progression of osteoarthritis. The optimal treatment strategies are determined by carefully correlating the patient's history and the findings of physical examination with detailed imaging studies. Surgery should be tailored to treat the individual patient's abnormal hip morphology and should address the major underlying impinging deformities. Future treatments may include cartilage grafting and computer-assisted surgery, further expanding the role of less invasive surgical techniques such as hip arthroscopy. Hip resurfacing is an additional tool for the treatment of young adults with hip pain and early stage osteoarthritis.

References

1. Ganz R, Parvizi J, Beck M, Leunig M, Nötzli H, Siebenrock KA: Femoroacetabular impingement: A cause for osteoarthritis of the hip. *Clin Orthop Relat Res* 2003;417:112-120.
2. Beck M, Kalhor M, Leunig M, Ganz R: Hip morphology influences the pattern of damage to the acetabular cartilage: Femoroacetabular impingement as a cause of early osteoarthritis of the hip. *J Bone Joint Surg Br* 2005;87:1012-1018.
3. Stulberg SD, Cordell LD, Harris WH, Ramsey PL, MacEwen GD: Unrecognized childhood hip disease: A major cause of idiopathic osteoarthritis of the hip, in *The Hip: Proceedings of the Third Open Scientific Meeting of the Hip Society*. St. Louis, MO, C.V. Mosby, 1975, pp 212-228.
4. Murray RO: The aetiology of primary osteoarthritis of the hip. *Br J Radiol* 1965;38:810-824.
5. Beck M, Leunig M, Parvizi J, Boutier V, Wyss D, Ganz R: Anterior femoroacetabular impingement: Part II. Midterm results of surgical treatment. *Clin Orthop Relat Res* 2004;418: 67-73.
6. Beaulé PE, Zaragoza E, Copelan N: Magnetic resonance imaging with gadolinium arthrography to assess acetabular cartilage delamination: A report of four cases. *J Bone Joint Surg Am* 2004;86:2294-2298.
7. Snow SW, Keret D, Scarangella S, Bowen JR: Anterior impingement of the femoral head: A late phenomenon of Legg-Calve-Perthes' disease. *J Pediatr Orthop* 1993;13:286-289.
8. Leunig M, Casillas MM, Hamlet M, et al: Slipped capital femoral epiphysis: Early mechanical damage to the acetabular cartilage by a prominent femoral metaphysis. *Acta Orthop Scand* 2000;71:370-375.
9. Rab GT: The geometry of slipped capital femoral epiphysis: Implications for movement, impingement, and corrective osteotomy. *J Pediatr Orthop* 1999;19:419-424.
10. Siebenrock KA, Wahab KH, Werlen S, Kalhor M, Leunig M, Ganz R: Abnormal extension of the femoral head epiphysis as a cause of cam impingement. *Clin Orthop Relat Res* 2004;418: 54-60.
11. Reynolds D, Lucas J, Klaue K: Retroversion of the acetabulum: A cause of hip pain. *J Bone Joint Surg Br* 1999;81: 281-288.
12. Siebenrock KA, Schoeniger R, Ganz R: Anterior femoro-acetabular impingement due to acetabular retroversion: Treatment with periacetabular osteotomy. *J Bone Joint Surg Am* 2003;85:278-286.
13. Li PL, Ganz R: Morphologic features of congenital acetabular dysplasia: One in six is retroverted. *Clin Orthop Relat Res* 2003;416:245-253.
14. Myers SR, Eijer H, Ganz R: Anterior femoroacetabular impingement after periacetabular osteotomy. *Clin Orthop Relat Res* 1999;363:93-99.
15. Beaulé PE, Zaragoza EJ: Femoroacetabular impingement: Diagnosis and treatment, in Beaulé PE (ed): *Young Adult With Hip Pain*. Rosemont, IL, American Academy of Orthopaedic Surgeons, 2007, pp 63-74.
16. Ganz R, Leunig M, Leunig-Ganz K, Harris WH: The etiology of osteoarthritis of the hip: An integrated mechanical concept. *Clin Orthop Relat Res* 2008;466:264-272.
17. Klaue K, Durnin CW, Ganz R: The acetabular rim syndrome: A clinical presentation of dysplasia of the hip. *J Bone Joint Surg Br* 1991;73:423-429.
18. Wyss TF, Clark JM, Weishaupt D, Notzli HP: Correlation between internal rotation and bony anatomy in the hip. *Clin Orthop Relat Res* 2007; 460:152-158.
19. Beaulé PE, Harvey N, Zaragoza E, Le Duff MJ, Dorey FJ: The femoral head/neck offset and hip resurfacing. *J Bone Joint Surg Br* 2007;89:9-15.
20. Meyer DC, Beck M, Ellis T, Ganz R, Leunig M: Comparison of six radiographic projections to assess femoral head/neck asphericity. *Clin Orthop Relat Res* 2006;445:181-185.
21. Eijer H, Leunig M, Mahomed N, Ganz R: Cross-table lateral radiographs for screening of anterior femoral head-neck offset in patients with femoroacetabular impingement. *Hip Int* 2001;11:37-41.
22. Notzli HP, Wyss TF, Stoecklin CH, Schmid MR, Treiber K, Hodler J: The contour of the femoral head-neck junction as a predictor for the risk of anterior impingement. *J Bone Joint Surg Br* 2002;84:556-560.
23. Beaulé PE, Zaragoza E, Motamedi K, Copelan N, Dorey FJ: Three-dimensional computed tomography of the hip in the assessment of femoroacetabular impingement. *J Orthop Res* 2005;23:1286-1292.
24. Siebenrock KA, Kalbermatten DF, Ganz R: Effect of pelvic tilt on acetabular retroversion: A study of pelves from cadavers. *Clin Orthop Relat Res* 2003;407:241-248.
25. Kalberer F, Sierra RJ, Madan SS, Ganz R, Leunig M: Ischial spine projection into the pelvis: A new sign for acetabular retroversion. *Clin Orthop Relat Res* 2008;466:677-683.
26. Kassarjian A, Yoon LS, Belzile E, Connolly SA, Millis MB, Palmer WE: Triad of MR arthrographic findings in patients with cam-type femoroacetabular impingement. *Radiology* 2005;236:588-592.
27. Leunig M, Werlen S, Ungersbock A, Ito K, Ganz R: Evaluation of the acetabular labrum by MR arthrography. *J Bone Joint Surg Br* 1997;79:230-234.
28. Leunig M, Podeszwa D, Beck M, Werlen S, Ganz R: Magnetic resonance arthrography of labral disorders in hips with dysplasia and impingement. *Clin Orthop Relat Res* 2004;418: 74-80.
29. Peters CL, Erickson JA: Treatment of femoro-acetabular impingement with surgical dislocation and débridement in young adults. *J Bone Joint Surg Am* 2006;88:1735-1741.
30. Beaulé PE, Le Duff MJ, Zaragoza E: Quality of life following femoral head-neck osteochondroplasty for femoroacetabular impingement. *J Bone Joint Surg Am* 2007;89:773-779.

31. Lavigne M, Parvizi J, Beck M, Siebenrock KA, Ganz R, Leunig M: Anterior femoroacetabular impingement: Part I. Techniques of joint preserving surgery. *Clin Orthop Relat Res* 2004; 418:61-66.

32. Murphy S, Tannast M, Kim YJ, Buly R, Millis MB: Debridement of the adult hip for femoroacetabular impingement: Indications and preliminary clinical results. *Clin Orthop Relat Res* 2004;429:178-181.

33. Ganz R, Gill TJ, Gautier E, Ganz K, Krugel N, Berlemann U: Surgical dislocation of the adult hip: A new technique with full access to the femoral head and acetabulum without the risk of avascular necrosis. *J Bone Joint Surg Br* 2001;83:1119-1124.

34. Gautier E, Ganz K, Krugel N, Gill T, Ganz R: Anatomy of the medial femoral circumflex artery and its surgical implications. *J Bone Joint Surg Br* 2000;82:679-683.

35. Espinosa N, Rothenfluh DA, Beck M, Ganz R, Leunig M: Treatment of femoro-acetabular impingement: Preliminary results of labral refixation. *J Bone Joint Surg Am* 2006;88: 925-935.

36. Jamali AA, Mladenov K, Meyer DC, et al: Anteroposterior pelvic radiographs to assess acetabular retroversion: High validity of the "cross-over-sign." *J Orthop Res* 2007;25:758-765.

37. Clohisy JC, McClure JT: Treatment of anterior femoroacetabular impingement with combined hip arthroscopy and limited anterior decompression. *Iowa Orthop J* 2005;25: 164-171.

38. Sampson TG: Arthroscopic treatment of femoroacetabular impingement: A proposed technique with clinical experience. *Instr Course Lect* 2006;55: 337-346.

39. Beaulé PE, Clohisy JC, Schoenecker PE, Kim YJ, Millis M, Trousdale RT: Hip arthroscopy: An emerging gold standard. *Arthroscopy* 2007; 23:682.

40. Ilizaliturri VM Jr, Orozco-Rodriguez L, Acosta-Rodríguez E, Camacho-Galindo J: Arthroscopic treatment of cam-type femoroacetabular impingement: Preliminary report at 2 years minimum follow-up. *J Arthroplasty* 2008;23:226-234.

41. Philippon MJ: New frontiers in hip arthroscopy: The role of arthroscopic hip labral repair and capsulorrhaphy in the treatment of hip disorders. *Instr Course Lect* 2006;55:309-316.

42. Peters CL, Erickson J: The etiology and treatment of hip pain in the young adult. *J Bone Joint Surg Am* 2006;88(suppl 4):20-26.

43. Beaulé P: A soft tissue-sparing approach to surface arthroplasty of the hip. *Oper Tech Orthop* 2004;14:75-84.

44. Beaulé PE, Poitras P: Femoral component sizing and positioning in hip resurfacing arthroplasty. *Instr Course Lect* 2007;56:163-169.

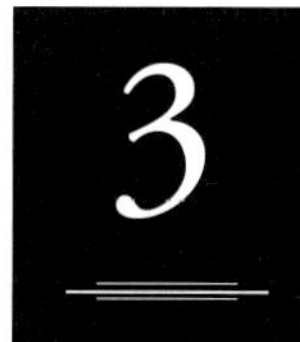

Arthroscopic Management of Hip Pathomorphology

Christopher M. Larson, MD

Abstract

The role for the arthroscopic correction of femoroacetabular impingement continues to evolve. As the understanding of hip pathomorphology improves and arthroscopic techniques for managing these disorders advance, the indications for arthroscopic femoroacetabular correction become clearer. Attention to detail with respect to diagnoses and surgical management is critical to optimize outcomes in this patient population. Studies have shown comparable outcomes for arthroscopic management and open surgical techniques. Further study is required to better define the role for arthroscopic versus open surgical management of selected pathomorphologies of the hip.

The body of literature regarding the arthroscopic management of hip pathomorphology, particularly femoroacetabular impingement (FAI), continues to grow[1-22] (CM Larson, MD, et al, San Francisco, CA, unpublished data presented at the Arthroscopy Association of North America annual meeting, 2011). There is a long learning curve for treating FAI arthroscopically, and specific techniques and indications continue to evolve. It is critical to identify those patients who are appropriate candidates for arthroscopic FAI correction.

Indications and Contraindications

Indications and contraindications for the arthroscopic management of FAI are based on a physician's ability to treat the underlying pathomorphology. Arthroscopic indications include focal anterior acetabular overcoverage, mild to moderate degrees of acetabular retroversion, coxa profunda, associated rim fractures and os acetabuli, and anterolaterally based cam lesions.[23] Relative contraindications for arthroscopic treatment include associated significant structural instability, extra-articular greater trochanteric impingement, posteriorly based cam lesions, and moderate to advanced degenerate arthritis.[23] More specifically, structural instability cannot be corrected with arthroscopy. Patients with center-edge angles less than 20°, evidence of femoral head lateralization, a break in the Shenton line, and more severe degrees of acetabular retroversion with a low volumetric acetabulum may be better treated with a corrective pelvic osteotomy. To more completely define instability in patients with milder degrees of structural instability, it is important to take into account other factors, such as acetabular inclination, the femoral neck-shaft angle, and femoral neck version. Although global rim resections can be performed for protrusio acetabuli, there are limitations associated with arthroscopic dynamic assessment. Ultimately, younger patients with more severe protrusio may be better treated with an open surgical dislocation.[23]

Surgical Technique Overview

When performing hip arthroscopy, the surgeon must be capable of treating a three-dimensional problem while viewing a two-dimensional image. Consequently, three-dimensional CT is valuable in better defining the pathology and correlating it with arthro-

Dr. Larson or an immediate family member is a member of a speakers' bureau or has made paid presentations on behalf of Smith & Nephew; serves as a paid consultant to Smith & Nephew and A2 Surgical; owns stock or stock options in A2 Surgical; and has received research or institutional support from Smith & Nephew.

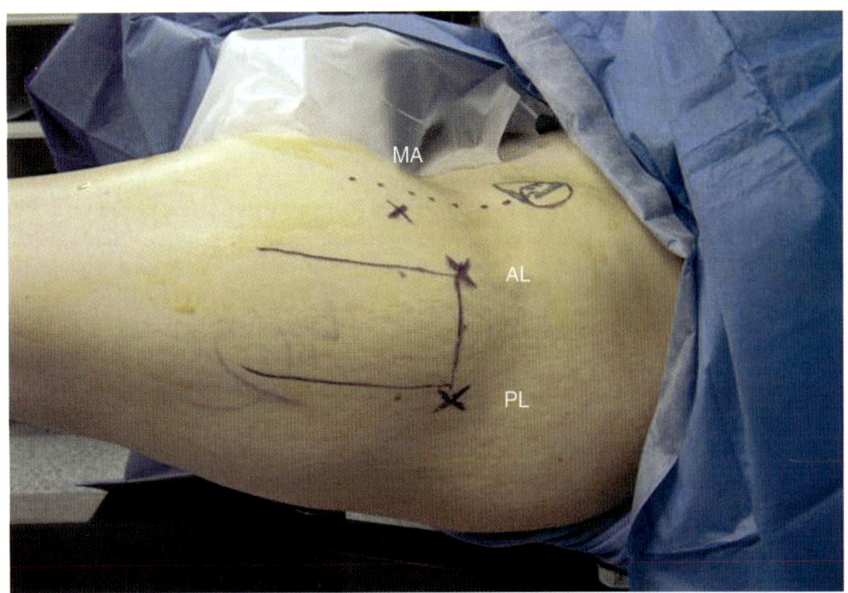

Figure 1 Typical portals used for hip arthroscopy (left hip shown) include the midanterior portal (MA), the anterolateral portal (AL), and the posterolateral portal (PL).

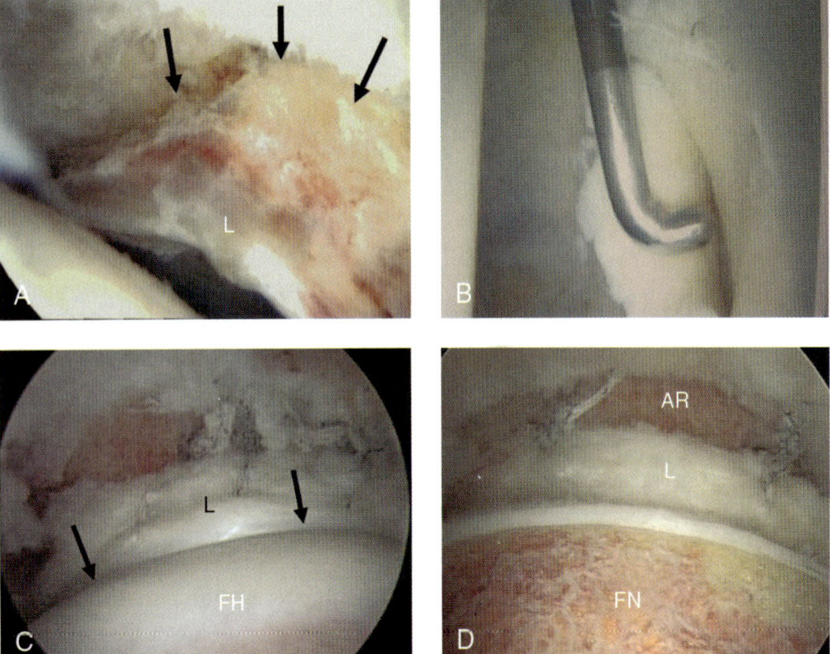

Figure 2 **A,** Arthroscopic image of the left hip shows labral bruising (L) and abnormal extension of the acetabular rim (arrows) beyond the labrochondral junction consistent with pincer-type impingement. **B,** Arthroscopic image of the left hip shows a chondral delamination with probing of the labrochondral junction. **C,** Arthroscopic image of the left hip after labral refixation (L) with mattress sutures shows maintenance of the labral seal (arrows) against the femoral head (FH). **D,** Arthroscopic image of the left hip after rim resection (AR), labral refixation (L), and femoral resection osteoplasty (FN) shows maintenance of the labral seal.

scopic findings. Most procedures can be performed using a two-portal technique, with anterolateral and midanterior portals. A posterolateral portal can be used when posterior acetabular rim pathology is treated (**Figure 1**). Initially, central compartment arthroscopy is performed with traction. Generous capsulotomies from the midanterior to anterolateral or posterolateral portals are created to access most of the acetabular rim and the anterolateral femoral head-neck junction. Inspection of the labrum, labrochondral junction, acetabulum, and femur should confirm the suspected pathomorphology and guide specific procedures (**Figure 2**). Labral ecchymosis, calcification, ossification, extension of the acetabular rim well beyond the labrochondral junction, and difficulty visualizing or accessing the central compartment despite adequate distraction on fluoroscopy are all consistent with pincer-type FAI (**Figure 2,** *A*). Labrochondral disruptions, with varying degrees of acetabular chondral delaminations, are consistent with cam-type FAI (**Figure 2,** *B*). Many patients will have a combination of these findings because of the presence of both cam- and pincer-type FAI. All the described findings should be correlated with preoperative imaging studies and evaluated with intraoperative dynamic assessment.

Rim resections for pincer-type FAI are typically performed with the hip in traction, with or without labral takedown. The labrum can be taken down from the acetabular rim with an arthroscopic knife along the area of the pincer-type impingement. Rim resection is then performed with a motorized burr. Alternatively, more focal areas of pincer-type FAI with an intact labrum can be resected peripheral to the labrum without labral takedown. Intraoperative fluoroscopy can help guide and confirm appropriate resections if the pelvis is properly aligned to re-create a well-centered, preoperative anteroposterior pelvic radiograph[24] (**Figure 3**). This is primarily achieved by aligning the anterior superior iliac spines parallel to the floor and ceiling.[24] The extent and degree of rim resection is ultimately based on intraoperative findings, dynamic assessment, and preoperative imaging studies (**Figure 4**). The labrum is then refixed with suture anchors placed approximately 1 cm apart. A mattress and labral base refixation may be preferred to a looparound refixation to preserve the sealing function of the labrum (**Figure 2**). Overresection of pincer-type pathology or resections in the setting of acetabular dysplasia should be avoided and can lead to iatrogenic postoperative instability.[25-27]

After treating the central compartment pathology, traction is released and the hip is flexed to approximately 40°. Portals can be maintained during traction release by withdrawing the arthroscope from the central compartment, which allows for visualization of the femoral head-neck junction. Dynamic assessment is then performed to evaluate for impingement secondary to cam-type FAI. Impingement is indicated by abnormal lifting of the acetabular labrum by the head-neck junction, levering of the femoral head out of the acetabulum, and/or limitations in hip range of motion with a firm end point during dynamic testing. The cam lesion is identified and correlated with preoperative imaging studies. Greater degrees of flexion and external rotation allow for visualization of the anteroinferior femoral head-neck junction and the medial synovial fold, whereas greater degrees of extension and internal rotation allow for visualization of the superoposterior femoral head-neck junction and the retinacular vessels.[5] A motorized burr is used to re-create a normal femoral-head neck junction; a repetition of dynamic assessment and intraoperative fluoroscopy can confirm appropriate femoral resection (**Figure 4**). A broader, more conservative resection is generally preferred over a more focal, aggressive resection because it may better maintain the labral seal. Resecting

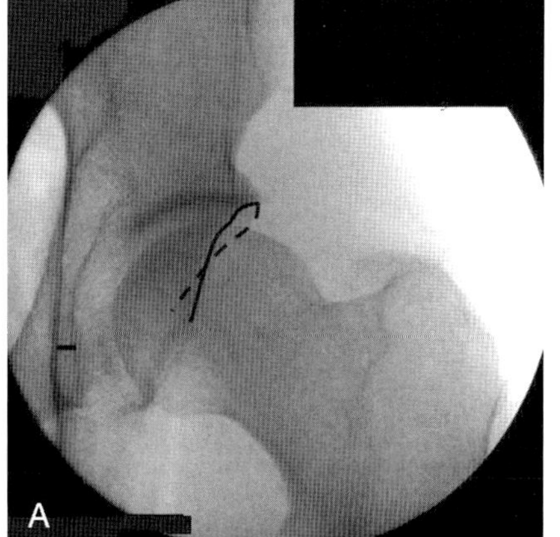

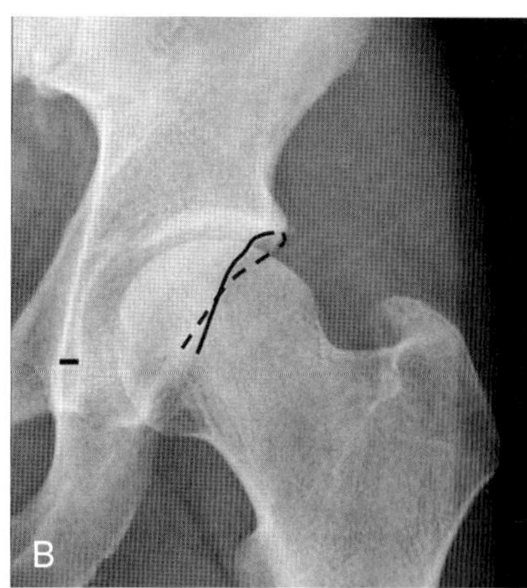

Figure 3 The intraoperative fluoroscopic image (**A**) of the left hip re-creates a well-centered preoperative AP pelvic radiograph (**B**) with respect to the relationship between the anterior (dashed line) and posterior acetabular walls (solid line), and between the ilioischial line and tear drop (horizontal line). (Reproduced with permission from Larson CM, Wulf CA: Intraoperative fluoroscopy for evaluation of bony resection during arthroscopic management of femoroacetabular impingement in the supine position. *Arthroscopy* 2009;25:1183-1192.)

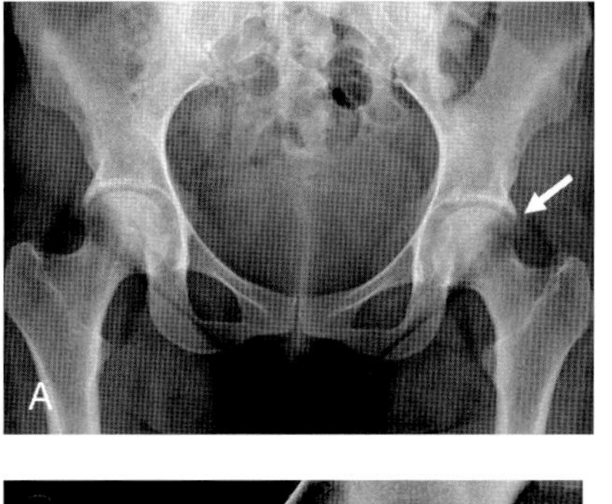

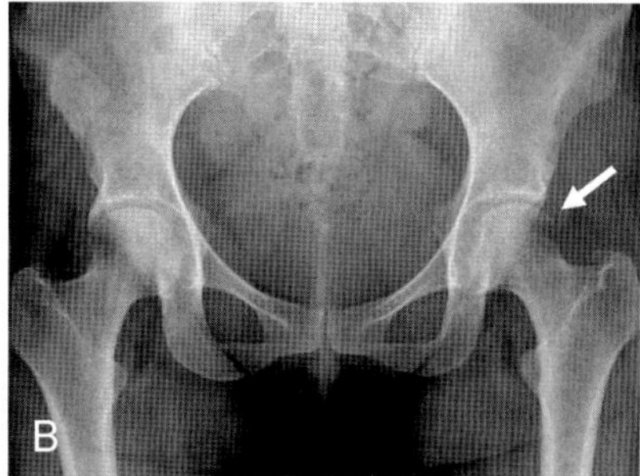

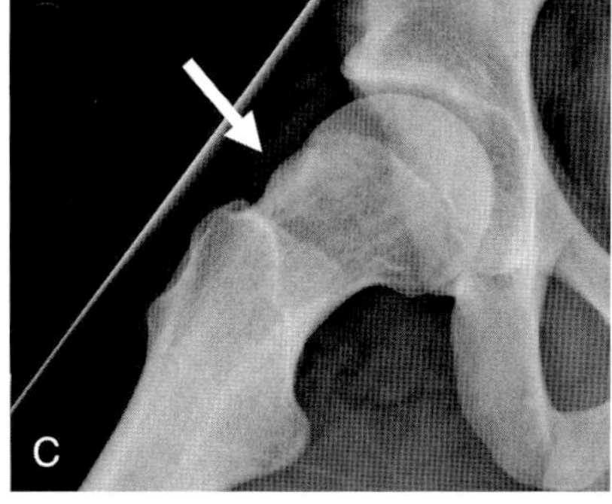

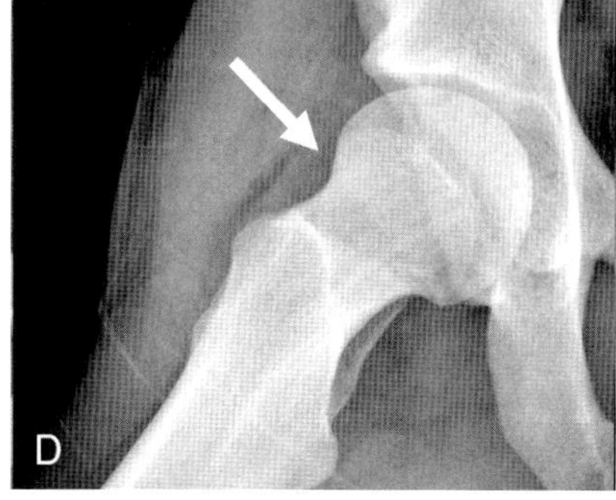

Figure 4 **A,** AP radiograph shows bilateral global acetabular overcoverage secondary to labral ossification (arrow). **B,** Postoperative radiograph after global anterior to posterior rim resection of the left hip (arrow). **C,** Lateral view of the right hip shows cam-type impingement (arrow). **D,** Postoperative radiograph of the right hip after femoral resection osteoplasty reveals improved head-neck offset.

Table 1
Clinical Outcomes After Arthroscopic Management of Femoroacetabular Impingement

Study	Hips	Mean Follow-up (Years)	Clinically Good or Excellent Outcomes
Brunner et al[12]	53	2.4	NA
Byrd et al[13]	200	1.6	95%
Byrd and Jones[1]	207	1.4	NA
Fabricant et a1[18]	27	1.5	NA
Gedouin et al[14]	111	0.8	NA
Horisberger et al[15]	20	3.0	NA
Ilizaliturri et al[19]	14	2.5	NA
Ilizaliturri et al[2]	19	2.4	NA
Larson and Giveans[4]	75	1.6	DB, 66.7%; LR, 89.7%
Larson et al[20]	227	2.2	NA
Larson et al[a]	100	3.5	DB, 68%; LR, 92%
Nho et al[17]	47	2.2	93%
Philippon et al[7]	112	2.3	NA
Philippon et al[21]	28	2.0	NA
Schilders et al[22]	101	2.44	NA
Singh and O'Donnell[16]	27	1.8	NA

[a]CM Larson, MD, et al, San Francisco, CA, unpublished data presented at the Arthroscopy Association of North America annual meeting, 2011.
ADL = activities of daily living; DB = débridement (labral resection); HHS = Harris Hip score; HOS = Hip Outcome score; LR = labral refixation; MHHS = modified Harris Hip score; NAHS = Nonarthritic Hip score; NA = not available; OA = osteoarthritis; RTP = return to play; SF-12 = Medical Outcomes Study 12-Item Short Form; THA = total hip arthroplasty; VAS = visual analog pain scale, WOMAC = Western Ontario and McMaster Universities Osteoarthritis Index.
(Courtesy of Asheesh Bedi, MD, and Bryan Kelly, MD, New York, NY.)

greater than 30% of the femoral neck width is reported to significantly increase the risk for postoperative femoral neck fractures.[28] Impingement is a unique condition, with each case varying with respect to the region and extent of bony resections. At the completion of the procedure, a motorized shaver is used to meticulously remove all residual bony debris to minimize the risk for postoperative heterotopic ossification. Closure of the capsulotomy is controversial and should be considered in patients with capsular laxity, generalized hypermobility, and borderline dysplasia.

Postoperative Management

Early postoperative range of motion begins on the day of surgery with well-leg cycling or a continuous passive range-of-motion machine. Limits are placed on the extremes of external rotation for patients with capsular repairs. Foot-flat weight bearing is advised for 2 to 3 weeks until the patient is able to ambulate with a nonantalgic gait. Weight-bearing restrictions are maintained for 4 to 8 weeks if microfracture is performed or osteopenic bone is encountered during bony resections. Nonsteroidal anti-inflammatory drugs are taken for 2 to 3 weeks postoperatively to decrease the risk of heterotopic bone formation.

Arthroscopic Outcomes and Complications

Reports and systematic reviews evaluating arthroscopic management of FAI in properly selected patients have noted significant improvements in pain and functional scores[1-22] (CM Larson, MD, et al, San Francisco, CA, unpublished data presented at the Arthroscopy Association of North America annual meeting, 2011) (**Table 1**). To date, there has been only

Table 1 *(continued)*

Clinical Outcomes After Arthroscopic Management of Femoroacetabular Impingement

Clinical Outcome Measure(s) and Mean Change in Hip Score (Points)	Failure Definition	Failure % (Number)
SF-12, 1.06; NAHS, 31.3; VAS, 4.1	NA	NA
MHHS, 21	Conversion to THA, inability to RTP	THA, 0.5%; professional RTP, 0.5%; intercollegiate RTP, 15%
MHHS, 20	NA	NA
HHS, 21; HOS, 16	NA	NA
WOMAC, 23	NA	NA
NAHS, 28; VAS, 4	Conversion to THA	THA, 8.6% (9)
WOMAC, 9.6	NA	0% (0)
WOMAC, 7	Advanced OA, recommended THA	5% (1)
DB: MHHS, 25; SF-12, 19; VAS, 5 LR: MHHA, 32; SF-12, 24; VAS, 5	MHHS less than 70, reconversion to THA, repeat débridement	DB, 11.1%; LR, 7.7%
No OA: MHHS, 22.8; SF-12, 20.9; VAS, 4.5 With OA: MHHS, 3.7; SF-12, 4.3; VAS, 2.6	No sustained improvement in MHHS	Failure rate, 12%; failure rate with mild joint-space narrowing, 33%; failure rate with OA, 82%
DB: MHHS, 20.2; SF-12, 18.4; VAS, 4.7 LR: MHHS, 26.1; SF-12, 28.1; VAS, 4.6	MHHS less than 70, reconversion to THA, repeat débridement	DB, 9.1%; LR, 8.0%
MHHS, 20; HOS, 13	Inability to RTP	7%
MHHS, 24; HOS-ADL, 17; HOS-Sport, 24; NAHS, 14	Conversion to THA	9% (10)
MHHS, 25	NA	NA
LR: HHS, 33; DB: HHS, 26	NA	NA
MHHS, 10; NAHS, 15	Continued hip pain or pain requiring surgical intervention	0% (0)

[a]CM Larson, MD, et al, San Francisco, CA, unpublished data presented at the Arthroscopy Association of North America annual meeting, 2011.

ADL = activities of daily living; DB = débridement (labral resection); HHS = Harris Hip score; HOS = Hip Outcome score; LR = labral refixation; MHHS = modified Harris Hip score; NAHS = Nonarthritic Hip score; NA = not available; OA = osteoarthritis; RTP = return to play; SF-12 = Medical Outcomes Study 12-Item Short Form; THA = total hip arthroplasty; VAS = visual analog pain scale, WOMAC = Western Ontario and McMaster Universities Osteoarthritis Index.

(Courtesy of Asheesh Bedi, MD, and Bryan Kelly, MD, New York, NY.)

one review article comparing arthroscopic and open surgical treatment of FAI.[11] This report found substantial improvement in outcomes after both open and arthroscopic approaches, but neither treatment was found to be clearly superior. Cadaver studies have shown that arthroscopic femoral resections for anteriorly based cam-type FAI are comparable to anterior femoral resections performed with an open surgical approach.[29,30]

Complications have been reported after arthroscopic management of FAI.[5,25-28,31,32] Specifically, underresection of bony impingement has been reported as a primary reason for failure in arthroscopic hip procedures.[31] Iatrogenic hip instability and femoral neck fractures also have been reported after hip arthroscopy; this emphasizes the importance of appropriate diagnosis, surgical technique, and the avoidance of bony overresection.[25-28,31,32] Hip joint preservation procedures in the presence of substantial osteoarthritis will lead to higher failure rates regardless of the surgical approach.[20]

Summary

The understanding of FAI is evolving, and new patterns of impingement are being identified. With appropriate patient selection, indications, and surgical technique, hip arthroscopy has been shown to be effective in treating these disorders. Published outcomes and systematic reviews support a role for hip arthroscopy in patients with FAI; however, further studies are required to better define the most appropriate surgical approach when treating the varying patterns of FAI.

References

1. Byrd JW, Jones KS: Arthroscopic femoroplasty in the management of cam-type femoroacetabular impingement. *Clin Orthop Relat Res* 2009;467(3):739-746.

2. Ilizaliturri VM Jr, Orozco-Rodriguez L, Acosta-Rodríguez E, Camacho-Galindo J: Arthroscopic treatment of cam-type femoroacetabular impingement: Preliminary report at 2 years minimum follow-up. *J Arthroplasty* 2008; 23(2):226-234.
3. Larson CM, Giveans MR: Arthroscopic management of femoroacetabular impingement: Early outcomes measures. *Arthroscopy* 2008;24(5):540-546.
4. Larson CM, Giveans MR: Arthroscopic debridement versus refixation of the acetabular labrum associated with femoroacetabular impingement. *Arthroscopy* 2009; 25(4):369-376.
5. Larson CM, Guanche CA, Kelly BT, Clohisy JC, Ranawat AS: Advanced techniques in hip arthroscopy. *Instr Course Lect* 2009; 58:423-436.
6. Ng VY, Arora N, Best TM, Pan X, Ellis TJ: Efficacy of surgery for femoroacetabular impingement: A systematic review. *Am J Sports Med* 2010;38(11):2337-2345.
7. Philippon MJ, Briggs KK, Yen YM, Kuppersmith DA: Outcomes following hip arthroscopy for femoroacetabular impingement with associated chondrolabral dysfunction: Minimum two-year follow-up. *J Bone Joint Surg Br* 2009;91(1):16-23.
8. Stevens MS, Legay DA, Glazebrook MA, Amirault D: The evidence for hip arthroscopy: Grading the current indications. *Arthroscopy* 2010;26(10):1370-1383.
9. Clohisy JC, St John LC, Schutz AL: Surgical treatment of femoroacetabular impingement: A systematic review of the literature. *Clin Orthop Relat Res* 2010; 468(2):555-564.
10. Lodhia P, Slobogean GP, Noonan VK, Gilbart MK: Patient-reported outcome instruments for femoroacetabular impingement and hip labral pathology: A systematic review of the clinimetric evidence. *Arthroscopy* 2011;27(2):279-286.
11. Botser IB, Smith TW Jr, Nasser R, Domb BG: Open surgical dislocation versus arthroscopy for femoroacetabular impingement: A comparison of clinical outcomes. *Arthroscopy* 2011;27(2):270-278.
12. Brunner A, Horisberger M, Herzog RF: Sports and recreation activity of patients with femoroacetabular impingement before and after arthroscopic osteoplasty. *Am J Sports Med* 2009;37(5):917-922.
13. Byrd JW, Jones KS: Arthroscopic management of femoroacetabular impingement in athletes. *Am J Sports Med* 2011;39(Suppl): 7S-13S.
14. Gedouin JE, May O, Bonin N, et al; French Arthroscopy Society: Assessment of arthroscopic management of femoroacetabular impingement: A prospective multicenter study. *Orthop Traumatol Surg Res* 2010;96(8, Suppl): S59-S67.
15. Horisberger M, Brunner A, Herzog RF: Arthroscopic treatment of femoral acetabular impingement in patients with preoperative generalized degenerative changes. *Arthroscopy* 2010;26(5):623-629.
16. Singh PJ, O'Donnell JM: The outcome of hip arthroscopy in Australian football league players: A review of 27 hips. *Arthroscopy* 2010;26(6):743-749.
17. Nho SJ, Magennis EM, Singh CK, Kelly BT: Outcomes after the arthroscopic treatment of femoroacetabular impingement in a mixed group of high-level athletes. *Am J Sports Med* 2011;39(Suppl): 14S-19S.
18. Fabricant PD, Heyworth BE, Kelly BT: Hip arthroscopy improves symptoms associated with FAI in selected adolescent athletes. *Clin Orthop Relat Res* 2007. http://www. springerlink.com/content/r475m171023133r0/fulltext.html. August 11, 2011. Accessed October 4, 2011.
19. Ilizaliturri VM Jr, Nossa-Barrera JM, Acosta-Rodriguez E, Camacho-Galindo J: Arthroscopic treatment of femoroacetabular impingement secondary to paediatric hip disorders. *J Bone Joint Surg Br* 2007;89(8):1025-1030.
20. Larson CM, Giveans MR, Taylor M: Does arthroscopic FAI correction improve function with radiographic arthritis? *Clin Orthop Relat Res* 2011;469(6):1667-1676.
21. Philippon MJ, Weiss DR, Kuppersmith DA, Briggs KK, Hay CJ: Arthroscopic labral repair and treatment of femoroacetabular impingement in professional hockey players. *Am J Sports Med* 2010;38(1):99-104.
22. Schilders E, Dimitrakopoulou A, Bismil Q, Marchant P, Cooke C: Arthroscopic treatment of labral tears in femoroacetabular impingement: A comparative study of refixation and resection with a minimum two-year follow-up. *J Bone Joint Surg Br* 2011;93(8): 1027-1032.
23. Larson CM: Arthroscopic management of pincer-type impingement. *Sports Med Arthrosc* 2010; 18(2):100-107.
24. Larson CM, Wulf CA: Intraoperative fluoroscopy for evaluation of bony resection during arthroscopic management of femoroacetabular impingement in the supine position. *Arthroscopy* 2009; 25(10):1183-1192.
25. Matsuda DK: Acute iatrogenic dislocation following hip impingement arthroscopic surgery. *Arthroscopy* 2009;25(4):400-404.
26. Ranawat AS, McClincy M, Sekiya JK: Anterior dislocation of the hip after arthroscopy in a patient with capsular laxity of the hip: A case report. *J Bone Joint Surg Am* 2009;91(1):192-197.
27. Benali Y, Katthagen BD: Hip subluxation as a complication of

arthroscopic debridement. *Arthroscopy* 2009;25(4):405-407.

28. Mardones RM, Gonzalez C, Chen Q, Zobitz M, Kaufman KR, Trousdale RT: Surgical treatment of femoroacetabular impingement: Evaluation of the effect of the size of the resection. Surgical technique. *J Bone Joint Surg Am* 2006;88(Suppl 1 Pt 1):84-91.

29. Mardones R, Lara J, Donndorff A, et al: Surgical correction of "cam-type" femoroacetabular impingement: A cadaveric comparison of open versus arthroscopic debridement. *Arthroscopy* 2009; 25(2):175-182.

30. Sussmann PS, Ranawat AS, Lipman J, Lorich DG, Padgett DE, Kelly BT: Arthroscopic versus open osteoplasty of the head-neck junction: A cadaveric investigation. *Arthroscopy* 2007;23(12): 1257-1264.

31. Heyworth BE, Shindle MK, Voos JE, Rudzki JR, Kelly BT: Radiologic and intraoperative findings in revision hip arthroscopy. *Arthroscopy* 2007;23(12):1295-1302.

32. Aveni OR, Bedi A, Lorich DG, Kelly BT: Femoral neck fracture after arthroscopic management of femoroacetabular impingement: A case report. *J Bone Joint Surg Am* 2010;93(9):e47. -

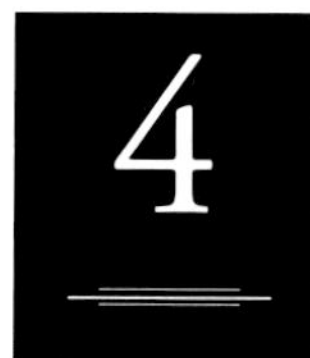

Open Surgical Dislocation for the Treatment of Femoroacetabular Impingement: Past, Present, and Future

Christopher L. Peters, MD
Benjamin M. Stronach, MD
Christopher E. Pelt, MD
Jill A. Erickson, PA-C

Abstract

Femoroacetabular impingement results from a lack of clearance between the femoral neck and the acetabulum. This condition is most commonly seen in the young adult presenting with hip pain after activity. There have been rapid advancements in the understanding of femoroacetabular impingement to include diagnostic, imaging, and treatment options. An open surgical dislocation approach has been developed that offers a safe and effective method to dislocate the hip and allow direct visualization and full access to treat the often complex intra-articular pathologies of femoroacetabular impingement. The ultimate goal of treatment in carefully selected patients is relief of hip pain and preservation of the hip joint.

Femoroacetabular impingement (FAI) is a clinical condition in which abutment of the femoral head-neck junction and the acetabular rim produces acetabular chondrolabral injury and results in a painful hip. The characteristic structural abnormalities associated with FAI include decreased femoral head-neck offset and/or acetabular overcoverage, such as acetabular retroversion and coxa profunda.[1-3] If left untreated, FAI can lead to labrum and articular cartilage damage, resulting in early-onset osteoarthritis.[2,4-11] Decreased clearance in the hip joint appears to be responsible for the development of osteoarthritis early in life; these patients were once classified as having primary or idiopathic osteoarthritis.[12] FAI may be caused by cam impingement, pincer impingement, or a combination of both types (mixed impingement).[4,13] There has been a great deal of interest in this topic recently, resulting in rapid advancements in imaging, diagnosis, and treatment methodologies. More information on cam and pincer impingement is in chapter 21.

Historic Perspective

Many patients with end-stage osteoarthritis with no known underlying cause for the disease process were considered to have primary osteoarthritis until the 1960s. In 1965, Murray[14] performed a radiographic study to find an explanation for hip degeneration in patients with a previous diagnosis of primary arthritis and recognized a deformity in 65% of the hips. He identified a proximal femur abnormality that was termed femoral head tilt. In 1976, Solomon[15] used radiographs and anatomic specimens obtained at the time of surgery to elucidate the underlying pathology in these patients. He identified an underlying cause for joint degeneration in 300 of the 327 study patients (92%) and found femoral head tilt in 59 patients.[15] Stulberg et al[16] performed a radiographic review of the hips of 75 adults with osteoarthritis and found that 79% of patients had

Dr. Peters or an immediate family member has received royalties from Biomet; is a member of a speakers' bureau or has made paid presentations on behalf of Biomet; serves as a paid consultant to Biomet; and serves as a board member, owner, officer, or committee member of the American Academy of Orthopaedic Surgeons. None of the following authors or any immediate family member has received anything of value from or owns stock in a commercial company or institution related directly or indirectly to the subject of this chapter: Dr. Stronach, Dr. Pelt, and Ms. Erickson.

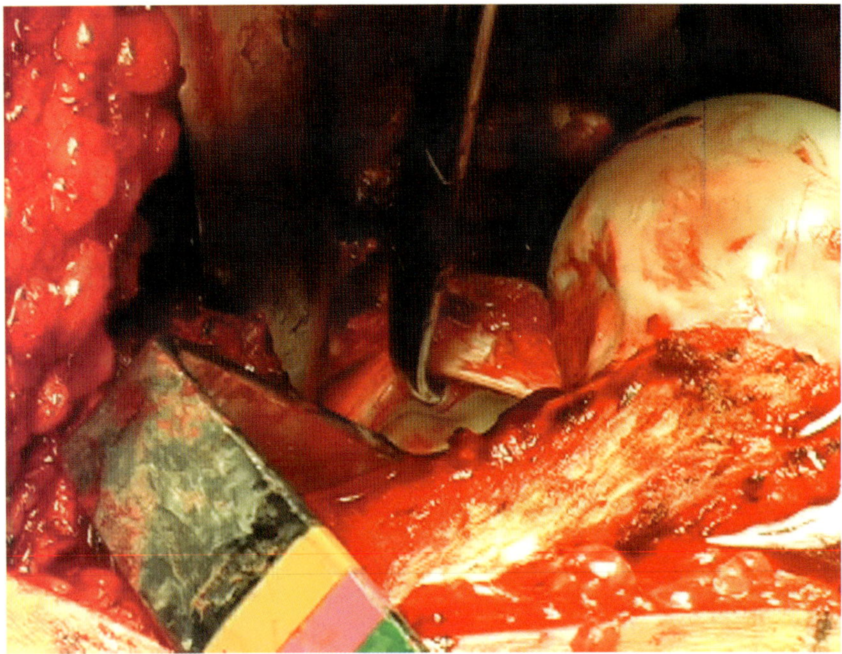

Figure 1 Image of the superior rim of the acetabulum with cartilage delamination lesion with hemostat inserted.

previously unidentified acetabular dysplasia or deformity of the femoral head and neck that was attributed to subtle Legg-Calvé-Perthes disease or slipped capital femoral epiphysis from childhood. This common finding in the proximal femur was termed a pistol grip deformity.[16] In each of these series, an underlying cause for some cases of osteoarthritis could not be found. It was hypothesized that these patients had a mechanical abnormality of the hip that could not be identified because of its subtle nature.[15-17]

Ganz et al[4] were able to identify subtle anatomic deformities that had not previously been described, likely providing an explanation for the small cohort of patients in previous investigations[15-17] with no identifiable mechanical abnormality. The authors noted continued anterior hip pain with decreased range of motion in a subset of their patients who had been treated with periacetabular osteotomy. On examination, the patients had a common finding of pain with flexion, internal rotation, and adduction. Surgical exploration showed that these patients had obvious impingement of the anterior femoral neck on the anterior rim of the acetabulum. This condition was corrected by performing an osteoplasty of the anterior femoral neck and was the initial work describing open surgical dislocation for FAI.[18] The concept of impingement was then considered as a possible mechanical cause of the previously described idiopathic hip pain in young patients. Magnetic resonance arthrograms with radial sequencing of the femoral head and neck were obtained and provided a better appreciation for the anatomic variations seen in these patients. The patients were treated with open surgical dislocation; the resultant clinical improvement further validated the mechanical model proposed for impingement. Ganz et al[19] noted two distinct patterns of morphologic abnormalities causing impingement and coined the terms cam and pincer impingement. This work became the foundation for the current understanding of FAI.[4,18]

Cam Impingement

Cam impingement results when an aspherical portion of the femoral head or the head-neck junction contacts the acetabulum during flexion and internal rotation of the hip, producing a shear force at the anterior chondrolabral junction, with subsequent labral and chondral injury. Decreased femoral head-neck offset had previously been described as a pistol grip deformity,[16] with more subtle variations now recognized as cam impingement.[2] Decreased femoral head-neck offset or a nonspherical head can result from multiple causes, including previous slipped capital femoral epiphysis, femoral neck fracture malunion, and decreased femoral anteversion.[20-22]

The pathomechanical shear stress on the anterosuperior chondrolabral junction resulting from cam impingement leads to acetabular cartilage damage, which typically presents as cartilage delamination from the underlying bone with a resultant chondral flap (**Figure 1**). Repetitive injury leads to failure of the articular margin of the labrum and progressive chondral damage. The capsular margin of the labrum is usually preserved until late in the disease process. The specific mechanism of damage to the acetabular cartilage is direct pressure from the aspherical femur during flexion and—to some degree—internal rotation. The process displaces the labrum from the acetabular margin, with resultant high tension and shear forces across this focused area. The rolling away of the labrum also exposes the osteochondral rim of the acetabulum to the impinging head-neck junction.[2,4,23]

Pincer Impingement

Pincer impingement is characterized by relative or absolute acetabular overcoverage of the femoral head. The result is premature abutment of the femoral head-neck junction against the acetabular rim, typically during flexion and internal rotation of the hip. Acetabular pathologic morphology associated with pincer impingement includes coxa profunda, coxa protrusio, acetabular retroversion, and calcified labra.[4,13,24,25] In pincer impingement, the femoral head-neck junction impinges against the prominent acetabular rim, which extends beyond the normal range of coverage. In contrast to cam impingement, the damage pattern in pincer impingement is characterized by direct labral compression, resulting in linear damage patterns to the labrum. There is evidence that the acetabular chondral surface is protected from damage with pincer impingement because the femur makes early contact with the acetabular rim and is prevented from entering the acetabulum.[23] Repeated labral compression leads to acetabular cartilage damage that is limited, with a mean of only 4 mm medial extension compared with 11 mm in cam impingement.[2] Ossification and cystic degeneration of the labrum can be pronounced in pincer impingement.[2,4,5] Secondary changes to the femoral head junction may be recognized as a so-called pincer groove or indentation.

Because most patients with FAI do not have isolated cam- or pincer-type impingement but have a combination of both impingement types,[2,26] the surgeon must have a thorough understanding of the specific hip pathomorphology to select the appropriate treatment for each patient. The available treatment options for FAI are evolving, and there is continued debate concerning which lesions are amenable to arthroscopic versus open procedures and which open procedure should be used in specific situations.

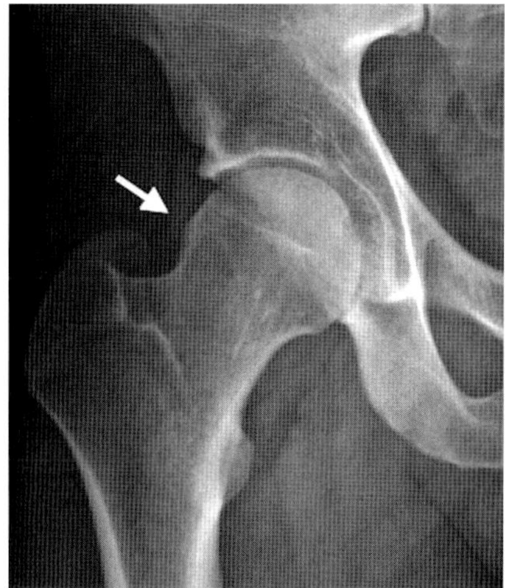

Figure 2 Preoperative AP radiograph of a right hip showing decreased femoral head-neck offset with a visible bump at the anterolateral femoral head-neck junction (arrow).

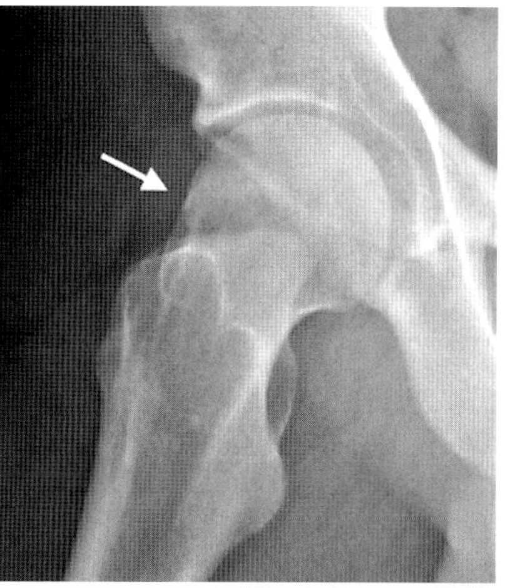

Figure 3 Preoperative frog-leg lateral radiograph of a right hip with decreased offset and visible anterolateral bump (arrow).

Presentation

Patients initially present for treatment because of pain and activity limitations. Most patients present with an insidious onset of hip pain that is frequently worsened with activity, but some patients present with an acute traumatic injury.[27,28] Specific activities that cause pain are associated with flexion, including rising from a sitting position, squatting, or sports that require high hip flexion, such as ballet, hockey, and soccer.[1,28] Pain is frequently localized to the groin but can also include regions proximal to the groin, such as the buttocks, the lateral hip, and the lower back.[28]

The physical examination includes an evaluation of gait for an antalgic or Trendelenburg gait pattern. Hip range of motion (adduction/abduction, flexion/extension, and internal/external rotation) should be documented. There is often decreased internal rotation of the affected hip(s) compared with patients with normal morphology.[27] The impingement test, which consists of flexing the hip to 90° with subsequent internal rotation and adduction, is useful in evaluating patients with suspected FAI.[4,7] One study reported a positive impingement test in all patients treated with open surgical dislocation,[1] and similar observations have been made in other patient populations.[29,30]

In some patients with hip pain, the source of the pain cannot be easily determined, and imaging is equivocal for intra-articular pathology. For these patients, this chapter's authors often use a fluoroscopically guided intra-articular hip injection with local anesthetic and corticosteroid as a diagnostic adjunct to determine if the pain generator is within the hip.

Imaging

Most FAI abnormalities can be detected on appropriately aligned AP pelvis and frog-leg lateral radiographs; however, the anterior bump seen in cam impingement can be missed on these views. Other views, such as the cross-table lateral, the false profile, and the Dunn view, may facilitate the diagnosis.[31] This chapter's authors obtain standing AP pelvis and hip (**Figure 2**), frog-leg lateral (**Figure 3**), and false profile lateral radiographs for all young

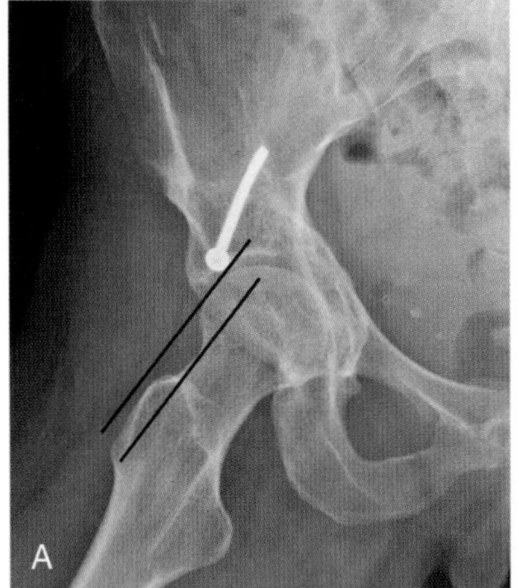

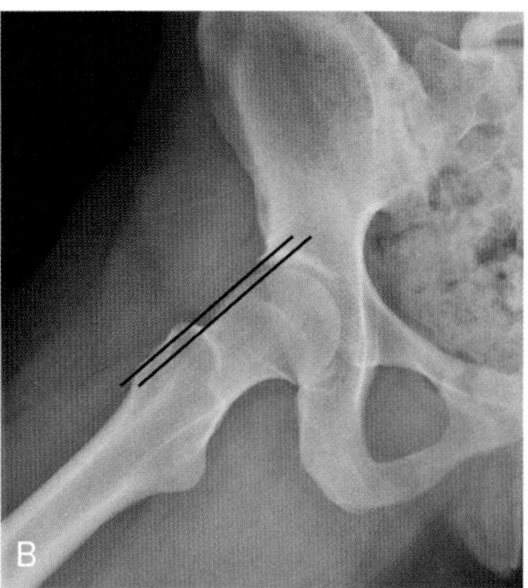

Figure 4 To determine the head-neck offset, the distance between a line drawn on a radiograph along the anteriormost portion of the femoral neck parallel to the neck axis and another line drawn parallel to this along the most anterior portion of the femoral head is measured. **A,** Radiograph of a hip with adequate head-neck offset. **B,** Radiograph of a hip with insufficient head-neck offset.

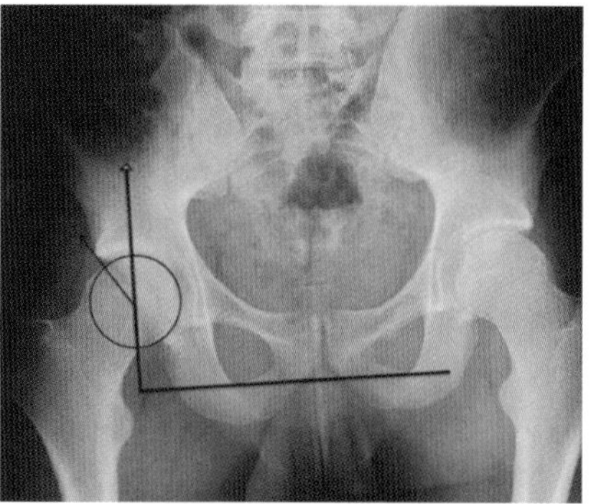

Figure 5 AP radiograph of the pelvis showing the lateral center-edge angle, which is determined by drawing a vertical line into the center of the femoral head with a connecting line from the femoral head center to the lateral rim of the acetabulum.

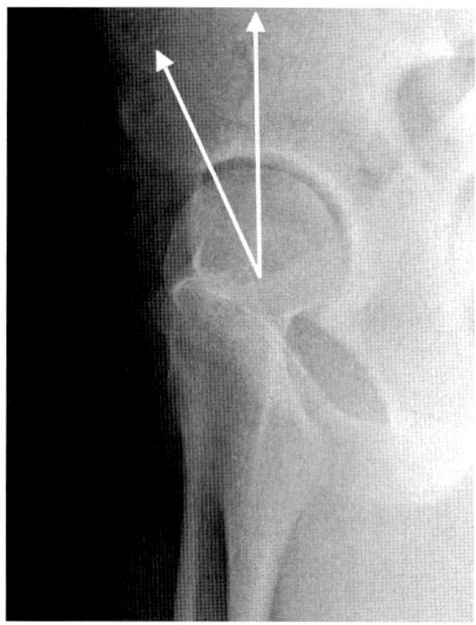

Figure 6 The lateral center-edge angle can be measured using a false-profile radiographic view of the hip.

adult patients being evaluated for hip pain. Other views as necessary are used to augment the diagnosis.

Several measurements are used to help identify FAI on radiographs. The femoral anterior offset has been defined to help determine the presence of cam pathology on a lateral radiograph (**Figure 4**). This is accomplished by drawing a line along the anteriormost portion of the femoral neck parallel to the neck axis and drawing another line parallel to this along the most anterior portion of the femoral head. The distance between these two lines is measured. Tannast et al[32] recommend using a measurement of 10 mm or less to clinically identify cam pathology. The anterior offset can be divided by the diameter of the femoral head to determine the femoral head-neck offset ratio, with a value less than 0.17 highly suspicious for cam deformity.[33] The α angle is another useful measurement to identify cam impingement on a lateral radiograph. It is determined by drawing a line down the center of the femoral neck and connecting this with a line drawn from the head center to the anterior point where the femoral head-neck contour becomes aspherical. An α angle greater than 50° is considered abnormal.[32,34] (See chapter 21, Figure 3 and chapter 27, Figure 15 for more information and an illustration of how the α angle is determined.)

Radiographic findings in pincer impingement reveal overcoverage of the femoral head. It is essential to obtain a true AP pelvis radiograph because pelvic tilt in an outlet or an inlet direction can give a false projection of overcoverage or undercoverage.[35,36] Coxa profunda (an acetabular fossa medial to the ilioischial line on an AP pelvis radiograph) and coxa protrusio (the femoral head is medial to the ilioischial line) result in a medialized femoral head with overcoverage.[32] The lateral center-edge angle is another measurement used for evaluating lateral acetabular coverage.[37] It is determined by drawing a vertical line into the center of the femoral head, with a connecting line from the femoral head center to the lateral rim of the acetabulum. A normal, lateral center-edge angle has been defined as 25° to 39°, with a value less than 25° defined as dysplasia[38] and a value greater than 39° indicative of overcoverage (**Figures 5** and **6**).[22]

Acetabular retroversion is a type of pincer impingement resulting in focal anterior overcoverage. The crossover sign (**Figure 7**) is used to identify retroversion on an AP pelvis radiograph by drawing a line along the lateral margin of anterior and posterior walls. In a normal, anteverted acetabulum, the posterior wall remains lateral to the anterior wall. In a retroverted acetabulum, the anterior wall crosses over the posterior wall, defining the crossover sign.[32,39] The posterior wall sign (**Figure 7**) is also useful in evaluating acetabular coverage. The posterior wall normally passes through the center of the femoral head. If the posterior wall is deficient, as is frequently seen in acetabular retroversion, the posterior wall is medial to the center of the femoral head. If the posterior wall crosses laterally to the femoral head, there is a prominent posterior wall with potential posterior overcoverage.[32]

MRI has become an important tool in the preoperative evaluation of FAI. It is useful in evaluating the hip for osteonecrosis, labral pathology, acetabular cartilage delamination lesions, and cam pathology. Magnetic resonance arthrography has become the gold standard for the detection of labral tears, with consistently good to excellent sensitivities (89% to 100%) and specificities (95% to 100%) in multiple studies.[40-44] Cartilage lesions can be difficult to detect with magnetic resonance arthrography because of the complex spherical shape of the hip and thinness of the cartilage.[44] MRI has shown fairly good sensitivities (47% to 93%) and specificities (66% to 89%) for detecting cartilage lesions[40,45-47] but is not yet effective enough to consistently detect acetabular delamination lesions (sensitivity, 22%).[23] MRI is currently the best noninvasive modality available for evaluating the cartilage despite these inherent shortcomings. Accuracy and detail in MRI continues to improve and helps the surgeon to fully appreciate the preoperative pathology and formulate a well-informed surgical plan.

CT arthrography is also a useful imaging modality in certain circumstances. A three-dimensional reconstruction of the joint can be obtained, which is helpful in understanding complex pathologic anatomy and is beneficial for surgical planning. This chapter's authors use CT arthrography on a select basis and do not believe this modality is necessary in evaluating all patients with FAI.

Treatment

A major challenge in treating FAI was finding a method to safely visualize the entire hip joint without damaging the cartilage or devascularizing the femoral head. A posterior approach to the hip risks damage to the medial femoral circumflex artery, which is the primary blood supply for the femoral head.[48,49] An anterior approach to the hip allows visualization of the anterior acetabular rim and the femoral head-neck junction but does not provide access to the superior femoral neck or the posterior acetabulum. This problem was solved by Ganz et al[19] when open surgical dislocation was first described. This procedure consisted of a lateral approach to the hip with a trochanteric flip osteotomy, which preserves the blood supply to the femoral head, followed by exposure of the anterior hip. An anterior capsulotomy and dislocation of the hip allows circumferential exposure of the acetabulum and most of the femoral head and neck.

The original procedure, which was described by Ganz et al[19] in 2001 has recently been updated with a comprehensive explanation of the surgery.[50] This chapter's authors use a similar exposure and surgical technique (**Figure 8**) with several minor modifications. After induction of anesthesia with complete relaxation, the patient is placed in the lateral decubitus position, and the pelvis is stabilized with an adjustable post system. After the patient is securely positioned and all nonsurgical regions are well padded, a wide surgical field from the ankle to the lower rib cage is prepared with an alcohol scrub, a chlorhexidine scrub, and an iodine-based sealant scrub. Sterile drapes are then placed to allow the operative leg to be manipulated, and a sterile pouch is positioned along the anterior portion of the patient. This allows the operative leg to remain sterile by placing it in the pouch during dislocation as it drops below the level of the surgical table.

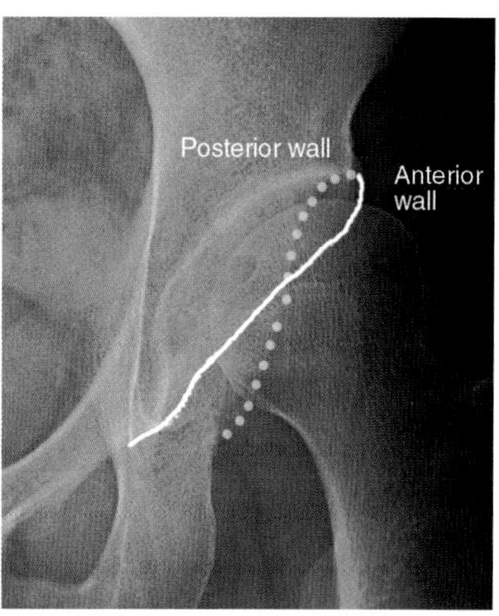

Figure 7 The posterior wall and crossover signs are shown on an AP pelvis radiograph.

The greater trochanter is fully palpated, and the incision is centered over this landmark in both the anterior-superior and the superior-inferior planes. Dissection is carried down through the subcutaneous fat to the level of the fascia overlying the gluteus maximus and the iliotibial band. At this point, the dissection is continued in a manner consistent with the initial portion of a posterior approach to the hip, which differs slightly from the Gibson approach used by Ganz et al[19] and Espinosa et al.[50] The midline of the femur is localized, the iliotibial band is incised, and dissection is performed superiorly through the anterior fibers of the gluteus maximus. A deep,

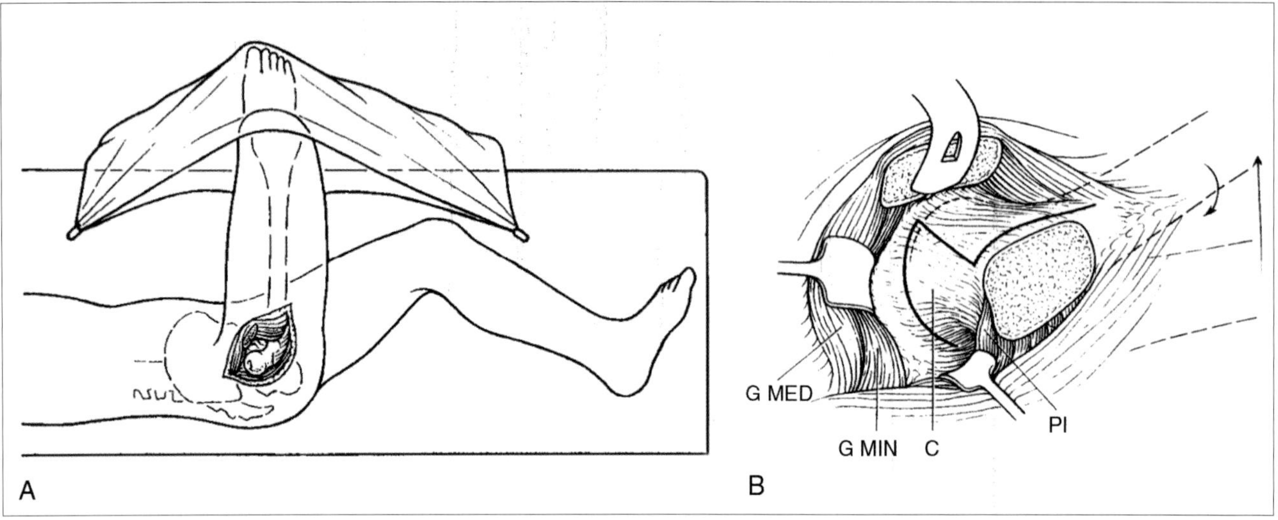

Figure 8 **A,** Illustration of patient positioning for surgical dislocation of the right hip. The patient is placed in the left lateral position with the right leg flexed and externally rotated until the hip dislocates anteriorly. The leg is then placed in a sterile anterior hip pouch. **B,** Illustration of the surgical approach as described by Ganz. G MED = gluteus medius, G MIN = gluteus minimus, C = capsule, PI = piriformis.

self-retaining retractor is placed, and the operative leg is then slightly internally rotated to visualize the posterior portion of the hip. It is critical at this point to understand the anatomic structures involved before proceeding to prevent injury to the blood supply to the femoral head. The posterior borders of the gluteus medius, greater trochanter, and vastus lateralis are identified. The fat overlying the external rotators is not disturbed, and no dissection should be performed in this specific region. The superior border of the piriformis is palpated, and the gluteus minimus is dissected from the capsule. No dissection is made inferiorly into the piriformis fossa, and the dissection always remains at or above the superior edge of the piriformis tendon. The joint capsule is now partially visualized, and a bent Hohmann retractor is placed in this interval deep to the gluteus minimus and superficial to the capsule. This chapter's authors have found that the definition of this interval before the trochanteric flip makes later dissection much easier and less traumatic to soft tissues. Attention is then turned to the inferior border of the greater trochanter, where the posterior border of the vastus lateralis is identified and elevated from the femur. A retractor is placed onto the anterior femur in this interval, allowing retraction of the vastus lateralis. The posterior margin of the greater trochanter is well visualized, and the precise location of the trochanteric osteotomy can be determined.

The osteotomy starts superiorly at the posterior border of the gluteus medius and is carried inferiorly to the posterior margin of the vastus lateralis. The level of resection is parallel to the calf to ensure the osteotomy site is parallel to the alignment of the femur. After the osteotomy is completed, granular collagen/thrombin is placed on the osteotomy site to improve visualization and decrease blood loss for the remaining portion of the procedure. The wafer of bone is approximately 1.5 cm thick; however, this will vary slightly based on the patient's body habitus and osseous anatomy. If the osteotomy is performed correctly, the vastus lateralis, gluteus medius, and gluteus minimus should be attached to the osteotomy fragment, allowing these structures to be retracted anteriorly. This is accomplished by placing a retractor onto the anterior border of the femur at the level of the remaining greater trochanter; the fragment is retracted anteriorly. The leg is then externally rotated gently to increase the exposure of the anterior capsule. The dissection is continued with electrocautery, releasing the adherent fibers of the rectus femoris and any remaining gluteus minimus. Once the capsule can be seen, the acetabular rim and the femoral head are palpated to ensure adequate exposure. The exposure is continued to include the anterior-inferior capsule and medially to the border of the iliopsoas tendon. After exposure of the capsule is complete, a Z-shaped capsulotomy is performed. The first incision is placed longitudinally down the anterior femoral neck. The second incision is started at the inferior margin of the first incision and carried anteriorly along the intertrochanteric line, releasing the inferior margin of the anterior capsule from

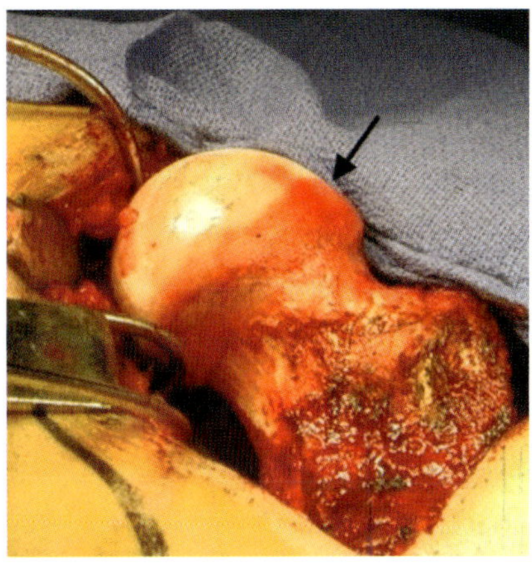

Figure 9 Photograph of the dislocated femoral head with decreased femoral head-neck offset and ecchymosis at the region of impingement against acetabulum (arrow).

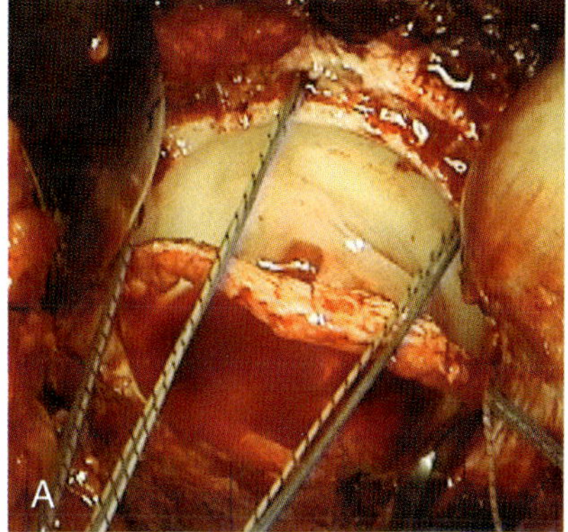

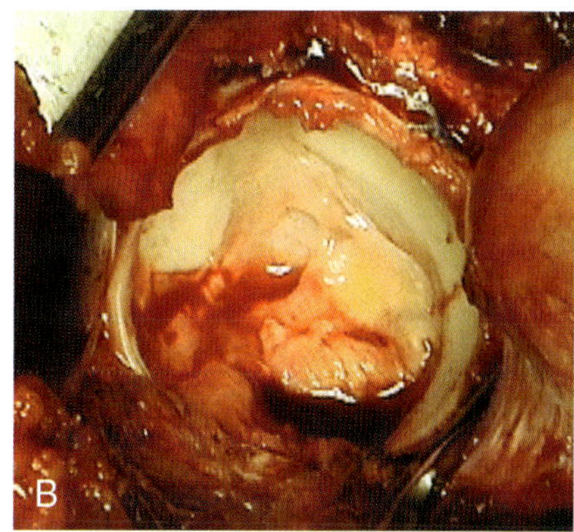

Figure 10 Intraoperative photographs of the left hip labrum. A, Suture anchors have been placed in the acetabular rim. **B,** The labrum has been reconstructed with the suture anchors fixed back to the acetabular rim.

the inferior neck. Returning to the superior margin of the first incision, this capsulotomy is continued superiorly with visualization of the labrum to prevent injury. Once this incision is superior to the labrum, the third incision is made by releasing the capsule from the acetabulum in a posterior direction.

The hip can then be flexed and internally rotated to identify the area of impingement. Frequently, there is visible damage on the anterior femoral neck that includes periosteal blushing consistent with ecchymosis and osseous reaction (**Figure 9**). This area is delineated for femoral osteochondroplasty. The hip is then dislocated with gentle flexion and external rotation. The ligamentum teres often must be released to completely dislocate the femoral head. The foot is placed into the anterior drape bag during the dislocation maneuver. A retractor is placed anteriorly to the acetabulum on the ilium, staying deep to the iliopsoas to avoid damage to the femoral vessels. A second retractor is placed anteriorly to the femoral neck and onto the posterior column. This is used to retract the proximal femur posteriorly and allows circumferential visualization of the acetabulum. The knee should be flexed during this portion of the procedure to decrease the tension on the sciatic nerve. The femoral head and acetabulum can be completely inspected for damage.

A labral takedown with subsequent repair is performed if required (**Figure 10**). This portion of the procedure is performed if there is a labral tear, cartilage damage on the acetabular rim, and/or a need for acetabuloplasty, which is often a necessary step to fully address the causative pathology. Acetabuloplasty is initiated with release of the labrum from the acetabular rim, usually from the anterior 4 o'clock position posteriorly to the 11 o'clock position. A high-speed burr is used for the acetabuloplasty, removing the amount of bone that was preoperatively templated. The amount of bone can be estimated by using the information provided by Philippon et al,[51] in which 1 mm of bone resection translates into a 2.4° decrease in the lateral center-edge angle, with each subsequent resected 1 mm of bone changing the center-edge angle by 0.6 mm. This translates into a bone resection of 5 mm, which decreases the center-edge angle by 5°.[51] This chapter's authors usually resect 3 to 5 mm of bone. If the patient has acetabular dysplasia (lateral center-edge angle < 25°), acetabuloplasty is not recommended because of the potential risk for hip instability or iatrogenic dysplasia. After the work on the acetabulum has been completed, small suture anchors are placed 2 to 3 mm from the articular surface, and the labrum is repaired to the acetabular rim with horizontal mattress sutures. The sutures should be arranged so that the knots are on the outer surface of the labrum instead of the inner surface, which places the labrum as a barrier between the knots and the articulating surface of the hip joint. The sutures are spaced at approximately 2 cm and can involve two to five anchors based on the amount of labrum that requires reattachment. Repair of the labrum to the acetabular rim is recommended if possible,[52] but occasionally the labrum is too damaged or too hypotrophic to retain a suture. In these instances, the labrum is resected. A labral reconstruction can be performed in these patients with the use of the ligamentum teres[53] or a section of iliotibial band.[54,55]

Attention is then turned to the femoral neck, and the region of bone causing impingement is removed. An osteotome is initially used to define the superior border of the femoroplasty,

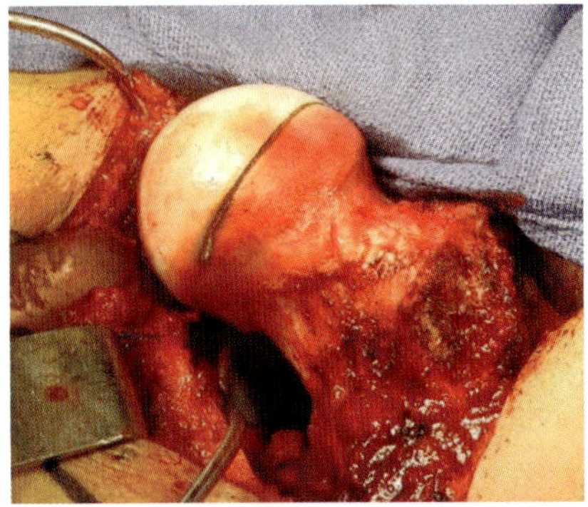

Figure 11 Image of a dislocated femoral head with the planned region of resection for femoroplasty delineated.

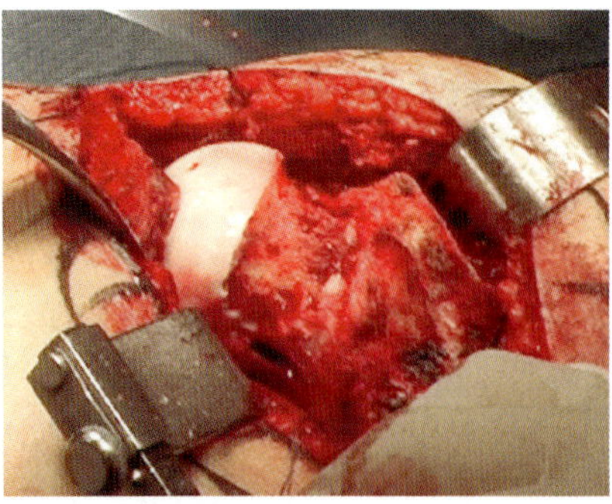

Figure 12 Image of a dislocated femoral head after completion of femoroplasty to restore femoral head-neck offset and remove the region of impingement.

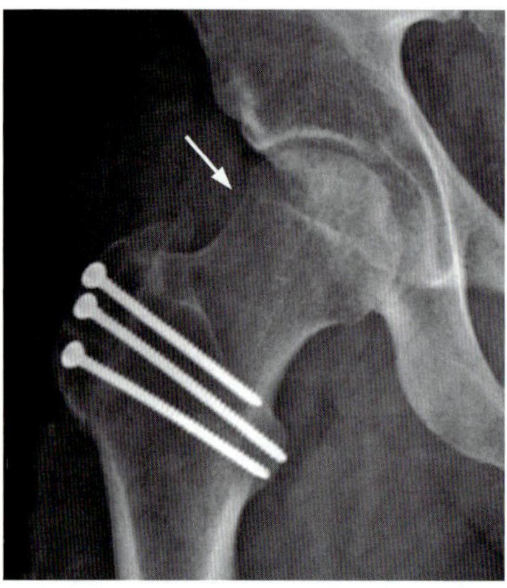

Figure 13 Postoperative AP radiograph of a right hip with trochanteric repair and the results of femoroplasty (arrow).

which is usually located proximal to the articular margin of the femoral head (**Figure 11**). The osteotome is directed distally and is used to remove periosteum with the assistance of a rongeur. The femoral osteochondroplasty is then completed with the use of a high-speed burr (**Figure 12**). The surgeon should strive to create a smooth transition from the articular surface of the femoral head to the femoral neck, with complete removal of the aspherical region. The final contour should be comparable to a ramp rather than a cliff to prevent the potential for a stress riser and allow for the restoration of a labral seal with normal fluid mechanics. Experience is needed to fully appreciate the amount of bone to remove; the amount may appear aggressive in a surgeon's initial experience. The assistant can now reduce the hip with gentle traction and internal rotation while the surgeon guides the head back into place. This chapter's authors have seen failure of the labral sutures on several occasions during this maneuver, requiring repeat dislocation and labral refixation. The number of dislocations should be minimized if possible. After the hip has been reduced, it can be taken through a range of motion to verify that no impingement occurs with flexion through an arc of 0° to 90° and internal rotation through an arc of 0° to 20° if obtainable. Dynamic and static fluorographic images can be obtained to radiographically confirm impingement-free motion and visualize the extent of the bony débridement. If there is continued impingement, dislocation should be performed with revision of the femoral osteochondroplasty.

Once the range of motion is satisfactory with no residual impingement, the hip is irrigated thoroughly with normal saline, and the capsule is then repaired with absorbable sutures. It is advisable to leave laxity in the capsule if possible and not overtighten this closure because this can place the perforating branches of the medial circumflex femoral vessels at risk, with the potential for osteonecrosis of the femoral head. The greater trochanter is next reapproximated and repaired with the use of cortical screws under fluoroscopic guidance. A final fluorographic image is obtained to verify adequate screw position (angled toward the lesser trochanter with flush seating of the screw head against the greater trochanter) and proper reduction of the trochanteric fragment. A relative femoral neck lengthening can be performed during reattachment of the greater trochanter fragment. This lengthening is performed in patients with coxa vara or a shortened neck as occurs in Legg-Calvé-Perthes disease, is accomplished by distalizing the fragment before reattachment, and results in increased tension on the hip abductors and thus improves mechanical function. The iliotibial band, subcutaneous layer, and skin are then closed with the suture material of choice. An intraoperative drain is not routinely placed. Postoperative radiographs can show the newly created contour on the femoral neck (**Figures 13** and **14**).

The average length of the patient's hospital stay is 3 days (range, 2 to 5 days).[1] This chapter's authors recommend compression stockings and mechanical foot compression pumps on the nonsurgical extremity during surgery and the placement of compression stockings and foot pumps bilaterally while the patient is in the hospital and in bed. All patients receive enoxaparin 30 mg subcutaneously twice a day while in the hospital unless contraindicated and are discharged on a regimen of 6 weeks of aspirin (325 mg once a day) to prevent deep venous thrombosis. Hip precautions for dislocation are not ordered for patients, but patients are required to observe 50% weight-bearing restrictions on the operated extremity for 6 weeks postoperatively to protect the trochanteric osteotomy site from excessive stress and prevent femoral neck fracture after femoral osteochondroplasty. Crutches are often sufficient ambulation aids in this young patient population. Radiographs are obtained at the 6-week postoperative visit, and weight bearing is progressed with the initiation of physical therapy at this time.

The described technique requires a thorough understanding of hip anatomy and is technically demanding. This procedure should not be used without proper preparation, which consists of spending time observing an experienced surgeon with a firm grasp of the technique and cadaveric study if possible.

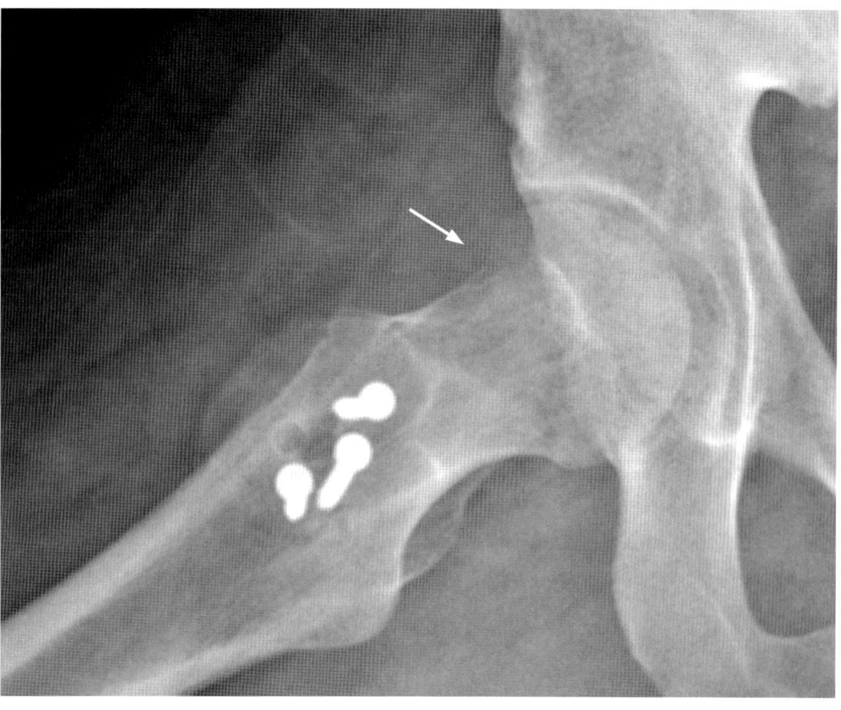

Figure 14 Postoperative frog-leg lateral radiograph of the right hip with restoration of the femoral head-neck offset (arrow).

Results

The treatment of FAI with open surgical dislocation has shown excellent functional outcomes and midterm survivorship in patients with no or minimal osteoarthritis[3,13,26,56] (**Table 1**). The first report of clinical results after surgical dislocation in 23 hips was encouraging, with 15 patients showing significant improvement in clinical outcomes at a minimum of 2 years postoperatively.[26] Similar findings were reported in 37 hips with an average follow-up of 3.1 years after surgical dislocation, with significant improvement in the average postoperative Western Ontario and McMaster Universities Osteoarthritis Index score compared with preoperative values.[56] A significant improvement in postoperative Harris hip scores in 96 hips with an average follow-up of 26 months was recently reported.[1]

In each of these studies, surgical failure, defined as no clinical improvement or conversion to hip arthroplasty, occurred in a small proportion of the patients. A common finding in these patients was moderate to severe arthritic changes at the time of surgery. In the first report documenting the results of open surgical dislocation, 15 of 23 patients had significant improvement with no further surgery, and 7 patients required conversion to total hip arthroplasty.[26] Five of those patients had significant preoperative arthritis, and the other two had residual, untreated acetabular dysplasia.[26] Beck et al[13] reported on 19 patients treated with open hip dislocation. In the five hips requiring total hip arthroplasty at a mean of 3.1 years, two of the patients had preoperative Tönnis grade 2 osteoarthritis, and the other three had Tönnis grade 1 or less preoperative arthritis; however, all were found to have severe arthritic changes intraoperatively, which were not always consistent with preoperative radiographs.[13] Two of this chapter's authors (CLP and JAE) initially reviewed 30 hips that had undergone open hip dislocation with an average follow-up of 32 months. There were four failures, with three patients requiring total hip arthroplasty.[3] This study was recently updated to include a total of 96 hips with an average follow-up of 26 months (range, 18 to 96 months). There were six failures defined as a decrease in the Harris hip score or conversion to arthroplasty. Four of the six patients were found to have severe acetabular cartilage damage (Outerbridge IV) at the time of surgery. Five of the 6 failures occurred in the initial 30 patients treated.[1] An improvement in the hip survival rate was seen when comparing the first group of 30 patients[3] treated with open surgical dislocation and the subsequent patients.[1] This improvement is attributed to the evolution in understanding the relationship of osteoarthritis and FAI and to greater patient selectivity in offering this surgical intervention. Philippon et al[57] also found a correlation between preexisting osteoarthritis and failure of

Table 1

Outcomes After Open Surgical Dislocation of the Hip for the Treatment of FAI

Study	No. of Patients	Average Age (Years)	Follow-up (Years)	Failures	Complications
Murphy et al[26]	23	35	2 to 12	7	0
Peters et al[3]	30	31	2.7	4	0
Beck et al[13]	19	36	4 to 5.2	5	0
Beaulé et al[56]	37	41	2.1 to 5	6	2
Peters et al[1]	96	28	2 to 9	6	2
Ganz et al[19]	213	34	2 to 7	NA	7

FAI = femoroacetabular impingement, NA = not available

arthroscopic femoroplasty. In the 10 procedures that failed, failure was directly correlated with intraoperative cartilage damage (6 with poor cartilage and 4 with moderate cartilage changes) and older patient age. It has become clear that patient selection has a critical effect on outcome results, especially in the presence of osteoarthritis. This has led to the development of improved preoperative imaging techniques to evaluate cartilage integrity and more selectivity in determining which patients should be offered the option of surgical dislocation.

Acetabular cartilage damage is frequently seen in patients with FAI.[13,23] These lesions are believed to be precursors to end-stage osteoarthritis that can eventually involve most of the hip joint. One important goal in the treatment of FAI is identifying these lesions early in the process and intervening in an attempt to halt the progression of joint degeneration. Cam impingement appears to be associated with a high prevalence of articular acetabular cartilage damage (specifically delamination). In a 2005 study, Beck et al[2] found acetabular cartilage damage in all 26 patients with a pure cam-type impingement pathology, with cartilage delamination in 10 of the patients. The acetabular lesions extended on average 11 mm medially toward the fovea. A study by Anderson et al[23] reported similar findings with acetabular cartilage delamination, which was strongly associated with cam impingement pathology (odds ratio, 11.9), in 44% of all patients who underwent surgical dislocation. The appropriate treatment of these lesions is unknown and evolving. This chapter's authors currently recommend excising the delamination and then trimming the acetabular rim to a stable base for labral reattachment if the patient has adequate preoperative acetabular coverage (no dysplasia). The cartilage in the delaminated lesions is currently being evaluated to determine if it is alive and reparable. Fibrin glue has been used to reattach large delamination lesions in several patients, with mixed results. Another option is microfracture to stimulate the production of fibrocartilage.[58]

Damage to the acetabular labrum is a consistent finding in most patients treated with surgical dislocation for FAI. All of the 19 patients in a study by Beck et al[13] had labral tears, and 18 of 19 patients were found to have cartilage lesions in proximity to the labral tears. All of the labral lesions were located in the anterosuperior quadrant of the acetabulum, which is the region of abutment between the neck and the acetabulum. In a 2010 study, labral abnormalities were found in 82 of 96 hips during surgical dislocation, with 44 labral detachments, 15 tears, 9 degenerative labra, 10 calcified labra, and 4 absent labra secondary to previous surgery.[1] Graves and Mast[59] classified labral lesions in 48 hips. They found undersurface tears in 14 hips, base tears in 20 hips, ossification in 11 hips, and thickening in 4 hips. Espinosa et al[52] evaluated the options for the treatment of a labral tear by comparing the functional results of 20 patients who had labral resection and 32 patients in whom the labrum was repaired after acetabuloplasty. They found improved clinical outcomes in the patients with labral refixation compared with patients who had labral débridement.[52] It has become apparent that the labrum is frequently damaged in FAI, and it is an important component that should be addressed at the time of surgery to ensure a successful outcome. It is also important to address the underlying bony abnormality causing impingement that initially led to the labral damage.[2]

Complications

The treatment of FAI with open surgical dislocation is a technically demanding procedure with concern for specific complications, including osteonecrosis of the femoral head, sciatic neurapraxia, heterotopic ossification, femoral neck fracture, and nonunion of the greater trochanter. Multiple studies have shown a low complication rate despite these concerns. In their initial study of open surgical dislocation, Ganz et al[19] reported 2 cases of sciatic neurapraxia, which completely resolved; 3 failures of trochanteric fixation requiring reoperation; and heterotopic ossification in 79 hips. The authors found that the rate of heterotopic ossification decreased as they gained experience with the procedure.[19] This high rate of heterotopic ossification has not occurred in more recent series.[1,56,59]

The only reported complications in a recently published study of 96 hips were 2 failures of trochanteric fixation; no osteonecrosis, infection, femoral neck fracture, or sciatic neurapraxia were reported.[1] One patient subsequently experienced a sciatic neurapraxia, which has since resolved. That patient's hip was dislocated for an extended period of time (approximately 60 minutes) because of the need for extensive surgery on the acetabulum and the femoral neck. In the 37 hips reviewed by Beaulé et al,[56] failure of trochanteric fixation requiring reoperation occurred in 1 patient, heterotopic ossification requiring excision developed in 1 patient, and 9 hips required hardware removal for bursal irritation from trochanteric screws. Another series reported similar findings with minimal heterotopic ossification in nine hips, which required no further surgery, and two patients with symptomatic trochanteric irritation requiring screw removal.[59]

Trochanteric-related complications are a common thread in the reviewed studies. Patients should be counseled on the small risk of nonunion or the need for subsequent hardware removal. Femoral neck fracture is also a potential risk after femoral osteochondroplasty and has been reported in the arthroscopic literature[60] but not in the open dislocation series reviewed.[1,13,19,56,59] Mardones et al[61] determined that up to 30% of the anterolateral neck could be removed before the proximal femur was at increased risk of fracture. This chapter's authors rarely remove an amount of bone approaching that limit and recommend against such an aggressive resection except in the most extreme circumstances. Postoperatively, patients are restricted to partial weight bearing for a period of 6 weeks as a precautionary measure to prevent femoral neck fracture.

Osteonecrosis of the femoral head remains a theoretic complication because it has not yet been reported in open surgical dislocation[1,13,19,56,59] or arthroscopic treatment of FAI.[62] This underscores the importance of meticulous surgical technique with protection of the medical circumflex femoral artery during the approach and the dislocation.

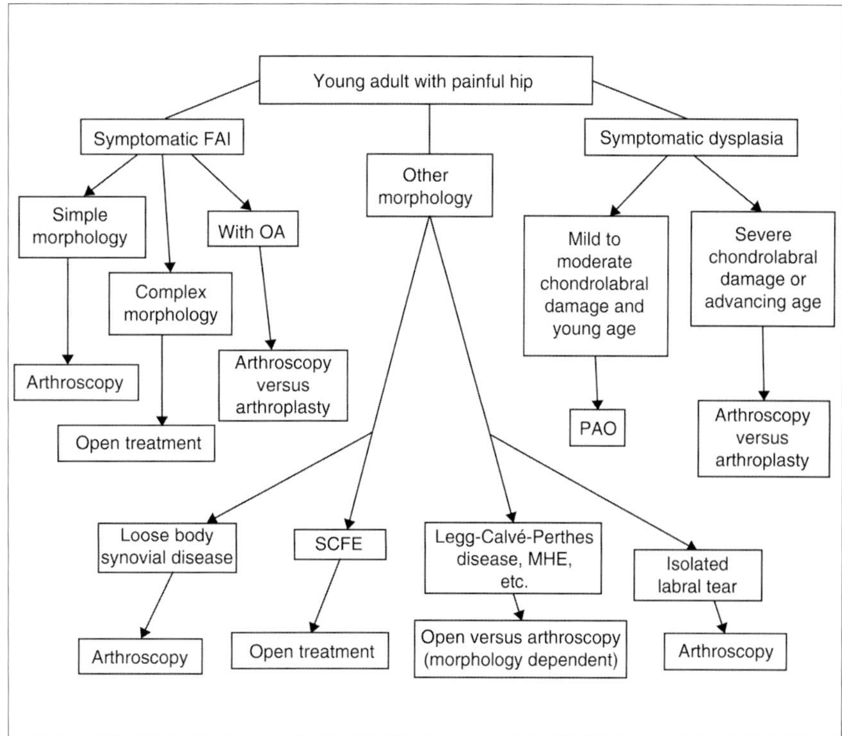

Figure 15 Treatment algorithm for the young patient with hip pain. OA = osteoarthritis, SCFE = slipped capital femoral epiphysis, PAO = periacetabular osteotomy, MHE = multiple hereditary exostoses.

Discussion and Future Directions

FAI has received a great deal of attention recently, and the understanding of this condition has rapidly evolved. This renewed interest began with the development of a surgical procedure that allows safe access to the entire articular field without damaging the blood supply to the femoral head. The specific concepts of pincer and cam impingement came out of this initial work and provided the foundation for one current treatment algorithm for FAI (**Figure 15**). The arthroscopic treatment of FAI has correspondingly evolved, and the indications for this procedure continue to expand. The future direction for treating FAI will be finding the boundaries for arthroscopic versus open management, improving imaging modalities to detect pathology earlier in the process, and potentially using preoperative computer modeling to precisely reshape the acetabulum and the femoral neck to prevent impingement. There is a need to improve treatment options for cartilage lesions in an effort to improve the survival of hips after surgical treatment of FAI. Whether this takes the form of cartilage repair or advanced technologies, such as cartilage transplantation, remains to be determined.

Another controversial topic in FAI is when surgery should be performed. A course of nonsurgical management with physical therapy and nonsteroidal anti-inflammatory medication remains as the initial course of treatment for symptomatic patients. This chapter's authors have found that nonsurgical modalities are rarely successful in the midterm or the long-term treatment of symptomatic patients. There is currently no indication to surgically treat an asymptomatic patient with radiographic findings of FAI. There is interest in but no active program in place for screening at-risk populations and providing counseling for these individuals so they can seek treatment earlier if pain develops.

Summary

Rapid advancements in the understanding of FAI have resulted in changes in diagnostic and imaging techniques and treatment options. Regardless of the approach used, surgical intervention should be focused on correcting the underlying pathomorphology as well as the resultant chondrolabral tissue damage. The approach using open surgical dislocation offers a safe and effective method to dislocate the hip and allows direct visualization and full access to treat the often complex intra-articular pathologies that may be present.

References

1. Peters CL, Schabel K, Anderson L, Erickson J: Open treatment of femoroacetabular impingement is associated with clinical improvement and low complication rate at short-term followup. *Clin Orthop Relat Res* 2010;468(2):504-510.
2. Beck M, Kalhor M, Leunig M, Ganz R: Hip morphology influences the pattern of damage to the acetabular cartilage: Femoroacetabular impingement as a cause of early osteoarthritis of the hip. *J Bone Joint Surg Br* 2005;87(7): 1012-1018.
3. Peters CL, Erickson JA: Treatment of femoro-acetabular impingement with surgical dislocation and débridement in young adults. *J Bone Joint Surg Am* 2006;88(8): 1735-1741.
4. Ganz R, Parvizi J, Beck M, Leunig M, Nötzli H, Siebenrock KA: Femoroacetabular impingement: A cause for osteoarthritis of the hip. *Clin Orthop Relat Res* 2003; 417:112-120.
5. Ito K, Leunig M, Ganz R: Histopathologic features of the acetabular labrum in femoroacetabular impingement. *Clin Orthop Relat Res* 2004;429:262-271.
6. Ito K, Minka MA II, Leunig M, Werlen S, Ganz R: Femoroacetabular impingement and the cam-effect: A MRI-based quantitative anatomical study of the femoral head-neck offset. *J Bone Joint Surg Br* 2001;83(2): 171-176.
7. Wagner S, Hofstetter W, Chiquet M, et al: Early osteoarthritic changes of human femoral head cartilage subsequent to femoroacetabular impingement. *Osteoarthritis Cartilage* 2003;11(7): 508-518.
8. Ecker TM, Tannast M, Puls M, Siebenrock KA, Murphy SB: Pathomorphologic alterations predict presence or absence of hip osteoarthrosis. *Clin Orthop Relat Res* 2007;465:46-52.
9. Leunig M, Beck M, Woo A, Dora C, Kerboull M, Ganz R: Acetabular rim degeneration: A constant finding in the aged hip. *Clin Orthop Relat Res* 2003;413:201-207.
10. Leunig M, Ganz R: Femoroacetabular impingement: A common cause of hip complaints leading to arthrosis. *Unfallchirurg* 2005;108(1):9-10, 12-17.
11. Tanzer M, Noiseux N: Osseous abnormalities and early osteoarthritis: The role of hip impingement. *Clin Orthop Relat Res* 2004; 429:170-177.
12. Ganz R, Leunig M, Leunig-Ganz K, Harris WH: The etiology of osteoarthritis of the hip: An integrated mechanical concept. *Clin Orthop Relat Res* 2008;466(2): 264-272.
13. Beck M, Leunig M, Parvizi J, Boutier V, Wyss D, Ganz R: Anterior femoroacetabular impingement: Part II. Midterm results of surgical treatment. *Clin Orthop Relat Res* 2004;418:67-73.
14. Murray RO: The aetiology of primary osteoarthritis of the hip. *Br J Radiol* 1965;38(455): 810-824.
15. Solomon L: Patterns of osteoarthritis of the hip. *J Bone Joint Surg Br* 1976;58(2):176-183.
16. Stulberg SD, Cordell LD, Harris WH, Ramsey PL, MacEwen GD: Unrecognized childhood hip disease: A major cause of idiopathic osteoarthritis of the hip. *Proceedings of the Third Open Scientific Meeting of the Hip Society.* St. Louis, MO, CV Mosby, 1975, pp 2112-2228.
17. Harris WH: Etiology of osteoarthritis of the hip. *Clin Orthop Relat Res* 1986;213:20-33.
18. Myers SR, Eijer H, Ganz R: Anterior femoroacetabular impingement after periacetabular osteotomy. *Clin Orthop Relat Res* 1999;363:93-99.
19. Ganz R, Gill TJ, Gautier E, Ganz K, Krügel N, Berlemann U: Surgical dislocation of the adult hip a technique with full access to the

femoral head and acetabulum without the risk of avascular necrosis. *J Bone Joint Surg Br* 2001; 83(8):1119-1124.

20. Leunig M, Casillas MM, Hamlet M, et al: Slipped capital femoral epiphysis: Early mechanical damage to the acetabular cartilage by a prominent femoral metaphysis. *Acta Orthop Scand* 2000;71(4): 370-375.
21. Eijer H, Myers SR, Ganz R: Anterior femoroacetabular impingement after femoral neck fractures. *J Orthop Trauma* 2001;15(7): 475-481.
22. Tönnis D, Heinecke A: Acetabular and femoral anteversion: Relationship with osteoarthritis of the hip. *J Bone Joint Surg Am* 1999; 81(12):1747-1770.
23. Anderson LA, Peters CL, Park BB, Stoddard GJ, Erickson JA, Crim JR: Acetabular cartilage delamination in femoroacetabular impingement: Risk factors and magnetic resonance imaging diagnosis. *J Bone Joint Surg Am* 2009;91(2): 305-313.
24. Reynolds D, Lucas J, Klaue K: Retroversion of the acetabulum: A cause of hip pain. *J Bone Joint Surg Br* 1999;81(2):281-288.
25. Siebenrock KA, Schoeniger R, Ganz R: Anterior femoroacetabular impingement due to acetabular retroversion: Treatment with periacetabular osteotomy. *J Bone Joint Surg Am* 2003;85-A(2):278-286.
26. Murphy S, Tannast M, Kim YJ, Buly R, Millis MB: Debridement of the adult hip for femoroacetabular impingement: Indications and preliminary clinical results. *Clin Orthop Relat Res* 2004; 429:178-181.
27. Beaulé PE, Allen DJ, Clohisy JC, Schoenecker P, Leunig M: The young adult with hip impingement: Deciding on the optimal intervention. *J Bone Joint Surg Am* 2009;91(1):210-221.
28. Clohisy JC, Knaus ER, Hunt DM, Lesher JM, Harris-Hayes M, Prather H: Clinical presentation of patients with symptomatic anterior hip impingement. *Clin Orthop Relat Res* 2009;467(3): 638-644.
29. Philippon MJ, Maxwell RB, Johnston TL, Schenker M, Briggs KK: Clinical presentation of femoroacetabular impingement. *Knee Surg Sports Traumatol Arthrosc* 2007; 15(8):1041-1047.
30. Siebenrock KA, Wahab KH, Werlen S, Kalhor M, Leunig M, Ganz R: Abnormal extension of the femoral head epiphysis as a cause of cam impingement. *Clin Orthop Relat Res* 2004;418:54-60.
31. Meyer DC, Beck M, Ellis T, Ganz R, Leunig M: Comparison of six radiographic projections to assess femoral head/neck asphericity. *Clin Orthop Relat Res* 2006;445: 181-185.
32. Tannast M, Siebenrock KA, Anderson SE: Femoroacetabular impingement: Radiographic diagnosis. What the radiologist should know. *AJR Am J Roentgenol* 2007; 188(6):1540-1552.
33. Peelle MW, Della Rocca GJ, Maloney WJ, Curry MC, Clohisy JC: Acetabular and femoral radiographic abnormalities associated with labral tears. *Clin Orthop Relat Res* 2005;441:327-333.
34. Nötzli HP, Wyss TF, Stoecklin CH, Schmid MR, Treiber K, Hodler J: The contour of the femoral head-neck junction as a predictor for the risk of anterior impingement. *J Bone Joint Surg Br* 2002;84(4):556-560.
35. Tannast M, Zheng G, Anderegg C, et al: Tilt and rotation correction of acetabular version on pelvic radiographs. *Clin Orthop Relat Res* 2005;438:182-190.
36. Siebenrock KA, Kalbermatten DF, Ganz R: Effect of pelvic tilt on acetabular retroversion: A study of pelves from cadavers. *Clin Orthop Relat Res* 2003;407: 241-248.
37. Murphy SB, Kijewski PK, Millis MB, Harless A: Acetabular dysplasia in the adolescent and young adult. *Clin Orthop Relat Res* 1990; 261:214-223.
38. Murphy SB, Ganz R, Müller ME: The prognosis in untreated dysplasia of the hip: A study of radiographic factors that predict the outcome. *J Bone Joint Surg Am* 1995;77(7):985-989.
39. Clohisy JC, Carlisle JC, Beaulé PE, et al: A systematic approach to the plain radiographic evaluation of the young adult hip. *J Bone Joint Surg Am* 2008; 90(Suppl 4):47-66.
40. Neumann G, Mendicuti AD, Zou KH, et al: Prevalence of labral tears and cartilage loss in patients with mechanical symptoms of the hip: Evaluation using MR arthrography. *Osteoarthritis Cartilage* 2007;15(8):909-917.
41. Chan YS, Lien LC, Hsu HL, et al: Evaluating hip labral tears using magnetic resonance arthrography: A prospective study comparing hip arthroscopy and magnetic resonance arthrography diagnosis. *Arthroscopy* 2005;21(10):1250.
42. Freedman BA, Potter BK, Dinauer PA, Giuliani JR, Kuklo TR, Murphy KP: Prognostic value of magnetic resonance arthrography for Czerny stage II and III acetabular labral tears. *Arthroscopy* 2006;22(7):742-747.
43. Toomayan GA, Holman WR, Major NM, Kozlowicz SM, Vail TP: Sensitivity of MR arthrography in the evaluation of acetabular labral tears. *AJR Am J Roentgenol* 2006;186(2):449-453.
44. Fadul DA, Carrino JA: Imaging of femoroacetabular impingement. *J Bone Joint Surg Am* 2009; 91(Suppl 1):138-143.
45. Keeney JA, Peelle MW, Jackson J, Rubin D, Maloney WJ, Clohisy JC: Magnetic resonance arthrogra-

phy versus arthroscopy in the evaluation of articular hip pathology. *Clin Orthop Relat Res* 2004;429: 163-169.

46. Mintz DN, Hooper T, Connell D, Buly R, Padgett DE, Potter HG: Magnetic resonance imaging of the hip: Detection of labral and chondral abnormalities using noncontrast imaging. *Arthroscopy* 2005;21(4):385-393.

47. Schmid MR, Nötzli HP, Zanetti M, Wyss TF, Hodler J: Cartilage lesions in the hip: Diagnostic effectiveness of MR arthrography. *Radiology* 2003;226(2):382-386.

48. Gautier E, Ganz K, Krügel N, Gill T, Ganz R: Anatomy of the medial femoral circumflex artery and its surgical implications. *J Bone Joint Surg Br* 2000;82(5): 679-683.

49. Sevitt S, Thompson RG: The distribution and anastomoses of arteries supplying the head and neck of the femur. *J Bone Joint Surg Br* 1965;47:560-573.

50. Espinosa N, Beck M, Rothenfluh DA, Ganz R, Leunig M: Treatment of femoro-acetabular impingement: Preliminary results of labral refixation. Surgical technique. *J Bone Joint Surg Am* 2007; 89(Suppl 2 Pt.1):36-53.

51. Philippon MJ, Wolff AB, Briggs KK, Zehms CT, Kuppersmith DA: Acetabular rim reduction for the treatment of femoroacetabular impingement correlates with preoperative and postoperative center-edge angle. *Arthroscopy* 2010;26(6):757-761.

52. Espinosa N, Rothenfluh DA, Beck M, Ganz R, Leunig M: Treatment of femoro-acetabular impingement: Preliminary results of labral refixation. *J Bone Joint Surg Am* 2006;88(5):925-935.

53. Sierra RJ, Trousdale RT: Labral reconstruction using the ligamentum teres capitis: Report of a new technique. *Clin Orthop Relat Res* 2009;467(3):753-759.

54. Philippon MJ, Briggs KK, Hay CJ, Kuppersmith DA, Dewing CB, Huang MJ: Arthroscopic labral reconstruction in the hip using iliotibial band autograft: Technique and early outcomes. *Arthroscopy* 2010;26(6):750-756.

55. Philippon MJ, Schroder e Souza BG, Briggs KK: Labrum: Resection, repair and reconstruction sports medicine and arthroscopy review. *Sports Med Arthrosc* 2010; 18(2):76-82.

56. Beaulé PE, Le Duff MJ, Zaragoza E: Quality of life following femoral head-neck osteochondroplasty for femoroacetabular impingement. *J Bone Joint Surg Am* 2007; 89(4):773-779.

57. Philippon MJ, Briggs KK, Yen YM, Kuppersmith DA: Outcomes following hip arthroscopy for femoroacetabular impingement with associated chondrolabral dysfunction: Minimum two-year follow-up. *J Bone Joint Surg Br* 2009;91(1):16-23.

58. Philippon MJ, Schenker ML, Briggs KK, Maxwell RB: Can microfracture produce repair tissue in acetabular chondral defects? *Arthroscopy* 2008;24(1):46-50.

59. Graves ML, Mast JW: Femoroacetabular impingement: Do outcomes reliably improve with surgical dislocations? *Clin Orthop Relat Res* 2009;467(3):717-723.

60. Sampson TG: Complications of hip arthroscopy. *Clin Sports Med* 2001;20(4):831-835.

61. Mardones RM, Gonzalez C, Chen Q, Zobitz M, Kaufman KR, Trousdale RT: Surgical treatment of femoroacetabular impingement: Evaluation of the effect of the size of the resection. Surgical technique. *J Bone Joint Surg Am* 2006;88(Suppl 1 Pt 1):84-91.

62. Ilizaliturri VM Jr: Complications of arthroscopic femoroacetabular impingement treatment: A review. *Clin Orthop Relat Res* 2009; 467(3):760-768.

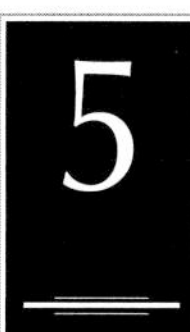

Femoroacetabular Impingement: Treatment of the Acetabular Side

Michael Leunig, MD
Thomas W. Huff, MD
Reinhold Ganz, MD

Abstract

Over the past decade, femoroacetabular impingement (FAI) has become an increasingly recognized pathomechanism that may explain why some hips that were previously considered to have normal morphology fail early in life. Subtle morphologic alterations in the acetabulum or femur, as well as the degree of hypermobility or impact on the hip, affect the potential for joint damage. The most frequent location of FAI is the anterosuperior acetabular rim, and the most critical motion is internal rotation of the hip in flexion. Because medication, activity restrictions, and physical therapy are rarely successful in treating symptoms caused by FAI, surgery has become a mainstay of treatment. Acetabular causes of FAI, called pincer FAI, can be treated by improving hip clearance. Independent of whether local or global overcoverage is present, rim reduction should be combined with labral preservation whenever possible.

Morphologic abnormalities in the osseous structures about the hip joint can lead to femoroacetabular impingement (FAI).[1,2] Repetitive impingement predisposes patients to the development of early osteoarthrosis.[2] The causative morphologic abnormality may exist on the femoral side, the acetabular side, or both. Structural abnormalities on the femoral side may result in asphericity, a decreased femoral head-neck ratio, leading to a cam-type impingement pattern. The primary injury is to the anterosuperior marginal articular cartilage and typically occurs during flexion and internal rotation. Shear forces at the junction of the labrum and articular cartilage first delaminate and then detach the cartilage. Labral injury and eventual detachment occur secondarily. Increased recognition and understanding of the consequences of these impinging structural abnormalities of the femur have led to treatment strategies aimed at improving the head-neck offset and preserving the native hip joint.[3,4]

Architectural abnormalities in the acetabulum that predispose to FAI can be described generally as patterns of overcoverage that lead to a pincer type of impingement. Patterns of overcoverage include anterior overcoverage with acetabular retroversion, coxa profunda, and protrusio acetabuli. In contrast to cam impingement, the primary injury mechanism is a repetitive, direct crush of the labrum and marginal articular cartilage. With time, the posteroinferior joint cartilage becomes abraded as a result of leverage of the head against the anterior rim. Overall, the degenerative process is much slower in pincer impingement than in the cam process. Similar to the approach to the femur in cam impingement, treatment strategies have been developed for correcting the acetabulum in pincer impingement. This chapter outlines an approach to the diagnosis and treatment of acetabular morphologies that predispose to impingement.

Diagnosis

Symptoms of the pincer type of FAI typically have a gradual onset and often are first noticed after vigorous physical activity (impact sports, sports demanding hypermobility) or, less commonly, after distortional trauma.[2,4] Pain is most commonly localized to the groin but may occur over the greater trochanter or in the gluteal region. The location of the pain often relates to the sites of impingement or the areas of overcoverage. Provocative maneuvers during physical examination will re-create the symptoms at the extremes of range of motion. For example, a maneuver that combines flexion, adduction, and internal rotation of the hip is provocative in patients with

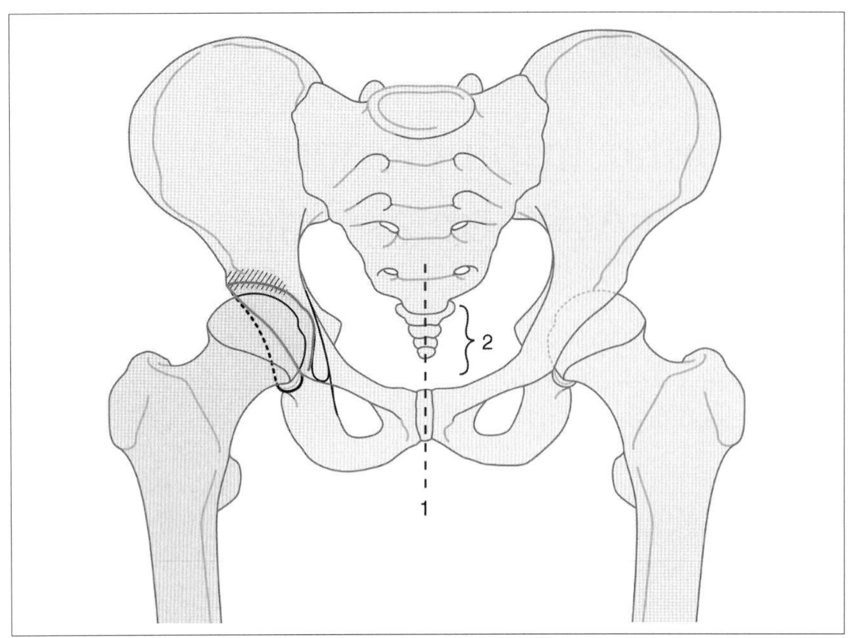

Figure 1 Accurate radiographic diagnosis is predicated on a standardized AP pelvic radiograph, as indicated. A proper orthograde AP pelvic radiograph must control flexion/extension and rotation of the pelvis. Criteria for an adequate radiograph include (1) a midline sacrum with the coccyx pointing to the symphysis pubis, and (2) the space between the sacrococcygeal joint and symphysis pubis should range between 2 and 4 cm (men) and 4 and 6 cm (women). Unless distorted by the disease process, the obturator foramina, teardrops, and iliac wings should appear symmetric.

anterolateral overcoverage, whereas extreme extension and external rotation are provocative in patients with posteroinferior overcoverage. Patients with coxa profunda or true protrusio may have impingement in all directions of hip motion. The clinical picture in these patients can include dramatic pain from the contused, inflamed, and sensitized labrum, in contrast to that of patients with cam impingement, where the labrum is not involved in the first stage of impingement.

The radiographic workup begins with a standardized set of plain radiographs. Radiographic features of FAI are also discussed in chapter 21. A correctly oriented AP pelvic radiograph (Figure 1) is evaluated for the acetabular index or Tönnis angle, the lateral center-edge angle, and posterior wall and crossover signs. The crossover sign is created when the projection of the superior portion of the anterior wall is lateral to the superior portion of the posterior wall. The crossover sign has been proposed as a sign of retroversion[5] but rather indicates anteversion of less than 4° on AP pelvic radiographs.[6] The anterior rim of the acetabulum courses medially, in a more horizontal direction than the vertically oriented posterior rim, creating the crossover. The posterior wall sign is present when the outline of the posterior wall lies medial to the center of the femoral head. The posterior wall sign is indicative of relative undercoverage posteriorly and may or may not be present with retroversion.[5] The radiographic diagnosis of protrusio is made when the femoral head lies medial to the Kohler line. Another parameter for quantification of femoral overcoverage is the femoral head extrusion index, which defines the percentage of the femoral head that is uncovered when a horizontal line is drawn parallel to the interteardrop line.[7,8] A normal extrusion index is less than 25%.[9] Although there is no defined minimal value for extrusion in the literature, less than 10% to 15% may indicate lateral overcoverage.

In a patient with a history, physical examination, and plain radiographs consistent with FAI, advanced imaging is warranted. High-resolution MRI of the hip with intra-articular gadolinium only is the imaging modality that provides the best visual representation of surrounding soft tissue structures.[10] Magnetic resonance arthrography of the hip is not only superior to plain pelvic hip MRI to detect labral pathology, it also is able to detect articular cartilage pathology that cannot be seen with plain radiographs.[11,12] MRI is less sensitive in detecting articular cartilage damage than it is for labral pathology, but it is specific. Radial cuts show bone appositions at the rim as well as potential contributions to the impingement by a femoral abnormality. Moreover, acetabular depth can be quantified based on radial sequences.[13] Considering all these aspects is crucial in developing a proper treatment plan. If there are still doubts whether all symptoms come from inside the joint, an intra-articular injection of local anesthetic can help to confirm the diagnosis.

Treatment

Impingement of hypermobile hips can occur without a specific morphologic abnormality. Patients with a type of extra-articular impingement are less likely to benefit from surgical intervention. Conversely, patients with anatomic intra-articular impingement are not likely to respond to nonsurgical treatment and are candidates for surgery. The surgical treatment of acetabular causes of impingement includes redirectional periacetabular osteotomy and trimming of the acetabular rim in combination with a labral refixation technique. The safety of these techniques is based on the results of detailed anatomic studies of the blood supply to the osseous structures of the hip.[14]

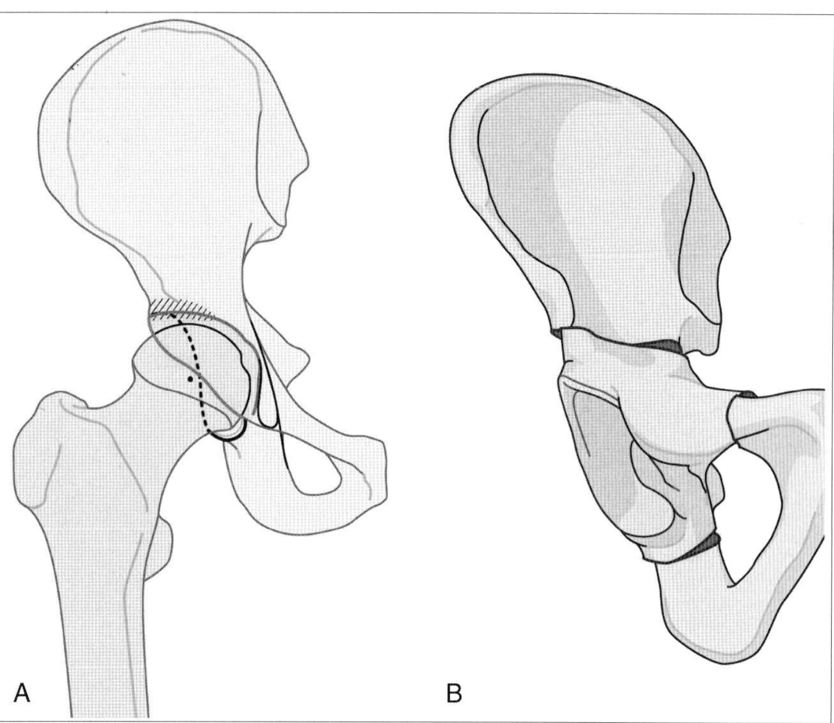

Figure 2 Local overcoverage: retroversion with a posterior wall sign is shown. **A,** Representation of a portion of an AP pelvic radiograph, showing a hip with the features of retroversion. The anterior wall (solid grey line) lies lateral to the posterior wall (dashed black line) in the cephalad portion of the acetabulum. The anterior wall courses in a more transverse direction than the vertically coursing posterior wall, creating the crossover sign. The center of the femoral head is marked (dot) and lies lateral to the posterior wall, creating the posterior wall sign. **B,** Reoriention of the retroverted acetabulum by periacetabular osteotomy (reverse PAO) with (flexion and) internal rotation can alleviate the anterior impingement and restore posterior coverage. Severe damage to the articular cartilage is a contraindication to this procedure.

Retroversion

Retroversion is defined as an acetabulum that opens with a partially (cephalad portion only) or totally posterior orientation relative to the sagittal plane.[5,15-17] Retroversion can exist as a primary deformity, in association with bladder exstrophy,[18] or with posttraumatic dysplasia.[19,20] It is also seen in all functional hips with proximal femoral focal deficiency,[21] those with Perthes disease,[22] and in combination with slipped capital femoral epiphysis.

The prominence of the anterolateral rim of the retroverted acetabulum predisposes to impingement with hip flexion, adduction, and internal rotation.[23,24] A diagnosis of retroversion can be confirmed by an orthograde plain AP pelvic radiograph by the presence of crossover and, sometimes, posterior wall signs.[25] Magnetic resonance arthrography is useful for assessing the extent of bony abnormality and the status of the labrum and articular cartilage. Special attention must be paid to the posteroinferior joint; sometimes the best information about this area comes from a false profile radiograph.[26]

Siebenrock and associates[24] reported the results of periacetabular osteotomy (PAO) for the treatment of FAI caused by retroversion. In their series, 26 of 29 patients had a good or excellent outcome at an average of 30 months after surgery. Failures reportedly were caused by overcorrection, undercorrection, and loss of reduction (one patient each), and were corrected to a good or excellent outcome with subsequent procedures using surgical dislocation of the joint. Capsulotomy at the time of PAO is recommended to allow labral pathology and femoral head-neck offset abnormalities to be corrected.

Although PAO can successfully treat symptomatic anterior impingement associated with acetabular retroversion and an insufficient posterior coverage of the femoral head (positive posterior wall sign; Figure 2), it is not required in all patients with this pathology. Patients with retroversion but adequate posterior wall coverage may benefit equally with surgical dislocation of the hip, combined with trimming of the anterolateral prominence with labral refixation (Figure 3). These patients can be identified radiographically with a positive crossover sign and a negative posterior wall sign. In these patients, PAO creating anteversion could create a posterior impingement. Similarly, if preoperative MRI demonstrates extensive

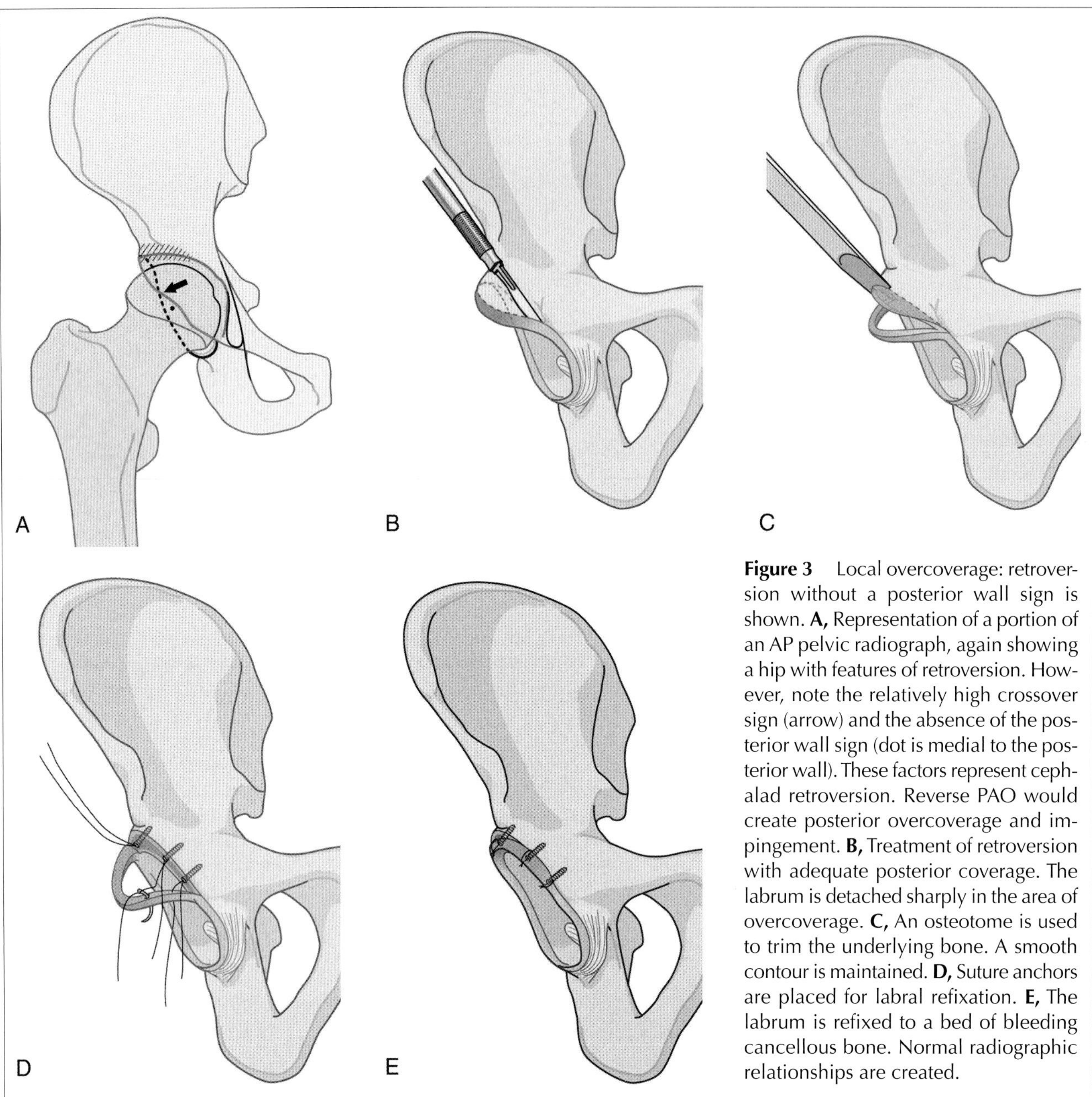

Figure 3 Local overcoverage: retroversion without a posterior wall sign is shown. **A,** Representation of a portion of an AP pelvic radiograph, again showing a hip with features of retroversion. However, note the relatively high crossover sign (arrow) and the absence of the posterior wall sign (dot is medial to the posterior wall). These factors represent cephalad retroversion. Reverse PAO would create posterior overcoverage and impingement. **B,** Treatment of retroversion with adequate posterior coverage. The labrum is detached sharply in the area of overcoverage. **C,** An osteotome is used to trim the underlying bone. A smooth contour is maintained. **D,** Suture anchors are placed for labral refixation. **E,** The labrum is refixed to a bed of bleeding cancellous bone. Normal radiographic relationships are created.

damage to the articular cartilage in the area of overcoverage, a reverse PAO would rotate this diseased area into the area of primary weight bearing and is, therefore, not indicated.

Coxa Profunda

Coxa profunda represents a global deepening of the acetabulum and a medialization of the femoral head. The ultimate pattern of the associated impingement is affected by the depth of medialization along with the orientation of the acetabular opening. In patients with coxa profunda, the surgical treatment of choice is trimming the bony rim of the acetabulum in areas of overcoverage while preserving the labrum (Figure 4). Knowing which area of the rim to reduce, and to what extent, is dictated by the degree of damage to the acetabular cartilage and the degree of overcoverage; however, excessive resection of the bony rim leading to undercoverage and its associated complications should be avoided.[27] With an open surgical dislocation technique, the impingement can be dynamically assessed under direct visualization, as can the adequacy of resection.

Preservation of the labrum is as

critical as making an appropriate bony resection. Espinosa and associates[27] emphasized the importance of the technique of labral refixation. They retrospectively reviewed and compared the results between patients treated with labral resection and those of patients treated with labral refixation. Two years after surgery, only 28% of the resection group had excellent results, compared with 80% of the refixation group. With labral refixation, the preserved labrum is repaired (or refixed) with suture anchors to a base of bleeding cancellous bone, where the bony rim has been resected. The suction seal and lubricating fluid film are dependent on an intact labrum.

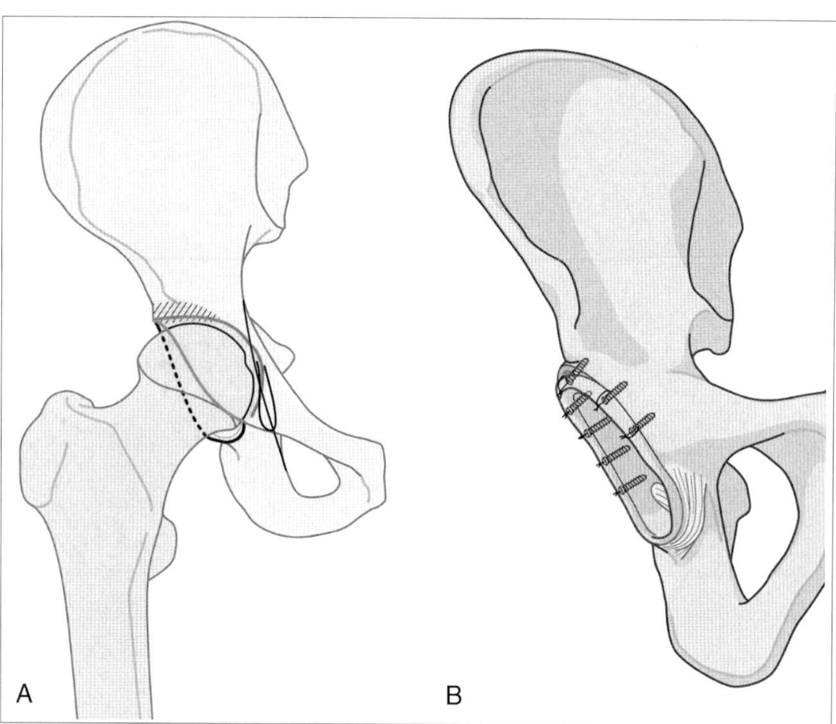

Figure 4 Global overcoverage: coxa profunda is shown. **A,** Medial femoral head and global overcoverage. The acetabular index is neutral. **B,** Treatment with near circumferential trimming of the acetabular rim and labral refixation. Normal radiographic relationships are created.

Protrusio

Coxa profunda may exist on a spectrum of pathology that ultimately becomes acetabular protrusio, with the femoral head migrating medial to the Kohler line. The medial migration of the femoral head is seen in patients with rheumatoid arthritis, osteomalacia, or Marfan syndrome and is believed to be the result of repeated stress fracture.[28] For protrusio associated with autoaggressive arthritis, total hip arthroplasty is indicated. However, protrusio also can be seen as a developmental or posttraumatic deformity in young people, with the articular cartilage in a healthy but prepathologic state. These patients are candidates for joint preservation if the posteroinferior joint space is maintained, but the surgery is challenging, especially if the acetabular roof inclination is negative. The mechanical situation must be normalized, the impingement alleviated, and the roof orientation corrected to between neutral and +5°.

The first step in the surgical treatment often is a circumferential trimming of the acetabular rim accessed by surgical dislocation of the hip (Figure 5), sometimes combined with relative lengthening of the femoral neck and distal advancement of the greater trochanter. In the absence of pelvitrochanteric impingement with the femur in varus, an intertrochanteric valgus osteotomy may be considered. The second step is a PAO that, if possible, is done during the same surgical session after repositioning of the patient from lateral decubitus to supine. During the first step of the procedure, with the patient in a lateral decubitus position, the first incomplete cut of the PAO into the ischium can be made with direct visual observation of the sciatic nerve. The goal is to lateralize the acetabular fragment and rotate it toward the midline (clockwise in a right hip; counterclockwise in a left hip) so that the roof angle and the acetabular version become normal. This is a technically difficult procedure, and the proximal displacement of the acetabular fragment can put the femoral nerve at risk of injury. As the femoral nerve courses with the iliopsoas tendon, these structures become draped over the step created by the rotation of the fragment, and the nerve is susceptible to a tension injury. Direct observation of the nerve and optimal rotation of the fragment are possible with an inguinal extension of the Smith-Peterson approach, allowing a ball spike to be placed onto the pubic portion of the acetabular fragment.[29] In this manner, the formation of a medial step is prevented while the osteotomized fragment is rotated with a supra-acetabular Schanz screw.

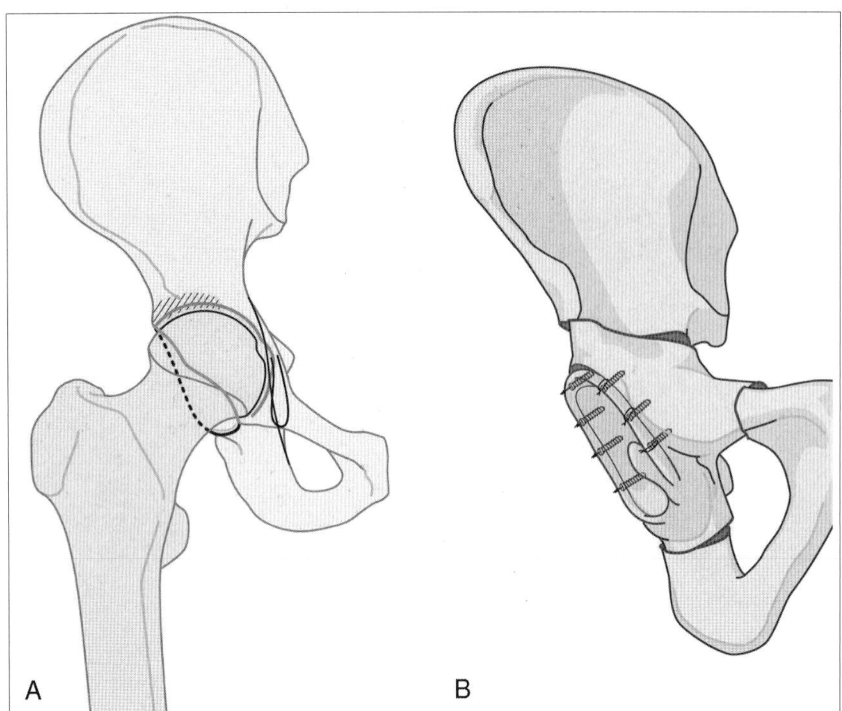

Figure 5 Global overcoverage: protrusio is shown. **A,** The head-extrusion index is approximately 10% to 15% only. The acetabular index is negative. **B,** The acetabular rim is trimmed circumferentially with labral refixation, and a PAO is used to correct the acetabular index to 0° to +5°. An intraoperative AP pelvic radiograph is obtained before definitive fixation. Trochanteric advancement is not shown.

Another important technical consideration is the horseshoe of articular cartilage in the acetabulum. The fact that there is global overcoverage does not mean that excess articular cartilage is present. In fact, often the opposite is true. The cotyloid fossa in patients with protrusio is typically enlarged, and the horseshoe may even be narrowed. In such patients, especially with a negative Tönnis angle, conservative trimming of the acetabular rim is indicated, and a PAO must be used to reposition and conserve the horseshoe.

Summary

This chapter presents a simplified, algorithmic approach to the diagnosis and treatment of acetabular causes of FAI. It is critical that individual treatment plans are based on the entire clinical picture of each patient. The understanding of these disease processes has evolved through experience with surgical dislocations, and the approach to the treatment of intra-articular impingement has been based on this technique. This is not meant to dismiss an emerging role for arthroscopy in some situations. The goals of treatment are the same regardless of approach: to safely and exactly correct morphologic abnormalities, to alleviate the symptomatology of FAI, and to stop or slow the progression to early osteoarthritis.

References

1. Beck M, Kalhor M, Leunig M, Ganz R: Hip morphology influences the pattern of damage to the acetabular cartilage: Femoroacetabular impingement as a cause of early osteoarthritis of the hip. *J Bone Joint Surg Br* 2005;87:1012-1018.
2. Ganz R, Parvizi J, Beck M, Leunig M, Notzli H, Siebenrock KA: Femoroacetabular impingement: A cause for osteoarthritis of the hip. *Clin Orthop Relat Res* 2003;417:112-120.
3. Ganz R, Gill TJ, Gautier E , Ganz K, Krugel N, Berlemann U: Surgical dislocation of the adult hip: A technique with full access to the femoral head and acetabulum without the risk of avascular necrosis. *J Bone Joint Surg Br* 2001;83:1119-1124.
4. Espinosa N, Rothenfluh D, Beck M, Ganz R, Leunig M: Treatment of femoroacetabular impingement: Preliminary results of labral refixation. *J Bone Joint Surg Am* 2006;88:925-935.
5. Reynolds D, Lucas J, Klaue K: Retroversion of the acetabulum: A cause of hip pain. *J Bone Joint Surg Br* 1999;81:281-288.
6. Jamali AA, Mladenov K, Meyer DC, et al: Anteroposterior pelvic radiographs to assess acetabular retroversion: High validity of the "cross-over-sign." *J Orthop Res* 2007;25:758-765.
7. Murphy SB, Kijewski PK, Millis MB, Harless A: Acetabular dysplasia in the adolescent and young adult. *Clin Orthop Relat Res* 1990;261:214-223.
8. Murphy SB, Ganz R, Müller ME: The prognosis in untreated dysplasia of the hip. *J Bone Joint Surg Am* 1995;77:985-989.
9. Li PLS, Ganz R: Morphologic features of congenital acetabular dysplasia. *Clin Orthop Relat Res* 2003;416:245-253.
10. Werlen S, Leunig M, Ganz R: Magnetic resonance arthrography of the hip: Evolution of the Bernese technique of radial sequencing. *Oper Tech Orthop* 2005;15:191-203.
11. Toomayan GA, Holman WR, Major NM, Kozlowicz SM, Vail TP: Sensitivity of MR arthrography in the evaluation of acetabular labral tears. *AJR Am J Roentgenol* 2006;186:449-453.

12. Schmid MR, Notzli HP, Zanetti M, Wyss TF, Hodler J: Cartilage lesions in the hip: Diagnostic effectiveness of MR arthrography. *Radiology* 2003;226: 382-386.

13. Pfirrmann CW, Mengiardi B, Dora C, Kalberer F, Zanetti M, Hodler J: Cam and pincer femoroacetabular impingement: Characteristic MR arthrographic findings in 50 patients. *Radiology* 2006;240:778-785.

14. Gautier E, Ganz K, Krugel N, Gill T, Ganz R: Anatomy of the medial femoral circumflex artery and its surgical implications. *J Bone Joint Surg Br* 2000;82:679-683.

15. Reikeras O, Bjerkreim I, Kolbenstvekt A: Anteversion of the acetabulum and femoral neck in normals and in patients with osteoarthritis of the hip. *Acta Orthop Scand* 1983;54:18-23.

16. Tonnis D: *Congenital Dysplasia and Dislocation of the Hip in Children and Adults.* New York, NY, Springer, 1987, pp 113-130, 156-161.

17. Tonnis D, Heinecke A: Acetabular and femoral anteversion: Relationship with osteoarthritis of the hip. *J Bone Joint Surg Am* 1999;81:1747-1770.

18. Sponseller PD, Bisson LJ, Gearhart JP, Jeffs RD, Magid D, Fishman E: The anatomy of the pelvis in the extrophy complex. *J Bone Joint Surg Am* 1995; 77:177-189.

19. Dora C, Zurback J, Hersche O, Ganz R: Pathomorphologic characteristics of posttraumatic acetabular dysplasia. *J Orthop Trauma* 2000;14: 483-489.

20. Murphy SB, Kijewski PK, Millis MB, Harless A: Acetabular dysplasia in the adolescent and young adult. *Clin Orthop Relat Res* 1990;261:214-223.

21. Dora C, Buhler M, Stover MD, Mahomed MN, Ganz R: Morphologic characteristics of acetabular dysplasia in proximal femoral focal deficiency. *J Pediatr Orthop B* 2004;13: 81-87.

22. Ezoe M, Naito M, Inoue T: The prevalence of acetabular retroversion among various disorders of the hip. *J Bone Joint Surg Am* 2006;88:372-379.

23. Myers SR, Eijer H, Ganz R: Anterior femoroacetabular impingement after periacetabular osteotomy. *Clin Orthop Relat Res* 1999;363:93-99.

24. Siebenrock KA, Schoeniger R, Ganz R: Anterior femoroacetabular impingement due to acetabular retroversion. *J Bone Joint Surg Am* 2003;85: 278-286.

25. Siebenrock KA, Kalbermatten DF, Ganz R: Effect of pelvic tilt on acetabular retroversion: A study of pelves from cadavers. *Clin Orthop Relat Res* 2003;407:241-248.

26. Lequesne M, deSeze S: Le faux profil du bassin: Nouvelle incidence radiographique pour l'étude de la hanche: Son utilité dans les dysplasies et les differentes coxopathies. *Rev Rhum* 1961;28:643-652.

27. Espinosa N, Beck M, Rothenfluh D, Ganz R, Leunig M: Treatment of femoroacetabular impingement: Preliminary results of labral refixation: Surgical technique. *J Bone Joint Surg Am* 2007;89:36-53.

28. Van De Velde S, Fillman R, Yandow S: The aetiology of protrusio acetabuli: Literature review from 1824 to 2006. *Acta Orthop Belg* 2006;72:524-529.

29. Letournel E: The treatment of acetabular fractures through the ilioinguinal approach. *Clin Orthop Relat Res* 1993;292:62-76.

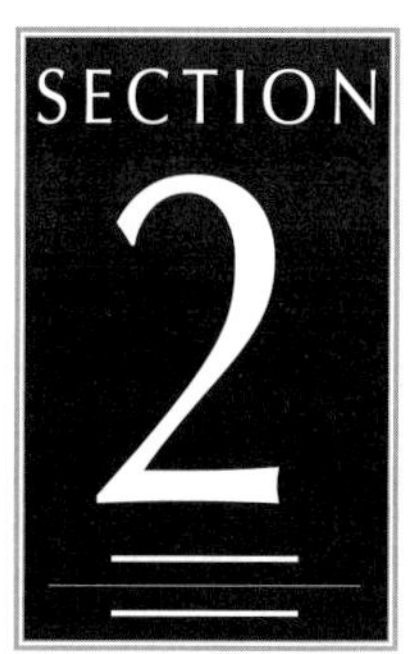

Fracture Care of the Hip

Fracture Care of the Hip

Fractures around the hip remain among the most common yet controversial injuries managed by orthopaedic surgeons. Given the enormous economic effect of these fractures, it is critical to have effective treatment algorithms that optimize outcomes and minimize complications. This section consists of five chapters that cover a broad range of hip fractures and disorders. The authors provide comprehensive reviews of many topics, including slipped capital femoral epiphysis (SCFE), femoral neck fractures, pertrochanteric fractures, and fractures of the acetabulum.

Anglen and associates present technical tips for treating hip fractures, with discussions of femoral neck and pertrochanteric fractures. After a basic discussion of patient demographics and general issues, a detailed discussion is provided on internal fixation techniques for femoral neck and pertrochanteric fractures. Several intraoperative and fluoroscopic images nicely illustrate reduction techniques and tricks, as well as ideal implant placement. Because a relatively cursory discussion of arthroplasty indications and techniques is provided, this review will be most beneficial to surgeons seeking more information regarding internal fixation of femoral neck fractures.

Karunakar and associates provide an excellent review of many of the nonsurgical issues involved in treating pertrochanteric hip fractures. A comprehensive discussion of preoperative clearance, anesthesia choices, medical management, and thromboembolic prophylaxis is provided. The data on the timing of hip fracture care are particularly well represented. The authors effectively use tables to summarize the available literature, which makes this useful chapter an "easy read." Implant selection theory is well covered; however, specific technical tips and tricks are lacking. Salvage of failed fixation is briefly discussed.

Moed and associates provide a true textbook-type review of the surgical treatment of acetabular fractures. The authors present a detailed discussion of imaging, classification, treatment indications, internal fixation techniques, complications, and results. This review should be required reading for trauma fellows and residents alike. The discussion of various surgical approaches and the specific methods for fixation of basic fracture patterns are well described and elegantly illustrated. The content is detailed and may be too comprehensive for surgeons who do not surgically treat acetabular fractures; however, the sections on nonsurgical treatment and indications for surgery can benefit any surgeon who actively takes trauma call and may need to make decisions about referring a patient to a higher level of care.

The chapter on intertrochanteric fractures, which I authored, primarily focuses on implant selection and provides specific surgical tips to avoid complications when performing open reduction and internal fixation of intertrochanteric fractures. This chapter nicely complements the chapters by Anglen and associates and Karunakar and associates by focusing specifically on fixation techniques rather than presenting an extensive literature review and information on nonsurgical issues. Following the 10 described principles in a checklist manner will provide the surgeon with guidelines to improve outcomes and minimize the risks for the most common complications.

In the chapter by Loder and associates, controversial issues for managing SCFE are discussed. The authors provide a thorough discussion of the basic science and animal data available on this disorder. This chapter may be somewhat tedious for orthopaedic surgeons who do not specialize in pediatrics. The most helpful content for general orthopaedic surgeons centers on the surgical management of SCFE, differentiation of stable and unstable slips, and preferred internal fixation constructs. Indications for contralateral fixation and endocrine issues are discussed, and information on osteotomies is particularly well covered. Overall, this chapter provides comprehensive coverage of SCFE, ranging from basic science to controversial state-of-the-art management.

George J. Haidukewych, MD
Academic Chairman
Chief of Orthopedic Trauma and Adult Reconstruction
Level One Orthopedics
University of Central Florida
Orlando, Florida

Dr. Haidukewych or an immediate family member has received royalties from DePuy; serves as a paid consultant to Smith & Nephew and Synthes; has stock or stock options held in OrthoPediatrics and the Institute for Better Bone Health; and serves as a board member, owner, officer, or committee member of the American Academy of Orthopaedic Surgeons.

6

Technical Tips in Fracture Care: Fractures of the Hip

*Jeffrey O. Anglen, MD
Michael R. Baumgaertner, MD
Wade R. Smith, MD
Paul Tornetta III, MD
*Bruce H. Ziran, MD

Abstract

Hip fracture is an increasingly common and clinically significant injury with substantial economic impact. Associated risk factors are age, gender, race, bone density, activity level, and medical disorders. Prevention efforts include treatment of osteoporosis and programs to reduce the risks of a fall.

Nondisplaced or impacted fractures of the femoral neck can be treated with screw fixation. Displaced femoral neck fractures in younger, more active patients may be treated with reduction and fixation. In physiologically older patients, joint arthroplasty is indicated for displaced fractures. In patients with systemic arthritis or preexisting hip disease, total hip arthroplasty may be an appropriate treatment choice.

Intertrochanteric fractures are treated with reduction and fixation using either a sliding hip screw and side plate or intramedullary nail with cephalic interlock. Key technical points for successful outcomes include proper patient positioning, using a correct starting point for the nail, achieving acceptable reduction before fixation, and the use of various reduction techniques and aids.

Fractures of the hip joint include fractures of the acetabulum, femoral head, and proximal femur. This chapter will examine fractures of the femoral neck and intertrochanteric area of the proximal femur.

Etiology, Incidence, and Risk Factors

Hip fracture can occur in patients of any age. In younger patients, such fractures are usually the result of high-energy trauma, such as a motor vehicle crash. In these patients, multiple system injuries or associated orthopaedic injuries often occur. In elderly patients, injury usually results from a lower energy mechanism such as a fall; older patients often have multiple medical comorbidities.

Hip fracture in elderly patients is extremely common. Current statistics show that more than 250,000 such injuries occur annually in the United States, with an expected increase to 350,000 by 2020.[1] Projections for the worldwide incidence of hip fracture are as high as 6.5 million annually by 2050.[2] A 50-year-old Caucasian woman currently has a 17.5% lifetime risk of hip fracture; for men of the same age, the risk is 6%. In the United States, the annual cost for the care of patients with hip fractures is more than $14 billion and may increase to $250 billion by 2040. Risk factors for hip fracture in elderly patients are shown in Table 1.

Outcome

Hip fracture is a significant event with potentially negative outcomes. Twenty percent of elderly patients with hip fractures die within 1 year of the fracture. The relative risk of death within that period is increased 3.3 times for women and 4.2 times for men with hip fracture, compared with age-matched control subjects who have not had a hip fracture. Ap-

Jeffrey Anglen, MD or the department with which he is affiliated has received royalties from EBI and serves as a consultant or employee for Eli Lilly. Bruce Ziran, MD or the department with which he is affiliated has received miscellaneous nonincome support, commercially derived honoraria, or other nonresearch-related funding from Stryker and Synthes.

Table 1
Risk Factors for Hip Fracture in Elderly Patients

Age: the incidence of hip fracture increases for each decade of life from the sixth to the ninth.
Gender: 80% of hip fractures occur in women, although the rate of increase may be higher in men according to some studies.
Race: Caucasian women have 2.4 times the risk of hip fracture compared with African-American women. The highest incidence of hip fracture occurs in Scandinavian women.
Bone mineral density: each standard deviation below the age-adjusted average doubles the risk of hip fracture.
Previous wrist fracture
Previous fall or other fracture
High transfer dependence
Dementia
Visual impairment
Neuromuscular impairment
Lower extremity weakness

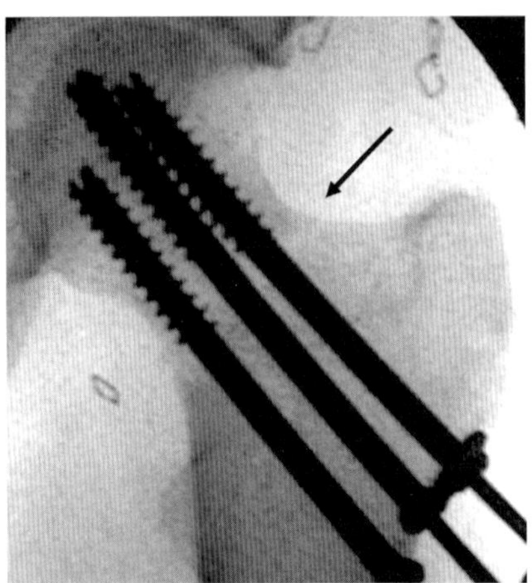

Figure 1 Placement of cannulated screws in parallel orientation with all threads crossing the fracture site results in compression of the fracture line (*arrow*). The use of washers in metaphyseal areas facilitates compression.

proximately one half of the patients with hip fracture never regain their premorbid level of ambulation, and approximately 17% who were community ambulators prior to the hip fracture will be institutionalized after the fracture.

Prevention

The prevention of hip fractures involves the use of dietary supplements and medications to treat patients with osteoporosis, reducing the risk of falls through exercise to improve balance and physical strength, behavioral instruction, environmental modifications, and the use of hip protectors in selected patients.[3-5] Information about reducing the risks of falls is available on the American Academy of Orthopaedic Surgeons Website.[6]

Treatment

In most patients, fractures of the hip require surgical treatment. Nonsurgical treatment is occasionally appropriate for bedridden or nonambulatory patients, those with extremely limited life expectancy, those with severe neurologic impairment, or patients who are unable to tolerate surgery.

Femoral Neck Fractures

The timing of surgery for a patient with a femoral neck fracture depends on many factors. In young patients, a femoral neck fracture is considered by most surgeons to be an emergent condition, with the risk of developing osteonecrosis of the femoral head increasing with any delay in treatment. However, a recent meta-analysis by Damany and associates[7] did not show strong evidence for this position. In elderly patients, optimization of the patient's medical condition may require surgery to be delayed; however, delays of more than 48 hours have been shown to increase the length of hospitalization, and delays in surgery of more than 4 to 5 days increase patient mortality.[8,9]

Fractures of the femoral neck have been classified by the Garden system into four types. In a Garden type 1 fracture, the femoral neck is impacted into the femoral head in a valgus position; a Garden type 2 fracture is a nondisplaced, nonimpacted fracture; a Garden type 3 is a displaced fracture with an offset of less than 50% of the neck width; and a Garden type 4 fracture has more than 50% displacement.

The appropriate surgical treatment for Garden type 1 and 2 fractures is fixation in situ with percutaneous, partially threaded, cannulated screws. The screws should be placed parallel and peripheral along the cortical bone of the neck to prevent postoperative displacement (Figure 1). Three screws are sufficient.[10] One screw is placed inferiorly along the medial aspect of the neck (calcar) and the other two screws are placed in an inverted triangular arrangement anterior and posterior. Correct positioning of the screws along the cortex of the femoral neck, particularly inferior and posterior, leads to a significant improvement in the rate of union. The more superior screws in the metaphysis should have washers to allow compression. Threads should not cross the fracture site.

For displaced fractures in younger patients, reduction and fixation preserve the hip joint. The most important surgeon-controlled factor in outcome is the quality of reduction. An open reduction is often required to achieve anatomic alignment. The patient is positioned supine on a fracture table to facilitate fluoroscopic visualization of the femoral neck. Good biplanar C-arm images should be confirmed before the patient is prepared for surgery. Either the Smith Petersen (anterior) or the Watson Jones (anterolateral) surgical approach can be used. The anterolateral approach makes it easier to insert fixation screws. An anterior arthrotomy is gently performed to preserve blood supply; it is done in a manner that allows closure of the capsule at the end.

Tips for achieving proper reduction include inducing full muscle relaxation in the patient and the use of joysticks. This procedure is commonly performed with a 4.5-mm Schanz screw in the femoral shaft, and a 2.5-mm terminally threaded Kirschner wire in the femoral head. Provisional reduction is held with multiple smooth Kirschner wires, while the reduction is evaluated with direct vision and fluoroscopy. The contour of the femoral head and neck should make a smooth, lazy S outline along superior, inferior, anterior, and posterior borders (Figure 2). Fixation is performed with three large, cannulated lag screws, as previously described.

In an elderly patient with a displaced femoral neck fracture, the surgeon and patient should discuss the options of treatment with open reduction and internal fixation or with hip joint arthroplasty. If joint replacement is chosen, hemiarthroplasty (bipolar or unipolar) or total hip arthroplasty may be performed. With either method, the stem may be cemented or cementless.

Internal fixation results in less blood loss, shorter surgical time, a lower infection rate, and a lower overall complication rate; however, the rate of resurgery is significantly higher.[11] Differences in the mortality rate have not been clearly established; however, a recent meta-analysis suggests a slightly higher mortality rate for patients treated with arthroplasty.[12] A study using cost analysis methodology suggested that arthroplasty was the most cost-effective treatment when complications, mortality, and the rate of resurgery were considered at 2 years postoperatively. However, the best functional results were obtained in patients with a healed femoral neck with no osteonecrosis after open reduction and internal fixation.[13] A reasonable approach is to perform arthroplasty in any patient older than 75 years, or older than 55 years if there are significant comorbidities, such as neurologic disease, lower extremity weakness, significant osteoporosis, and preexisting arthritis, or if the patient is sedentary with a limited activity level. Reduction and fixation may be a worthwhile treatment choice in healthy, active patients who are younger than 60 years, do not have arthritis, have good bone quality, and have limited comminution. For patients who do not fit into either group, treatment options should be carefully discussed with the patient.

If arthroplasty is selected, total hip arthroplasty is indicated in patients with preexisting arthritis, acetabular damage, or in patients with systemic arthritic disease, even if the hip is relatively spared. Some surgeons believe that better functional results are achieved with total hip arthroplasty for all patients.[14] In a recent prospective, randomized study of 81 elderly patients with displaced femoral neck fractures, patients treated with total hip arthroplasty reported walking farther and had better hip scores than patients treated with hemiarthroplasty. There were no significant differences in mortality rates or complications in the two groups.[15] Dislocations occurred in three patients treated with total hip arthroplasty. Some studies have shown higher dislocation rates with total hip arthroplasty (more than 10% in some studies).[16] No consistent clinical differences have been found in several studies comparing bipolar with unipolar hemiarthroplasty; however, bipolar prostheses have a significantly higher cost.[17-20] In studies comparing cemented with cementless stems, results showed better functional results and less pain with the use of cemented stems, although most of these studies included patients with older stem designs.[21-24] The comparison of posterior and lateral surgical approaches have shown no differences in outcome.[25] The use of general and regional an-

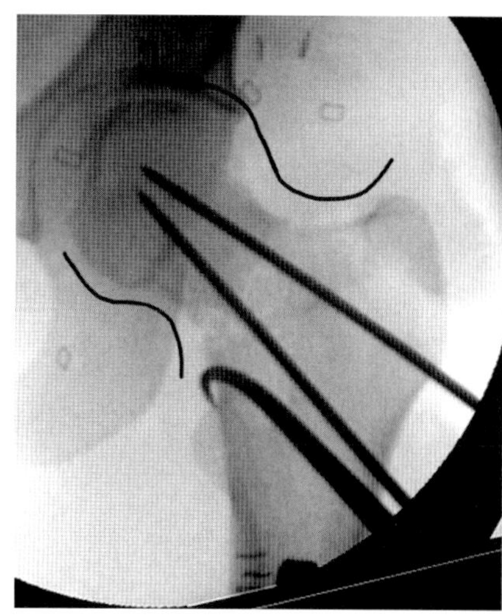

Figure 2 Accurate reduction of the femoral neck results in a smooth S outline of the head and neck in both AP and lateral projections.

esthesia has also resulted in similar outcomes.[26,27]

Intertrochanteric Fractures

Intertrochanteric (pertrochanteric) fractures in ambulatory patients are treated with reduction and fixation. This procedure is best performed on a fracture table (Figure 3). Verification of C-arm visualization is recommended before the patient is prepared and draped for surgery. Reduction is performed with longitudinal traction and rotation, which is usually internal. The use of crutch support of the distal fragment is often helpful (Figure 4); occasionally, a percutaneous ball-tipped spike or Schanz screw is used to assist in the reduction (Figures 5 and 6). These devices are often placed through a small anterior stab incision to correct a flexed proximal fragment.

Fixation options for these fractures include a sliding compression screw and side plate, intramedullary hip screws, 95°-blade plates or a screw and side plates, and specialized plates such as the Medoff plate or a locking proximal femur plate. In most instances, a sliding compression screw or an intramedullary screw will be equally effective, and both can be placed through relatively small incisions. A sliding compression screw with a two-hole side plate is adequate fixation for simple two-part fractures. A meta-analysis of the literature suggests that intraoperative complications and postoperative femoral fractures more commonly occur with intramedullary hip screws; however, the more recent literature suggests that intramedullary screws may allow earlier ambulation.[28-30] If there is comminution of the lateral cortex,

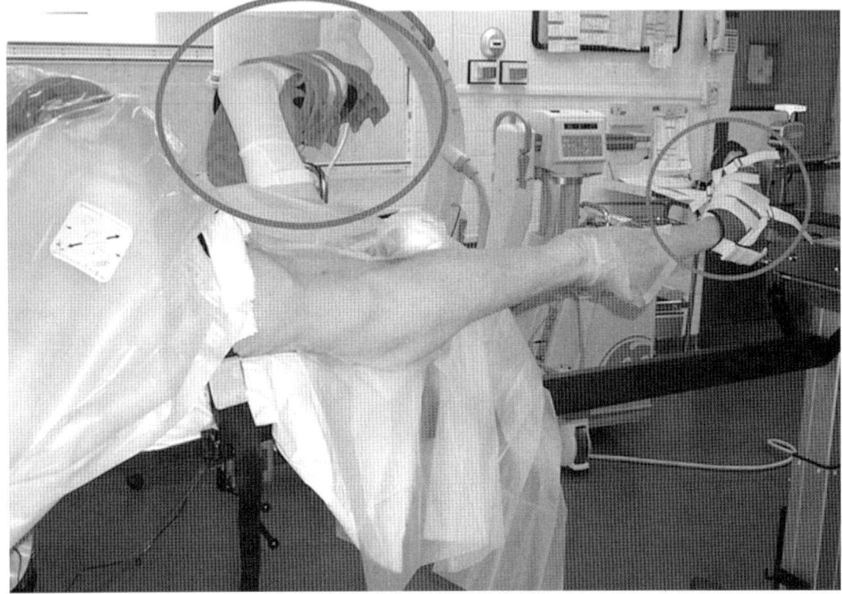

Figure 3 The patient is positioned on the fracture table with the foot (on the injured side) slightly internally rotated to facilitate reduction. Note the position of the leg and foot (*circled areas*). The hemilithotomy position, which should only be used for short periods (< 2 hours), is shown.

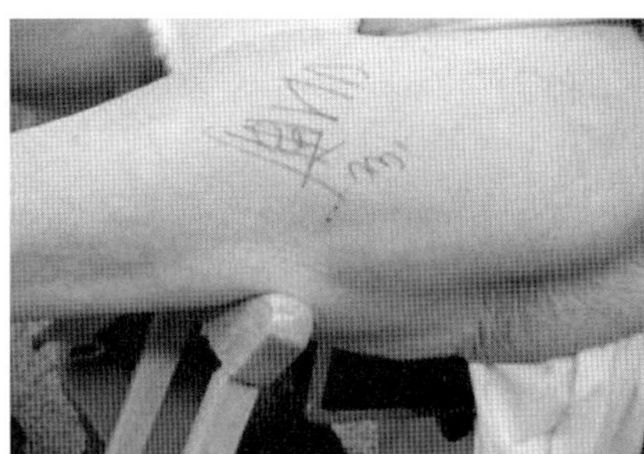

Figure 4 A crutch can be used to support the leg and reduce posterior sag.

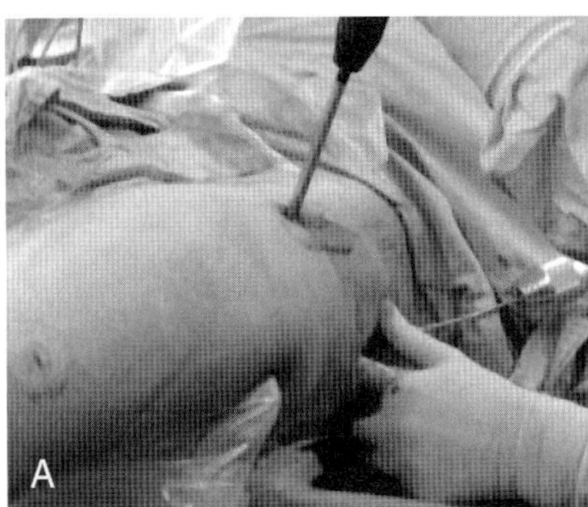

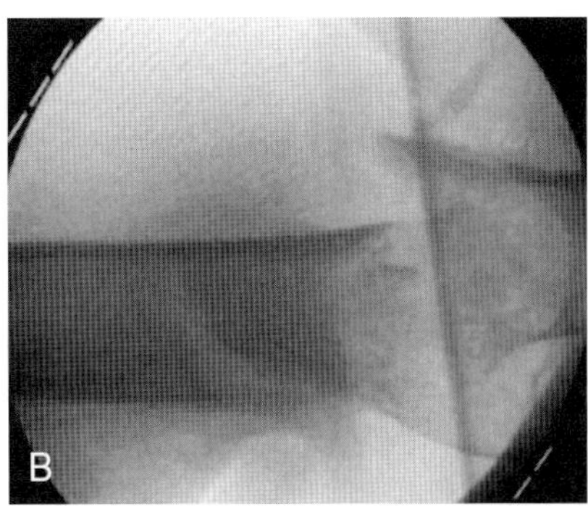

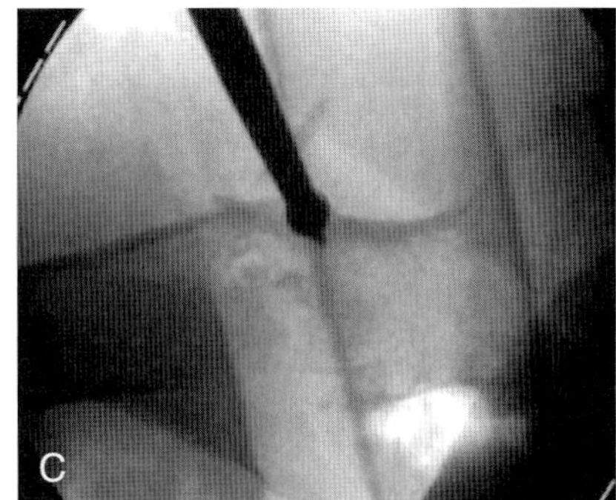

Figure 5 **A,** A percutaneous ball-tipped spike is used to improve reduction by resisting flexion of the proximal fragment. **B,** Fluoroscopic view showing apex anterior angulation at the fracture site caused by flexion of the proximal fragment. **C,** Fluoroscopic view showing correction of the malreduction using a percutaneous ball-tipped spike.

or reverse obliquity of the fracture line, an intramedullary screw or 95°-device is necessary to resist displacement.[31,32] Use of a standard compression hip screw in fractures of this type will often result in shortening and medial displacement.

A sliding compression hip screw can be placed through a minimal incision for simple, stable (lateral cortex intact) fractures. The guide pin is placed percutaneously through a poke hole with fluoroscopic control, using a 130° or larger angle guide that is determined based on preoperative planning. The ideal position of the guide pin is central and deep on both views. This placement results in a final screw position with a tip-apex distance of less than 2 cm, which decreases the risk of screw cutout.[33] An incision from skin to bone is made from the guidewire distally 2 or 3 cm. Reaming, measuring, tapping, and screw placement are done in standard fashion through this incision. A two-hole short barrel plate is inserted through the incision and bluntly worked to the bone; after verification of position, it is attached with cortical screws (Figure 7).

Intramedullary hip screw or nail placement begins with proper positioning to allow access to the starting point without introducing varus malalignment. The trunk of the patient should be leaned or angled toward the opposite side. An adequate incision must be made in obese patients to allow the insertion handle to be used without undue lateral pressure from the soft tissues proximal to the hip; this results in fracture distraction (Figure 8). As with any intramedullary device, the starting point is the key factor in good technique. The most common error is using a starting point too far lateral, which results in varus malalign-

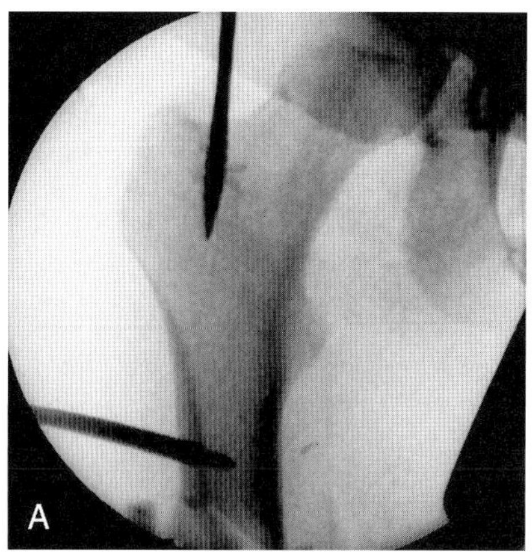

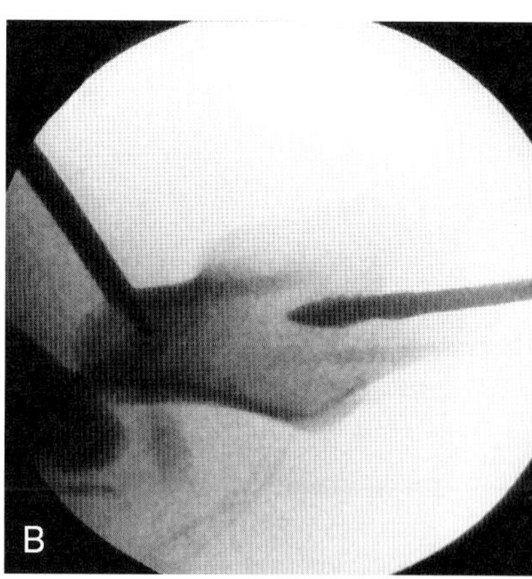

Figure 6 Percutaneous placement of a Schanz pin may be useful in controlling the proximal fragment in many fractures of the proximal femur. **A,** AP fluoroscopic view showing use of a percutaneous unicortical Schanz pin to resist abduction of the short proximal fragment. **B,** Lateral fluoroscopic view showing correct alignment of the T-handled awl.

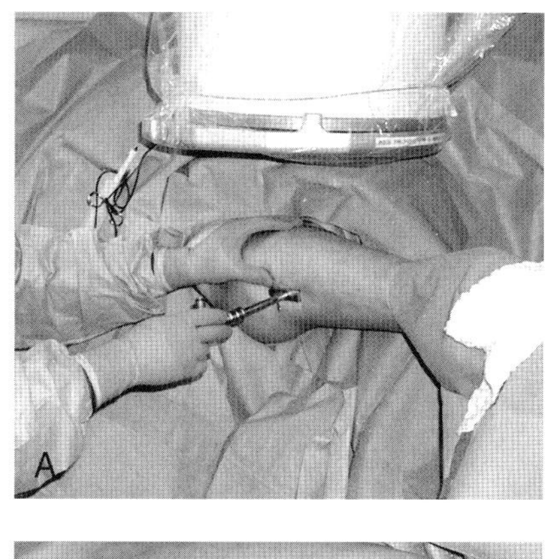

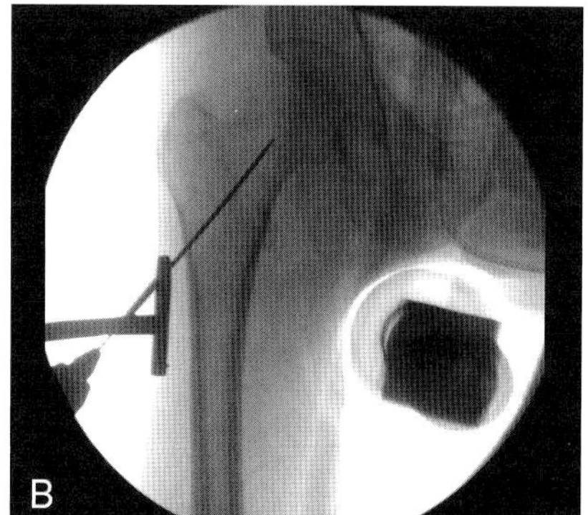

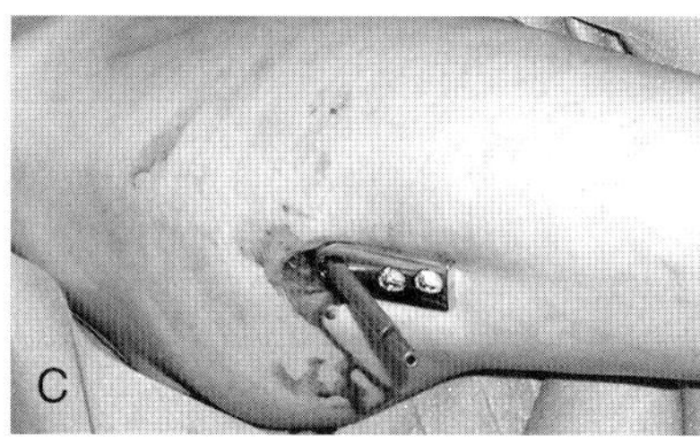

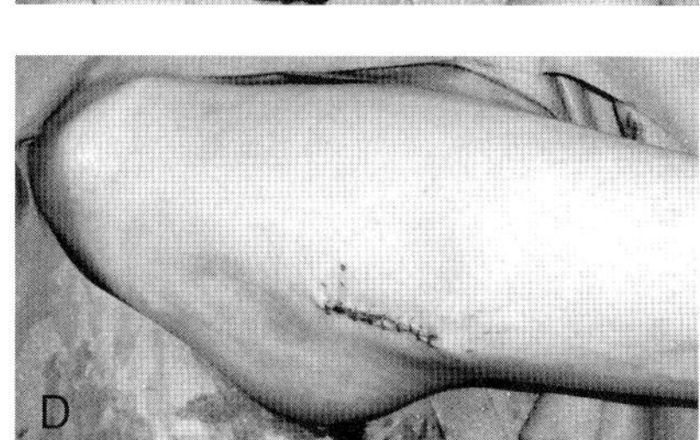

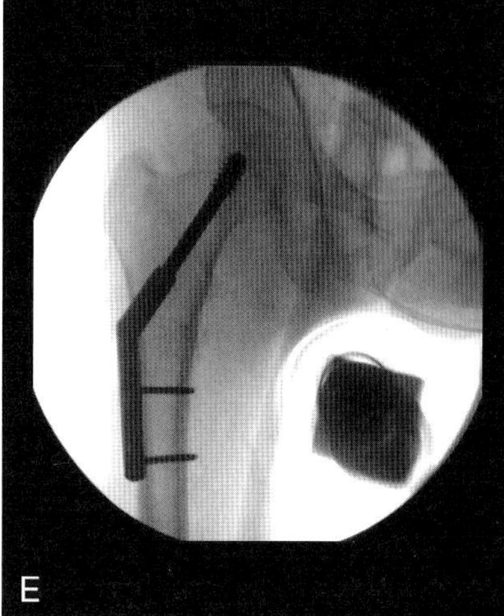

Figure 7 Photograph **(A)** and fluoroscopic view **(B)** showing placement of a percutaneous guide pin for minimal incision hip screw insertion. **C,** After reaming and placement of the lag screw through a small (4 cm) incision, the two-hole plate can be inserted and attached by mobilizing the skin and soft tissues. **D,** Final incision for a three-hole plate. **E,** Fluoroscopic view showing the final reduction and plate position.

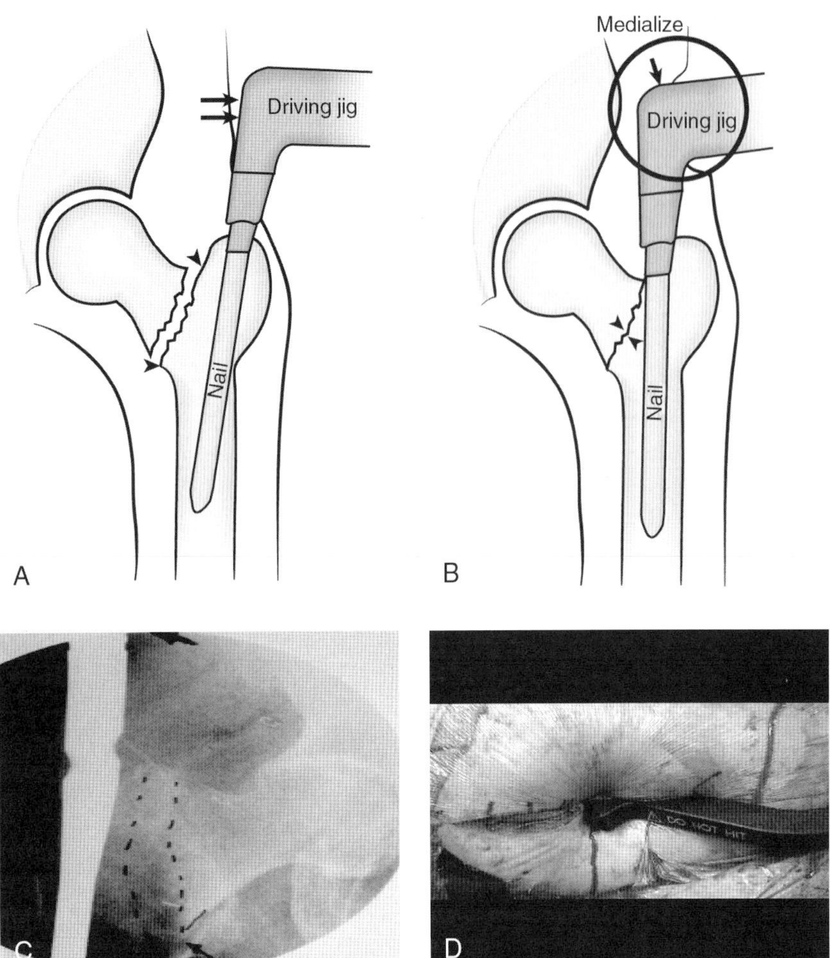

Figure 8 Illustration showing a potential complication that may occur during intramedullary nail placement in patients with large hips. **A,** A small incision in the hip allows only the nail to go through the skin and subcutaneous tissue. In patients with large hips, this causes the soft tissue to resist the medial positioning of the insertion driving handle. This lateral force is indicated by the two arrows. That resistance forces the nail laterally and can create a distraction force at the intertrochanteric fracture site resulting in a gap (*arrowheads*). **B,** To prevent this complication, a larger skin incision has been made in the hip, and the subcutaneous tissue is divided. This larger incision allows the driving handle to move through and past the skin level, to go more medially, and prevents lateral pressure against the intertrochanteric region. The distraction force at the fracture site is relaxed. Note that the gap has been closed at the intertrochanteric fracture site (*arrowheads*). Lateral distraction is caused by impingement of soft tissues on the driving handle and can be prevented by making an adequate incision. **C,** Fluoroscopic image showing lateral distraction of the fracture site. **D,** Clinical photograph showing the insertion handle in the soft tissues.

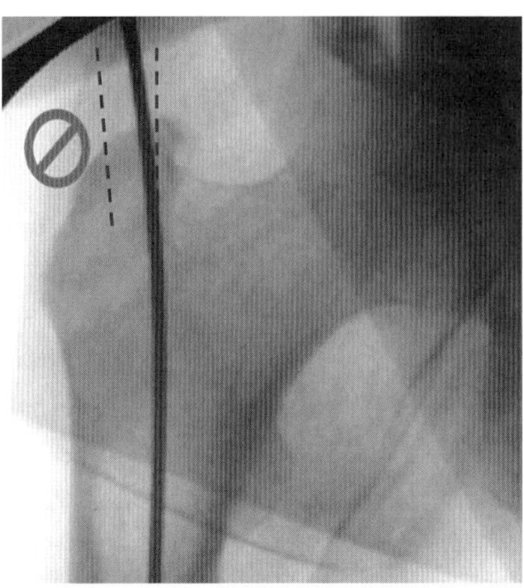

Figure 9 An excessively lateral starting point, which will result in varus, should be avoided. This fluoroscopic view shows a guidewire in good position. Dashed lines indicate the correct entry window. The circle with a bar indicates a starting zone that is too far lateral.

ment (Figure 9). Adequate reduction of the fracture before fixation is essential; the device will not correct malreduction. Some techniques to achieve reduction include percutaneous placement of ball-tipped spikes or Schanz pins used as a joystick. Temporary Kirschner wire stabilization of the fragments in reduced position may be helpful. In some very unstable fractures, temporarily pinning the proximal fragment to the acetabulum with transarticular smooth pins may be necessary (Figure 10). Care should be taken to keep all joysticks or temporary fixation out of the path of the definitive fixation hardware.

Hip screws, whether connected to the shaft by means of a plate or an intramedullary nail, have the common complication of screw cutout of the head and subsequent loss of fixation and joint destruction (Figure 11). The risk of this complication is reduced by correct screw placement in the head, which is central and deep in both AP and lateral radiographic views. This position is described by the tip-to-apex distance.[33] The sum of the measured distances from the tip of the screw to the apex of the femoral head on both views should be less than 2 cm.

Summary

Hip fractures, which can occur in patients of any age, are common and have a significant economic and per-

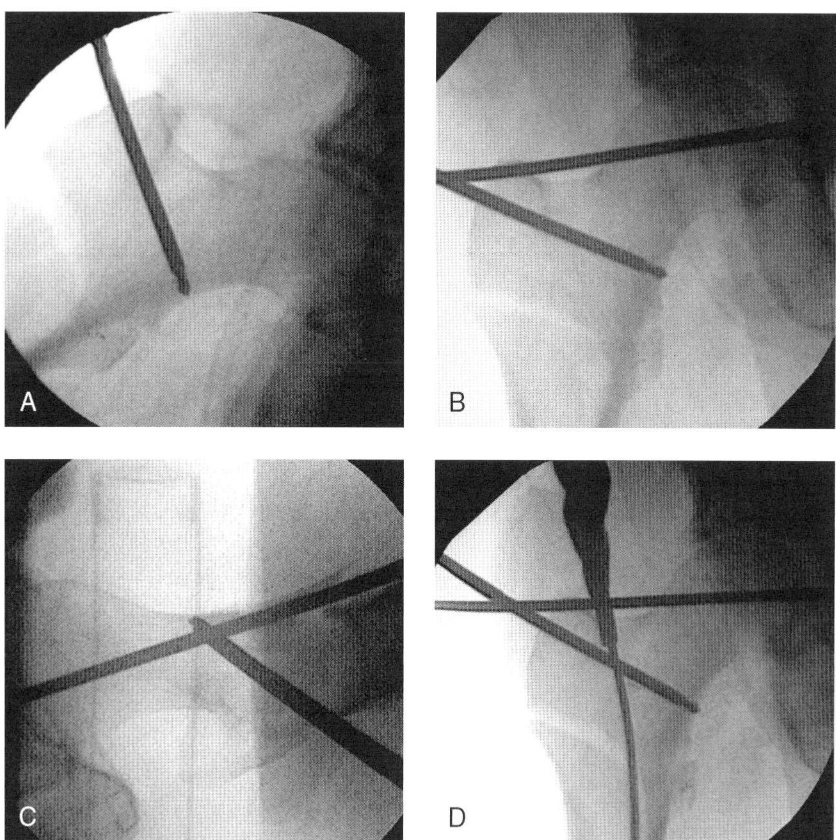

Figure 10 **A,** A very unstable proximal fragment is controlled with a Schanz pin as a joystick. After using the joystick for reduction, the proximal fragment is pinned to the acetabulum with a smooth pin placed out of the way of definitive intramedullary fixation. AP **(B)** and lateral **(C)** fluoroscopic views of the short proximal fragment pinned to the pelvis. **D,** The guidewire and reamer are passed with the temporary stabilization in place.

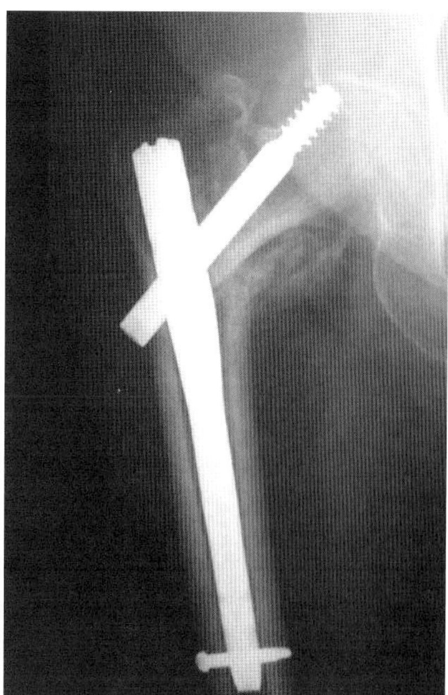

Figure 11 Lag screw cutout is prevented by placing the screw central and deep, as indicated by a cumulative tip-apex distance of less than 2.5 cm.

sonal impact on the patient. Treatment is based on the type of fracture, the location of the fracture, and the patient's age and medical comorbidities. Nondisplaced or impacted fractures of the femoral neck can be treated with screw fixation, and displaced femoral neck fractures can be treated with reduction and fixation or with hip arthroplasty. Intertrochanteric fractures are treated with reduction and fixation. To ensure the best outcomes for patients, various techniques and aids should be used, including proper patient positioning, choosing the correct starting point for nail insertion, and achieving acceptable reduction before fixation.

References

1. National Center for Injury Prevention and Control Website. Available at: http://www.cdc.gov/ncipc/factsheets/falls.htm. Accessed November 2006.
2. Riggs BL, Melton L: The worldwide problem of osteoporosis: Insights afforded by epidemiology. *Bone* 1995; 17:505S-511S.
3. Chapuy MC, Arlot ME, Duboeuf F, et al: Vitamin D_3 and calcium to prevent hip fractures in the elderly women. *N Engl J Med* 1992;327:1637-1642.
4. Tinetti ME, Baker DI, McAvay G, et al: A multifactorial intervention to reduce the risk of falling among elderly people living in the community. *N Engl J Med* 1994;331:821-827.
5. Kannus P, Parkkari J, Niemi S, et al: Prevention of hip fracture in elderly people with use of a hip protector. *N Engl J Med* 2000;343:1506-1513.
6. How to reduce your risks of falling. American Academy of Orthopaedic Surgeons Website. Available at: http://orthoinfo.aaos.org/fact/thr_report.cfm?thread_id=78&topcategory=Injury%20Prevention. Accessed June 13, 2007.
7. Damany DS, Parker MJ, Chojnowski A: Complications after intracapsular hip fractures in young adults: A meta-analysis of 18 published studies involving 564 fractures. *Injury* 2005;36: 131-141.
8. Siegmeth AW, Guruswamy K, Parker MJ: Delay to surgery prolongs hospital stay in patients with fractures of the proximal femur. *J Bone Joint Surg Br* 2005;87:1123-1126.
9. Moran CG, Wenn RT, Sikand M, Taylor AM: Early mortality after hip fracture: Is delay before surgery im-

portant? *J Bone Joint Surg Am* 2005;87: 483-489.

10. Swiantkowski MF, Harrington RM, Kella TS, Van Patten PK: Torsion and bending analysis of internal fixation techniques for femoral neck fractures: The role of implant design and bone density. *J Orthop Res* 1987;3:433-444.
11. Masson M, Parker MJ, Fleischer S: Internal fixation versus arthroplasty for intracapsular proximal femoral fractures in adults. *Cochrane Database Syst Rev* 2003;2:CD001708.
12. Bhandari M, Devereaux PJ, Swiontkowski MF, et al: Internal fixation compared with arthroplasty for displaced fractures of the femoral neck: A meta-analysis. *J Bone Joint Surg Am* 2003;85-A:1673-1681.
13. Iorio R, Healy WL, Lemos DW, Appleby D, Lucchesi CA, Saleh KJ: Displaced femoral neck fractures in the elderly: Outcomes and cost effectiveness. *Clin Orthop Relat Res* 2001;383: 229-242.
14. Healy WL, Iorio R: Total hip arthroplasty: Optimal treatment for displaced femoral neck fractures in elderly patients. *Clin Orthop Relat Res* 2004;429:43-48.
15. Baker RP, Squires B, Gargan MF, Bannista GC: Total hip arthroplasty and hemiarthroplasty in mobile, independent patients with a displaced intracapsular fracture of the femoral neck: A randomized controlled trial. *J Bone Joint Surg Am* 2006;88:2583-2589.
16. Lee BP, Berry DJ, Harmsen WS, Sim FH: Total hip arthroplasty for the treatment of an acute fracture of the femoral neck: Long-term results. *J Bone Joint Surg Am* 1998;80:70-75.
17. Calder SJ, Anderson GH, Jagger C, Harper WM, Gregg PJ: Unipolar or bipolar prosthesis for displaced intracapsular hip fracture in octogenarians: A randomized prospective study. *J Bone Joint Surg Br* 1996;78: 391-394.
18. Raia FJ, Chapman CB, Herrera MF, Schweppe MW, Michelson CB, Rosenwasser MP: Unipolar or bipolar hemiarthroplasty for femoral neck fractures in the elderly? *Clin Orthop Relat Res* 2003;414:259-265.
19. Wathne RA, Koval KJ, Aharenoff GB, Zuckerman JD, Jones DA: Modular unipolar versus bipolar prosthesis: A prospective evaluation of functional outcomes after femoral neck fracture. *J Orthop Trauma* 1995;9:298-302.
20. Cornell CN, Levine D, O'Doherty J, Lyden J: Unipolar versus bipolar hemiarthroplasty for the treatment of femoral neck fractures in the elderly. *Clin Orthop Relat Res* 1998;348:67-71.
21. Emery RJ, Broughton NS, Desai K, Bulstrode CJ, Thomas TL: Bipolar hemiarthroplasty for subcapital fracture of the femoral neck: A prospective randomized trial of cemented Thompson and uncemented Moore stems. *J Bone Joint Surg Br* 1991;73: 322-324.
22. Lo WH, Chen WM, Huang CK, Chen TH, Chiu FY, Chen CM: Bateman bipolar hemiarthroplasty for displaced intracapsular femoral neck fractures: Cemented versus uncemented. *Clin Orthop Relat Res* 1994; 302:75-82.
23. Khan RJK, MacDowell A, Crossman P, Keene GS: Cemented or uncemented hemiarthroplasty for displaced intracapsular fractures of the hip: A systematic review. *Injury* 2002; 33:13-17.
24. Parker MJ, Gurusamy K: Arthroplasties (with and without bone cement) for proximal femoral fractures in adults. *Cochrane Database Syst Rev* 2004;2:CD001706.
25. Parker MJ, Pervez H: Surgical approaches for inserting hemiarthroplasty of the hip. *Cochrane Database Syst Rev* 2002;3:CD001707.
26. O'Hara DA, Duff A, Berlin JA, et al: The effect of anesthetic technique on postoperative outcomes in hip fracture repair. *Anesthesiology* 2000;92: 947-957.
27. Felsenthal G, Magaziner J: Spinal anesthesia versus general anesthesia for hip fracture repair: A longitudinal observation of 741 elderly patients during 2-year follow-up. *Am J Orthop* 2000;29:25-35.
28. Utrilla AL, Reig JS, Munoz FM, Tufanisco CB: Trochanteric gamma nail and compression hip screw for trochanteric fractures: A randomized, prospective, comparative study in 210 elderly patients with a new design of the gamma nail. *J Orthop Trauma* 2005;19:229-233.
29. Pajarinen J, Lindahl J, Michelsson O, Savolainen V, Hirvensalo E: Pertrochanteric femoral fractures treated with a dynamic hip screw or a proximal femoral nail: A randomized study comparing post-operative rehabilitation. *J Bone Joint Surg Br* 2005;87: 76-81.
30. Parker MJ, Handoll H: Gamma and other cephalocondylic intramedullary nails versus extramedullary implants for extracapsular hip fractures in adults. *Cochrane Database Syst Rev* 2005;4:CD000093.
31. Templeman D, Baumgaertner MR, Leighton RK, Lindsey RW, Moed BR: Reducing complications in the surgical treatment of intertrochanteric fractures. *Instr Course Lect* 2005; 54:409-415.
32. Sadowski C, Lubbeke A, Saudan M, Riand N, Stern R, Hoffmeyer P: Treatment of reverse oblique and transverse intertrochanteric fractures with use of an intramedullary nail or a 95 degrees screw-plate: A prospective, randomized study. *J Bone Joint Surg Am* 2002;84-A:372-381.
33. Baumgaertner MR, Solberg BD: Awareness of tip-apex distance reduces failure of fixation of trochanteric fractures of the hip. *J Bone Joint Surg Br* 1997;79:969-971.

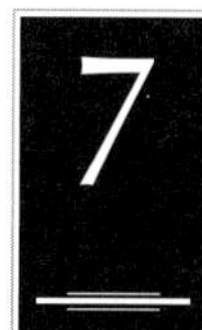

Improving Outcomes After Pertrochanteric Hip Fractures

Madhav Karunakar, MD
Toni M. McLaurin, MD
Steven J. Morgan, MD
*Kenneth A. Egol, MD

Abstract

Complex pertrochanteric fractures, such as those with reverse obliquity and subtrochanteric extension, represent a subset of hip fractures that sometimes is difficult to treat. Critical assessment of the available literature and a review of treatment indications, implant recommendations, and technical pitfalls will provide insight to physicians to enable better care of patients with these complex injuries.

Surgical stabilization of hip fractures in geriatric patients continues to be the standard of care. Surgical repair allows early mobilization, limits the period of recumbency, and allows patients to return more rapidly to functional activity. Nonsurgical management of hip fractures in geriatric patients has been associated with high rates of medical morbidity and mortality and usually is reserved for patients with medical conditions that preclude surgical treatment. Mobilizing elderly patients after fracture fixation aids in preventing the complications of prolonged recumbency, such as decubiti, urinary tract infections, atelectasis and respiratory infections, venous thromboembolism (VTE), and pulmonary embolism (PE).

Nonsurgical treatment is associated with increased rates of mortality at 6 months and 1 year after fracture, and in those who survive, there is a significant loss of functional status and ambulatory ability.[1] Although there is clear evidence that most pertrochanteric hip fractures should be stabilized surgically, the influence of age, sex, medical comorbidities, mental status, and the preinjury level of function on postoperative function, complication rates, and patient mortality remains unclear.

Timing of Surgery

Once surgical treatment is chosen for a geriatric patient with a hip fracture, it should be performed as soon as possible. Many studies have shown an association between a surgical delay of more than 24 to 48 hours and a higher 1-year mortality rate.[2-7] However, there is an important balance between the optimization of medical issues and expeditious surgical management. Table 1 summarizes the existing literature regarding the timing of hip fracture fixation.[2,5-11] In general, hip fracture surgery should be done as soon as possible after the stabilization of all comorbid medical conditions, especially cardiopulmonary problems and fluid and electrolyte imbalances.

Medical Evaluation

Although advanced age itself is not an independent risk factor for complications after surgery, older patients tend to have more coexisting medical conditions that affect surgical risks. Many elderly patients have pulmonary, renal, cardiovascular, or

**Kenneth A. Egol, MD or the department with which he is affiliated has received research or institutional support from Stryker, Synthes, and Biomet.*

Table 1
Summary of Literature Regarding Timing of Hip Fracture Fixation

Study Authors (Year)	Number of Patients	Time to Surgical Repair	Findings
Kenzora et al[8] (1984)	399	96 patients operated on < 24 hours	One-year mortality rate of 34%, which was significantly higher than that reported in patients operated on 2 to 5 days after injury
Zuckerman et al[2] (1995)	367	> 48 hours	Mortality nearly doubles compared with those operated on within 2 hospital days (hazard ratio of 1.76)
Hamlet et al[6] (1997)	168	> 24 hours	Three-year mortality rate of 50%, compared with 20% rate for patients operated on within 24 hours
Doruk et al[9] (2004)	65	> 5 days	Late cohort had longer hospital stay, longer time to functional recovery, lower activities of daily living scores at 6 months postoperatively, and higher mortality at 1 year
Orosz et al[5] (2004)	1,206	> 24 hours	Cohort had significantly less pain, shorter hospital stay, and lower incidence of postoperative complications; no difference in function or 6-month mortality rate
Gdalevich et al[10] (2004)	651	> 48 hours	One-year mortality rate of 25.7%, compared with a rate of 14.1% for patients operated on within 48 hours
McGuire et al[7] (2004)	18,209	> 48 hours	Delayed surgery led to a 17% higher chance of mortality by postoperative day 30
Moran et al[11] (2005)	2,660	> 4 days	Increased risk of mortality at 90 days and 1 year, compared with those operated on within 4 days (hazard ratios of 2.25 and 2.4, respectively)

neurologic disorders concurrent with the normal aging process and may be taking multiple medications for these conditions. Good perioperative care is important. The anesthesiologist frequently assumes care for chronically ill patients who have recently experienced an acute traumatic episode with associated pain, anemia, and hypovolemia. The American Society of Anesthesiologists classification, which is a measure of a patient's acute medical condition at the time of surgery, is predictive of increased mortality risk after hip fracture surgery. American Society of Anesthesiologists class III and class IV patients have a significantly increased risk of death after hip fracture.[12]

Cardiac Conditions

In one study, congestive heart failure, angina, and chronic pulmonary disease were all found to be independent risk factors for mortality at 30 days after injury.[13] Sixty-three percent of inpatient mortalities were attributable to cardiovascular events. The American College of Cardiology and the American Heart Association have developed guidelines for patients undergoing noncardiac surgery, including orthopaedic procedures. Perioperative stress testing is indicated for patients with unstable cardiac conditions and those with either new-onset angina or a change in the anginal pattern. A preoperative echocardiogram is recommended for patients with a history of angina pectoris and any condition in which there is a known decrease in left ventricular function. The more extensive work-up potentially required for older patients with hip fractures and known cardiac disease will provide the anesthesiologist with important physiologic information. Postoperative cardiac complications are the most common medical complications after hip fracture repair.

Pulmonary Conditions

Important factors in determining the risk of postoperative pulmonary complications include a history of smoking, a history of chronic obstructive pulmonary disease, and low oxygen levels on arterial blood gas analysis. The value of routine preoperative pulmonary function testing in pulmonary risk assessment remains controversial. Smetana[14] reviewed the importance of preoperative pulmonary function testing and found that most studies in the medical literature suggested that a forced expiratory volume (FEV_1) or forced vital capacity (FVC) of less than 70% of the predictive value and an FEV_1/FVC ratio of less than 65% are associated with an increased risk of postoperative pulmonary complications.[14] Elderly hip fracture patients are at high risk for postoperative pulmonary complications; efforts to minimize these complications, such as early mobilization, pulmonary toilet, and prevention of VTE, are essential.

Diabetes

Diabetes mellitus is a frequent comorbidity in elderly patients. Oral

Table 2
Summary of Literature Regarding Type of Anesthesia for Hip Fracture Patients

Study Authors (Year)	Number of Patients	Type of Anesthesia	Findings
Koval et al[18] (1998)	631	354 general; 277 regional	No difference in length of hospital stay, recovery of ambulatory ability, or percentage of functional recovery at 3, 6, and 12 months
Gilbert et al[19] (2000)	741	311 general; 430 regional	No difference in mortality rate at 2 years or incidence of postoperative complications; general anesthesia group had slightly better ambulatory function at the 2-year time point
Urwin et al[20] (2000)	Meta-analysis of 15 studies (2,162 patients)	General versus regional	Lower 30-day mortality rate and lower incidence of DVT with regional anesthesia
Parker et al[17] (2004)	Meta-analysis of 22 studies (2,567 patients)	General versus regional	Regional anesthesia associated with lower incidence of DVT and a lower 30-day mortality rate compared with general anesthesia; no difference in mortality rates at 90 days postoperatively

DVT = deep vein thrombosis

hypoglycemic agents usually are stopped the morning of surgery. Serum glucose levels are checked every 4 to 6 hours, and sliding-scale, low-dose regular insulin is given to blunt severe hyperglycemia. Intravenous fluids should not contain glucose. Oral hypoglycemic agents are resumed when the patient is eating well. For patients who require insulin, a general rule is to give one third to one half of the usual dose of long-acting insulin the morning of surgery, with an intravenous drip containing dextrose. A sliding scale of insulin coverage also is required.

Anemia

Elderly patients frequently are anemic because of coexisting medical conditions or bleeding at the fracture site. A reasonable rule is that otherwise healthy elderly people can tolerate a hemoglobin as low as 8.0, whereas those with cardiac or pulmonary disease should maintain a hemoglobin above 9 or 10. Allogeneic blood transfusion should be used judiciously because of the risk of disease transmission. Koval and associates[15] reported a prospective study of 687 community-dwelling, ambulatory, surgically treated geriatric patients with hip fractures. The authors found that allogeneic red blood cell transfusion was associated with an increased incidence of postoperative infection. No studies have defined an acceptable hematocrit level before surgery; the accepted preoperative hemoglobin level should be based on the expected blood loss.[16]

Type of Anesthesia

Although many physicians believe that spinal anesthesia is safer for patients, this has not been proven in the literature. Currently, no consensus exists as to which method of anesthesia is superior in hip fracture surgery[17-20] (Table 2). The choice of anesthesia typically is based on the preference of the anesthesiologist and the patient's medical status and preference. Induction is a crucial time during administration of general anesthesia. Slower circulation may result in overdose, low intravascular volume can lead to hypotension, and cardiac disease can present as ischemic electrocardiogram changes or arrhythmias. Factors especially important in managing geriatric patients with hip fractures undergoing general anesthesia include decreasing the dose of induction agents and having vasopressors on hand in the event of hypotension. Recent evidence suggests that for hip fracture surgery, general anesthesia with controlled hypotension may reduce intraoperative blood loss.[21]

In a Cochrane review of 22 trials involving 2,567 geriatric patients with hip fractures, Parker and associates[17] pooled data from eight trials to compare outcomes after general and regional anesthesia. They found that regional anesthesia was associated with a mild reduction in the incidence of deep vein thrombosis (DVT) and a lower mortality rate at 1 month after surgery; however, there was no significant difference in 3-month mortality rates between the two anesthesia methods. The authors concluded that, based on the available data, there was insufficient evidence to determine the superiority of general or regional anesthesia.

Local anesthesia techniques, such as lateral femoral cutaneous nerve blocks, may have a limited role in the treatment of femoral neck fractures, but there appears to be no role for this modality in pertrochanteric hip fractures.

Table 3
Summary of Literature Regarding VTE Prophylaxis

Study Authors (Year)	Number of Patients	VTE Prophylaxis Agent Studied	Findings
Pulmonary Embolism Prevention Trial Collaborative Group[24] (2000)	13,356	Aspirin versus placebo	Aspirin significantly reduced incidence of symptomatic DVT by 30% and PE by 43%, compared with placebo
Turpie et al[25] (2002)	7,344	Fondaparinux (factor Xa inhibitor) versus enoxaparin (LMWH)	Fondaparinux significantly reduced the incidence of DVT (6.8%), compared with enoxaparin (13.7%), by postoperative day 11
Handoll et al[23] (2002)	Cochrane review of 31 clinical trials	Unfractionated heparin, LMWH, and mechanical prophylaxis	Heparins provided significant protection against DVT; insufficient evidence to confirm protection against PE; mechanical prophylaxis protective, but compliance is problematic
Ennis et al[22] (2003)	1,000	Aspirin versus LMWH (enoxaparin)	Aspirin group had three cases of DVT and one PE, enoxaparin group had two cases of DVT and no PE; slight increase in risk of postoperative bleeding complications with enoxaparin
Eriksson et al[26] (2003)	656	Fondaparinux for 6 to 8 days versus fondaparinux for 1 month postoperatively	Extension of prophylaxis reduced incidence of DVT from 35% to 1.4%

VTE = venous thromboembolism, DVT = deep vein thrombosis, PE = pulmonary embolism, LMWH = low-molecular-weight heparin.

VTE Prophylaxis

Patients with lower extremity fractures, including pertrochanteric hip fractures, are at increased risk for thrombophlebitis. The reported incidence of DVT after hip fracture is 36% to 60%, whereas thrombi involving the proximal venous system have been reported in up to 36%.[22] According to the available literature, the incidence of PE after hip fracture ranges between 4.3% and 24%, while the incidence of fatal PE ranges from 3.6% to 12.9%[22-26] (Table 3). Thrombi limited to the calf veins rarely are associated with PE. Popliteal and more proximal venous thrombi carry a much higher embolic risk; however, most above-knee deep vein thrombi represent extension of thrombi from the calf venous system.

The two basic forms of prophylaxis are chemical and mechanical. In a Cochrane review of different methods of thromboprophylaxis after hip fracture surgery, Handoll and associates[23] compiled data from 31 clinical trials covering 2,958 cases. Based on the pooled data, the authors found that unfractionated and low-molecular-weight heparin protected against the development of lower extremity venous thrombosis, but there was insufficient evidence to confirm a protective effect against the development of PE. Mechanical methods of prophylaxis with foot or calf pumps provide significant protection against the development of DVT and PE and reduce overall mortality, but compliance remains an issue.[23] Although different prophylaxis techniques are effective in preventing thrombotic complications after hip fracture surgery, data are insufficient in the orthopaedic literature to form a consensus protocol with regard to prophylaxis.

Inferior vena cava filters offer the advantage of preventing PE in hip fracture patients when anticoagulation or compression devices are contraindicated or when the patients are at elevated risk despite prophylaxis. Filters may prevent PE when DVT is already present and prevent further emboli in patients who have PE despite anticoagulation therapy. Recently, retrievable filters have been developed to minimize the complications that occur with permanent indwelling inferior vena cava filters.

Pain Issues

Elderly patients, especially cognitively impaired elderly patients, usually receive substantially less pain medication than younger adults.[27] Many elderly patients have medical comorbidities that may influence the choice and dosage of selected analgesics. Drug interactions and potential complications must be considered when choosing an analgesic. In general, elderly patients receive greater peak dosing and have longer duration of action than younger patients because of slower clearance. Elderly patients with hip fractures should be started at lower doses than younger patients and titrated up slowly, based on pain reduction ratings.

Multidisciplinary Approach

The surgical treatment of fractures in elderly patients often is successful; however, the patients are unable to achieve their preinjury level of function. In the mid-1990s, the American Orthopaedic Association developed a task force to serve elderly orthopaedic patients. This task force developed several recommendations, including the use of a collaborative approach.[28]

Collaborative practice, or the multidisciplinary approach, involves the coordination of multiple services within an institution to manage certain nonsurgical patient care issues that can affect outcome. Historically, these programs have begun after surgery, but there is now an initiative to implement these programs as soon as the patient is admitted to the hospital. These programs involve orthopaedic surgeons, geriatricians, physiatrists, therapists, pharmacists, nutritionists, pain specialists, and nurses, with each acting on specific issues to reduce comorbidities and complications in the perioperative period. Reducing potential complications benefits patients, physicians, and hospitals with improved functional outcomes, decreased costs per admission, reduced lengths of hospital stays, and appropriate discharges.

Classification and Fracture Stability

The most commonly used classification systems for intertrochanteric hip fractures are based on fracture stability. The integrity of the posteromedial cortex is a key component for assessing fracture stability in all classifications. Greater involvement of the posteromedial cortex results in a more unstable fracture. The reverse oblique fracture is an inherently unstable pertrochanteric fracture pattern because of the tendency of the adductors to medially displace the femoral shaft. The unstable fracture patterns in the AO/Orthopaedic Trauma Association (OTA) classification (A2.2-A3.3) also are characterized by increasing comminution in the posteromedial cortex and intertrochanteric region (Figure 1). This classification also recognizes the instability of the reverse oblique and transverse intertrochanteric fracture patterns.[29]

Recently, the concept of the lateral femoral wall, defined anatomically as the lateral femoral cortex distal to the vastus ridge, has received more recognition as a factor in determining fracture stability. Gotfried[30] described this concept in a report on 24 patients who required reoperation after failure of fixation of intertrochanteric fractures treated with a sliding hip screw. He concluded that a fracture of the lateral femoral wall resulted in sliding hip screw failures, and that in some patients the fracture occurred during the surgical procedure. Many intraoperative fractures of the lateral wall occur when a large-diameter hole is drilled into the lateral femoral wall for insertion of the sliding hip screw.[31] In a study of 214 patients with intertrochanteric anterior fractures reported by Palm and associates,[32] a lateral wall fracture occurred in one third of AO/OTA type 31-A.2.2 and A2.3 fractures, which are characterized by trochanteric comminution and a thinner lateral cortex, making them more susceptible to lateral wall fractures. The intraoperative fracture of the lateral femoral wall created in these fracture patterns is similar to a reverse oblique or transverse intertrochanteric fracture (AO/OTA A3.1-3.3). The authors concluded that, if the lateral wall or greater trochanter is fractured, a sliding hip screw alone should not be used for fracture fixation.

In the most simplistic terms, intertrochanteric fractures may be classified as stable or unstable based on the integrity of the posteromedial cortex and the lateral wall.[33] The recognition of fracture stability is critical because it directs implant selection. Stable fractures have an intact posteromedial cortex and lateral wall and may be treated with a sliding hip screw, whereas unstable fracture patterns have comminution of the posteromedial cortex, greater trochanteric comminution with loss of the lateral buttress, or reverse and transverse intertrochanteric fracture extension and should not be treated with a sliding hip screw.

Implant Selection and Recommendations

Selection

Compression hip screws have long been considered the gold standard for the treatment of pertrochanteric fractures. The devices currently in use evolved from designs first introduced in the 1950s and have produced reliable results.[34] In stable fracture patterns, the hip screw acts as a lateral tension band; in unstable fractures, it allows the controlled collapse and impaction of the fracture fragments. This collapse shortens the lever arm acting on the implant, which decreases the bending moment, thus decreasing the risk of mechanical failure and screw cutout. Telescoping of a 135° sliding hip screw by 10 and 20 mm improves implant strength by 28% and 80%, respectively, because of the shortened lever arm. This allows the fracture to achieve a position of stability while maintaining a constant neck-shaft angle.[35]

Groups:
Femur, proximal trochanteric (31-A)
1. Pertrochanteric simple (31-A1)

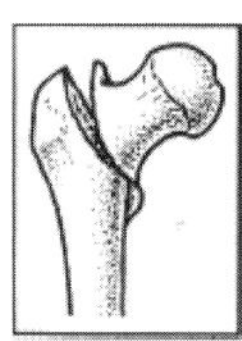

2. Pertrochanteric multifragmentary (31-A2)

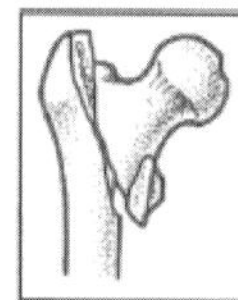

3. Intertrochanteric (31-A3)

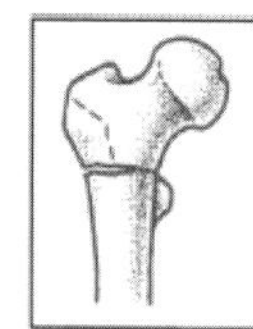

Subgroups and Qualifications:
Femur, proximal, pertrochanteric simple (31-A1; only 2 fragments)
1. Along intertrochanteric line (31-A1.1)

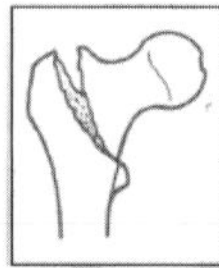

2. Through the greater trochanter (31-A1.2)
(1) nonimpacted
(2) impacted

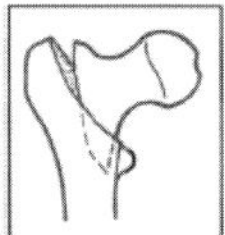

3. Below lesser trochanter (31-A1.3)
(1) high variety, medial fracture line at lower limit of lesser trochanter
(2) low variety, medial fracture line in diaphysis below lesser trochanter

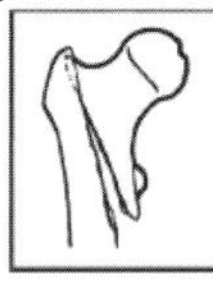

Femur, proximal, trochanteric fracture, pertrochanteric multifragmentary (always have posteromedial fragment with lesser trochanter and adjacent medial cortex; 31-A2)
1. With one intermediate fragment (31-A2.1)

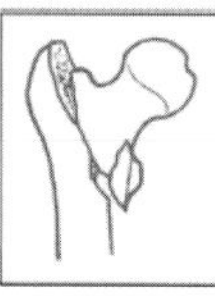

2. With several intermediate fragments (31-A2.2)

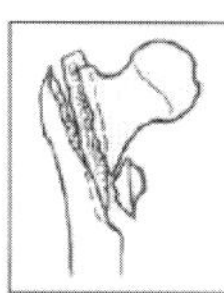

3. Extending more than 1 cm below lesser trochanter (31-A2.3)

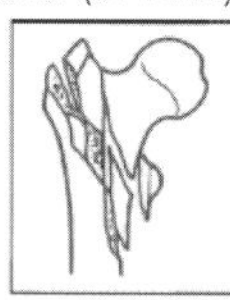

Femur, proximal, trochanteric area, intertrochanteric fracture (31-A3)
1. Simple oblique (31-A3.1)

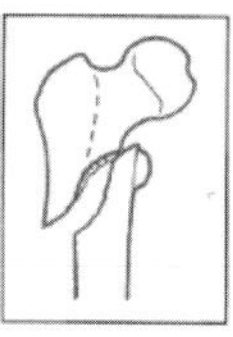

2. Simple transverse (31-A3.2)

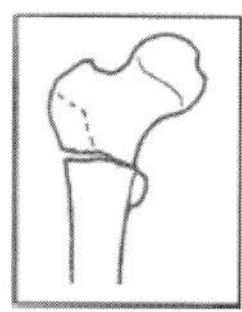

3. Multifragmentary (31-A3.3)
(1) extending to greater trochanter
(2) extending to neck

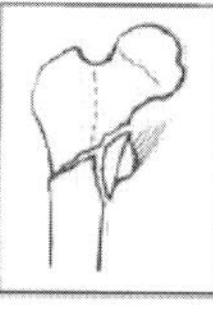

Figure 1 AO/OTA classification of trochanteric fractures. (Adapted with permission from Marsh JL, Slongo TF, Agel JN, et al: Fracture and Dislocation Classification Compendium 2007: Orthopaedic Trauma Association Classification Database and Outcomes Committee. *J Orthop Trauma* 2007;21(suppl 10):S1-S6.)

Reported failure rates of compression hip screws range from 6% to 56%, with screw cutout being the most common mode of failure.[34,36,37] The incidence of screw cutout increases with unstable fracture patterns and has been reported to be as high as 19%.[34] Other reported modes of failure include fatigue failure of the lag screw, implant disassembly, and, rarely, pullout or breakage of the side plate.[30,38] The characteristics of the implant that allow it to maintain implant stability despite loss of reduction because of sliding also contribute to fixation failure. Although sliding of the lag screw increases implant strength, sliding of more than 15 mm increases the rate of fixation failure[35] (Figure 2). Excessive sliding in unstable fractures can result in medialization of the femoral shaft. This can lead to a more stable configuration initially, but medialization of more than one third of the shaft diameter results in a sevenfold increase in fixation failure.[39] Recent studies have shown an association between fracture settling and pain, as well as an association between increased sliding and decreased postoperative mobility.[35,40]

These complications prompted attempts to improve on the compression hip screw, which led to in-

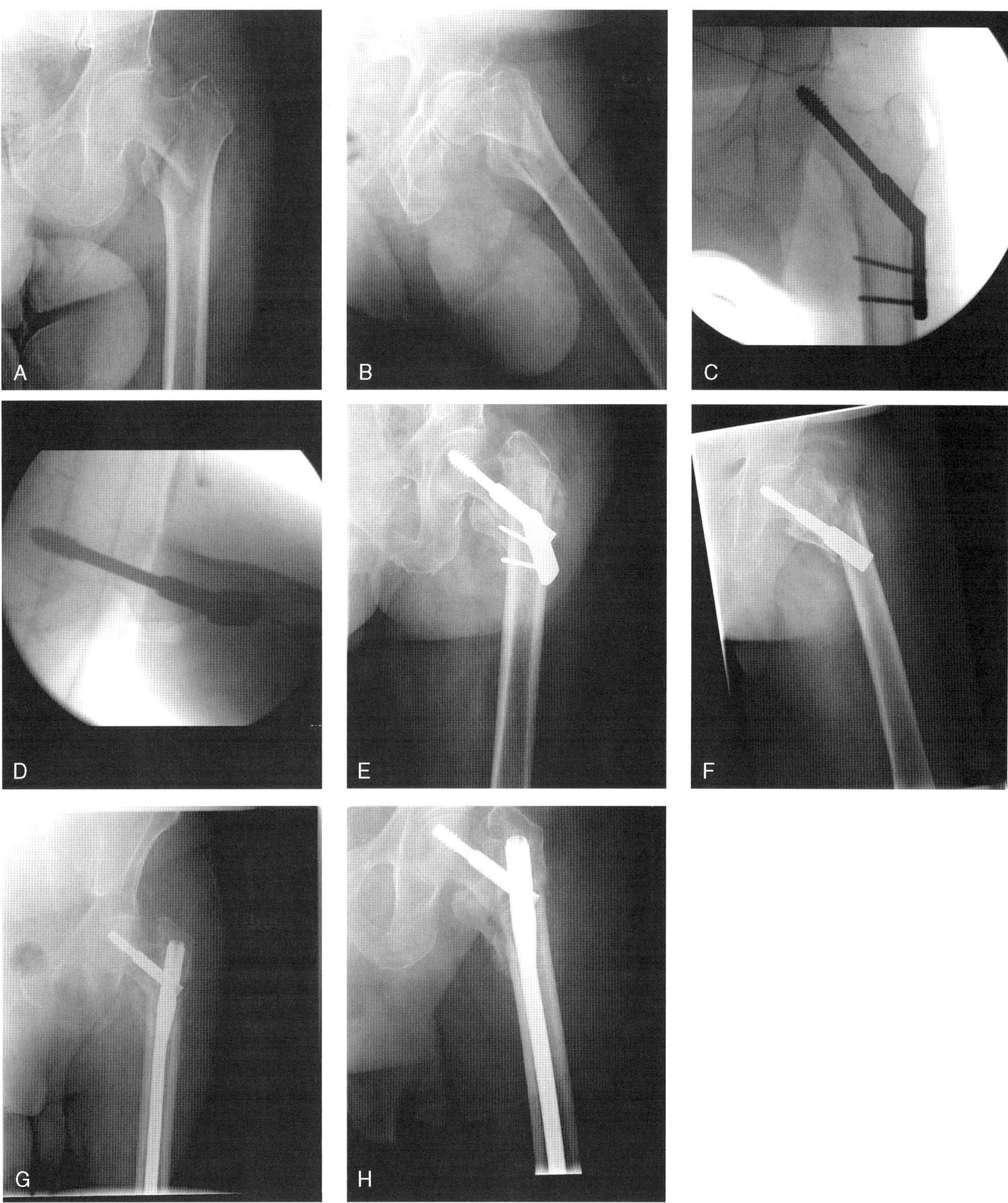

Figure 2 Radiographic views of a pertrochanteric fracture in an 82-year-old man. **A** and **B,** Traction AP and frog-leg lateral preoperative views, respectively, are shown. The fracture was believed to be stable, and the patient was treated with a screw and sideplate device; AP and lateral intraoperative views are shown in **C** and **D,** respectively. The patient reported increasing pain with ambulation, and at 6 weeks presented with implant failure. **E** and **F,** AP and lateral radiographs, respectively, showing implant failure and fracture displacement. The patient had a revision to a long intramedullary implant. **G,** AP view. **H**, Frog-leg lateral view.

creasing use of intramedullary hip screw devices. The intramedullary hip nail is an appealing design because it combines the advantages of intramedullary fixation with those of a sliding hip screw. The most obvious biomechanical advantage of an intramedullary nail over a sliding hip screw is that the nail is a load-sharing device rather than a load-bearing device. Another biomechanical advantage is the location of the nail closer to the hip center than the side plate of the sliding hip screw, which translates to a shorter lever arm with the nail, decreasing tensile strain on the implant.[33,34] This also results in a decreased bending moment on the lag screw, causing a reduction of bending stress and decreasing the rate of implant failure. In fracture patterns where excessive collapse may cause complications, the nail acts as an intramedullary buttress, allowing less collapse to a stable configuration because of the presence of the nail in the medullary canal.[33] None of these biomechanical advantages, however, have translated into clinical advantages.[33,34]

Suggested clinical advantages include shorter surgical time, decreased fluoroscopy time, a smaller incision resulting in decreased soft-tissue trauma, a closed insertion technique resulting in decreased blood loss and decreased transfusion requirements, and decreased intraoperative complications, leading to decreased mortality, improved ambulatory ability, and improved functional outcomes. Only in unstable fractures did Baumgaertner and associates[41] show a decrease in surgical time with intramedullary nails; other studies showed either no significant difference or increased surgical time with intramedullary nails.[33,34]

Some studies comparing intramedullary nails with compression hip screws have shown a higher intraoperative complication rate with nails, but these were based on earlier nail designs that had up to a 20% occurrence of intraoperative and postoperative femoral fractures.[34,41] Problems with early nail designs included long, large-diameter nails and large distal interlocking screws with no or inaccurate targeting; one of the most significant design flaws was a 10° valgus bend in the nail. This resulted in stress shielding of the medial calcar, with load transfer and concentration of the stress at the distal tip of the nail onto the lateral cortex, increasing the risk of femoral fracture at the tip of the nail. Newer nail designs have corrected these problems by decreasing the valgus bend to 4°, decreasing the nail diameter and length, and decreasing the size of the distal interlocking screws while improving the targeting devices.[34,35] Femoral fractures are still reported with the newer intramedullary nail designs, but at a much lower rate.[33] An additional complication of intramedullary nail fixation is cortical hypertrophy distally, which is associated with more frequent thigh pain.[33] However, as with the compression hip screw, the most common cause of failure remains lag screw cutout.[34,41]

Another common but less often reported complication with long intramedullary nails is the result of mismatching of the nail-femur radius of curvature. In general, most nail designs are straighter than the average human femur.[42] Care must be taken when implanting a long intramedullary nail for a pertrochanteric fracture because distal perforation can lead to a stress riser and the potential for peri-implant fracture.

Recommendations

Review of the literature to determine the best implant shows that many studies mix stable and unstable pertrochanteric fractures and use different definitions of unstable. For all fracture patterns, no clinical or functional benefits of the theorized biomechanical advantages of intramedullary nails have been shown.

For stable 31-AO/OTA type A1 pertrochanteric fractures, no studies have shown any improvement in clinical or functional outcomes with intramedullary nails compared with compression hip screws. Studies vary as to which implant is most advantageous regarding operating time, fluoroscopy time, and blood loss and transfusion requirements; however, all show no differences in mortality, ambulatory ability, return to preinjury level of function, need for assistive devices, or overall functional recovery. There are no findings to recommend intramedullary nails over compression hip screws in stable fractures.

The results of treatment of 31-A2 fractures can be difficult to sort out in the literature because they are combined with only A1 fractures in some studies and with A1 or A3 fractures in others. No studies have shown a significant difference in the rates of fixation failure when comparing the sliding hip screw with intramedullary nails in A2 fractures. The frequency and amount of pain are comparable with both implants, but the location of the pain changes, with lateral thigh and groin pain reported with compression hip screws and mid- to distal-thigh pain with intramedullary nails.[43] No significant differences have been proven in rates of functional recovery, return to preinjury level of function, and level of ambulatory independence achieved. Although better mobility scores in the early postoperative period have been reported with intramedullary nails, there was no difference in the total mobility score at 1 year. The ability to ambulate outside was significantly better at 6 and 12 months with intramedullary nails.[33] Hardy and associates[33] also found significant differences in the amount of lag screw sliding in A2 fractures, with compression hip screws showing more sliding than intramedullary nails. This sliding resulted in a significant difference in limb-length discrepancies between the two implants, although the functional significance of this finding was not well defined.[33] Long term, no-compensatory walking strategies have been shown to be used with a limb-length discrepancy of less than 20 mm. A limb-length discrepancy of less than 30 mm has little effect on overall hip biomechanics, so this may not actually contribute notably to mobility differences.[44] Therefore, for 31-A2 fractures, there is no clear indication for choosing intramedullary fixation over a compression hip screw.

Unstable 31-A3 pertrochanteric fractures include fractures with subtrochanteric extension and reverse oblique intertrochanteric fractures. Reverse oblique fractures have not only lost the medial buttress, but the fracture line is parallel to the direction of the lag screw sliding. These fractures represent the only pertrochanteric fracture pattern in which implant choice affects outcomes. Up to 56% loss of fixation has been reported with compression hip screws in the treatment of reverse obliquity fractures.[37] The location of the fracture line distal to the lag screw results in fewer points of fixation in the distal fragment. Sliding of the proximal fragment along the lag screw barrel then results in medialization of the distal fragment. This malalignment can lead to fracture distraction, resulting in nonunion. It also can result in failure of fixation with superior screw cutout.[37] The use of an intramedullary nail in this fracture pattern does not rely on the presence of an intact medial buttress nor does it allow medialization of the distal fragment because the nail itself acts as an intramedullary buttress. This is true not only for reverse oblique intertrochanteric fractures, but also for those with subtrochanteric extension. There is a paucity of literature evaluating treatment of 31-A3 fractures, but improved clinical outcomes are seen in A3 fractures treated with intramedullary nailing compared with compression hip screws.[45] However, no differences in functional outcomes have yet been shown.

No evidence in the literature confirms that using intramedullary devices leads to a decrease in intraoperative or postoperative complications or postoperative mortality, improved mobility, or improved patient and hip function outcomes compared with compression hip screws in A1 and A2 pertrochanteric fractures. It is significant that the primary mode of failure for both types of implants is screw cutout, which is based on screw position rather than the device used and is a function of tip-apex distance. Some authors have concluded that intramedullary nails are the better or preferred implant despite results that do not support this conclusion, and meta-analyses have concluded that the routine use of intramedullary nails for A1 and most A2 fractures is neither indicated nor evidence based.[39,46] In the treatment of A3 fractures, decreased complications and improved clinical outcomes have been reported with intramedullary nails, but there is still no evidence of significant functional differences.

Common Pitfalls

Recognition and avoidance of the common pitfalls associated with the treatment of pertrochanteric hip fractures are the best methods to prevent complications. A failure to recognize complicating underlying conditions, inappropriate decision making regarding implant selection, and failure to obtain an adequate reduction with correct placement of the implants account for most of the common complications associated with pertrochanteric fractures.

Initial evaluation of injury radiographs should focus on the fracture pattern and bone quality. A careful assessment for the presence of metastatic disease is mandatory because metastatic lesions are unlikely to heal and normal union may be compromised. Implant selection for patients with metastatic disease must be based on the ability of the implant to withstand long-term cyclical loading; the implant should splint the entire femur to bridge other potential areas of unrecognized or future metastatic disease. A long intramedullary implant that provides fixation into the femoral head and distal interlocking is best used in these patients. When metastatic disease extends into the femoral neck, internal fixation should be avoided, and hemiarthroplasty should be considered. If metastatic disease is extensive in the area of the medial calcar, a calcar-replacing prosthesis should be considered. In either case, a long-stem prosthesis should be used to splint the femur to the greatest possible extent.

In patients with significant osteoporosis, similar recommendations apply to implant selection. Using an

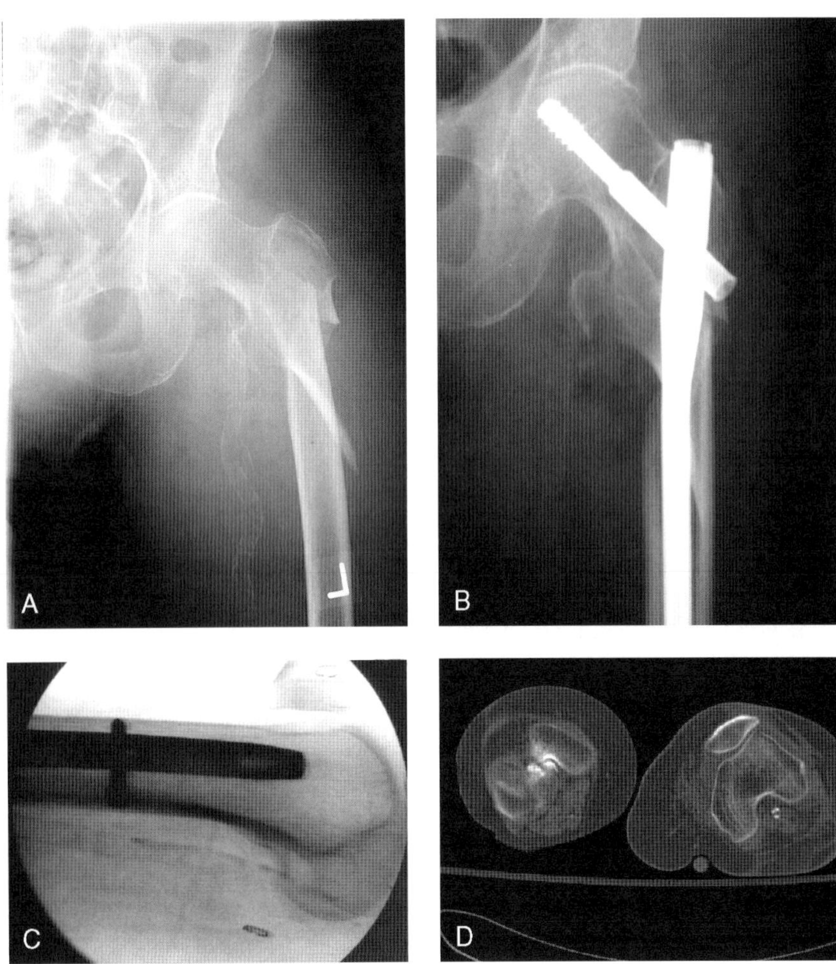

Figure 3 **A,** Preoperative AP radiograph of the proximal femur showing a comminuted intertrochanteric-subtrochanteric femoral fracture in a 90-year-old woman. **B**, Postoperative AP radiograph. **C,** Postoperative lateral radiograph of the distal shaft; a long intramedullary locked nail device is shown. **D,** Malrotation was noted clinically and confirmed with a postoperative CT scanogram.

intramedullary device with a compression hip screw for proximal fixation minimizes the risk of failure at the implant-bone interface distal to the fracture. In contrast, using a cephalomedullary nail-screw device may increase the chance of femoral head cutout because controlled collapse to a stable position is limited by the shaft of the intramedullary device, increasing the deforming varus force at the tip of the screw. Central placement of the screw in the femoral head is paramount to limiting failure. In some patients with significant bone loss from osteoporosis, augmentation of femoral head fixation with bone cement injected into the femoral head may limit cutout. Alternatively, proximal fixation devices focused on increasing implant surface area or minimizing bone loss during insertion have been developed to prevent femoral head cutout, but their effectiveness remains controversial.

Stable fracture patterns can be treated with any implant without undue risk of failure. Unstable fracture patterns are best treated with intramedullary fixation devices that limit fracture collapse and prevent limb-length discrepancy and subsequent abductor weakness. Reverse obliquity intertrochanteric fractures or subtrochanteric femoral fractures should be treated only with intramedullary devices to limit lateral displacement of the proximal fracture fragment that will cause failure of hip screw and side-plate devices. Alternatively, plate fixation with fixed-angle devices (blade plate, dynamic condylar screw, or locking plates) also can be used effectively and can adequately resist lateral displacement of the proximal fragment; however, the extended approach and blood loss with the primary implantation make this a second line option if intramedullary nail fixation is feasible. Regardless of the implant chosen, it is imperative that the proximal fixation be placed in the area of the subchondral bone in the center of the femoral head, as described by Baumgartner and associates.[47] Failure to limit the tip-apex distance to less than 25 mm is a strong predictor of failure at the implant-femoral head interface.

Nonanatomic reduction of pertrochanteric fractures can lead to deformity and delayed union or nonunion. The deforming forces acting at the level of the proximal femur commonly lead to varus, apex-posterior angulation or translation, and rotational malalignment. Although reduction on a fracture table can correct most of these complications, additional careful manipulation can further improve fracture reduction and avoid deformity.[48] Percutaneously placed clamps and ball spike pushers can help reduce posterior sag and translation. Alternatively, external devices can be used to reduce posterior displacement. In fractures with subtrochanteric ex-

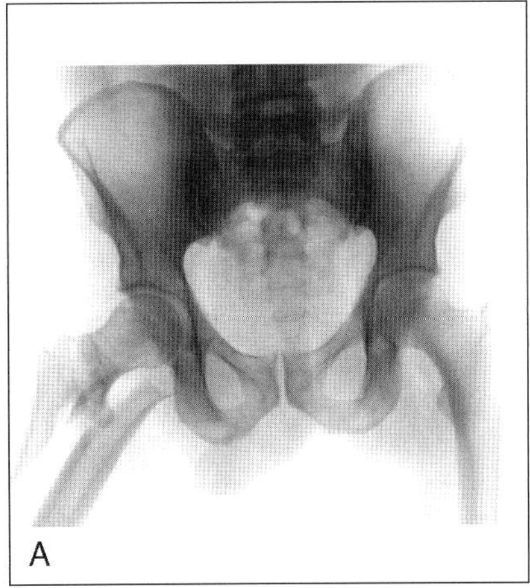

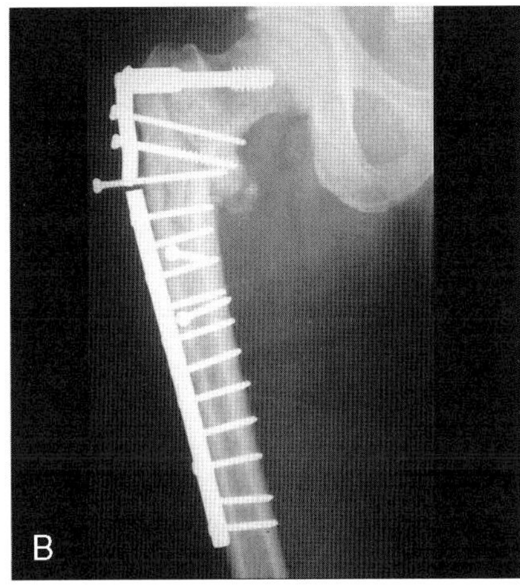

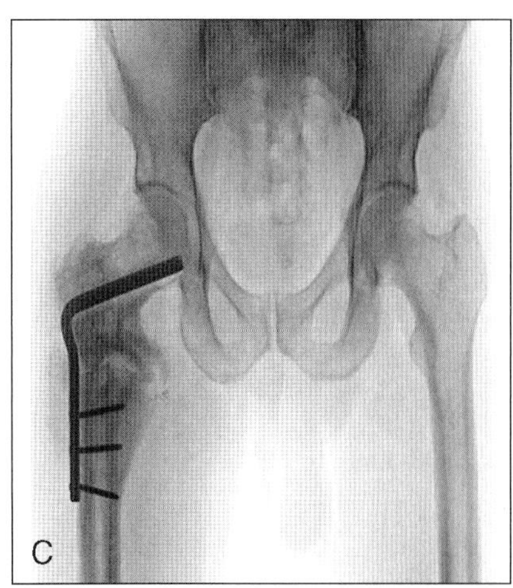

Figure 4 **A,** Radiograph of a right pertrochanteric hip fracture sustained by a 50-year-old man in a high-speed motor vehicle collision. **B,** At 6 months, the fracture was not united, and the hardware had failed. **C,** After hardware removal, the nonunion was repaired with a compression blade plate.

tension, care must be taken to avoid malrotation of the femur because reduction keys may be absent (Figure 3). When intramedullary devices are used, eccentric reaming of the lateral femoral cortex also should be avoided to prevent varus deformity.

Salvage After Treatment Failures

Identification of the reason for failure is paramount in selecting the best salvage option to avoid future failure while providing an acceptable functional result (Figure 4). The most common reasons for failed treatment of pertrochanteric femoral fractures are use of the wrong implant, poor implant placement, poor bone quality, limited biologic potential for healing, infection, and patient-related risk factors such as underlying systemic diseases or smoking. Other considerations include the viability of the proximal femoral bone segment, its related healing potential, and the functional demands of the patient. Salvage options consist of either revision of internal fixation or proximal femoral replacement with or without acetabular resurfacing.

Criteria for the revision of internal fixation are viability of the proximal bone segment and the femoral head as shown by bone scans or intraoperative assessment of bleeding potential, reasonable bone quality, no destruction of the femoral head articular surface, and a patient with high or moderate functional demands. For revision of failed internal fixation, the goal is to choose an implant that provides maximal stability and improves the mechanical environment of the fracture, principally with valgus osteotomy.[49] Blade plate fixation allows for planned correction and improvement of the deformity, and valgus osteotomies diminish the varus load at the site of nonunion and convert the tension into compression. Alternatively, locking plates and 95° dynamic condylar screw plates can improve the rigidity of the fixation but provide less correction of deformity or alteration of the mechanical forces at the nonunion site.[50] Bone grafting can be used to improve union when extensive medial soft-tissue stripping is required or for atrophic nonunion. Bone grafting for hypertrophic nonunion is not generally required.

When the criteria for the revision of internal fixation are not met, or when the patient has preexisting arthritis, advanced age, and low functional demands, proximal femoral replacement with or without acetabular resurfacing generally is the best reconstructive option in the absence of infection. When the medial calcar is destroyed or absent, a calcar-replacing prosthesis is required, with tension-band fixation of the greater trochanter to improve hip abductor function (Figure 5). Care must be taken to ensure that cement is not extruded from preexisting sites of internal fixation. Bone wax can be used to seal areas with a cortical defect to prevent cement extrusion. Acetabular resurfacing should be considered in patients with preexisting arthritis or when the articular surface has been destroyed by an extruded implant. In younger, higher-demand patients, recent reports suggest improved function with acetabular resurfacing as opposed to hemiarthroplasty alone.[51,52]

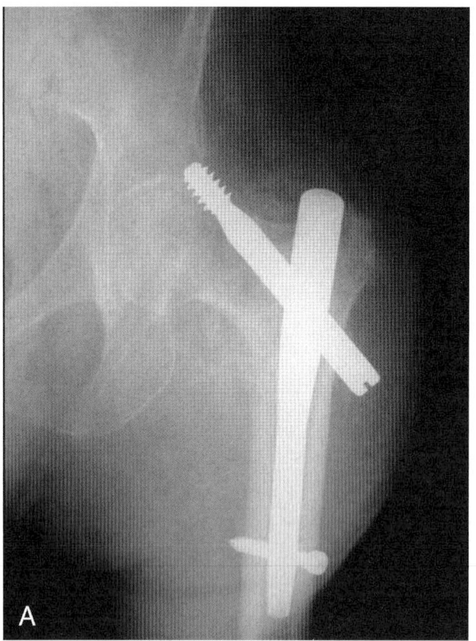

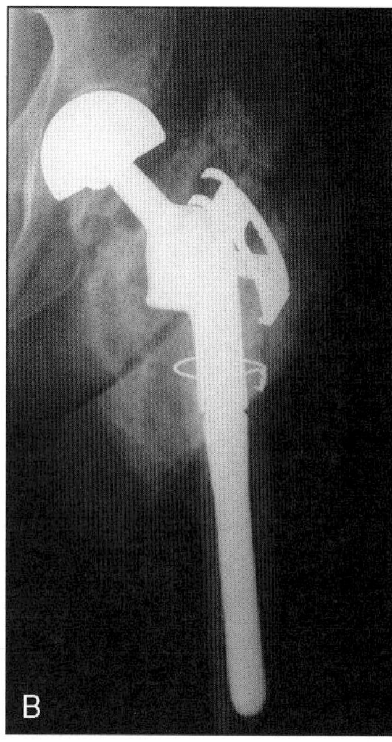

Figure 5 **A,** Radiograph of an unstable intertrochanteric hip fracture treated with a short intramedullary nail device in a 75-year-old woman. At 4 months, there was screw cutout and failure. **B,** Because of the bone quality and functional status of the patient, a calcar-replacing hemiarthroplasty was done.

Infection

Salvage in the presence of infection remains difficult. When analyzing initial treatment failure, infection should remain in the differential diagnosis as a root cause of treatment failure. When considering revision of internal fixation, preoperative laboratory analysis with a white blood cell count, erythrocyte sedimentation rate, and C-reactive protein level should be obtained as baseline tests. Positive values should be further investigated with an indium bone scan or joint aspiration. If salvage with arthroplasty is considered a treatment option, preoperative hip aspiration should be performed, and a staged reconstruction should be considered, with explantation of implanted hardware and culture testing being done first. If cultures are positive, the infection should be eradicated with débridement and antibiotic therapy with antibiotic-impregnated cement before arthroplasty. Revision internal fixation can proceed in the absence of gross purulence, but deep cultures should be obtained at the time of revision surgery. Positive cultures should initiate treatment with organism-specific antibiotics, and implants should be retained as long as they provide stability.

Summary

Improving outcomes in patients with pertrochanteric fractures involves maximizing the perioperative environment and understanding the fracture patterns and classification that ultimately guide treatment and it implant selection. The process begins with the identification of surgical candidates and medical optimization before surgery. It continues with the choice of anesthesia and thromboembolic prophylaxis, and culminates with proper implant selection and the prevention of postoperative complications. Strategies aimed at avoiding pitfalls minimize the potential for complications. Prompt recognition of complications allows salvage and recovery.

References

1. Ooi LH, Wong TH, Toh CL, Wong HP: Hip fractures in nonagenarioans: A study on operative and nonoperative management. *Injury* 2005;36:142-147.
2. Zuckerman JD, Skovron ML, Koval KJ, Aharonoff G, Frankel VH: Postoperative complications and mortality associated with operative delay in older patients who have a fracture of the hip. *J Bone Joint Surg Am* 1995;77:1551-1556.
3. Dorotka R, Schoechtner H, Buchinger W: The influence of immediate surgical treatment of proximal femoral fractures on mortality and quality of life: Operation within six hours of the fracture versus later than six hours. *J Bone Joint Surg Br* 2003;85:1107-1113.
4. Sexson SB, Lehner JT: Factors affecting hip fracture mortality. *J Orthop Trauma* 1987;1:298-305.
5. Orosz GM, Magaziner J, Hannan EL, et al: Association of timing of surgery for hip fracture and patient outcomes. *JAMA* 2004;291:1738-1743.
6. Hamlet WP, Lieberman JR, Freedman EL, Dorey FJ, Fletcher A, Johnson EE: Influence of health status and the timing of surgery on mortality in hip fracture patients. *Am J Orthop* 1997;26:621-627.
7. McGuire KJ, Bernstein J, Polsky D, Silber JH: Delays until surgery after hip fracture increases mortality. *Clin Orthop Relat Res* 2004;428:294-301.
8. Kenzora JE, McCarthy RE, Lowell JD, Sledge CB: Hip fracture mortality: Relation to age, treatment, preoperative illness, time of surgery, and complications. *Clin Orthop Relat Res* 1984;186:45-56.

9. Doruk H, Mas MR, Yildiz C, Sonmez A, Kýrdemir V: The effect of the timing of hip fracture surgery on the activity of daily living and mortality in elderly. *Arch Gerontol Geriatr* 2004;39: 179-185.

10. Gdalevich M, Cohen D, Yosef D, Tauber C: Morbidity and mortality after hip fracture: The impact of operative delay. *Arch Orthop Trauma Surg* 2004;124:334-340.

11. Moran CG, Wenn RT, Sikand M, Taylor AM: Early mortality after hip fracture: Is delay before surgery important? *J Bone Joint Surg Am* 2005;87: 483-489.

12. Richmond J, Aharonoff GB, Zuckerman JD, Koval KJ: Mortality risk after hip fracture. *J Orthop Trauma* 2003;17: 53-56.

13. Nettleman MD, Alsip J, Schrader M, Schulte M: Predictors of mortality after acute hip fracture. *J Gen Intern Med* 1996;11:765-767.

14. Smetana GW: Preoperative pulmonary assessment of the older adult. *Clin Geriatr Med* 2003;19:35-55.

15. Koval KJ, Rosenberg AD, Zuckerman JD, et al: Does blood transfusion increase the risk of infection after hip fracture? *J Orthop Trauma* 1997;11: 260-265.

16. Egol KA, Koval KJ, Zuckerman JD: Functional recovery following hip fracture in the elderly. *J Orthop Trauma* 1997;11:594-599.

17. Parker MJ, Handoll HH, Griffiths R: Anaesthesia for hip fracture surgery in adults. *Cochrane Database Syst Rev* 2004;4:CD000521.

18. Koval KJ, Aharonoff GB, Rosenberg AD, Bernstein RL, Zuckerman JD: Functional outcome after hip fracture: Effect of general versus regional anesthesia. *Clin Orthop Relat Res* 1998;348:37-41.

19. Gilbert TB, Hawkes WG, Hebel JR, et al: Spinal anesthesia versus general anesthesia for hip fracture repair: A longitudinal observation of 741 elderly patients during 2-year follow-up. *Am J Orthop* 2000;29:25-35.

20. Urwin SC, Parker MJ, Griffiths R: General versus regional anaesthesia for hip fracture surgery: A meta-analysis of randomized trials. *Br J Anaesth* 2000;84:450-455.

21. Covert CR, Fox GS: Anaesthesia for hip surgery in the elderly. *Can J Anaesth* 1989;36:311-319.

22. Ennis RS: Postoperative deep vein thrombosis prophylaxis: A retrospective analysis in 1000 consecutive hip fracture patients treated in a community hospital setting. *J South Orthop Assoc* 2003;12:10-17.

23. Handoll HH, Farrar MJ, McBirnie J, Tytherleigh-Strong G, Milne AA, Gillespie WJ: Heparin, low molecular weight heparin and physical methods for preventing deep vein thrombosis and pulmonary embolism following surgery for hip fractures. *Cochrane Database Syst Rev* 2002;4:CD000305.

24. Prevention of pulmonary embolism and deep vein thrombosis with low dose aspirin: Pulmonary Embolism Prevention (PEP) trial. *Lancet* 2000; 355:1295-1302.

25. Turpie AG, Eriksson BI, Lassen MR, Bauer KA: A meta-analysis of fondaparinux versus enoxaparin in the prevention of venous thromboembolism after major orthopaedic surgery. *J South Orthop Assoc* 2002;11:182-188.

26. Eriksson BI: Improvements in the prevention of postoperative venous thromboembolism in hip fracture patients. *Orthopedics* 2003;26(suppl 8): 851-858.

27. Horgas AL, Tsai PF: Analgesic drug prescription and use in cognitively impaired nursing home residents. *Nurs Res* 1998;47:235-242.

28. Koval KJ, Schemitsch E, Liporace F, Strauss E, Zuckerman JD: An AOA critical issue. Geriatric trauma: Young ideas. *J Bone Joint Surg Am* 2003;85: 1380-1388.

29. Browner WS, Pressman AR, Nevitt MC, Cummings SR: Mortality following fractures in older women: The study of osteoporotic fractures. *Arch Intern Med* 1996;156:1521-1525.

30. Gotfried Y: The lateral trochanteric wall: A key element in the reconstruction of unstable pertrochanteric hip fractures. *Clin Orthop Relat Res* 2004;425:82-86.

31. Audige L, Hanson B, Swiontkowski MF: Implant-related complications in the treatment of unstable intertrochanteric fractures: Meta-analysis of dynamic screw-plate versus dynamic screw-intramedullary nail devices. *Int Orthop* 2003;27: 197-203.

32. Palm H, Jacobsen S, Sonne-Holm S, et al: Integrity of the lateral femoral wall in intertrochanteric hip fractures: An important predictor of a reoperation. *J Bone Joint Surg Am* 2007;89: 470-475.

33. Hardy DC, Descamps PY, Krallis P, et al: Use of an intramedullary hip-screw compared with a compression hip-screw with a plate for intertrochanteric femoral fractures: A prospective, randomized study of one hundred patients. *J Bone Joint Surg Am* 1998;80:618-630.

34. Adams CI, Robinson CM, Court-Brown CM, McQueen MM: Prospective randomized controlled trial of an intramedullary nail versus dynamic screw and plate for intertrochanteric fractures of the femur. *J Orthop Trauma* 2001;15:394-400.

35. Lorich DG, Geller DS, Nielson JH: Osteoporotic pertrochanteric hip fractures: Management and current controversies. *Instr Course Lect* 2004; 53:441-454.

36. Butt MS, Krikler SJ, Nafie S, Ali MS: Comparison of dynamic hip screw and gamma nail: A prospective, randomized, controlled trial. *Injury* 1995; 26:615-618.

37. Haidukewych GJ, Israel TA, Berry DJ: Reverse obliquity fractures of the intertrochanteric region of the femur. *J Bone Joint Surg Am* 2001;83: 643-650.

38. Bolhofner BR, Russo PR, Carmen B: Results of intertrochanteric femur fractures treated with a 135-degree

sliding screw with a two-hole side plate. *J Orthop Trauma* 1999;13:5-8.

39. Parker MJ, Gillespie LD, Gillespie WJ: Hip protectors for preventing hip fractures in the elderly. *Cochrane Database Syst Rev* 2004;3:CD001255.

40. Bendo JA, Weiner LS, Strauss E, Yang E: Collapse of intertrochanteric hip fractures fixed with sliding screws. *Orthop Rev* 1994;23(suppl): 30-37.

41. Baumgaertner MR, Curtin SL, Lindskog DM: Intramedullary versus extramedullary fixation for the treatment of intertrochanteric hip fractures. *Clin Orthop Relat Res* 1998; 348 :87-94.

42. Egol KA, Chang EY, Cvitkovic J, Kummer FJ, Koval KJ: Mismatch of current intramedullary nails with the anterior bow of the femur. *J Orthop Trauma* 2004;18:410-415.

43. Saudan M, Lubbeke A, Sadowski C, Riand N, Stern R, Hoffmeyer P: Pertrochanteric fractures: Is there an advantage to an intramedullary nail? A randomized, prospective study of 206 patients comparing the dynamic hip screw and proximal femoral nail. *J Orthop Trauma* 2002;16:386-393.

44. Olsson O, Ceder L, Hauggaard A: Femoral shortening in intertrochanteric fractures: A comparison between the Medoff sliding plate and the compression hip screw. *J Bone Joint Surg Br* 2001;83:572-578.

45. Kregor PJ, Obremskey WT, Kreder HJ, Swiontkowski MF: Evidence-Based Orthopaedic Trauma Working Group: Unstable pertrochanteric femoral fractures. *J Orthop Trauma* 2005;19:63-66.

46. Parker MJ, Pryor GA: Gamma versus DHS nailing for extracapsular femoral fractures: Meta-analysis of ten randomised trials. *Int Orthop* 1996;20: 163-168.

47. Baumgaertner MR, Curtin SL, Lindskog DM, Keggi JM: The value of the tip-apex distance in predicting failure of fixation of peritrochanteric fractures of the hip. *J Bone Joint Surg Am* 1995;77:1058-1064.

48. Vaidya SV, Dholakia DB, Chatterjee A: The use of a dynamic condylar screw and biological reduction techniques for subtrochanteric femur fracture. *Injury* 2003;34:123-128.

49. Haidukewych GJ, Berry DJ: Hip arthroplasty for salvage of failed treatment of intertrochanteric hip fractures. *J Bone Joint Surg Am* 2003;85: 899-904.

50. Marti RK, Schuller HM, Raaymakers EL: Intertrochanteric osteotomy for non-union of the femoral neck. *J Bone Joint Surg Br* 1989;71:782-787.

51. Macaulay W, Nellans KW, Garvin KL, Iorio R, Healy WL, Rosenwasser MP; other members of the DFACTO Consortium: Prospective randomized clinical trial comparing hemiarthroplasty to total hip arthroplasty in the treatment of displaced femoral neck fractures: Winner of the Dorr Award. *J Arthroplasty* 2008;23(6, suppl 1):2-8.

52. Keating JF, Grant A, Masson M, Scott NW, Forbes JF: Randomized comparison of reduction and fixation, bipolar hemiarthroplasty, and total hip arthroplasty: Treatment of displaced intracapsular hip fractures in healthy older patients. *J Bone Joint Surg Am* 2006;88:249-260.

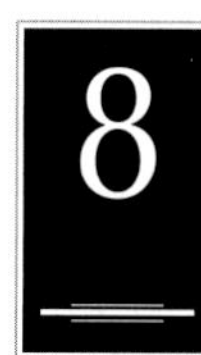

The Surgical Treatment of Acetabular Fractures

Berton R. Moed, MD
Kyle F. Dickson, MD, MBA
Philip J. Kregor, MD
Mark C. Reilly, MD
Mark S. Vrahas, MD

Abstract

The goals of treating an acetabular fracture are to restore the congruity and stability of the hip joint. Some fracture types may not require surgery for a satisfactory outcome, but a displaced fracture in the weight-bearing area of the acetabulum generally should be treated with open reduction and internal fixation. The surgery is complex and demanding, and the fracture reduction must be anatomic to obtain the best result. There is no doubt, however, that an experienced surgeon can achieve an excellent result. Usually a poor result is related to residual fracture displacement or a perioperative complication. The evaluation and treatment protocols initially developed by Letournel and Judet continue to be important; in addition, the surgeon should be aware of the progress made during the past decade.

An acetabular fracture routinely requires surgical intervention. The literature from the 1950s and 1960s offered conflicting recommendations for both nonsurgical and surgical treatment regimens.[1,2] It was agreed, however, that no matter the treatment, the result would be poor after a hip injury with residual joint instability or incongruity between the femoral head and the weight-bearing area of the acetabulum.[1-4] In 1964, Judet and associates[5] described the radiographic findings for acetabular fracture and outlined a plan of treatment. These authors refined several aspects of their seminal publication during the next three decades, but their basic principles did not change. These principles can be summarized as the need for the surgeon to understand the surgical anatomy of the innominate bone, define the injury through appropriate radiographic assessment, and use these findings to determine a suitable treatment plan. The results published by Letournel and Judet[6] in their definitive 1993 text still are considered optimal. Little new information appeared in the subsequent years,[7] however, during the past 5 to 10 years emerging trends have expanded the management of fractures of the acetabulum.

Imaging and Classification

Judet and associates[5] recognized that the plane of the ilium is approximately 90° to the plane of the obturator foramen and that both of these structures are oriented roughly 45° to the frontal plane. They proposed, therefore, that the AP view and two 45° oblique views of the pelvis be used to study the radiographic anatomy of the acetabulum, and they derived the

Dr. Moed or an immediate family member has received royalties from DePuy and has received research or institutional support from DePuy, Smith & Nephew, Stryker, and Synthes. Neither Dr. Dickson nor an immediate family member has received anything of value from or owns stock in a commercial company or institution related directly or indirectly to the subject of this article. Dr. Kregor or an immediate family member has received research or institutional support from the AO Foundation and Synthes. Dr. Reilly or an immediate family member serves as a board member, owner, officer, or committee member of the AO Foundation; is a member of a speakers' bureau or has made paid presentations on behalf of Synthes and Smith & Nephew; and has received research or institutional support from Biomet, EBI, the Musculoskeletal Transplant Foundation, Smith & Nephew, Stryker, Synthes, and Wright Medical Technology. Dr. Vrahas or an immediate family member has received research or institutional support from DePuy, Synthes, Zimmer, and AO and has stock or stock options held in Pioneer Medical.

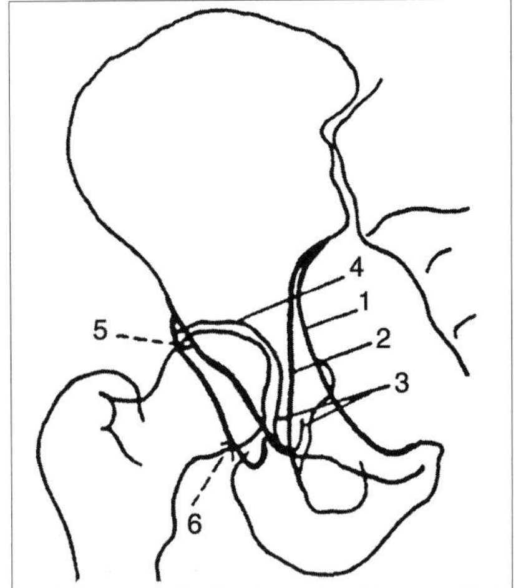

Figure 1 Schematic diagram showing the six acetabular landmarks seen on an AP radiograph: iliopectineal line (1), ilioischial line (2), U or teardrop (3), roof (4), anterior rim (5), and posterior rim (6). (Reproduced from Templeman D, Olson S, Moed BR, Duwelius P, Matta JM: Surgical treatment of acetabular fractures. *Instr Course Lect* 1999;48:481-496.)

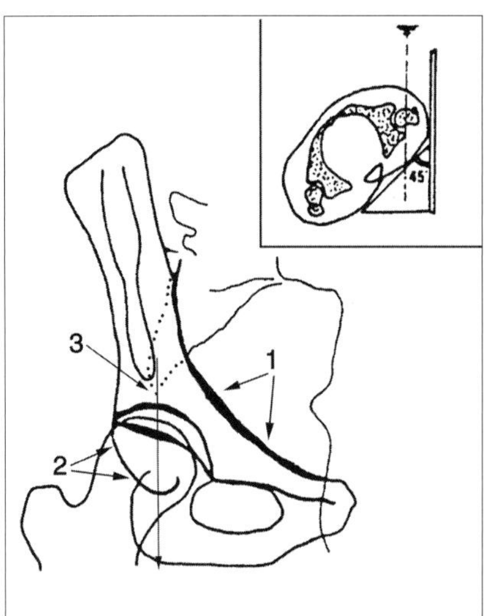

Figure 2 Schematic diagram showing the iliopectineal line (1) and posterior rim (2) as seen on an obturator oblique radiograph. The obturator ring is seen en face. The proper amount of rotation for the obturator oblique view (inset) is present when the tip of the coccyx lies just above the center of the ipsilateral femoral head (3). (Adapted from Templeman D, Olson S, Moed BR, Duwelius P, Matta JM: Surgical treatment of acetabular fractures. *Instr Course Lect* 1999;48:481-496.)

first systematic classification of acetabular fractures based on the anatomic pattern of the fracture. This analysis was expanded to include preoperative two-dimensional CT.[6] Subsequent advances in CT technology have improved the information provided by the two-dimensional images and offer the promise of useful three-dimensional images. These newer imaging studies enhance but do not replace the use of the three plain radiographic projections. Accurate interpretation of the plain radiographs requires correlation of the normal anatomy of the innominate bone with the pertinent radiographic landmarks seen on each view of the pelvis.

AP Radiograph

The AP view shows six basic radiographic landmarks (Figure 1). The iliopectineal line is the major landmark of the anterior column.[6] The inferior three quarters of the iliopectineal line are directly correlated with the pelvic brim on the innominate bone. However, the superior one quarter of the iliopectineal line is formed by the x-ray beam tangent to the superior quadrilateral surface and the posterosuperior aspect of the greater sciatic notch. The ilioischial line, extending from the posterosuperior greater sciatic notch to the ischial tuberosity, generally is considered a radiographic landmark of the posterior column;[6] this radiographic landmark is formed by the x-ray beam tangent to the posterior portion of the quadrilateral surface of the innominate bone. The radiographic U, or teardrop, consists of a lateral and a medial limb;[6] the lateral limb represents the inferior aspect of the anterior wall of the acetabulum, and the medial limb is formed by the obturator canal and the anteroinferior portion of the quadrilateral surface. The teardrop and ilioischial lines always are superimposed on the AP view because these landmarks are from different parts of the quadrilateral plate;[6] therefore, dissociation of the teardrop from the ilioischial line suggests that the innominate bone is rotated or there has been displacement of the quadrilateral surface. The dense line of the superior articular surface of the acetabulum on the AP view is known as the roof; it results from the tangency of the x-ray beam to the subchondral bone in the superior acetabulum. The anterior and posterior rims of the acetabulum represent, respectively, the peripheral contours of the anterior and posterior walls of the acetabulum.

Obturator Oblique Radiograph

The obturator oblique radiograph is taken with the patient placed so that the injured hemipelvis is rotated 45° toward the x-ray beam (Figure 2). This view shows the obturator foramen in its largest dimension and profiles the anterior column. The iliopectineal line has the same relationship to the pelvic brim as on the AP radiograph. The posterior rim of the acetabulum is best seen in this view, as is a fracture involving the posterior wall. A comparison of the relationship between the femoral head and the posterior wall can reveal subtle posterior subluxation.

Iliac Oblique Radiograph

The iliac oblique radiograph is taken with the patient placed so that the injured hemipelvis is rotated 45° away from the x-ray beam (Figure 3). This view shows the iliac wing in its largest dimension and

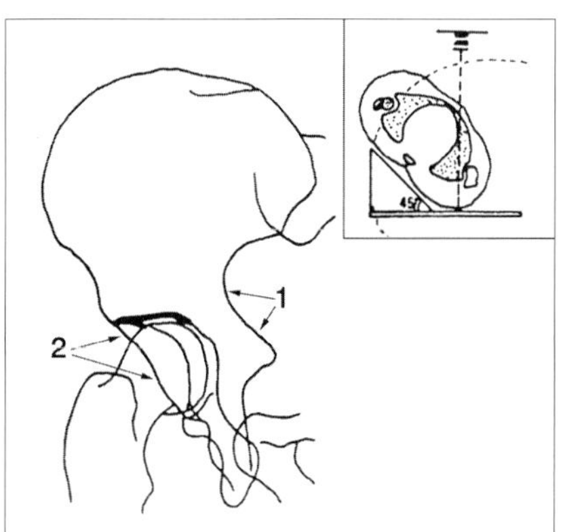

Figure 3 Schematic diagram showing the posterior border of the innominate bone (1) and anterior rim of the acetabulum (2) as seen on an iliac oblique radiograph. The iliac wing is seen en face. The anterior rim of the acetabulum can best be seen on this view. The proper amount of rotation for the iliac oblique view (inset) is present when the tip of the coccyx lies just above the center of the contralateral femoral head. (Adapted from Templeman D, Olson S, Moed BR, Duwelius P, Matta JM: Surgical treatment of acetabular fractures. *Instr Course Lect* 1999;48:481-496.)

profiles the greater and lesser sciatic notches as well as the anterior rim of the acetabulum. Involvement of the posterior column often can best be seen on this view. Fractures of the anterior column traversing the iliac wing also can be detected.

Computed Tomography

CT is a helpful adjunct to the three plain radiographic projections to further define the fracture pattern and assess for associated injuries. The most reliable and useful information is obtained from contiguous CT sections of no more than 3 mm in thickness. After studying the plain radiographs, the surgeon should use CT scans to resolve specific unanswered questions about the fracture (Figure 4). Two-dimensional axial CT images are superior to plain radiographs in showing the extent and location of acetabular wall fractures, the presence of intra-articular free fragments or injury to the femoral head, the orientation of the fracture lines, the presence of any additional fracture lines (such as the vertical portion of a T-shaped fracture), the rotation of fracture fragments, and the status of the posterior pelvic ring. The orientation of one or more fracture lines can be helpful in distinguishing among fracture types.

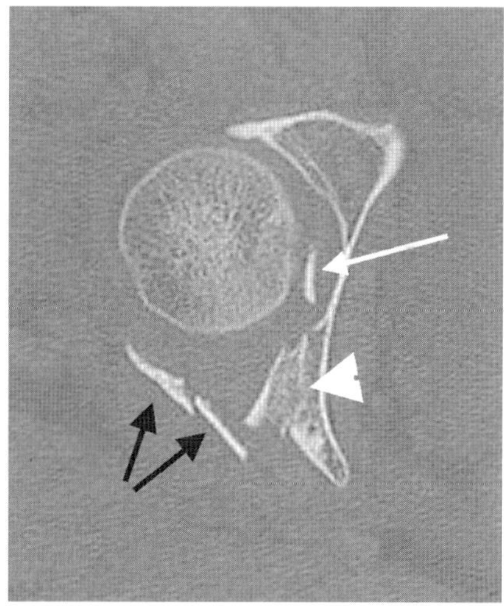

Figure 4 Axial CT scan showing a section through the acetabulum in which the posterior wall is fractured (*black arrows*) with marginal impaction (*white arrowhead*). An intra-articular loose body appears between the femoral head and acetabulum (*white arrow*). (Copyright Berton R. Moed, MD, St. Louis, MO.)

CT also can help in identifying fractures of the quadrilateral plate that cannot be seen on the radiographs. Marginal impaction, which is defined as depression of the articular surface of the joint, is best seen using two-dimensional axial CT.[6] Two-dimensional CT was found to be superior to plain radiography for the detection of fracture step and fracture gap deformities.[8] However, displacements in the plane of CT imaging may be underappreciated or averaged out. Two-dimensional CT has proved unreliable for determining hip joint stability.[9]

Improvements in three-dimensional CT technology have made it a useful tool for further defining the fracture pattern and thereby assisting in preoperative planning. However, three-dimensional CT does not provide as much diagnostic detail as two-dimensional CT. Three-dimensional CT scans can help a surgeon who is inexperienced in interpreting plain radiographs to better understand the fracture pattern. The understanding of the fracture pattern can be further enhanced by drawing the fracture lines taken from the radiographic landmarks onto a plastic bone model or by making a line drawing of the pelvis as seen on each radiographic view. The fracture pattern can be fully appreciated only by understanding the location and orientation of each fracture line.

Fracture Classification

The AO[10] and Orthopaedic Trauma Association[11] comprehensive fracture classification systems use a basic alphanumeric coding of the acetabular fracture classification developed by Judet and Letournel.[5,6] and offer no clinical advantage. Therefore, the so-called Letournel acetabular fracture classification is preferred internationally by most surgeons treating these complex injuries. The classification is based on the anatomy of the fracture pattern and has 10 categories, including 5 elementary and 5 associated patterns (Figure 5). The five elementary fracture patterns are the anterior wall, anterior column, posterior wall, posterior column, and transverse. Each of the associated patterns is either a combination of elementary patterns or an elementary pattern with an additional fracture component. The five associated fracture patterns are the

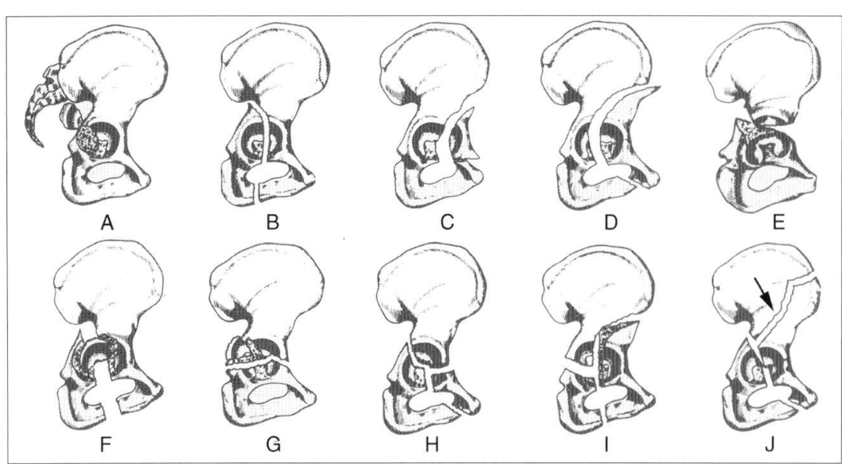

Figure 5 Schematic diagram showing the classification of acetabular fractures. **A,** Posterior wall fracture. **B,** Posterior column fracture. **C,** Anterior wall fracture. **D,** Anterior column fracture. **E,** Transverse fracture. **F,** Associated posterior column and posterior wall fracture. **G,** Associated transverse and posterior wall fracture. **H,** Associated T-shaped fracture. **I,** Associated anterior column and posterior hemitransverse fracture. **J,** Associated both-column fracture, with the supra-acetabular fracture line (*arrow*). (Adapted from Fitzgerald RH Jr, ed: Trauma: Pelvis and acetabulum, in *Orthopaedic Knowledge Update 2*. Park Ridge, IL, American Academy of Orthopaedic Surgeons, 1987, p 341-356.)

posterior column and posterior wall, anterior column (or wall) and posterior hemitransverse, transverse and posterior wall, T-shaped, and both-column. A variant pattern occasionally is seen, but usually it can easily be integrated into the system.

The Letournel system both describes the fracture and serves as a guide for subsequent surgical treatment. The fracture types are straightforward, with high rates of interobserver and intraobserver reliability.[12] However, those inexperienced with the system may be confused by the differentiation of the both-column type from the types with two-column fracture involvement (transverse, anterior column [or wall] and posterior hemitransverse, transverse and posterior wall, T-shaped). The both-column fracture is unique because it has both a displaced supra-acetabular fracture and a fracture line separating the anterior and posterior column components; no portion of the acetabular articular surface remains intact to the innominate bone (Figure 5, *J*).

Fracture Evaluation

Most fractures can be classified by using the information gleaned from high-quality plain radiographs. An organized approach must be used for examining the AP and oblique radiographs and the CT scan, so that each of the fracture types can be sequentially ruled in or ruled out. One useful method begins with a careful sequential analysis of each line on the AP radiograph (Figure 1). If the iliopectineal line is disrupted, the possible fracture types include the anterior wall, anterior column, transverse, transverse and posterior wall, T-shaped, anterior column and posterior hemitransverse, and both-column. If the ilioischial line is disrupted, the possible fracture types include the posterior column, transverse, transverse and posterior wall, T-shaped, anterior column and posterior hemitransverse, and both-column. If both lines are disrupted, the possible types are limited to the transverse, transverse and posterior wall, T-shaped, anterior column and posterior hemitransverse, and both-column. If the line along the posterior rim is disrupted, the possibility of a posterior wall fracture must be considered. Displacement of the ilioischial line from its normal relationship to the teardrop usually indicates that the two columns are separated from each other.

The obturator oblique radiograph is next examined to refine the diagnosis. A suspected posterior wall component will become obvious, as will a disruption involving the anterior wall or column. A fractured obturator ring suggests that the two columns are separated from each other. The presence of a supra-acetabular fracture line (the spur sign) is pathognomonic for a both-column fracture (Figure 6). The iliac oblique radiograph is examined to further define the injury to the posterior column and the possible presence and location of a fracture involving the iliac wing (anterior column, anterior column and posterior hemitransverse, or both-column).

Finally, the CT scan is studied for additional information (Figure 4). After this analysis, the plain radiographs are revisited to determine the fracture subtype, such as the level of a transverse fracture or the path of the stem of a T-shaped fracture. If the diagnosis still is unclear, three-dimensional CT can be helpful. However, three-dimensional CT has limitations (Figure 6, *B* and *C*).

Indications for Nonsurgical and Surgical Treatment

Nonsurgical Treatment

A stable, concentrically reduced acetabular fracture that does not in-

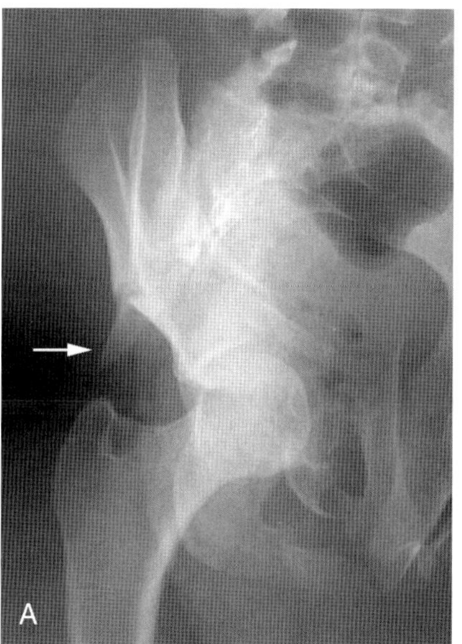

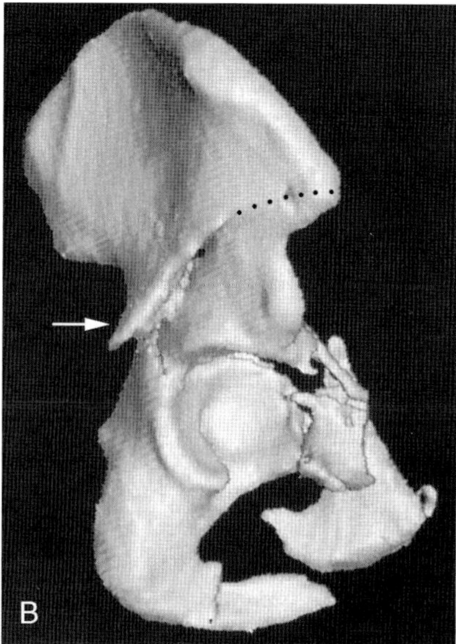

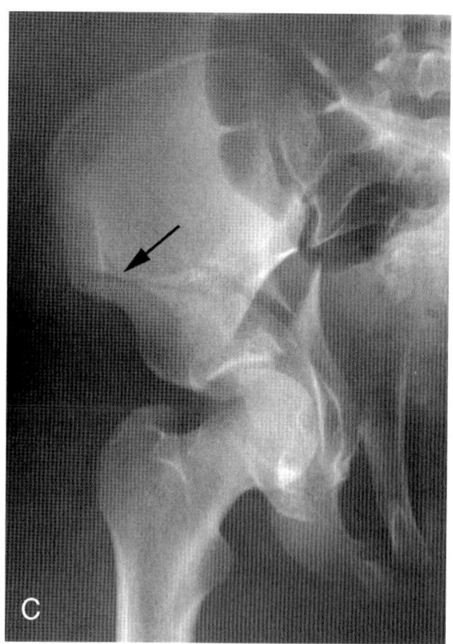

Figure 6 **A,** Obturator oblique radiograph showing a both-column fracture with the spur sign (arrow). **B,** Three-dimensional CT scan showing a supra-acetabular fracture (arrow), which creates the spur sign. The continuation of the anterior column fracture line (dotted line) cannot be seen on three-dimensional CT but was clearly visible (arrow) on a plain radiograph **(C)** and two-dimensional CT. (Copyright Berton R. Moed, MD, St. Louis, MO.)

volve the superior acetabular dome generally can be treated nonsurgically.[2,13-16] This group of fractures includes nondisplaced and minimally displaced fractures, fractures in which the intact part of the acetabulum is large enough to maintain stability and congruity, and both-column fractures in which the displaced articular fragments remain congruent with the femoral head without the application of skeletal traction (so-called secondary congruity[6]). Nonsurgical treatment also may be selected for a patient with severe osteoporosis or a severe comorbidity that precludes surgical intervention. There are relatively few such patients, most of whom are elderly.

Matta and associates[14] developed roof arc measurements to be used in deciding whether an acetabular fracture violates the weight-bearing dome. This measurement has been used to determine whether the remaining intact acetabulum is sufficient to maintain a stable and congruent relationship with the femoral head. Nonsurgical or surgical treatment can then be selected. The acetabular roof arc is measured on all three radiographic views with the leg out of traction. The AP view is used to measure the medial roof arc; the obturator oblique view, to measure the anterior roof arc; and the iliac oblique view, to measure the posterior roof arc. The measurements are obtained by drawing a vertical line through the center of the femoral head and a second line from the center of the femoral head to the fracture location at the articular surface (Figure 7, *A* through *C*). Initially, it was believed that roof arc values of greater than 45° on all three views indicated that the hip would remain stable and congruent.[17] However, these values have been revised.[18] Fractures with a medial roof arc angle greater than 45°, an anterior roof arc angle greater than 25°, and a posterior roof arc angle greater than 70° are currently believed to have sufficient intact acetabulum for nonsurgical treatment[18] (Figure 7, *D*). Therefore, displaced low anterior column, low transverse, and low T-shaped acetabular fractures are amenable to nonsurgical treatment, if, as expected, the fracture position is stable and the joint remains congruent.[2,6,15,19] These measurements are not applicable to both-column fractures or fractures involving the posterior wall.

Although it is generally recommended that all nondisplaced and minimally displaced acetabular fractures be considered for nonsurgical management, some authors believe that patients with such a fracture should be treated with percutaneous fracture fixation.[20-22] Their concern centers on the questionable stability of these fractures and the possibility that some of them later will become displaced. Early percutaneous fixation of these fractures with oc-

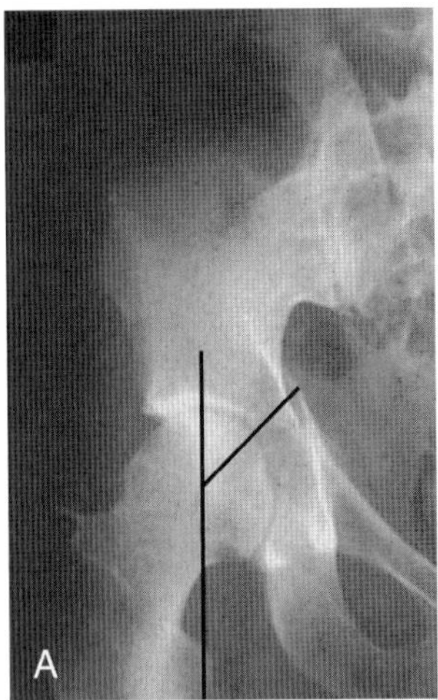

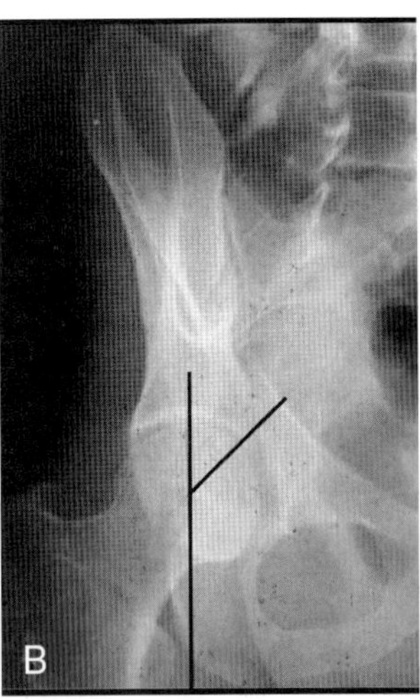

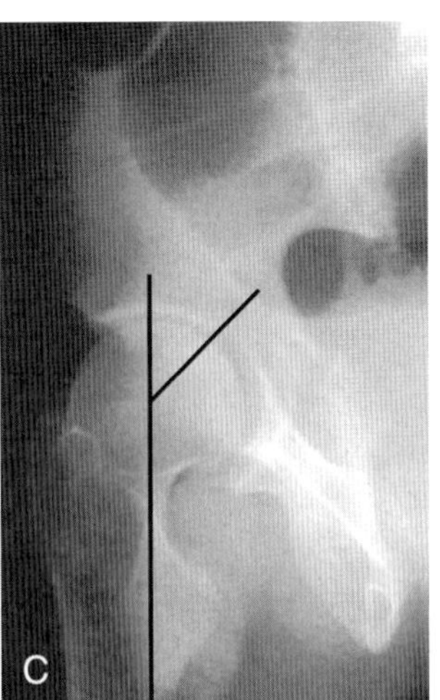

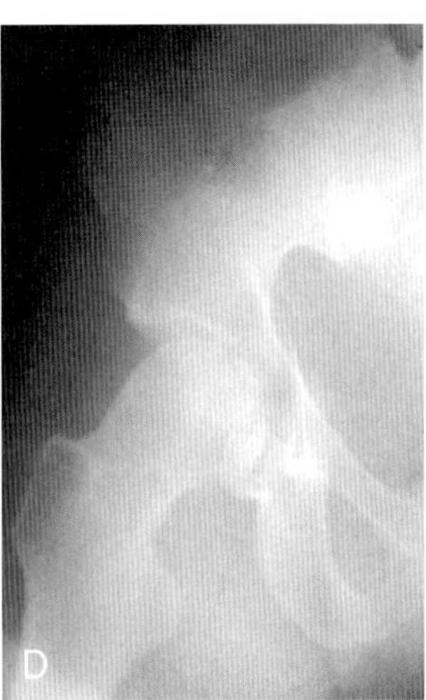

Figure 7 AP (**A**), obturator oblique (**B**), and iliac oblique (**C**) radiographs of the hip of a 35-year-old man treated approximately 15 years ago for a transverse fracture of the acetabulum. The lines in all views show roof arc measurements of approximately 50°, according to the initial recommendations of Matta and Merritt,[17] the hip joint is considered stable. **D,** AP radiograph taken 3 weeks later, showing gross medial subluxation of the hip, as could be predicted by using the criteria of Vrahas and associates.[18] (Copyright Berton R. Moed, MD, St. Louis, MO.)

cult instability may avoid a later, more extensive open procedure or prevent early traumatic arthritis (if the patient is not treated for the later displacement). However, fewer than 7% of nondisplaced or minimally displaced fractures have the potential to become significantly displaced without traction.[23] To avoid unnecessary surgical treatment of a large number of fractures in the interest of preventing displacement in a few, it is worthwhile to attempt to identify the fractures at risk for displacement. Dynamic fluoroscopic stress examination, done with the patient under general anesthesia, has been proposed for identifying these fractures at risk for displacement.[23] However, the exact technique for this examination is ill defined for fractures other than an isolated posterior wall fracture. Another method is close observation of every patient with a fracture suitable for nonsurgical treatment. Weekly radiographic follow-up is accompanied by readiness to shift immediately to percutaneous or open surgical treatment if joint instability or incongruity is detected.[13]

In summary, the prerequisites for nonsurgical treatment of an acetabular fracture include measurements indicating an intact roof arc and congruity of the femoral head to the intact acetabulum; both are evaluated on AP and oblique (also known as Judet) radiographs taken without traction applied to the leg. The patient's age, preinjury activity level, functional demands, and medical comorbidities also must be considered in deciding whether the patient is better served by surgical or nonsurgical treatment. Nonsurgical treatment may be appropriate for an elderly or infirm patient, particularly if the fracture displacement is minimal, with a plan for arthroplasty if symptomatic arthritis develops.[24-26]

Surgical Treatment

Surgical treatment is indicated for all acetabular fractures that result in hip joint instability or incongruity, regardless of how the fracture is classified or whether it is displaced or has occult instability. Fracture displacement of 2 mm or more in the weight-bearing dome results in joint incongruity, and it is one of the main indications for open reduction and internal fixation.[17,27] Posterior and anterior wall fractures with instability of the hip joint require surgical fixation. A fragment of bone or soft tissue incarcerated within the hip joint also can cause joint incongruity. Open reduction and removal of the loose body or obstructing tissue are indicated to prevent the early onset of traumatic arthritis. Recurrent dislocation, with disastrous consequences for the hip joint, is inevitable if stability is not restored.[28] Two-dimensional CT is unreliable for determining hip joint stability,[9] and therefore it should be assumed that all posterior wall fractures are unstable unless dynamic stress examination proves otherwise.[9] There is no need for dynamic stress examination of an obviously unstable hip. A both-column fracture may be significantly displaced but not require surgical treatment; however, surgi-

Table 1
Acetabular Fracture Patterns and Preferred Surgical Approaches

	Preferred Surgical Approach					
Fracture Pattern	**Kocher-Langenbeck**	**Ilioinguinal**	**Iliofemoral**	**Extended Iliofemoral**	**Modified Stoppa**	**Triradiate**
Posterior column	X					
Anterior column		X	X		X	
Posterior wall	X					
Anterior wall		X			X	
Transverse	X	X		X	X	X
T-shaped	X	X		X	X	X
Anterior column and posterior hemitransverse		X		X		X
Transverse and posterior wall	X			X		X
Posterior column and posterior wall	X					
Both-column		X		X		X

cal treatment is required if a loss of parallelism between the femoral head and acetabular articular surface is noted on any of the three radiographic views, indicating an incongruous hip joint.

Surgical Approaches

The main surgical approaches to the acetabulum, as described by Letournel and Judet,[6] are the Kocher-Langenbeck, ilioinguinal, iliofemoral, and extended iliofemoral approaches. The surgical approach usually is selected with the expectation that it will allow the entire fracture reduction and fixation[6,27,29] (Table 1). The Kocher-Langenbeck approach provides direct access only to the posterior column of the acetabulum, and the ilioinguinal and iliofemoral approaches provide direct access only to the anterior column. These three approaches rely on indirect manipulation for reduction of any fracture lines that traverse the opposite column. The extended iliofemoral approach allows almost complete direct access to all aspects of the acetabulum. This approach most often is used for an associated fracture that is surgically treated more than 21 days after injury or for a transverse, T-shaped or both-column fracture with a complicating feature that is not amenable to treatment by one of the more limited approaches.

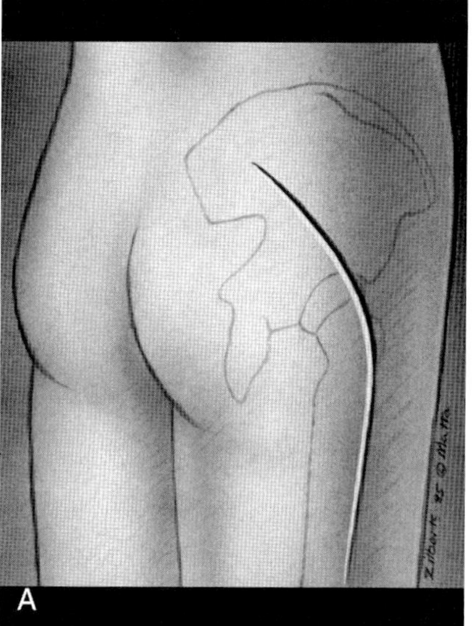

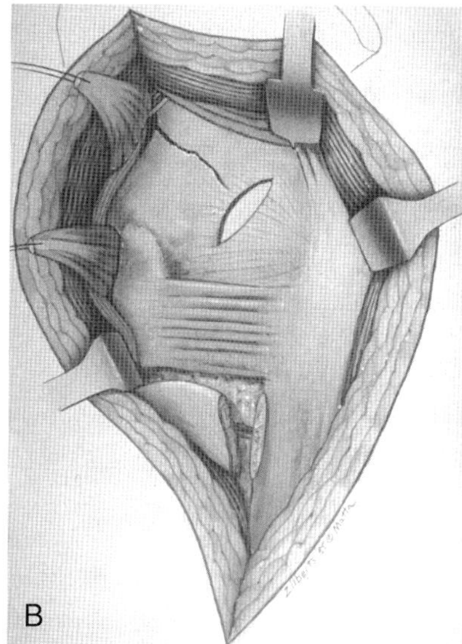

Figure 8 Schematic diagrams showing the Kocher-Langenbeck approach. **A,** Surgical incision. **B,** Final exposure of the retroacetabular surface. (Reproduced from Matta JM, Letournel E, Browner BD: Surgical management of acetabular fractures. *Instr Course Lect* 1986;35:382-397.)

Kocher-Langenbeck Approach

The Kocher-Langenbeck approach (Figure 8) is ideal for a posterior wall fracture or a posterior column fracture with or without an associated posterior wall fracture. A transverse or T-shaped fracture also is amena-

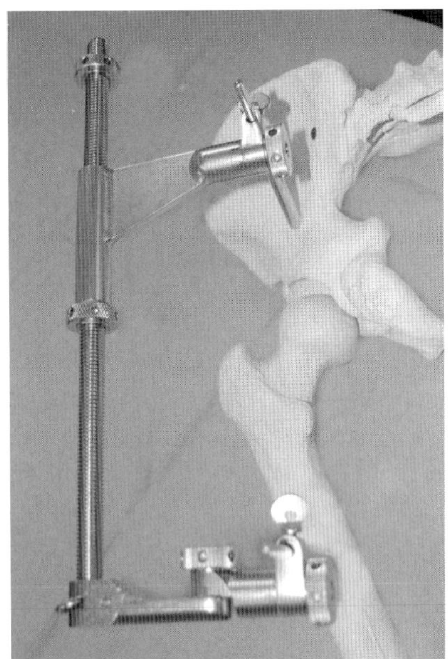

Figure 9 The application of a universal distractor, shown on a plastic bone model. (Copyright Berton R. Moed, MD, St. Louis, MO, and Mark S. Vrahas, MD, Boston, MA.)

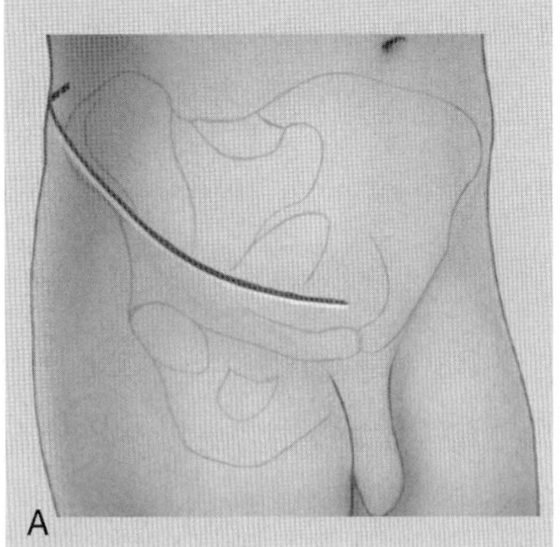

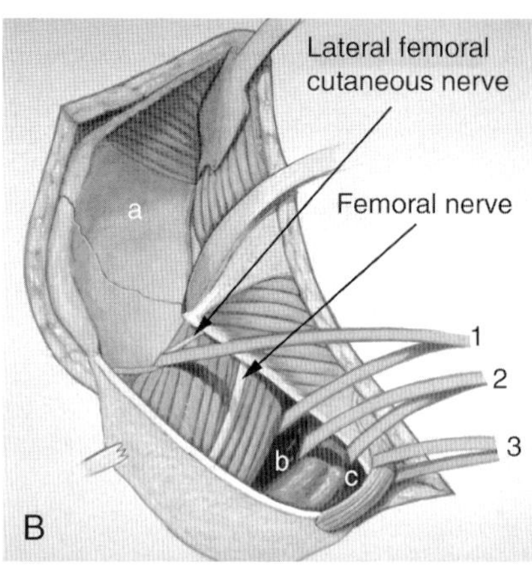

Figure 10 Schematic diagrams showing the ilioinguinal approach. **A,** Surgical incision. (Reproduced from Matta JM, Letournel E, Browner BD: Surgical management of acetabular fractures. *Instr Course Lect* 1986;35:382-397.) **B,** Final exposure, with isolation of the iliopsoas femoral and lateral femoral cutaneous nerves (1), external iliac vessels (2), and the spermatic cord in a male patient or round ligament in a female patient (3). Through the windows thus created, the surgeon gains access to the lateral (a), middle (b), and medial (c) innominate bone. (Adapted from Reilly MC, Olson SA: Treatment considerations for surgical and nonsurgical management of acetabular fractures, in Olson SA, Reilly MC, eds: *Acetabular and Pelvic Fractures.* Rosemont, IL, American Academy of Orthopaedic Surgeons, 2006, pp 43-66.)

ble to this surgical approach within 15 days of injury. In a T-shaped fracture, the major displacement should be posterior, with only minor anterior displacement at the pelvic brim. The patient can be in the lateral or prone position. Surgeons often choose to operate on posterior wall fractures with the patient lateral, allowing easier patient positioning, better visualization for the assistants, and a more familiar orientation. However, the patient should be positioned prone if the fracture involves the posterior column; in the lateral position, the weight of the leg displaces the femoral head medially and makes reduction of the column more difficult. The Kocher-Langenbeck approach is best used with a specialized fracture traction table. Such a table may not be available, however, and some means must be used to distract the femoral head from the acetabulum for fracture reduction. A universal distractor is a useful alternative to a specialized table (Figure 9).

Ilioinguinal Approach

The ilioinguinal approach (Figure 10) is indicated for anterior wall or anterior column fractures as well as most anterior column and posterior hemitransverse fractures. Transverse fractures in which the displacement is primarily anterior, with minimal posterior displacement, and both-column fractures having a noncomminuted posterior column fragment also can be treated using the ilioinguinal approach. Fractures of these complex types must have no displacement in the acetabular roof, and they must be treated within 15 days of injury. Both-column fractures that extend into the sacroiliac joint and have a fracture-dislocation component are not amenable to reduction through the ilioinguinal approach.

The ilioinguinal approach allows access to the internal aspect of the innominate bone from the sacroiliac joint to the symphysis pubis. The internal iliac fossa, pelvic brim, superior pubic ramus, and a portion of the quadrilateral surface can be directly visualized. Indirect access to the inferior portion of the quadrilateral surface is obtained using a palpating finger or special instruments. Limited access to the external aspect of the iliac wing is possible if the abductor origin is released. It is best to avoid dissection on the outer aspect of the pelvis. If this dissection is necessary, the sartorius origin always should be left intact to prevent overzealous exposure. Although the ilioinguinal approach offers extensive exposure, it is not convenient. The surgeon must work through small windows between major nerves and vessels to view the fracture (Figure 10, *B*). Many of the necessary reduction and fixation techniques are not intu-

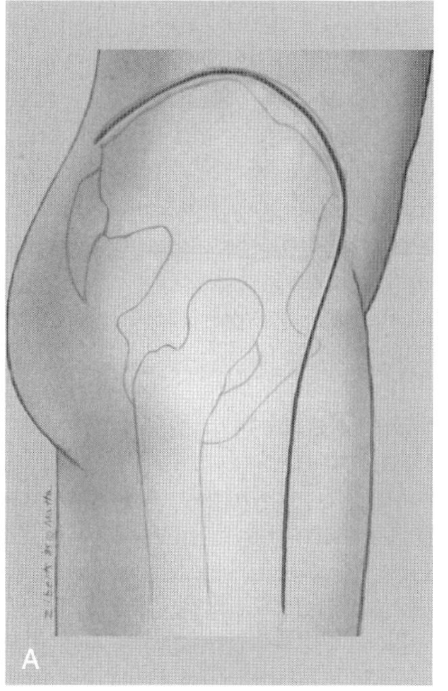

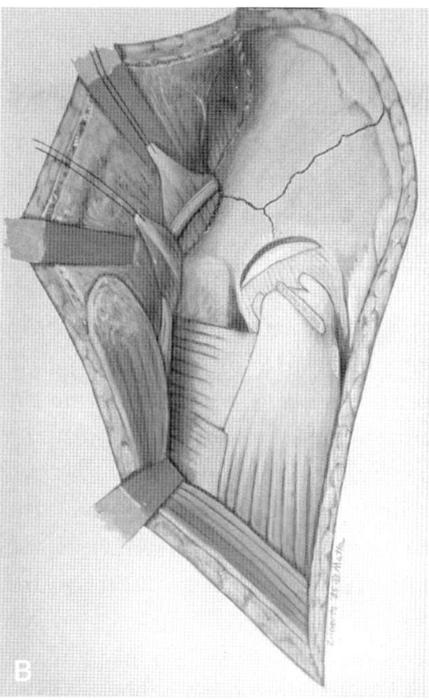

Figure 11 Schematic diagrams showing the extended iliofemoral approach. **A,** Surgical incision. **B,** Final exposure of the external aspect of the innominate bone. (Reproduced from Matta JM, Letournel E, Browner BD: Surgical management of acetabular fractures. *Instr Course Lect* 1986;35:382-397.)

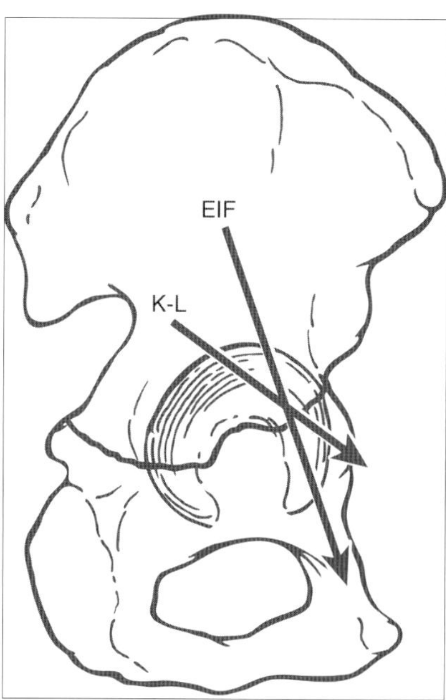

Figure 12 Schematic diagram showing the angles for insertion of an anterior column lag screw using the Kocher-Langenbeck (K-L) and extended iliofemoral (EIF) approaches. The angle shown for the extended iliofemoral approach also can be obtained with percutaneous techniques. (Copyright Berton R. Moed, MD, St. Louis, MO.)

itive when the ilioinguinal approach is used; the work of an experienced pelvic surgeon should be closely observed before fracture fixation is attempted through this approach.

Iliofemoral Approach

The iliofemoral approach exposes the iliac fossa but does not allow access medial to the iliopectineal eminence. This approach has limited application. Although the ilioinguinal approach usually is preferable, the iliofemoral approach may be sufficient for a high anterior column fracture in which the main displacement is cephalad to the hip joint.

Extended Iliofemoral Approach

The extended iliofemoral approach (Figure 11) is used for selected complex acetabular fracture types and for surgery delayed more than 2 to 3 weeks following injury. These include transverse plus posterior wall fractures if the surgeon expects unusual difficulties with reduction.[6,27] Examples include a transtectal transverse component with an extended posterior wall fracture (those involving the posterior border of the bone), a T-shaped and posterior wall fracture, and fractures associated with dislocation of the symphysis pubis or fracture of the contralateral pubis ramus.[6,27] A suitable T-shaped fracture has a transtectal transverse component, a wide separation along the vertical stem of the T, or an association with dislocation of the symphysis pubis or fracture of the contralateral pubic ramus.[6,27] A suitable both-column fracture has a complex fracture of the posterior column, a displaced fracture line crossing the sacroiliac joint, or a wide separation of the anterior and posterior columns at the rim of the acetabulum.[27]

The extended iliofemoral approach provides maximal simultaneous access to both columns of the acetabulum. The entire lateral aspect of the iliac wing, the anterior column to the level of the iliopectineal eminence, the retroacetabular surface, and the interior of the hip joint are accessible. Unlike the Kocher-Langenbeck approach, the extended iliofemoral approach allows for a long screw to be placed down the anterior column under direct visualization (Figure 12). It is possible to expose the entire internal iliac fossa, however, this maneuver risks devascularizing the iliac wing.

Other Approaches

Modified Stoppa Intrapelvic Approach

The modified Stoppa intrapelvic approach has been advocated for treating anterior wall, anterior column, transverse, T-shaped, anterior column (or wall) and posterior hemitransverse, and both-column fractures.[30] Although this approach has not gained wide acceptance, it is especially useful for fractures that require buttress plating of the quadrilateral plate.[31] The pure modified Stoppa approach exposes only the true pelvis. Therefore, a second approach often is necessary for fracture reduction or hardware insertion. Combining these two approaches functions as the equivalent of using the lateral and medial windows of the ilioinguinal approach. As with the ilioinguinal approach, indirect reduction is required for posterior fracture lines. The advantage of the modified Stoppa approach over the ilioinguinal approach is that dissection of the iliac vessels is not required. However, this lack of access to the middle window of the ilioinguinal approach also is a disadvantage of the modified Stoppa approach.

Triradiate Approach

The triradiate approach described by Mears and Rubash[32] is used for many of the same fractures as the extended iliofemoral approach. However, the exposure is more limited, and the iliac crest cannot be completely seen. The skin incision is Y shaped, with a posterior limb nearly identical to that of the Kocher-Langenbeck incision. The anterior limb of the incision extends from the greater trochanter to the anterosuperior iliac spine. The skin incision is deepened through the fascia. The posterior portion of the triradiate approach is the same as that of the Kocher-Langenbeck approach. The triradiate approach is useful for transverse, transverse and posterior wall, and T-shaped fractures, especially for late fractures and those with substantial displacement of both the anterior and posterior columns. It is not ideal for fractures that exit high in the anterior column because only the anterior portion of the iliac crest is exposed.

The standard triradiate approach includes a trochanteric osteotomy, which provides more exposure than usually is necessary. Completing the anterior and posterior limbs of the approach without removing the trochanter allows visualization of the anterior and posterior columns and avoids extensive dissection of the abductors. The triradiate approach is similar to simultaneous anterior and posterior approaches, except that it allows both anterior and posterior column fractures to be treated from one side of the operating table.

Trochanteric Flip Osteotomy

The trochanteric flip osteotomy is used with the Kocher-Langenbeck approach to obtain greater anterosuperior exposure and facilitate intraoperative dislocation of the femoral head for inspection of the joint.[33,34] Although the patient is usually in the lateral position for this approach, the patient also can be placed in the prone position.[33] Indications for the use of this approach potentially include combined femoral head/posterior wall acetabular fractures, posterior wall fractures with anterosuperior extension, posterior wall and column fracture patterns, as well as certain transverse or T-shaped fractures.[34]

Simultaneous Anterior and Posterior Approaches

Many surgeons prefer to use an anterior (ilioinguinal or iliofemoral) and posterior (Kocher-Langenbeck) approach simultaneously as an alternative to the more extensive triradiate or extended iliofemoral approach or as the primary approach for transverse, T-shaped, and some both-column fractures. Although this combined approach is not generally considered the best method, excellent results have been obtained when two experienced surgical teams work together.[35]

Open Reduction and Internal Fixation of Specific Types of Fractures Grouped According to Common Features

The protocols developed by Letournel and Judet[6] call for strict adherence to patient positioning and the use of a fracture table. Fracture reduction is the most difficult and critical element of the surgical procedure. Before surgical intervention, the surgeon must use plain radiographs and two-dimensional CT to ascertain the pattern of displacement and fracture fragment malrotation. Drawing the fracture on paper or a plastic pelvic bone model is extremely helpful to establish a careful preoperative plan and determine the approximate clamp position required to achieve anatomic joint reduction. Intraoperative traction, which reduces the deforming force of the femoral head, permits a precise reduction of the fracture with the use of special clamps. Traction is best achieved by using a specialized fracture table, although alternative methods can be used (Figure 9). Obtaining an anatomic reduction is critical to consistently achieving a good clinical result.[27]

The fracture usually is fixed with 3.5-mm hardware; however, smaller screw sizes often are needed for fixation of a posterior wall or osteochondral fracture fragment.[36-38] The standard fracture fixation constructs (Figure 13) often must be modified to accommodate the individual fracture morphology, as determined during preoperative planning. However, posterior wall fracture fixation always should include a buttress plate[37,38] (Figure 13, *A*). After fracture reduction and fixation are completed, the quality of the reduction and the hardware position should be assessed using intraoperative fluoroscopy through a 180° arc. Both the absence of a subchondral fracture gap or step-off and the congruity of the femoral head with the acetabular roof should be seen on the fluoroscopic images. Additional axial and tangential views can be used to ensure that all screws are extra-articular[39] (Figure 14). The acetabulum is a concave joint; therefore, only one projection showing extra-articular position of the entire screw is required. If this one projection cannot be found for a particular screw, then the screw should be removed.[39]

The three standard radiographs should be obtained postoperatively. Any concern generated from the review of these radiographs should be further evaluated with two-dimensional CT. Plain radiographs cannot adequately assess the posterior wall,[6,40] and therefore postoperative two-dimensional CT is required for fractures involving the posterior wall.

Posterior Wall, Posterior Column, and Posterior Column and Posterior Wall Fractures

Posterior Wall Fracture

Although a posterior wall fracture often is considered simple (Figure 5, *A*), an uncomplicated one-fragment posterior wall fracture rarely occurs.[6,37,40] Complicating factors in a posterior wall fracture include fragmentation of the wall, marginal impaction, the presence of intra-articular fragments, and femoral head damage.[27,37,40] Moed and associates[40] found that the quality of the reduction must be as anatomic as possible because imperfections are correlated with a poorer clinical outcome. The common mistakes in surgical treatment of a posterior wall fracture include an inadequate understanding of the complexity of the fracture, an inability to retrieve intra-articular fragments, difficulty in reducing and fixing small osteochondral fragments or marginal impaction, and poor reduction or fixation of the posterior wall fragment.

Appropriate fixation of a posterior wall fracture requires a well-executed Kocher-Langenbeck approach. The surgeon must minimize surgical devitalization of the abductors, preserve the vascular supply of the femoral head, maintain the capsular attachments to the posterior wall, and carefully débride the edges of the fracture and cancellous recipient bed of the posterior wall. Distraction of the hip joint is helpful for completely visualizing and débriding the hip joint. A specially designed fracture table that provides traction through a distal femoral pin allows flexion of the hip and approximately 1.5 cm of hip joint distraction, which enables removal of the torn ligamentum teres and any other small intra-articular fragments. Alternatively, a femoral distractor can be used across the hip joint, with one Schanz pin placed in the sciatic buttress region (1.5 cm lateral and 1.5 to 2 cm caudal to the sciatic notch) and another pin placed in the proximal femur (Figure 9).

After adequate débridement of the hip joint, the traction is released to allow the femoral head to assume its normal position against the intact articular surface of the acetabulum. The femoral head then can be used as a template for reducing the posterior wall. Often, there are multiple free osteochondral fragments that need to be reduced into position and held by mini-fragment screws.[36,37] Any marginal impaction should be reduced into position, possibly held with screws, and supported by bone graft placed into the void behind the elevated fragment. The key to the reduction is to elevate the marginal impaction as one fragment; this usually is best accomplished using a Freer elevator beneath the impacted fragment. A minifragment screw can be used to secure a fragment of adequate size that is unstable after being impacted into place.[36] After the osteochondral fragments and marginal impaction have been reduced into position, the posterior wall is reduced and fixed (Figure 13, *A*). The common errors in posterior wall fixation include overcontouring the plate so it does not adequately buttress the wall; failing to bring the plate sufficiently peripheral; and bringing the plate high above the greater sciatic notch, thereby placing the superior gluteal nerve at risk.

Posterior Column Fracture

The Kocher-Langenbeck approach is used for a posterior column fracture (Figure 5, *B*). The congruity of the hip joint is highly dependent on appropriate reduction of the posterior column, and obtaining a perfect reduction may be difficult. Therefore, placing the patient prone is preferred. The most common deformity is slight gapping superiorly and cephalad translation of the posterior column. Rotational mismatch of the posterior column is common and can best be assessed by palpation through the greater sciatic notch. Rotational control of the posterior column can be obtained with a

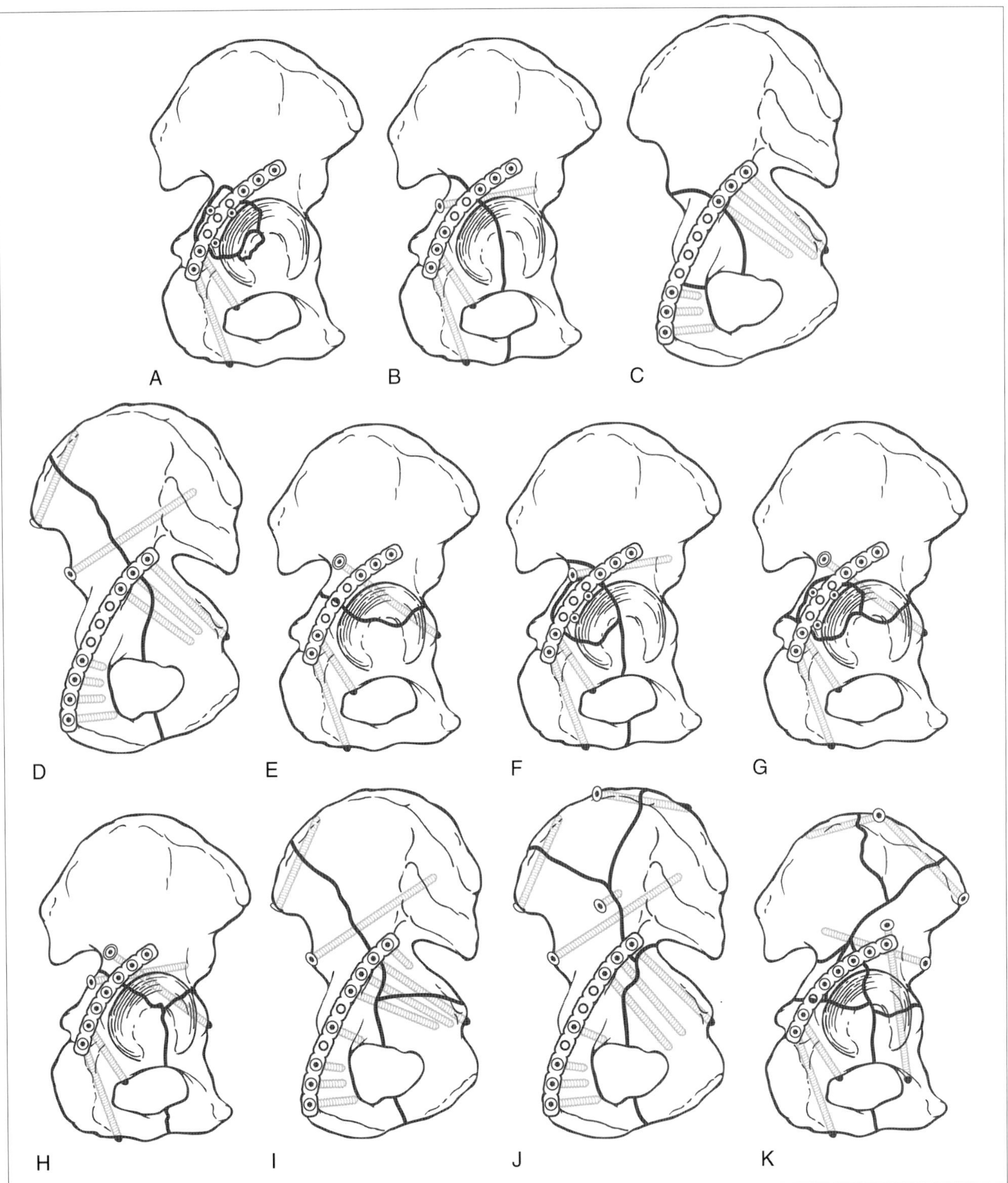

Figure 13 Schematic diagrams showing the 10 acetabular fracture types, with typical fixation constructs. (*A* through *E* show elementary types; *F* through *K* show associated types.) **A,** Multifragmented posterior wall fracture with intra-articular comminution. **B,** Posterior column fracture. **C,** Anterior wall fracture. **D,** High anterior column fracture. **E,** Juxtatectal transverse fracture. **F,** Posterior column and posterior wall fracture. **G,** Transverse and posterior wall fracture. **H,** T-shaped fracture. **I,** Anterior column and posterior hemitransverse fracture. **J,** Both-column fracture; the ilioinguinal approach was used. **K,** Both-column fracture with posterior column comminution; the extended iliofemoral approach was used. (Copyright Berton R. Moed, MD, St. Louis, MO.)

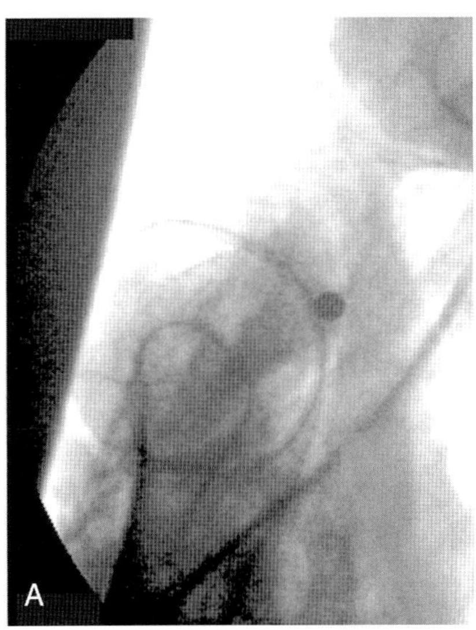

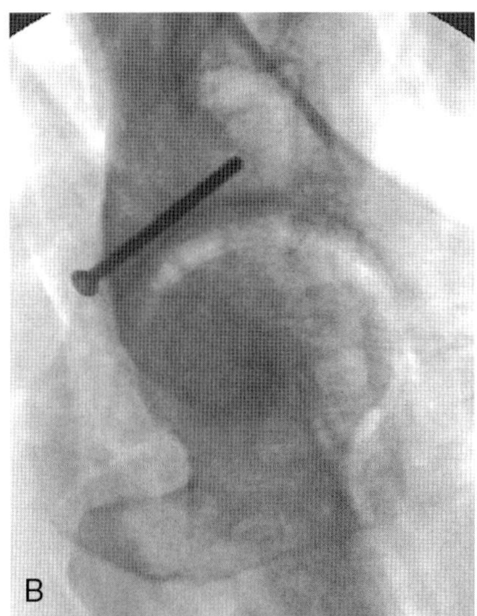

Figure 14 Axial **(A)** and tangential **(B)** fluoroscopic views of a cadaver specimen showing an extra-articular screw position. (Copyright Berton R. Moed, MD, St. Louis, MO.)

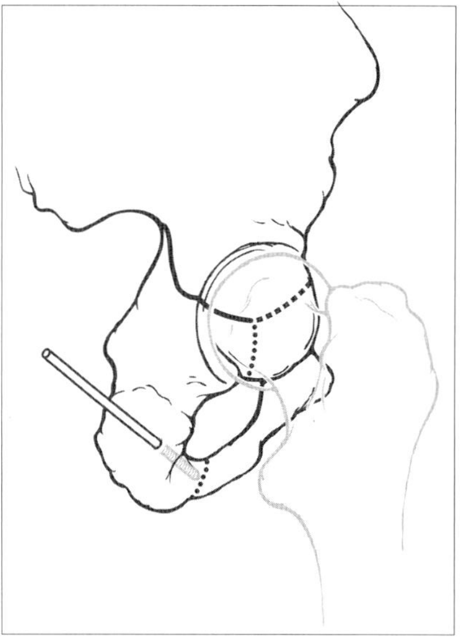

Figure 15 Schematic diagram of a hemipelvis with a Schanz screw in the ischium. A Schanz screw is used to control the rotational and translational displacement of the posterior column that occurs in several types of fractures. (Copyright Berton R. Moed, MD, St. Louis, MO.)

6.0-mm Schanz screw driven into the ischium (Figure 15). The posterior column then is reduced through the greater sciatic notch using an angled-jaw bone forceps, a pointed reduction clamp, or a clamp applied to two temporary screws located on either side of the fracture. It may be helpful to use a ball spike pusher to push the posterior column from posterior to anterior. It is important that the surgeon not simply look at the posterior column reduction on the posterior aspect but also assess the rotation of the posterior column by palpation through the greater sciatic notch. After the posterior column is reduced, a lag screw from posterior to anterior is placed, keeping in mind the frontal plane nature of the fracture. A posterior column neutralization plate is then placed (Figure 13, *B*).

Posterior Column and Posterior Wall Fracture

The Kocher-Langenbeck approach is preferred for an associated posterior column and posterior wall fracture (Figure 5, *F*), with the patient in the prone position. The posterior column is reduced first. This reduction is facilitated by retracting the posterior wall fragment so that the joint can be inspected. After lag screw fixation of the posterior column fracture, the posterior wall is reduced and fixed. The fracture fixation construct is completed by the application of a buttress plate (Figure 13, *F*).

Anterior Wall and Anterior Column Fractures

Anterior Wall Fracture

The surgical treatment of an anterior wall fracture (Figure 5, *C*) usually requires all or part of the ilioinguinal surgical approach, with the patient in the supine position. A Pfannenstiel extension of the medial aspect of the ilioinguinal incision can be used to expose the entire quadrilateral surface to the sacroiliac joint; the exposure is similar to that obtained using a modified Stoppa approach.[30] Reduction of the anterior wall fracture starts with traction and internal rotation of the femur. Occasionally, intraoperative lateral traction with a Schanz pin placed in the greater trochanter aids reduction of the fractured anterior wall. The fracture usually can be reduced by direct posterior lateral force applied with a ball spike or a bone clamp positioned with one tine on the anterior wall fragment and the other lateral to the anteroinferior iliac spine. A curved buttress plate is placed along the pelvic brim, extending from the superior pubic ramus to the internal iliac fossa (Figure 13, *C*). This construct can be augmented by two lag screws inserted from the brim to the quadrilateral surface, with care to avoid penetrating the joint. Medial subluxation of the femoral head cannot occur if the anterior and posterior articular surfaces are intact or have been reconstructed, and any quadrilateral fracture fragments

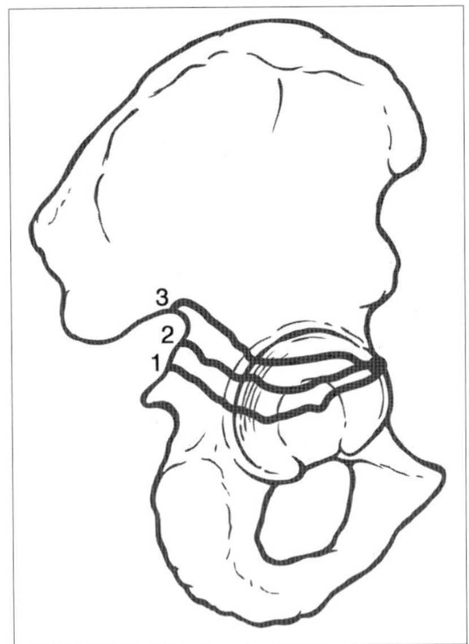

Figure 16 Schematic diagram of a hemipelvis showing the infratectal (1), juxtatectal (2), and transtectal (3) levels of the transverse fracture component and the component's exit at the iliopectineal eminence (dot). (Copyright Berton R. Moed, MD, St. Louis, MO, and Mark S. Vrahas, MD, Boston, MA.)

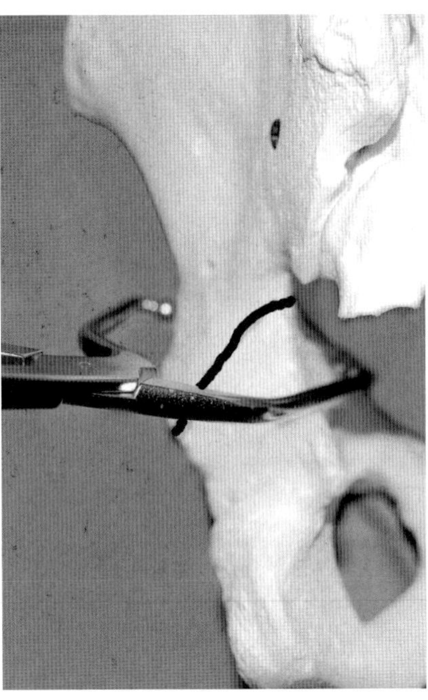

Figure 17 A clamp placed through the sciatic notch to stabilize a transverse fracture (line), shown on a plastic bone model. (Copyright Berton R. Moed, MD, St. Louis, MO, and Mark S. Vrahas, MD, Boston, MA.)

without articular involvement can be ignored.

Anterior Column Fracture

The treatment of an anterior column fracture (Figure 5, *D*) is similar to that of an anterior wall fracture. A complete or partial ilioinguinal approach is used, with the patient in the supine position. The anterior column fracture fragment usually is malrotated, and maximal displacement is observed at the pelvic brim. The reduction requires lateral traction on the femoral head and derotation of the anterior column. Traction and internal rotation places the femoral head on the intact posterior wall, often reducing the anterior column. Lateral traction through a Schanz pin placed from lateral to medial into the neck of the femur occasionally is helpful for reduction.

In a high anterior column fracture (including the anterior border of the iliac wing), rotational control of the fracture can be obtained by gripping the anterior border of the bone with a clamp in the interspinous region. A second clamp can be placed across the fracture line at the iliac crest. The fracture usually is fixed with lag screws and a buttress plate (Figure 13, *D*).

Transverse, Transverse and Posterior Wall, and T-Shaped Fractures

In a transverse, transverse and posterior wall, or T-shaped fracture, the transverse fracture component commonly exits the anterior column at the iliopectineal eminence. The level at which it crosses the articular surface and exits the posterior column determines the effect on the joint (Figure 16). An infratectal fracture crosses below the acetabular roof and does not affect the weight-bearing surface, a juxtatectal fracture crosses just below the roof, and a transtectal fracture crosses the weight-bearing surface. Fracture reduction is most critical for a transtectal fracture; however, a juxtatectal fracture in many ways is the most difficult to reduce and stabilize.

Transverse Fracture

In a transverse fracture (Figure 5, *E*), the inferior (ischiopubic) segment is in one piece, and reduction requires the simultaneous control of the displacement and malrotation of the entire segment. The posterior column usually is the site of greatest fracture displacement, and therefore, the Kocher-Langenbeck approach is used. A reduction clamp is placed across the posterior column fracture to reduce the displacement, and a Schanz pin is secured near the ischial tuberosity to control the malrotation (Figure 15). Alternatively, a clamp can be placed across the fracture through the greater sciatic notch (Figure 17). The reduction is confirmed by palpation of the quadrilateral surface through the sciatic notch. A lag screw is directed from the retroacetabular surface across the fracture toward the anterior column. A neutralization plate is placed on the retroacetabular surface to complete the construct (Figure 13, *E*).

Transverse and Posterior Wall Fracture

The posterior wall component of an associated transverse and posterior wall fracture requires a posterior exposure (Figure 5, *G*). The choice of an extended iliofemoral or Kocher-Langenbeck approach is dictated by the configuration of the transverse component or the length of time from injury to surgical treatment. The transverse component is reduced first. Placing a reduction clamp across the posterior column fracture line with a posterior wall fracture present may be challenging; however, retraction of a posterior wall fracture improves visualization of the acetabular articular surface. After the transverse fracture component is fixed with a lag screw across the anterior column and plating or lag screw fixation across the posterior column, the posterior wall fracture is fixed (Figure 13, *G*).

T-Shaped Fracture

The Kocher-Langenbeck approach is used for most T-shaped fractures (Figure 5, *H*). Prone patient positioning on a fracture table is preferred. The anterior column fracture is exposed with longitudinal traction and retraction of the posterior column. As for a transverse fracture, the anterior column is reduced with a clamp (Figure 17) and fixed with a lag screw. The traction is released, the femoral head is repositioned, and the posterior column is reduced. The reduction is confirmed by palpation of the quadrilateral surface through the sciatic notch. A lag screw is inserted across the posterior column, and a plate is placed on the retroacetabular surface to complete the construct (Figure 13, *H*). If this strategy does not allow reduction of the anterior column, the posterior column is reduced and fixed, and the patient is repositioned for a second-stage anterior approach (usually the ilioinguinal approach). If a second-stage anterior approach is required, the posterior column fixation must not cross into the anterior column. Otherwise, independent manipulation of the anterior column fracture fragment will be impossible, and subsequent reduction maneuvers will be blocked.

Anterior Column and Posterior Hemitransverse and Both-Column Fractures

Anterior Column and Posterior Hemitransverse Fracture

In an associated anterior column and posterior hemitransverse fracture (Figure 5, *I*), the primary fracture line involves an anterior wall or column fracture. An associated transverse fracture component originates from the anterior fracture across the articular surface and extends to the posterior border of the innominate bone. The posterior hemitransverse fracture line is identical to the posterior half of a transverse fracture and usually is juxtatectal or infratectal. This fracture almost always is amenable to surgical treatment through the ilioinguinal approach. However, if there is segmental comminution or combined rotational and translational displacement of the posterior column fracture, the extended iliofemoral or staged combined approach is best used. The patient is positioned supine on the fracture table, with traction through a transcondylar femoral pin; or on the radiolucent table with the leg draped free. Sufficient flexion at the hip is necessary to relax the iliopsoas and allow dissection beneath the muscle.

The anterior column or wall is reduced and fixed first, as for an isolated anterior wall or column fracture. A plate is applied along the pelvic brim, leaving holes for subsequent lag screw fixation of the posterior column. The posterior column fracture is reduced using an angled clamp coursing around the iliopsoas; one tine is placed through the middle window onto the quadrilateral surface of the posterior column fragment, and the other tine is placed at the supra-acetabular ilium. An intrapelvic rotational reduction of the posterior column is achieved. The posterior column reduction to both the intact ilium and anterior column is assessed by visualization and fluoroscopic evaluation. However, the reduction of the articular surface can never be directly seen. The fixation construct is completed by screws placed from the internal iliac fossa and directed down the length of the posterior column to exit the ischium or lesser sciatic notch (Figure 13, *I*). In addition, a screw can be placed percutaneously from the outer cortex of the ilium to the quadrilateral surface to fix the posterior column. Screws often can be used alone for fixation of an anterior column and posterior hemitransverse fracture. However, buttress plates along the pelvic brim contribute additional stability, and they always should be used if there is any question about the stability of the screw-only construct, as in a comminuted fracture or a fracture in a patient with osteoporosis. An anterior wall fracture component may require additional buttress plate fixation.

Both-Column Fracture

The ilioinguinal approach is used for most associated both-column fractures (Figure 5, *J*), with the patient in the supine position. Frequently, the technique is similar to that of an anterior column and posterior hemitransverse fracture. The anterior column is first reduced and fixed with lag screws. A plate then is applied along the pelvic brim, with holes left for subsequent lag screw fixation of the posterior column. The posterior column fracture is reduced and fixed to complete the construct (Figure 13, *J*). Like some

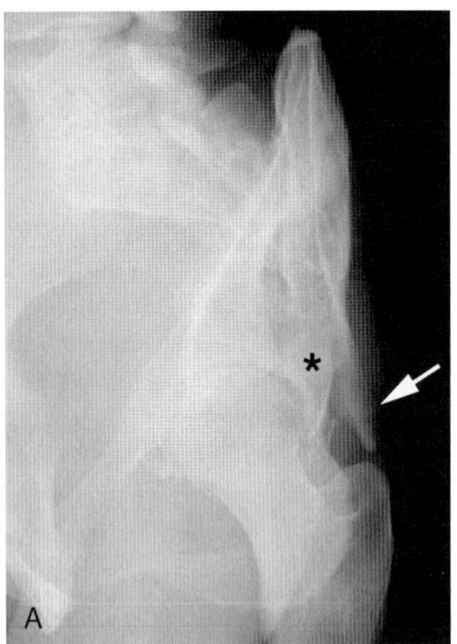

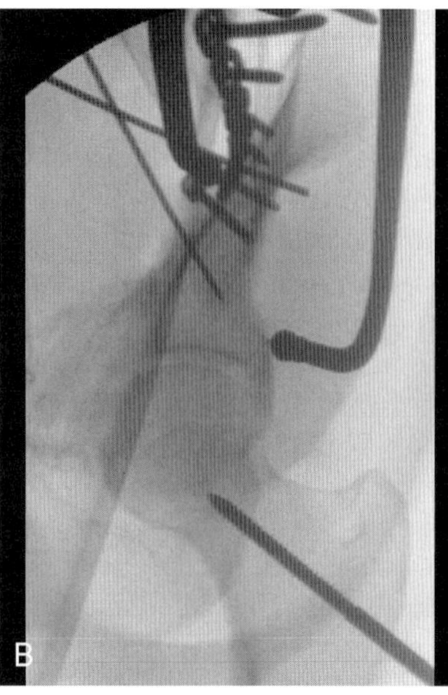

Figure 18 **A,** A preoperative obturator oblique radiograph showing the spur sign (arrow) and a large posterosuperior wall fracture fragment (asterisk). **B,** Intraoperative fluoroscopic view after reduction of the anterior column to the innominate bone; the spur sign is no longer evident, and the wall fracture has been reduced using a large clamp. (Copyright Berton R. Moed, MD, St. Louis, MO.)

anterior column and posterior hemitransverse fractures, many both-column fractures are amenable to lag screw fixation alone.

The extended iliofemoral approach commonly is used if there is a posterior wall fracture, comminution of the posterior column, or involvement of the sacroiliac joint (Figure 13, *K*). However, a posterior wall component of a both-column fracture differs from an isolated posterior wall fracture. The fragment is created at the junction of the anterior and posterior column fracture fragments, and frequently has a large cranial spike of cortical bone associated with it. Even in very comminuted both-column fractures, the acetabular labrum usually remains intact. Therefore, the fragment often can be manipulated by developing a small window of exposure through the interspinous region or over the iliac crest to the lateral surface of the ilium. A reduction clamp is used to reduce the posterior wall (Figure 18). The fracture then can be fixed by obliquely oriented screws inserted just lateral to the pelvic brim and directed posteriorly toward the superior iliac extension of the wall fragment. Buttress plate fixation of the fragment generally is not necessary because the intact capsule and labrum prevent posterior femoral head subluxation.

Acetabular Fracture Treatment With Associated Injuries

A fracture of the acetabulum usually is caused by high-energy blunt trauma. Surgery through a compromised soft-tissue envelope is ill advised because of the increased risk of infection. Therefore, the surrounding soft tissues should be carefully evaluated. Open wounds usually require débridement followed by delayed closure. Closed degloving soft-tissue injuries over the trochanteric region associated with underlying hematoma formation and fat necrosis (the Morel-Lavallé lesion) are associated with the presence of pathogenic bacteria.[41] Débridement followed by delayed wound closure and subsequent delayed fracture fixation often is required.[6,41] Recently, a percutaneous method has been reported, using a plastic brush to débride the injured fatty tissue.[42] A closed-suction drain is placed within the lesion and removed when drainage is less than 30 mL over 24 hours. Fracture fixation is deferred until at least 24 hours after drain removal.

An associated nonacetabular fracture can occur locally about the hip, distal to the hip at the location of the applied traumatic axial load, or at any location between these two points. Its initial treatment often affects later treatment of the acetabular fracture. A displaced fracture of the femoral head may be present, especially in association with a posterior fracture-dislocation, and usually is treated at the time of acetabular fracture fixation.[43] Treatment of a proximal femur fracture may compromise the optimal surgical approach to the acetabulum. This dilemma can be avoided if the proximal femur fracture is treated at the same time as acetabular fracture fixation or if a staged surgical procedure is planned so as not to interfere with optimal acetabular fracture care. A femoral neck fracture often requires immediate surgery, and it would be unusual to treat the acetabular fracture at the same time.[43] The acetabular fracture can be treated later, as required, through a separate, optimal approach. In contrast, an intertrochanteric or subtrochanteric femur fracture does not require urgent surgical treatment. Therefore, the treating physician can choose a staged procedure (proximal femur fracture fixation followed by acetabular fracture fixation) or an appropriately timed delayed fixation of both fractures during a single surgical procedure, using one or more separate incisions. Any treatment scheme should be planned to optimize the treatment of the acetabular fracture.

If both acetabular and femoral shaft fractures are present, the femur usually is stabilized first. Again, staged treatment should be planned for optimal acetabular fracture treatment. If an incision for antegrade nailing would compromise the surgical approach to the acetabulum, an alternative femoral shaft fracture treatment method, such as retrograde nailing, should be selected. When the femoral shaft and acetabular fracture surgeries are performed as sequential procedures during the same anesthesia, antegrade femoral nailing may not be the best choice. Compromised access to the proximal femur, which may occur with a severely displaced both-column fracture, or an irreducible dislocation of the femoral head that precludes satisfactory femoral shaft fracture reduction are two such situations. The alternatives to antegrade nailing include plating or retrograde nailing.

Prevention and Treatment of Postoperative Complications

The rate of infection is approximately 5% after surgical treatment of an acetabular fracture.[6,27,44] The adverse effects of a deep postoperative intra-articular wound infection cannot be minimized. Complete joint destruction occurs in approximately half of such infections.[27,44] The best preventive measures are perioperative antibiotic prophylaxis and meticulous surgical technique, including avoidance of operating through a compromised soft-tissue envelope. The treatment of infection in the acetabular region is similar to treatment in other anatomic regions. In an early infection, the hardware is preserved, if possible, until union to maintain the stability of the hip, and it is then removed. Late infection is treated with hardware removal. Long-term, culture-specific antibiotics are required for all infections, usually as an empiric course of 6 weeks.

Although the superior gluteal, inferior gluteal, obturator, and femoral nerves may be injured during acetabular surgery, these injuries appear to have a low prevalence. However, iatrogenic damage to the sciatic nerve is one of the most clinically important complications of acetabular fracture management, occurring in approximately 3% of cases.[27] These injuries usually are associated with the posterior and extended surgical approaches that involve direct exposure and retraction of the sciatic nerve.[6,45] Injury also can occur through an anterior surgical approach used for indirect reduction of posterior column displacement.[6,46,47] Although intraoperative nerve monitoring has been promoted, no data clearly indicate that nerve monitoring reduces the overall rate of iatrogenic sciatic nerve injury. There is no substitute for attention to detail in the operating room with respect to positioning the patient, maintaining the knee flexed to relax the sciatic nerve (for a posterior approach), placing retractors cautiously, and limiting traction on the nerve during fracture reduction.

Intra-articular placement of screws is a documented, destructive complication of acetabular fracture surgery. Letournel and Judet[6] originally proposed detecting intra-articular hardware by listening for crepitus as the hip is taken through the range of motion in the operating room, under conditions of complete silence. Anglen and DiPasquale[48] recommended using a sterile esophageal stethoscope for the same purpose. Other authors have recommended intraoperative and postoperative radiography to ensure that the hardware has been placed outside the joint.[49,50] Currently, intraoperative fluoroscopy appears to be the best method[39] (Figure 14). If hardware has been placed within the joint, removal of the implant is imperative.

Magnetic resonance venography identified proximal deep venous thrombosis in 34% of patients with an acetabular fracture.[51] Letournel and Judet[6] reported that 13 of 565 patients (2.3%) died after acetabular fracture surgery, and that 4 of these deaths were caused by massive pulmonary embolism. Some form of mechanical or chemical prophylaxis is recommended to decrease the risk of thromboembolic complications. The use of mechanical prophylaxis with a foot pump beginning at the time of hospital admission, with the addition of enoxaparin 5 days after all acute bleeding from the blunt trauma had resolved, was found to be successful for prophylaxis against venous thromboembolic disease after serious musculoskeletal injury.[52] The prevalence of large or occlusive deep venous thromboses among patients who had been managed with this protocol was significantly less than that among patients who had been managed with enoxaparin alone, initiated 24 to 48 hours after blunt trauma.[52] Enoxaparin was discontinued the night before surgery and resumed within 12 hours after surgery. Despite prophylactic treatment, the rate of posttraumatic and postoperative thromboembolism is approximately 11%.[52-54] Screening with Doppler ultrasonography or magnetic resonance venography remains controversial.[54] The placement of prophylactic vena cava filters is controversial, but it may be indicated for some high-risk patients.[54,55] The risk continues after discharge from the hospital, and it is prudent to continue postoperative prophylaxis until the patient is fully ambulatory.[6,56]

Severe heterotopic ossification of the hip is clinically defined as involving a loss of motion of at least 20%.[27] Using this criterion, Matta[27] reported its prevalence as 20% using the extended iliofemoral approach, 8% for the Kocher-Langenbeck, and 2% for the ilioinguinal. The most important risk factor for heterotopic ossification is the stripping of the gluteal muscles from the external surface of the ilium.[6,27,32,57,58] Although heterotopic ossification is an important postoperative complication, the risks associated with the available prophylactic treatments, their potential for failure, and the actual risk of occurrence must be weighed for each individual patient. A study of patients with acetabular fracture found that the use of indomethacin increases the risk of long-bone nonunion.[59] Induced malignant disease is a possible consequence of low-dose radiation therapy.[60] One study of a cohort of 2,067 women receiving 2.6 to 5.3 Gy of midline radiation for the benign condition metropathia hemorrhagica and followed for an average of 28 years found an increase in mortality from cancers of the irradiated pelvic sites.[60] However, for the radiation dosage and methods used for the prophylaxis of heterotopic ossification about the hip, the likelihood of induced malignancy is very low.[61] In deciding on prophylactic therapy, the clinician must keep in mind the actual rates of functionally important heterotopic ossification. Delayed excision of mature, functionally significant heterotopic ossification is a viable treatment option after unsuccessful prophylactic therapy and an alternative to prophylaxis. Functional improvement can be expected in patients with congruent joint surfaces, and Letournel and Judet[6] reported only one poor result in 14 patients. Delayed excision surgery is a relatively low risk procedure with good results, and a return to more than 80% of normal motion can be expected.[6,32,62]

Posttraumatic arthritis is the most common complication after an acetabular fracture. The quality of the fracture reduction appears to be the main determinant for clinical outcome and for the risk of late traumatic arthritis..[6,27,44] Damage to the femoral head at the time of initial injury is another important factor.[27] Osteonecrosis of the femoral head is known to result from acetabular fracture associated with hip dislocation and can also result in posttraumatic arthritis.[27,37] However, posttraumatic arthritis is more commonly caused by wear of the femoral head against a malreduced fracture.[6,27] Total hip arthroplasty or arthrodesis is indicated for patients who have disabling pain from posttraumatic arthritis.

Results of Surgical Treatment

The three largest studies of the outcome of acetabular fractures treated within 3 weeks of injury found a 75% to 81% rate of good or excellent results at long-term follow-up.[6,27,44] The most important objective of surgical treatment is to obtain an anatomic reduction of the articular surface, and the clinical outcome is strongly correlated with the adequacy of fracture reduction.[6,27] Letournel and Judet[6] studied 492 acetabular fractures followed for at least 1 year and found that anatomic reduction was achieved in 366 (74%), of which 316 (86%) had a good to excellent result. However, only 64% of those with an imperfect reduction (81 of 126 patients) had a good to excellent result. Among patients who had posttraumatic arthritis after a perfect articular reduction (10%), 50% had arthritis appearing 10 to 25 years after the injury. In contrast, among those who had posttraumatic arthritis after an imperfect reduction (36%), 80% had arthritis appearing within the first 10 years after injury.[6] Matta[27] found that achieving an anatomic reduction (defined 1 mm or less of residual displacement) is the most important determinant of the outcome of acetabular fracture surgery. Therefore, the surgeon must strive for a so-called inframillimetric reduction of every fracture to maximize the patient's quality of life after the injury.

The rate of anatomic reduction decreases with greater fracture complexity, patient age, and delay from injury to fixation.[27] The time from injury to fracture fixation has a dramatic effect on the outcome. Letournel and Judet[6] found that among 138 patients who were treated after a 3-week delay, the rate of good to excellent results was only 54%; Johnson and associates[63] found that 65% of 187 such patients had a good to excellent result. In a study of 237 patients, Madhu and associates[64] found that a fracture of an elementary type was more likely to be anatomically reduced and have a good to excellent clinical outcome if surgery was performed within 15 days; a fracture of an associated type was more likely to be anatomically reduced if the surgery was performed within 5 days and was more likely to have a good to excellent clinical outcome if the surgery was performed within 10 days.

Fractures of some types appear to have better outcomes after surgical treatment than fractures of other types. Both-column fractures are complex injuries and technically demanding; however, their outcome generally is better than that of many other fracture types despite a higher rate of nonanatomic reduction. Matta[27] obtained anatomic reduction in only 57% of these cases; nonetheless, 77% of patients had a good to excellent result. The treatment of posterior wall fractures is straightforward, with reported rates of anatomic reduction as high as 100%.[27] However, Matta[27] reported a 32% clinical failure rate in 22 treated fractures, despite having obtained anatomic reduction in every fracture. This rate was higher than that of any other fracture type. Aho and associates[65] and Chiu and associates[66] reported similar results. However, other researchers reported results of posterior wall fractures similar to those of other types of acetabular fractures (more than 80% good to excellent clinical outcomes).[6,36,37] Letournel and Judet[6] suggested and Moed and associates[40] later established that the disparity between apparent anatomic reduction, as determined by plain radiography, and clinical results is largely attributable to the inadequacy of radiographs for assessing the quality of the postoperative posterior wall reduction. Postoperative CT appears to be a more accurate means of documenting articular reduction after a posterior wall fracture.[40]

Summary

The goals of treating an acetabular fracture are to restore hip joint congruity and stability. Although some fracture types may not require surgery for a satisfactory outcome, in general a patient with a displaced fracture in the weight-bearing area of the acetabulum should be treated with open reduction and internal fixation. The surgery is complex and demanding, and fracture reduction must be anatomic to obtain the best results. However, there is no doubt that an experienced surgeon can obtain an excellent result. Poor results are related mainly to residual fracture displacement and perioperative complications. When treating an acetabular fracture, the surgeon must be cognizant of the importance of the evaluation and treatment protocols initially developed by Letournel and Judet, as well as the progress made during the past decade.

References

1. Knight RA, Smith H: Central fractures of the acetabulum. *J Bone Joint Surg Am* 1958;40:1-16.
2. Rowe CR, Lowell JD: Prognosis of fractures of the acetabulum. *J Bone Joint Surg Am* 1961;43A:30-59.
3. Stewart MJ: Discussion: Prognosis of fractures of the acetabulum. *J Bone Joint Surg Am* 1961;43A:59.
4. Stewart MJ, Milford LW: Fracture-dislocation of the hip: An end-result study. *J Bone Joint Surg Am* 1954;36:315-342.
5. Judet R, Judet J, Letournel E: Fractures of the acetabulum: Classification and surgical approaches for open reduction. Preliminary report. *J Bone Joint Surg Am* 1964;46:1615-1646.
6. Letournel E, Judet R: *Fractures of the Acetabulum*, ed 2. New York, NY, Springer-Verlag, 1993.
7. Templeman DC, Olson S, Moed BR, Duwelius P, Matta JM: Surgical treatment of acetabular fractures. *Instr Course Lect* 1999;48:481-496.
8. Borrelli J Jr, Goldfarb C, Catalano L, Evanoff BA: Assessment of articular fragment displacement in acetabular fractures: A comparison of computerized tomography and plain radiographs. *J Orthop Trauma* 2002;16:449-456.
9. Moed BR, Ajibade DA, Israel H: Computed tomography as a predictor of hip stability status in posterior wall fractures of the acetabulum. *J Orthop Trauma* 2009;23:7-15.
10. Helfet DL, Bartlett CS III: Acetabular fractures: Evaluation/classification/treatment concepts and approaches, in Ruedi TP, Murphy WM, eds: *AO Principles of Fracture Management*, New York, NY, Thieme, 2001, pp 419-442.
11. Marsh JL, Slongo TF, Agel J, et al: Fracture and dislocation classification compendium, 2007: Orthopaedic Trauma Association classification, database and outcomes committee. *J Orthop Trauma* 2007;21:S1-S133.
12. Beaulé PE, Dorey FJ, Matta JM: Letournel classification for acetabular fractures: Assessment of interobserver and intraobserver reliability. *J Bone Joint Surg Am* 2003;85:1704-1709.
13. Heeg M, Oostvogel HJ, Klasen HJ: Conservative treatment of acetabular fractures: The role of the weight-bearing dome and anatomic reduction in the ultimate results. *J Trauma* 1987;27:555-559.
14. Matta JM, Anderson LM, Epstein HC, Hendricks P: Fractures of the acetabulum: A retrospective analysis. *Clin Orthop Relat Res* 1986;205:230-240.
15. Olsen SA, Matta JM: The computerized tomography subchondral arc: A new method of assessing acetabular articular continuity after fracture. A preliminary report. *J Orthop Trauma* 1993;7:402-413.
16. Tile M, Helfet DL, Kellam JF: *Fractures of the Pelvis and Acetabulum*. Philadelphia, PA, Lippincott Williams and Wilkins, 2003.
17. Matta JM, Merritt PO: Displaced acetabular fractures. *Clin Orthop Relat Res* 1988;230:83-97.

18. Vrahas MS, Widding KK, Thomas KA: The effects of simulated transverse, anterior column, and posterior column fractures of the acetabulum on the stability of the hip joint. *J Bone Joint Surg Am* 1999;81:966-974.

19. Heeg M, Otter N, Klasen HJ: Anterior column fractures of the acetabulum. *J Bone Joint Surg Br* 1992;74: 554-557.

20. Crowl AC, Kahler DM: Closed reduction and percutaneous fixation of anterior column acetabular fractures. *Comput Aided Surg* 2002;7:169-178.

21. Kahler DM, DeGrange D, Wang G-J: Percutaneous fixation of selected acetabular fractures using computed tomographic guidance. *Orthop Trans* 1996;20:83.

22. Starr AJ, Reinert CM, Jones AL: Percutaneous fixation of columns of the acetabulum: A new technique. *J Orthop Trauma* 1998;12:51-58.

23. Tornetta P III: Non-operative management of acetabular fractures: The use of dynamic stress views. *J Bone Joint Surg Br* 1999;81:67-70.

24. Helfet DL, Borrelli J Jr, DiPasquale T, Sanders R: Stabilization of acetabular fractures in elderly patients. *J Bone Joint Surg Am* 1992;74: 753-765.

25. Sermon A, Broos P, Vanderschot P: Total hip replacement for acetabular fractures: Results in 121 patients operated between 1983 and 2003. *Injury* 2008;39:914-921.

26. Spencer RF: Acetabular fractures in older patients. *J Bone Joint Surg Br* 1989;71:774-776.

27. Matta J: Fractures of the acetabulum: Accuracy of reduction and clinical results in patients managed operatively within three weeks after the injury. *J Bone Joint Surg Am* 1996;78:1632-1645.

28. Dean DB, Moed BR: Late salvage of failed open reduction and internal fixation of posterior wall fractures of the acetabulum. *J Orthop Trauma* 2009;23: 180-185.

29. Helfet DL, Schmeling GJ: Management of complex acetabular fractures through single nonextensile exposures. *Clin Orthop Relat Res* 1994;305: 58-68.

30. Cole JD, Bolhofner BR: Acetabular fracture fixation via a modified Stoppa limited intrapelvic approach: Description of operative technique and preliminary treatment results. *Clin Orthop Relat Res* 1994;305: 112-123.

31. Qureshi AA, Archdeacon MT, Jenkins MA, Infante A, DiPasquale T, Bolhofner BR: Infrapectineal plating for acetabular fractures: A technical adjunct to internal fixation. *J Orthop Trauma* 2004;18:175-178.

32. Mears DC, Rubash H: *Pelvic and Acetabular Fractures*. Thorofare, NJ, Slack, 1986.

33. Ellis TJ, Beck M: Trochanteric osteotomy for acetabular fractures and proximal femur fractures. *Orthop Clin North Am* 2004;35:457-461.

34. Siebenrock KA, Gautier E, Ziran BH, Ganz R: Trochanteric flip osteotomy for cranial extension and muscle protection in acetabular fracture fixation using the Kocher-Langenbeck approach. *J Orthop Trauma* 1998;12: 387-391.

35. Harris MA, Althausen P, Kellam JF, Bosse MJ: Simultaneous anterior and posterior approaches for complex acetabular fractures. *J Orthop Trauma* 2008;22:494-497.

36. Giannoudis PV, Tzioupis CC, Moed BR: Two-level reconstruction of comminuted posterior-wall fractures of the acetabulum. *J Bone Joint Surg Br* 2007;89:503-509.

37. Moed BR, WillsonCarr SE, Watson JT: Results of operative treatment of fractures of the posterior wall of the acetabulum. *J Bone Joint Surg Am* 2002;84:752-758.

38. Moed BR, McMichael JC: Outcomes of posterior wall fractures of the acetabulum: Surgical technique. *J Bone Joint Surg Am* 2008;90:87-107.

39. Carmack DB, Moed BR, McCarroll K, Freccero D: Accuracy of detecting screw penetration of the acetabulum with intraoperative fluoroscopy and computed tomography. *J Bone Joint Surg Am* 2001;83: 1370-1375.

40. Moed BR, Carr SE, Gruson KI, Watson JT, Craig JG: Computed tomography assessment of fractures of the posterior wall of the acetabulum after operative treatment. *J Bone Joint Surg Am* 2003;85:512-522.

41. Hak DJ, Olson SA, Matta JM: Diagnosis and management of closed internal degloving injuries associated with pelvic and acetabular fractures: The Morel-Lavallée lesion. *J Trauma* 1997;42:1046-1051.

42. Tseng S, Tornetta P III: Percutaneous management of Morel-Lavallee lesions. *J Bone Joint Surg Am* 2006;88: 92-96.

43. Kregor PJ, Templeman D: Associated injuries complicating the management of acetabular fractures: Review and case studies. *Orthop Clin North Am* 2002;33:73-95.

44. Mayo KA: Open reduction and internal fixation of fractures of the acetabulum: Results in 163 fractures. *Clin Orthop Relat Res* 1994;305:31-37.

45. Vrahas M, Gordon RG, Mears DC, Krieger D, Sclabassi RJ: Intraoperative somatosensory evoked potential monitoring of pelvic and acetabular fractures. *J Orthop Trauma* 1992;6: 50-58.

46. Dunbar RP Jr, Gardner MJ, Cunningham B, Routt ML Jr: Sciatic nerve entrapment in associated both-column acetabular fractures: A report of 2 cases and review of the literature. *J Orthop Trauma* 2009;23:80-83.

47. Helfet DL, Schmeling GJ: Somatosensory evoked potential monitoring in the surgical treatment of acute, displaced acetabular fractures: Results of a prospective study. *Clin Orthop Relat Res* 1994;301:213-220.

48. Anglen JO, DiPasquale T: The reliability of detecting screw penetration of the acetabulum by intraoperative auscultation. *J Orthop Trauma* 1994;8: 404-408.

49. Ebraheim NA, Savolaine ER, Hoeflinger MJ, Jackson WT: Radiological

diagnosis of screw penetration of the hip joint in acetabular fracture reconstruction. *J Orthop Trauma* 1989;3: 196-201.

50. Norris BL, Hahn DH, Bosse MJ, Kellam JF, Sims SH: Intraoperative fluoroscopy to evaluate fracture reduction and hardware placement during acetabular surgery. *J Orthop Trauma* 1999;13:414-417.

51. Montgomery KD, Potter HG, Helfet DL: The detection and management of proximal deep vein thrombosis in patients with acute acetabular fractures: A follow-up report. *J Orthop Trauma* 1997;11:330-336.

52. Stannard JP, Lopez-Ben RR, Volgas DA, et al: Prophylaxis against deep-vein thrombosis following trauma: A prospective, randomized comparison of mechanical and pharmacologic prophylaxis. *J Bone Joint Surg Am* 2006;88:261-266.

53. Stannard JP, Singhania AK, Lopez-Ben RR, et al: Deep-vein thrombosis in high-energy skeletal trauma despite thromboprophylaxis. *J Bone Joint Surg Br* 2005;87:965-968.

54. Borer DS, Starr AJ, Reinert CM, et al: The effect of screening for deep vein thrombosis on the prevalence of pulmonary embolism in patients with fractures of the pelvis or acetabulum: A review of 973 patients. *J Orthop Trauma* 2005;19:92-95.

55. Rogers FB, Shackford SR, Ricci MA, Huber BM, Atkins T: Prophylactic vena cava filter insertion in selected high-risk orthopaedic trauma patients. *J Orthop Trauma* 1997;11: 267-272.

56. Bjørnarå BT, Gudmundsen TE, Dahl OE: Frequency and timing of clinical venous thromboembolism after major joint surgery. *J Bone Joint Surg Br* 2006;88:386-391.

57. Bosse MJ, Poka A, Reinert CM, Ellwanger F, Slawson R, McDevitt ER: Heterotopic ossification as a complication of acetabular fracture: Prophylaxis with low-dose irradiation. *J Bone Joint Surg Am* 1988;70:1231-1237.

58. Moed BR, Maxey JW: The effect of indomethacin on heterotopic ossification following acetabular fracture surgery. *J Orthop Trauma* 1993;7:33-38.

59. Burd TA, Hughes MS, Anglen JO: Heterotopic ossification prophylaxis with indomethacin increases the risk of long-bone nonunion. *J Bone Joint Surg Br* 2003;85:700-705.

60. Darby SC, Reeves G, Key T, Doll R, Stovall M: Mortality in a cohort of women given x-ray therapy for metropathia haemorrhagica. *Int J Cancer* 1994;56:793-801.

61. Haas ML, Kennedy AS, Copeland CC, Ames JW, Scarboro M, Slawson RG: Utility of radiation in the prevention of heterotopic ossification following repair of traumatic acetabular fracture. *Int J Radiat Oncol Biol Phys* 1999;45: 461-468.

62. Webb LX, Bosse MJ, Mayo KA, Lange RH, Miller ME, Swiontkowski MF: Results in patients with craniocerebral trauma and an operatively managed acetabular fracture. *J Orthop Trauma* 1990;4:376-382.

63. Johnson EE, Matta JM, Mast JW, Letournel E: Delayed reconstruction of acetabular fractures 21-120 days following injury. *Clin Orthop Relat Res* 1994;305:20-30.

64. Madhu R, Kotnis R, Al-Mousawi A, et al: Outcome of surgery for reconstruction of fractures of the acetabulum: The time dependent effect of delay. *J Bone Joint Surg Br* 2006;88: 1197-1203.

65. Aho AJ, Isberg UK, Katevuo VK: Acetabular posterior wall fracture: 38 cases followed for 5 years. *Acta Orthop Scand* 1986;57:101-105.

66. Chiu FY, Lo WH, Chen TH, Chen CM, Huang CK, Ma HL: Fractures of posterior wall of acetabulum. *Arch Orthop Trauma Surg* 1996;115: 273-275.

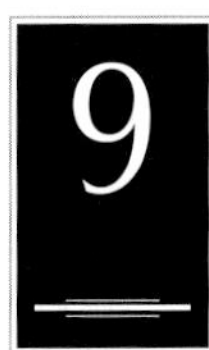

Intertrochanteric Fractures: Ten Tips to Improve Results

George J. Haidukewych, MD

Abstract

Intertrochanteric hip fractures are among the most common types of fractures, and the numbers are increasing as the population ages. Most intertrochanteric fractures are treated surgically. It is therefore important that the treatment methods are effective and have a minimal risk of complications. The goals of treatment include a predictable union, unrestricted early weight bearing, and avoidance of fixation failure or excessive deformity of the proximal femur. Careful attention to the fracture pattern (obliquity or other hallmarks implying instability) can guide fixation device selection. Regardless of the device, accurate reduction and implant placement are important to a good outcome.

Intertrochanteric hip fractures are becoming increasingly common as the population ages. These fractures typically occur in frail patients with multiple medical comorbidities and often result in loss of the patient's functional independence. The all-too-often problematic dispositions and prolonged hospital stays result in a tremendous cost to patients, their families, and society. Effective treatment strategies that result in high rates of union of these fractures and low rates of complications are important. Orthopaedic surgeons cannot control the quality of the bone, patient compliance, or comorbidities, but they should be able to minimize the morbidity associated with the fracture. Doing so requires choosing the appropriate fixation device for the fracture pattern, recognizing the problem fracture patterns, and performing accurate reductions with ideal implant placement while being conscious of implant costs. If these fractures are treated expeditiously, fixation failures minimized, and underlying osteoporosis is recognized and treated accordingly, patients outcomes will improve and the cost of treatment will decrease. The purpose of this review is to summarize 10 simple tips to help minimize failures and improve outcomes when treating intertrochanteric fractures.

Tip 1: Use the Tip-to-Apex Distance

The tip-to-apex distance has been described by Baumgaertner and associates[1,2] as a useful intraoperative indicator of deep and central placement of the lag screw in the femoral head, regardless of whether a nail or a plate is chosen to fix the fracture (Figure 1). This is perhaps the most important measurement of accurate hardware placement and has been shown in multiple studies to be predictive of success after the treatment of standard obliquity intertrochanteric fractures. Older theories about screw placement favored a low and occasionally a posterior position of the lag screw, thereby leaving more bone superior and anterior to the screw. This position effectively lengthens the tip-to-apex distance and should be avoided. The ideal position for a lag screw in both planes is deep and central in the femoral head within 10 mm of the subchondral bone[3,4] (Figure 2). A

Dr. Haidukewych or an immediate family member serves as a board member, owner, officer, or committee member of the Florida Orthopaedic Institute; has received royalties from DePuy and Zimmer; is a member of a speakers' bureau or has made paid presentations on behalf of DePuy; serves as a paid consultant to or is an employee of DePuy and Surmodics; has received research or institutional support from DePuy; and has stock or stock options held in Surmodics.

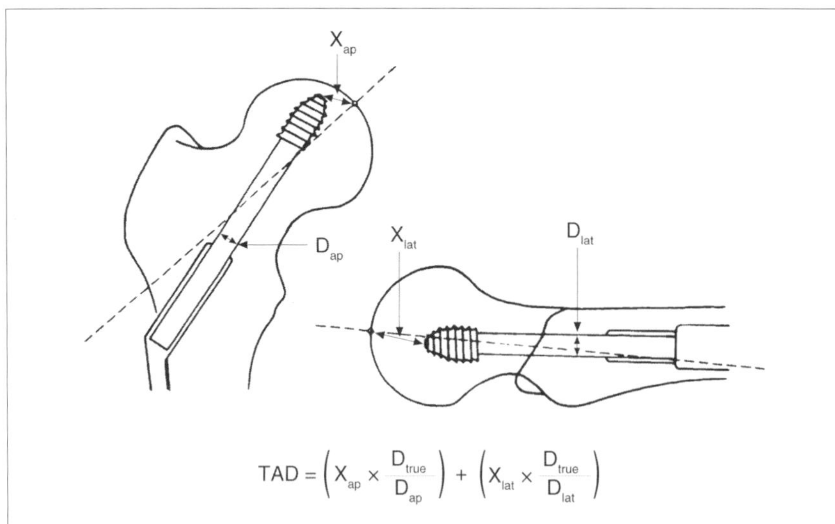

Figure 1 The technique for calculating the tip-to-apex distance (TAD). For clarity, a peripherally placed screw is depicted in the anteroposterior (ap) view, and a shallowly placed screw is depicted in the lateral (lat) view. D_{true} = known diameter of the lag screw. (Reproduced with permission from Baumgaertner MR, Curtin SL, Lindskog DM, Keggi JM: The value of the tip-apex distance in predicting failure of fixation of peritrochanteric fractures of the hip. *J Bone Joint Surg Am* 1995;77:1059.)

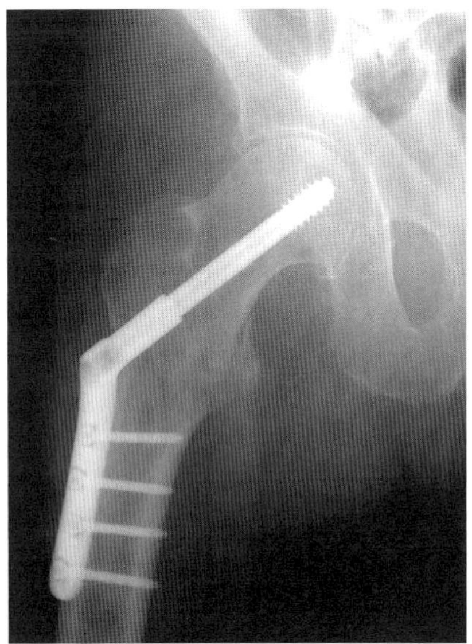

Figure 2 Radiograph showing excellent reduction and deep, central placement of the lag screw in the femoral head.

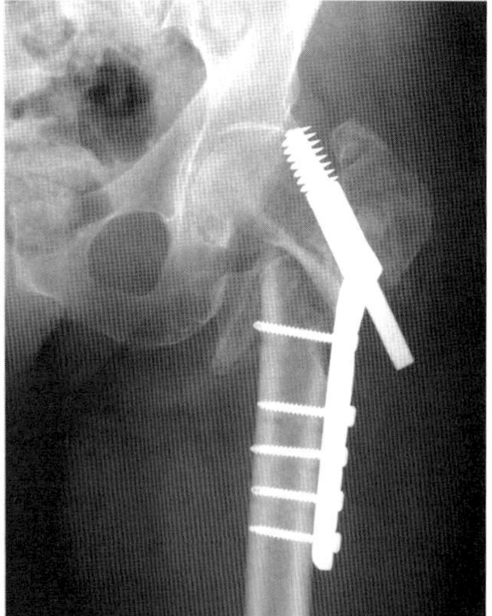

Figure 3 Radiograph showing failed fixation of a reverse obliquity fracture with lateralization of the proximal fragment and screw cutout.

tip-to-apex distance of less than 25 mm has been shown to be generally predictive of a successful result; however, most traumatologists aim for a tip-to-apex distance of less than 20 mm.

Tip 2: No Lateral Wall, No Hip Screw

Fractures that involve the lateral wall of the proximal part of the femur are, by definition, either reverse obliquity fractures or transtrochanteric fractures. These fractures do not have any lateral osseous buttress, and therefore, if a sliding hip screw is used, medial translation of the femoral shaft and lateralization of the proximal femoral fragment can occur. The result is deformity, nonunion, and screw cutout (Figure 3). Haidukewych and associates[5] found a 56% failure rate when a sliding hip screw had been used for reverse obliquity fractures of the proximal part of the femur. Although devices with a trochanteric stabilizing plate, those with a proximal trochanteric flare, and those that allow axial compression and locking of the sliding hip screw (such as the Medoff device) are reported to have reasonably good results, a hip screw should not be used if there is no lateral wall.[3-9] Locking plates and 95-degree condylar blade plates may function as prosthetic lateral cortices, but the results of using these devices for more problematic fractures of the proximal part of the femur are not available.[9-11] Intramedullary nails seem to be superior to dynamic condylar screws for reverse obliquity fractures, but comparative studies of intramedullary nails and proximal femoral locking plates are not available.

Tip 3: Know the Unstable Intertrochanteric Fracture Patterns and Nail Them

There are four classic intertrochanteric fracture patterns that signify instability. When internally fixed, the osseous fragments of these unstable fractures are not able to share the weight-bearing loads, and therefore the loads are predominantly borne by the internal fixation device. The unstable patterns include reverse obliquity fractures, transtrochanteric fractures, fractures with a large posteromedial fragment implying loss of the calcar buttress, and fractures with subtrochanteric extension[3-5,9,12-16] (Figures 4 through 7). These fractures, in general, should be treated with an intramedullary nail because of the more favorable biomechanical properties of an intramedullary nail compared with a sliding hip screw. An intramedullary nail is located closer to the center of gravity than is a sliding hip screw, and therefore the lever arm on the femoral fixation is shorter. Intramedullary nails can more reliably resist the relatively high forces across the medial calcar that are typically borne by the implant in an unstable fracture. The intramedullary position of the implant also prevents shaft medialization, which is a common complication associated with the transtrochanteric and reverse obliquity fracture patterns. Recognizing the unstable patterns preoperatively and choosing to use an intramedullary nail decrease the risk of fixation failure. A simple fracture of the lesser trochanter does not, in itself, automatically imply an unstable fracture, as many three-part and four-part fractures can include a small, relatively unimportant fracture of the lesser trochanter and yet have a primary fracture line that will tolerate compression well. It is not known how large the posteromedial fragment must be to be mechanically important. When there is doubt about the status of the calcar, however, an intramedullary nail is preferable to a sliding hip screw.

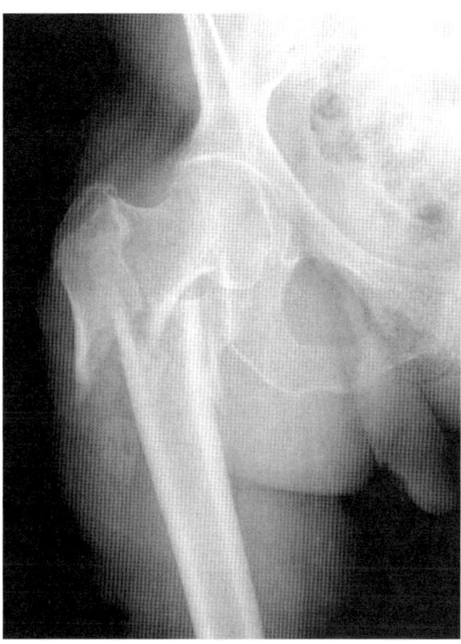

Figure 4 Radiograph showing a reverse obliquity fracture.

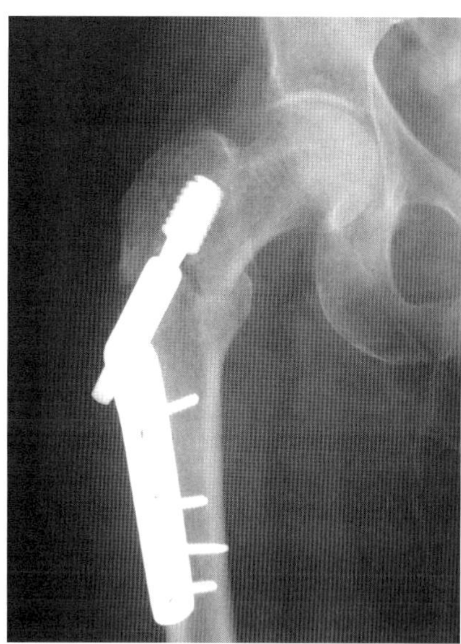

Figure 5 Radiograph showing a transtrochanteric fracture.

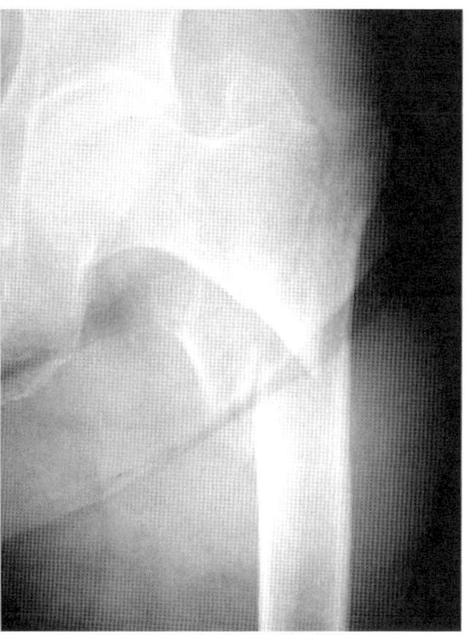

Figure 6 Radiograph showing a four-part fracture with a large posteromedial fragment.

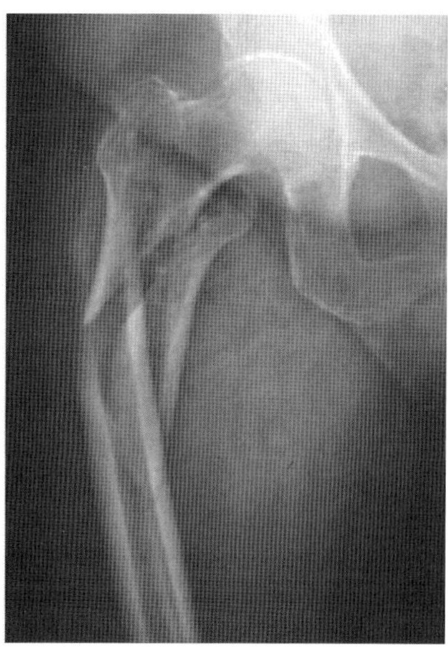

Figure 7 Radiograph showing a fracture with subtrochanteric extension.

Tip 4: Beware of the Anterior Bow of the Femoral Shaft

As a person ages, the femoral diaphysis enlarges, and the femoral bow increases.[17] Most commercial intramedullary nails have gradually evolved into a more bowed design, and many of them now have a radius of curvature of less than 2 m. The concern with using a straight intramedullary nail in a bowed osteopenic femur is that the nail can impinge on, and in some cases even perforate, the anterior femoral metaphyseal cortex distally (Figure 8). Additionally, when the nail hugs the anterior femoral cortex, any locking screws placed in the distal part of the femur may cause a stress riser in this area, which may lead to a fracture during the postoperative rehabilitation period. It is wise to know the radius of curvature of the particular device, which ideally should be no more than 2 m. Most commercially available in-

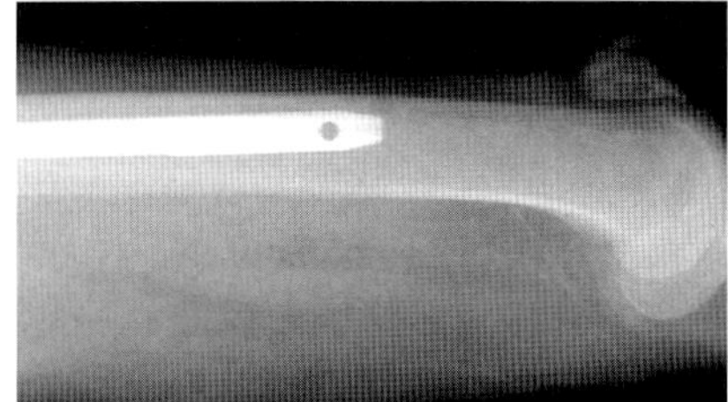

Figure 8 Radiograph showing a straight nail inserted into a bowed femur. Vigorous impaction or a bow mismatch may lead to perforation of the distal anterior femoral cortex.

tramedullary nails have a radius of curvature of between 1.5 and 2.2 m. It is also important to recognize that, if resistance is encountered during insertion of a long intramedullary nail for fixation of an intertrochanteric fracture, the surgeon should obtain a lateral radiograph of the distal part of the femur rather than trying to impact the device with a hammer. Hammering in a long intramedullary nail that is impinging on the anterior cortex can produce an iatrogenic fracture.

Tip 5: When Using a Trochanteric Entry Nail, Start Slightly Medial to the Exact Tip of the Greater Trochanter

The patient's soft-tissue mass, the surgical drapes, the trajectory of the reamer insertion and of the reaming, and the nail insertion can gradually enlarge the pilot hole in the greater trochanter laterally. This enlargement leads to more lateral placement of the intramedullary nail than intended. In turn, this can result in a varus reduction of the proximal fragment or a high lag-screw position in the femoral head, both of which are undesirable. A starting point slightly medial to the exact tip of the trochanter is recommended[18] (Figure 9). The starter reamer is used while it is observed with fluoroscopy, and subsequent reaming is performed very carefully. Use of the reamers should not be started until they are well contained in the proximal part of the femur. This avoids any gradual lateral enlargement of the pilot hole.

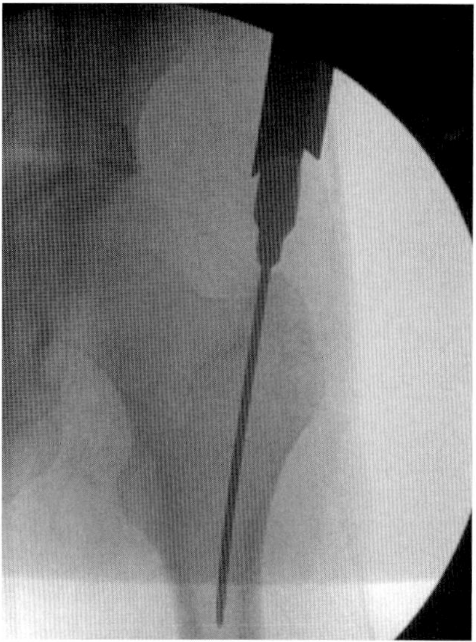

Figure 9 Fluoroscopic image showing the ideal starting point slightly medial to the exact tip of the greater trochanter. Note the good position of the guidewire distally.

Tip 6: Do Not Ream an Unreduced Fracture

In sharp contradistinction to diaphyseal fractures of the femur, which may be reamed in a position that is not necessarily well reduced because the interference fit in the diaphysis aligns the fracture as the intramedullary nail is passed, a misaligned intertrochanteric fracture cannot be reduced simply by passing the intramedullary nail across it. The intertrochanteric fracture should be reduced to an aligned position before reaming and passing of the intramedullary nail. One must remember that the way that these fractures look during reaming will not change after the nail has been inserted.

It is not possible to make a starting point in the proximal fragment and then manipulate this fragment with a reduction tool or even the intramedullary nail because the bone is too soft and the medullary canal is too large. Obtaining good muscle relaxation and then performing a gentle closed reduction with the patient on a fracture table while observing the fracture with fluoroscopy is recommended. If reduction cannot be obtained by closed means, then some form of percutaneous or miniopen reduction is recommended. A bone hook placed along the lesser trochanter, or even percutaneous joysticks or clamps, can be used to reduce the fragment without the need for substantial periosteal stripping or evacuation of the fracture hematoma (Figure 10). The fragment can then be reamed, and the intramedullary nail can be inserted.

Tip 7: Be Cautious About the Nail Insertion Trajectory and Do Not Use a Hammer to Seat the Nail

It is important to achieve a vertical trajectory with nail insertion. This can be difficult in obese patients. Even if care was taken with the starting point and the subsequent reaming, if the intramedullary nail is inserted at an oblique angle, the nail itself can impact the relatively soft bone of the lateral aspect of the greater trochanter and lead to a relatively oval entry point and a lateral position of the intramedullary nail in the proximal fragment. It is critical that the nail be inserted by hand with slight rotational motions. A hammer is not recommended because its use can lead to iatrogenic femoral fracture. It is safe to tap the jig with a mallet for the final seating; this is an easy way to fine-tune the final position of the intramedullary nail. The mallet should not be used if difficulty is encountered when inserting the intramedullary nail by hand. The variety of diameters at the distal end and valgus angles at the proximal end of modern intramedullary nail systems have decreased the frequency of iatrogenic femoral fractures.[19] It is still important to realize that, if a hammer is needed to advance the nail (as opposed to simply tapping it in a few final millimeters), there is a problem. The femoral shaft may need to be reamed further to prevent nail incarceration (this is not uncommon in younger patients), or there may be impingement on the anterior femoral cortex with a mismatch between the bows of the femur and the intramedullary nail. The cause of the difficulty should be identified and corrected because the intramedullary nail should be passed by hand. The suggested procedure is to ream the intramedullary canal to a diameter that is 1 mm larger than the diameter of the selected intramedullary nail and to ensure that the starter reamer has been inserted to the recommended depth. This prevents the funnel shape of the proximal nail from impinging on the endosteum proximally and preventing final seating.

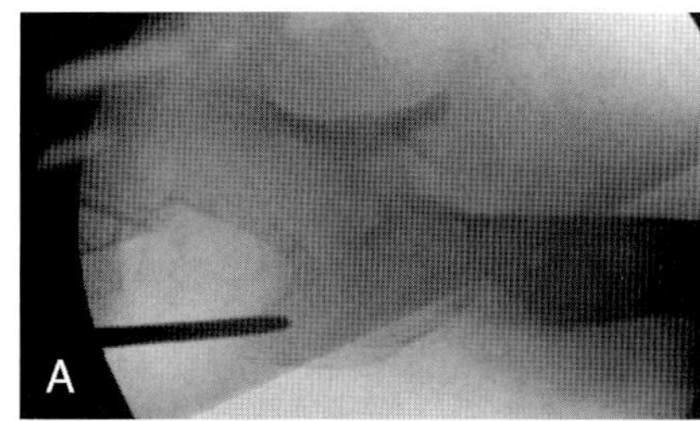

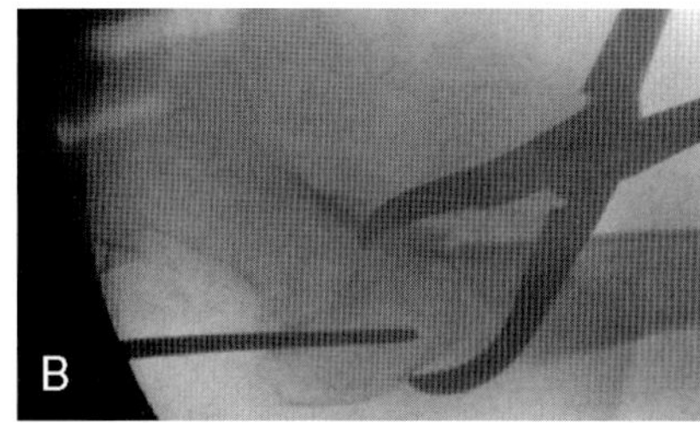

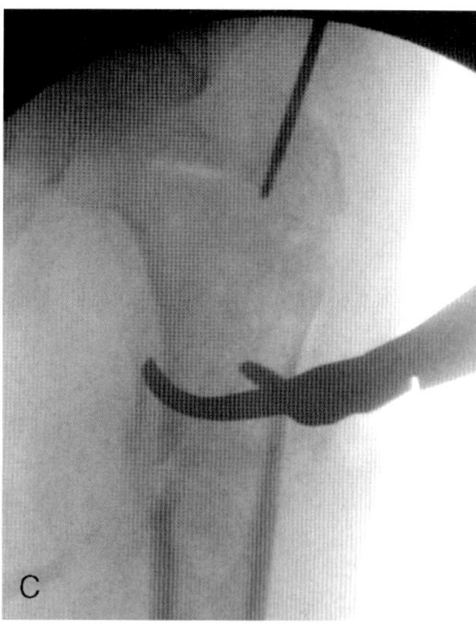

Figure 10 Fluoroscopic images of an unreduced fracture. **A,** An unreduced fracture cannot be reduced with nail passage because of the capacious metaphysis typically found in most patients with osteopenia. **B,** Reduction has been achieved with a clamp placed through a small lateral incision. **C,** A clamp is used to reduce a fracture with a subtrochanteric extension. Clamps can be inserted without evacuation of the fracture hematoma and with minimal soft-tissue disruption.

Tip 8: Avoid Varus Angulation of the Proximal Fragment—Use the Relationship Between the Tip of the Trochanter and the Center of the Femoral Head

Varus angulation of the proximal fragment increases the lever arm on the fixation because it makes the femoral neck more horizontal and therefore functionally longer when body weight is applied. This also results in the femoral head fixation being placed more superiorly in the head than is ideal and increases the risk of the device cutting out of the femoral head. It can be difficult to determine the appropriate femoral neck-shaft angle in a patient with an intertrochanteric fracture. When using an intramedullary nail for fixation of an intertrochanteric fracture, most surgeons choose a nail with a 130° neck-shaft configuration (Figure 11). It is important to know the neck-shaft angle of the device that is being used. One way to assess varus or valgus position during surgery is to look at the relationship between the tip of the greater trochanter and the center of the femoral head. These two points should be coplanar. If the center of the femoral head is distal to the tip of the greater trochanter, the reduction is in varus. If the center of the head is proximal to the greater trochanter, the reduction is in valgus. Preoperative plain radiographs of the uninjured hip can be used to assess the patient's normal neck-shaft angle because the two sides are normally symmetric. Varus and high lag screw placement are associated with an increased frequency of failure of fixation with an intramedullary nail and sliding hip screw.[20,21]

Tip 9: When Nailing, Lock the Nail Distally if the Fracture is Axially or Rotationally Unstable

Most unstable fractures of the proximal part of the femur require a long intramedullary nail. If there is any question about the stability of a fracture, then a long nail should be chosen and, in most instances, it should be locked distally.[15,22-24] Although short nails may be used for minimally displaced or nondisplaced fractures or very stable patterns, they can be associated with a subsequent fracture in the subtrochanteric area. Although most modern short nail designs have smaller diameter locking screws in this high-stress area to prevent the fractures that were en-

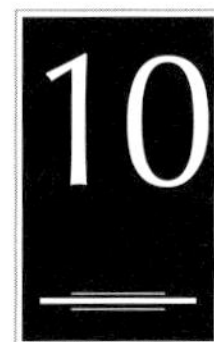

Slipped Capital Femoral Epiphysis

Randall T. Loder, MD
David D. Aronsson, MD
Stuart L. Weinstein, MD
Gert J. Breur, DVM, PhD
Reinhold Ganz, MD
Michael Leunig, MD

Abstract

Slipped capital femoral epiphysis (SCFE) is a common adolescent hip disorder. The etiology of SCFE includes biomechanical and biochemical factors. SCFEs are classified as stable and unstable and are more common in boys than girls and in certain racial groups; most children with SCFEs are obese. Bilateral SCFEs may have a simultaneous or sequential presentation.

Imaging studies show a posterior slip of the epiphysis relative to the metaphysis, seen early on lateral radiographs. The most common and effective initial treatment for stable SCFEs is in situ central single-screw fixation; other options include epiphysiodesis, and osteotomy with or without surgical dislocation of the hip. Later reconstruction options, typically reserved for the child with functional abnormalities, include proximal femoral osteotomy, or surgical dislocation of the hip with removal of metaphyseal prominent bone to remove the source of femoroacetabular impingement. Unstable SCFEs have an increased risk of osteonecrosis; the role of reduction, methods of fixation, and decompression are controversial. The natural history of untreated SCFEs is associated with the risk of progression and later degenerative joint disease.

Based on treatment methods of 30 to 40 years ago, in situ fixation provided the best long-term function with the lowest risk of complications and the most effective delay of degenerative arthritis regardless of the severity of the SCFE. Newer technologies and techniques are allowing the reevaluation of the role of either acute or later reconstructive osteotomy. It has not yet been determined if these improved techniques will result in better outcomes than in the past. Surgical dislocation of the hip with epiphyseal orientation is a considered treatment option for those technically adept at the procedure; however, the long-term outcome compared with in situ fixation is still unknown.

Slipped capital femoral epiphysis (SCFE) is an adolescent hip disorder in which there is a displacement of the capital femoral epiphysis from the metaphysis through the physis. The term SCFE is a misnomer because it is actually the metaphysis that moves superiorly and anteriorly, with the epiphysis held in the acetabulum by the ligamentum teres (Figure 1). An apparent varus relationship between the epiphysis and metaphysis exists in most patients, but occasionally the epiphysis displaces laterally and superiorly in relation to the metaphysis (valgus SCFE).[1-4] Most SCFEs have an idiopathic etiology, although they also can occur from a known endocrine disorder, renal failure osteodystrophy, or previous radiation therapy.[5-10] This chapter is limited to a discussion of idiopathic SCFE.

Epidemiology and Demographics

The incidence of SCFE is not completely known. The reported incidence ranges from 0.2 per 100,000 people in eastern Japan, 2.13 per 100,000 in the southwestern United States, and 10.08 per 100,000 people in the northeastern United States.[11,12] Recent studies indicate that the overall incidence of SCFE in the United States is 10.8 per 100,000 people, but in Japan has increased to 2.22 per 100,000 for boys and 0.76 per 100,000 for girls.[13,14] Although most studies show a male predominance, as seen early in this century when 90% of all SCFE incidents occurred in males, recent studies show that males account for only 60% of patients with SCFE.[15] The average duration of symptoms for children with chronic SCFEs, with no difference noted by gender, is 5 months; however, two recent

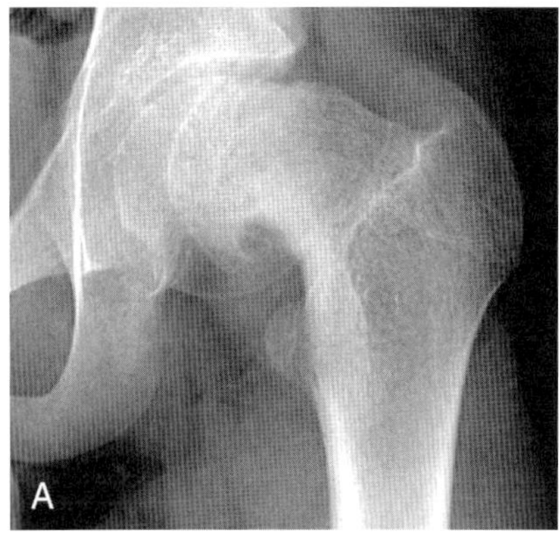

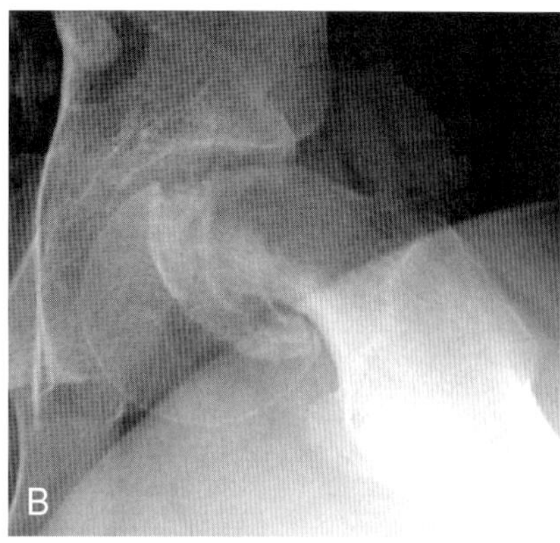

Figure 1 AP **(A)** and frog-lateral **(B)** radiographs of a left SCFE in a boy age 13 years, 7 months. Note the superior and anterior displacement of the metaphysis relative to the epiphysis and the remodeling with a bony callus/buttress inferiorly and posteriorly.

studies noted a decrease to between 2 and 3 months.[16,17] The average age at diagnosis is 13.5 years for boys and 12.0 years for girls, with a typical range for both genders from 9 to 16 years.[18] Newer data indicate a younger age at diagnosis for children with SCFE, likely a result of the earlier maturation of children.[13] Most children with SCFE are obese; at least 50% of the children with SCFE are above the 95th percentile for weight based on age.[18,19] Using body mass index to evaluate body habitus, more recent studies have shown an average body mass index of between 25 and 30 kg/m2 (above the 85th percentile).[17,20-24] Children with bilateral SCFE have an even greater average body mass index (31.1 kg/m2) than children with unilateral SCFE (26.8 kg/m2).[22] The age of onset decreases with increasing obesity; onset occurs at 12.4 years for those above the 95th percentile for weight based on age, and at 14.3 years for those under the 10th percentile for weight based on age.[18] Although variability in chronologic age exists, SCFE occurs in a more narrow physiologic age range—the "narrow window" of bone age.[25,26] In latitudes north of 40°, SCFE presents more frequently in the late summer and fall months[27-33] (Figure 2, *A*).

The reported incidence of bilateral SCFE is variable and depends on the study, method of radiographic measurement, the child's race, and treatment method. Most studies report an incidence of between 18% and 50%; however, recent studies with follow-up into adulthood describe the incidence of bilaterality as high as 63%.[18,30,34,35] The percentage of bilaterality is higher in blacks (34%) than in Hispanics (17%), whites (17%), or Asians (18%).[18] Treatment may affect the incidence of bilaterality; the prevalence of bilaterality in those treated with in situ fixation in one study was 36%, and 7% in those treated with a spica cast.[36] Therefore, close attention to the opposite normal hip is mandatory in those children with a unilateral SCFE treated with in situ fixation. Children who are physiologically younger at the initial presentation of unilateral SCFE are at higher risk for development of a contralateral SCFE. In a study of 50 children with unilateral SCFE, Stasikelis and associates[37] used a modified Oxford hip score to correlate bone age with the subsequent development of a contralateral SCFE and found an occurrence of 85% in hips with a score of 16, 11% in hips with a score of 21, and no occurrence of contralateral SCFE with a score of 22 or more.

Of those with bilateral SCFE, 50% to 60% of patients present with bilateral involvement. In the 40% with sequential bilateral progression, 80% to 90% of the second SCFEs occur within the first 18 months after the first SCFE.[18,30,38-41] The age at presentation is younger in children who present with a unilateral SCFE and have later development of bilateral SCFEs compared with those with a unilateral SCFE who do not have later development of bilateral SCFEs.[27,37,40-42] This age difference is seen in both the chronologic age (12 versus 13 years of age) as well as in the pelvic bone age. Of those with unilateral SCFEs, 60% occur in the left hip.

There is racial variability in the incidence of SCFE. The relative racial frequency of SCFE is 1.0 for whites, 4.5 for Pacific Islanders, 2.2 for blacks, 1.05 for Amerindian peoples (Native Americans and Hispanics), 0.5 for Indonesian-Malay (such as Chinese, Japanese, Thai, Vietnamese), and 0.1 for Indo-Mediterranean people (Near East, North African, or Indian subcontinent ancestry).[18] More recent data indicate that these numbers, relative to occurrence in whites (1.0) is 5.6 for Polynesians, 3.9 for blacks, and 2.5 for Hispanics[13,43] (Figure 2, *B*). These racial differences most likely reflect the average body weights for each racial group and further support the major role that obesity and mechanical stress play in the etiology of SCFE.[18] A less likely explanation for the differences is racial variability in acetabular depth and femoral head coverage. One study showed that the acetabular depth in black children was greater than in white children; however, another study did not support this finding.[44,45]

Classification

SCFE is classified both by its clinical nature and by its magnitude. The traditional clinical classification is preslip, acute, chronic, and acute-on-chronic and is based on the patient's history, physical examination, and radiographs.[46-50]

In the preslip stage, patients usually report weakness in the leg, limping, or exertional pain in the groin or the knee, which are further provoked by prolonged standing or walking. On physical examination, the most consistent positive finding is lack of internal rotation. On radiographs, generalized bone atrophy of the hemipelvis and upper femur is noted in patients with limited activity or limp, as well as potential for widening and irregularity of the physis.[51]

An acute SCFE is defined as that occurring in patients with symptoms for fewer than 3 weeks with an abrupt displacement through the proximal physis in which there was a preexisting epiphyseolysis.[46] In 67% of patients with acute SCFEs, a 1- to 3-month history of mild prodromal symptoms occurs before an acute episode, indicating that a preslip or a mild SCFE existed before the acute episode.[1,46,49,50,52] The acute episode may consist of an activity as trivial as turning over in bed. Physical examination shows an external rotation deformity, shortening, and marked limitation of motion secondary to pain that is usually severe enough to prevent weight bearing. Acute SCFEs represent

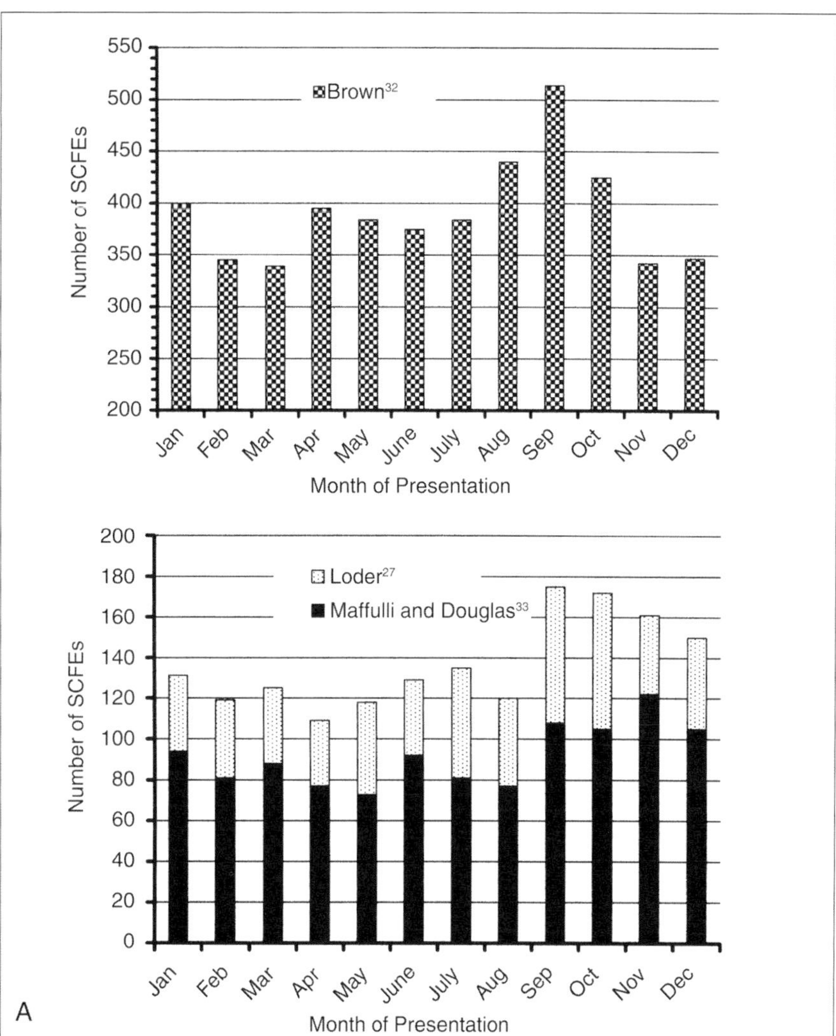

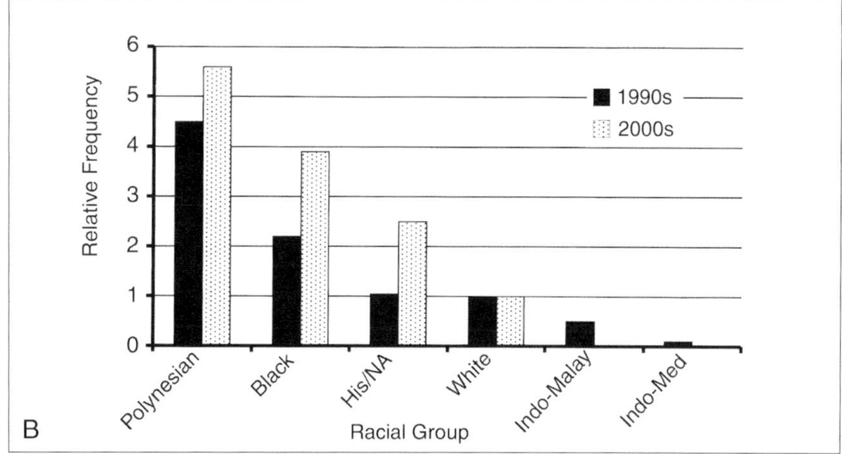

Figure 2 **A,** Seasonal variation in the month of presentation of children with SCFE north of the 40 N° latitude; data combined from three recent studies. **B,** The relative racial frequency of children with SCFE using the white population as a norm of 1.0. The studies were either published in the 1990s or 2000s; note the increase in frequency in the Polynesian, black, and Hispanic/Native American groups between the 1990s and the first decade of the 21st century.

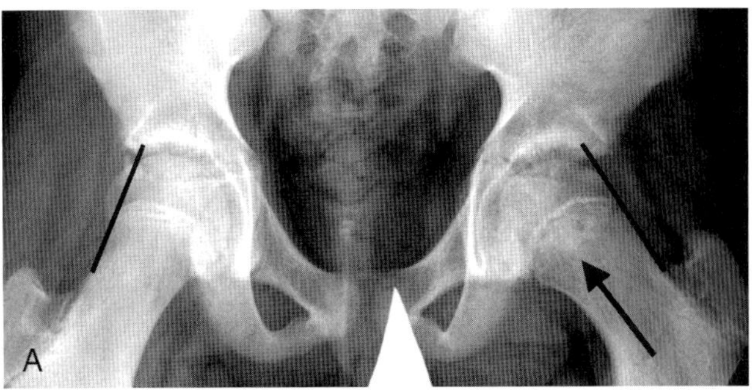

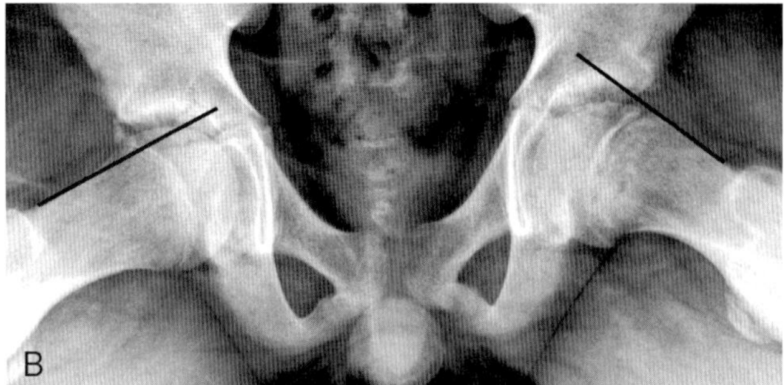

Figure 3 Radiographs of a 15-year-old boy with a mild left SCFE. **A,** The metaphyseal blanch sign is a radiographic double density seen on the AP view at the level of the metaphysis (*arrow*); this double density reflects the posterior cortical lip of the epiphysis as it is beginning to slip posteriorly and is radiographically superimposed on the metaphyseal density. Klein's line is a line along the anterior or superior aspect of the femoral neck; the epiphysis should normally intersect this line (right hip). In an early SCFE the epiphysis will be flush with or even below this line (left hip). **B,** The frog-lateral radiograph shows early slipping and step-off at the physeal level and also an abnormal Klein's line on the left compared with the right.

10% to 15% of SCFEs in most large studies.[41,50]

Chronic SCFEs account for 85% of all slips; patients usually present with more than 3 weeks of groin, thigh, and knee pain and often have a history of exacerbations and remissions of the pain and limp.[41] The initial symptom is frequently knee or lower thigh pain, emphasizing the importance of a hip examination in a child reporting knee pain.[16,53,54] Physical examination shows an antalgic gait, with loss of internal rotation, abduction, and flexion of the hip.[55] In severe instances, there is a limb-length discrepancy with the lower extremity in external rotation. As the hip is flexed, the lower extremity spontaneously assumes an increased external rotation position. Acute-on-chronic SCFEs are those with initial chronic symptoms and the subsequent development of acute symptoms.

The traditional classification is based on the memory of the child and parent and may be inaccurate. Newer, more clinically useful classifications are based on physeal stability, which provide a prognosis regarding subsequent hip osteonecrosis. There are two such classifications: clinical and radiographic. The clinical classification is based on the degree to which the child is able to ambulate.[56] A stable SCFE is defined as one in which the child is able to ambulate with or without crutches, whereas an unstable SCFE is defined as one in which the child cannot ambulate with or without crutches. By contrast, the radiographic classification system is based on the presence or absence of a hip effusion on ultrasonography.[57,58] The absence of metaphyseal remodeling and the presence of an effusion define an unstable SCFE; the presence of metaphyseal remodeling and the absence of an effusion define a stable SCFE.

Unstable SCFEs have a much higher incidence of osteonecrosis (up to 50% in some studies) compared with stable SCFEs (nearly 0%).[56] The high complication rates associated with unstable slip are most likely secondary to vascular injury caused at the time of the initial displacement.[56,59] Osteonecrosis correlates with results of pretreatment bone scans. A "cold" bone scan (showing the absence of vascularity) essentially is seen with unstable SCFEs. When a cold bone scan is present, the subsequent development of osteonecrosis is 80% to 100%.[60] A child with unstable SCFE has symptoms similar to those of a child with a hip fracture, and the SCFE may be considered as a type of Salter-Harris I fracture. The child is in severe pain and resists any passive or active attempts to move the lower extremity, which is held in a flexed and externally rotated position.

Imaging

Radiographs of SCFEs show an inferior and posterior slip of the proximal femoral epiphysis relative to the metaphysis. In a gradual slip, radiographic signs of remodeling on the superior and anterior femoral metaphysis are present along with periosteal new bone formation at the epiphyseal-metaphyseal junction posteriorly and inferiorly. In the early SCFE, the changes can be subtle with only posterior displacement.[55] As such, it is often only seen early on the lateral view, and both AP and lateral radiographs must be obtained. Other radiographic signs of an early SCFE are the metaphyseal blanch sign of Steel and Klein's line[61,62] (Figure 3). The metaphyseal blanch sign of Steel is a radio-

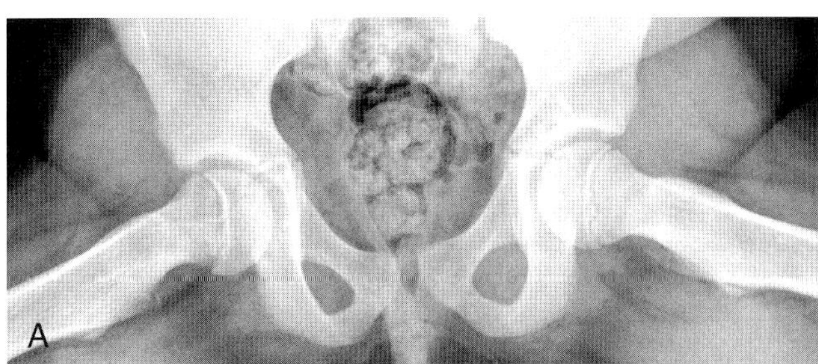

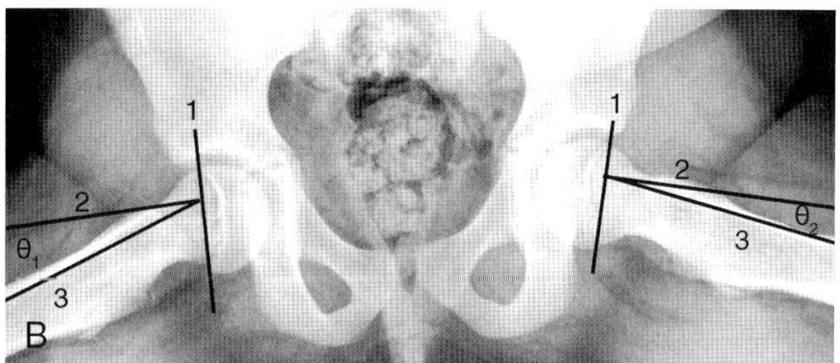

Figure 4 The lateral epiphyseal-shaft angle of the Southwick angle is measured on a frog-lateral radiograph. **A,** Frog-lateral radiograph of a 9-year-old girl with a mild right SCFE. **B,** Line 1 is drawn between the anterior and posterior physis; line 2 is perpendicular to line 1; line 3 is an axial line along the shaft of the femur. The angle defined by the intersection of line 2 and 3 is the lateral epiphyseal shaft angle (θ). The slip angle is calculated by subtracting the lateral epiphyseal shaft angle of the normal hip from the slip side. In this example, the angle on the right hip (θ_1) created by lines 2 and 3 is 20°, and on the angle (θ_2) on the left hip is 7°. The magnitude of the SCFE is 20° – 7° = 13° (a mild SCFE).

graphic double density seen on the AP view at the level of the metaphysis; this double density reflects the posterior cortical lip of the epiphysis as it is beginning to slip posteriorly and is radiographically superimposed on the metaphyseal density. Klein's line is drawn along the anterior or superior aspect of the femoral neck; the epiphysis should normally intersect this line, whereas in an early SCFE, the epiphysis will be level with or even below the level of this line.

Other imaging methods are occasionally used in children with SCFE. Bone scans and MRI scans allow earlier diagnosis of osteonecrosis and chondrolysis, whereas ultrasonography allows early visualization of an effusion in the hip.[60] The CT scan has improved the three-dimensional understanding of a SCFE and can be used in preoperative planning of an osteotomy and when determining whether there is joint penetration by internal fixation.[63]

SCFE magnitude is described by two different methods. The first describes magnitude by the amount of displacement of the epiphysis on the metaphysis. A mild SCFE is defined as epiphyseal-metaphyseal displacement less than one third the width of the metaphysis, a moderate SCFE is defined as displacement one third to one half the width of the metaphysis, and a severe SCFE is defined as greater than one half the width of the metaphysis.[54] This first method to describe SCFE magnitude by degree of displacement is less accurate because distinct landmarks are difficult to determine as a result of metaphyseal remodeling in the gradually stable SCFE.[64] Angular measurement, the second method, is more accurate. The epiphyseal-shaft angle on the frog-lateral radiograph is measured and categorized into three groups: mild, less than 30°; moderate, 30° to 50°; and severe, greater than 50°[50,65] (Figure 4). This classification is important for long-term prognosis because mild and moderate slips have a much better long-term prognosis than severe slips, in which degenerative hip disease more rapidly develops.[53,66]

Etiology

The etiology of idiopathic SCFE is a combination of both biomechanical and biochemical factors, the combined effect of which results in a weakened physis with subsequent failure[67] (Figure 5). Mechanical factors associated with SCFE are obesity, femoral retroversion, and increased physeal obliquity.[18,19,68-71] Obesity and femoral retroversion increase shear stress across the physis.[70] The average anteversion in adolescents of normal weight is 10.6° and 0.4° in obese adolescents.[68] Children with SCFE also have a more vertical proximal femoral physis, even in the contralateral normal hip (8° to 11° increase compared with children without SCFE). The increase in physeal shear force resulting from femoral retroversion and increased physeal slope is enough to cause a SCFE.[70] The average shear load to failure of the proximal femoral physis in adolescents of normal weight is 4.0 times body weight; the average shear load to failure in obese adolescents with neutral version and who are running is 5.1 times body weight, higher than the 4.0 body weight threshold. Similarly, finite element analysis studies have shown that a varus load on the proximal femoral physis in an overweight child with femoral retroversion creates physeal shear strains above the yield point and can result in a slip.[72] In one study, children with SCFE were found to have greater acetabula depth than a group

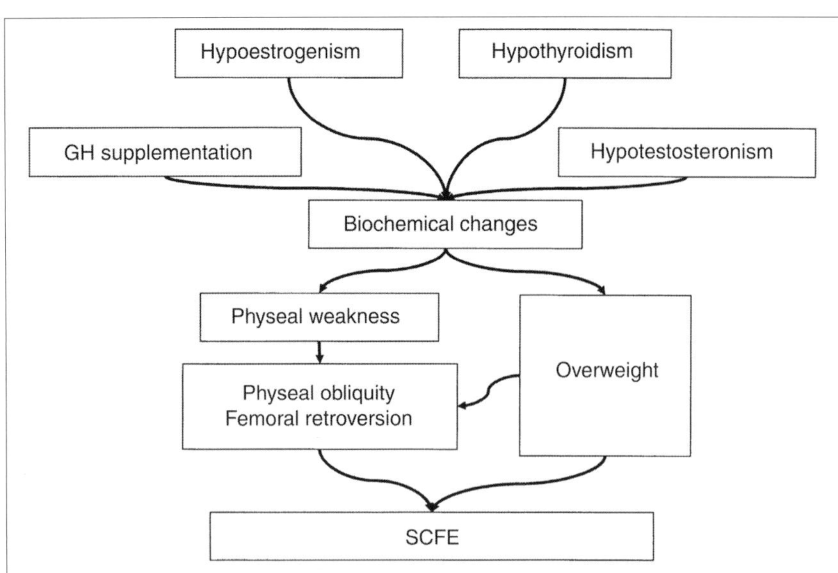

Figure 5 Proposed pathophysiology of SCFE across all species, including humans. GH = growth hormone.

of children without SCFE (center-edge angle of Wiberg 37° versus 33°, respectively), demonstrating greater coverage of the femoral head yields more shearing stress across the physis.[44] However, this concept recently has been questioned.[45]

Biochemical and endocrine factors also are components of the disorder. SCFE is a disease of puberty, with rapid longitudinal growth occurring in response to growth hormone.[73] This growth is a result of increased physiologic activity of the physis and is associated with widening of the physis. Decreased physeal strength also occurs at puberty; the cause is not clear but may result from increased cartilage width of the zones of hypertrophy and provisional calcification.[29,74]

Many other hormonal changes occur during this time.[29] The increased incidence of SCFE in children with hypothyroidism, during growth hormone supplementation, and hypogonadal states also suggests an association between SCFE and endocrine dysfunction. The effects of the gonadotropins on the physis may explain the male predominance in SCFE, given that testosterone reduces physeal strength, whereas estrogen reduces physeal width and increases physeal strength.[29,75] This effect explains why the incidence of SCFE is extremely rare in girls after the onset of menarche.[39] Although most children with SCFE do not have demonstrable endocrine disorders, a subtle but as-yet undiagnosable endocrinopathy may be present.[76-81] In some children there is a delay in bone age compared with chronologic age, further supporting this concept.[29,39]

The role of genetics and heredity is variable. Rennie[82] discovered that the risk of SCFE to a second family member was 7.1% and that 14.5% of patients with SCFE were related to a close relative who also had SCFE. In a few families with members who have SCFE, there may be an autosomal dominant inheritance with incomplete penetrance.[82] Tightly knit communities (such as the Amish community) with little change in gene pools may have more familial tendencies in SCFE.[83] Human leukocyte antigen typing in children with SCFE is variable.[84-87]

Routine histology and electron microscopy show both cellular and matrical abnormalities in the proliferative and hypertrophic zones. Cellular abnormalities consist of a decreased number of chondrocytes and chondrocyte clustering and disarray; this decrease in chondrocyte number is the result of an abnormal frequency and distribution of chondrocytes undergoing apoptosis.[88-90] Reported histologic changes in the matrix include deficiency and abnormality in the supporting collagenous and proteoglycan framework of the physis. Changes in proteoglycan and glycoprotein concentrations with an increased glycoprotein staining in the territorial matrix and increased proteoglycan staining in the interterritorial matrix were seen in the proliferative zone. Ultrastructural studies have shown defective collagen fibrils and defects in collagen banding in the matrix of the hypertrophic zone.[91] Whether these abnormalities represent the cause or effect of the SCFE is not known.

SCFE in Animals and Insights Into Etiology

Naturally occurring SCFE has been reported in cats, pigs, dogs, coypus, and cattle. These occurrences of SCFE in animal models suggest that biochemical changes precede both physeal changes and subsequent SCFE; animal models may further elucidate the pathophysiology of SCFE.

Cats

SCFE has been reported in cats.[92-94] In the most detailed study, 26 cases with spontaneous, often insidious, femoral capital physeal fractures were examined, 9 of which were bilateral (35%).[92] The mean age of the cats was 22.5 months; 25 of 26 were neutered males with an average weight of 5.6 kg compared with a weight of 4.5 kg in an age- and sex-matched control group. Of the 16 cats with a recorded age at the time of neutering, 14 had been neutered before 6 months of age (prepubescent). Radiographically, more severe metaphyseal osteolysis and sclerosis scores were seen in chronic separations; 72% had radiographically open femoral capital physes. Histopathologically, the capital epiphysis contained cartilage and bone. Physeal tissue attached to the capital epiphysis lacked the normal chondrocyte columnar arrangement, and chondrocytes were clustered within the extracellular matrix. It was concluded that this feline condition mimics SCFE in children. Collectively, these studies identified obesity, gender (male), castration (particularly prepubescent castration), and delayed physeal closure as risk factors for feline SCFE.[92,93] Prepubertal or postpubertal castration in cats results in delayed physeal closure in a set of steps that are hypothesized to begin with hypotestosteronism resulting from castration with subsequent delayed physeal closure, followed by increased shear forces to the capital physis, resulting in a spontaneous, nontraumatic slippage of the capital femoral epiphysis[95,96] (Figure 6).

Pigs

Separation of the femoral head also occurs in sows and boars (epiphysiolysis capitis femoris), and morphologic changes of the femoral head and neck have been described.[97,98] Although epiphysiolysis in pigs does not mimic SCFE in children, the condition may provide insight into the mechanisms of growth plate weakening, metaphyseal slippage and separation, and the effect of obesity on hip development. The associated lameness varies from moderate to severe in unilateral lesions, to an inability to rise or walk in bilaterally affected animals. It has been suggested that osteochondritis weakens the growth plate, which ultimately results in slippage and separation. Causative factors of osteochondrosis (genetics, rapid growth) and trauma (such as fighting, copulation,) are considered risk factors for epiphysiolysis.

Coypus

SCFE in the coypu *(Myocastor coypus)*, a large rodent (approximately 8 to 10 kg) commercially raised for fur, has been reported as a cause of lameness. In two reports, the onset of SCFE occurred during puberty (8 of 10 cases), and gross pathologic and histologic changes were consistent with SCFE in children.[99,100] These studies suggest that gender (female), pregnancy, and being overweight are risk factors for SCFE in coypus but do not explain whether the risk associated with pregnancy is a result of endocrine-related or mechanical factors. Because the incidence of SCFE in the coypu is low, and basic endocrine and skeletal physiology information is lacking, the coypu is not a good animal model for the study of SCFE.

Dogs and Cattle

Recently, bilateral SCFE was reported in five dogs.[101,102] SCFE may also have caused other reported canine cases of capital femoral physeal fractures with insidious onset.[103] SCFE also has been reported in calves.[104] However, in 21 of 29 of the affected calves, the separation was attributed to difficult parturition and forced traction delivery. More recently, bovine SCFE was reported in older calves and young adult cattle without a history of trauma.[105] The limited number of reported cases and limited information about canine and bovine SCFE currently make either animal model unsuitable for future investigations.

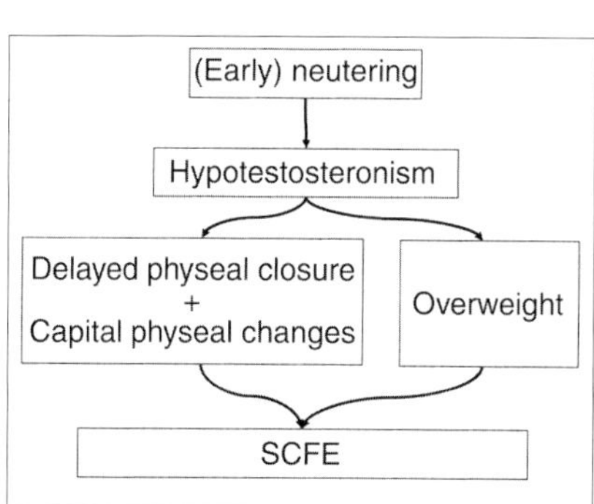

Figure 6 Proposed pathophysiology of SCFE in the cat.

Although the pathologic changes of SCFE across species are the same, it appears that the etiology and pathophysiology are different. Common findings are trauma and physeal changes. In children these physeal changes include physeal obliquity and femoral retroversion, both the result of asymmetric physeal growth during development, which is the result of physeal trauma secondary to obesity. Slippage appears to occur during a limited bone age window when the perichondrial ring of the proximal capital femoral epiphysis is weakened.[25,26] Biochemical changes include endocrine alterations. Whereas in children no direct relationship has been established between SCFE and biochemical and mechanical changes, a very clear relationship between endocrine (hypotestosteronism) and physeal (delayed closure) changes exists in the cat model. It is not known why delayed physeal closure in cats can result in increased vulnerability and whether this vulnerability is a result of increased physeal obliquity, femoral retroversion, and perichondrial weakness. It is possible that physeal changes in children are also the result of both biochemical changes and obesity, which result in asymmetric physeal growth (Figure 5). Because biochemical changes are often minimal, and the time of onset of physeal closure is difficult to determine, weight control may be the most important measure to prevent SCFE. Further studies regarding the genesis of the physeal changes are needed.

Treatment

Once a diagnosis of SCFE is made, treatment is indicated to prevent slip progression and to avoid complications, especially osteonecrosis and chondrolysis.[16,17,106] Several treatment methods exist, each characterized by particular advantages and disadvantages.

The treatment of SCFE has changed with improvements in imaging techniques. The development of intraoperative fluoroscopy to assist in the placement of internal fixation has markedly lowered the complication rate of internal fixation. Previously, patients were often treated by in situ multiple pin fixation using intraoperative spot radiographs to control pin placement. Using this technique, pin placement was not always ideal, and malpositioned pins were associated with complications including further slippage, chondrolysis, and osteonecrosis in 20% to 40% of patients. This high complication rate led to increased use of the hip spica cast, open epiphysiodesis, or femoral osteotomy as treatment. The hip spica cast, multiple pins, and, to a large extent, epiphysiodesis currently are treatments of historic interest only.[47,48,107-109]

Stable SCFE

Treatment methods for a patient with a stable (chronic) SCFE include (1) in situ stabilization with a single screw,[47,48,110,111] (2) epiphysiodesis,[108,112,113] (3) open reduction with corrective osteotomy through the physis and internal fixation,[114-117] (4) treatment with a bilateral hip spica cast, (5) in situ fixation with multiple pins, (6) basilar neck osteotomy,[118,119] (7) intertrochanteric osteotomy,[63,65,120-122] and (8) surgical dislocation of the hip with transphyseal callus removal, reduction, and fixation.[123-127]

In Situ Fixation Using a Single Central Screw

Since O'Brien and Fahey[128] reported on the remodeling potential of the proximal femur in patients with SCFE, internal fixation in situ has been the most popular treatment method. Long-term follow-up studies have shown that postoperative remodeling occurs, and the loss of internal rotation of the hip after in situ fixation in many patients is not clinically relevant.[129,130]

Because of femoral head vascularity and the blind spot, the ideal position for a screw is in the center of the epiphysis (Figure 7). The major contribution of the blood supply to the femoral head is derived from the lateral epiphyseal vessels, which enter the femoral head in the posterosuperior quadrant and anastomose with vessels from the round ligament at the junction of the medial and central thirds of the femoral head.[131,132] If fixation is placed in the posterosuperior quadrant, there is an increased risk of damage to the epiphyseal blood supply. This risk is minimized by a single screw in the center of the epiphysis and perpendicular to the physis.[47]

The blind spot is the area in which fixation devices radiographically appear to be within the femoral head but in reality are penetrating into the joint. [133] Often unrecognized pin protrusion results in subsequent development of chondrolysis and degenerative changes. The use of multiple pins increases the possibility that one or more pins will protrude into the joint; this risk is lowered by using a single screw.[48,134,135] Because single-screw fixation is 77% as stable as double-screw fixation in a calf model, single-screw fixation is recommended because the small gains in stiffness with a second screw do not offset the increased risk of joint penetration.[136]

The technique for the percutaneous insertion of a single screw has been described.[47,135] The patient is positioned supine on a fracture or radiolucent table to allow simultaneous biplane AP and lateral fluoroscopic imaging. The authors prefer a fracture table for single screw fixation, although others report good results and reduced surgical time on a radiolucent table.[137,138] It is important to emphasize that the technique is image dependent; therefore, excellent visualization of the femoral head and neck is required before beginning the procedure. Because the procedure is performed percutaneously through a small skin incision using a cannulated screw, it is critical to locate the proper starting position for the guide pin. To determine the starting point, a guide pin is placed on the skin overlying the proximal femur and, under anteroposterior fluoroscopic guidance, the pin is positioned such that it projects over the center of the femoral epiphysis, crossing the physis in a perpendicular fashion. Once this pin position has been obtained, a marking pen is used to draw a line on the skin that reflects the pin position on the AP image. The same procedure is used for the lateral fluoroscopic image, and a 1-cm skin incision is made at the intersection of the two lines. The guide pin is advanced in a freehand manner through the soft tissues to the anterolateral femoral cortex. Using fluoroscopic guidance, the position and angulation of the guide pin are adjusted to obtain the proper alignment before the guide pin is drilled into the bone. It is ideal to advance the guide pin into the center of the epiphysis, perpendicular to the physis, on both the AP and lateral fluoroscopic images on the first attempt because multiple drill holes can weaken the bone, causing a fracture through an unused hole.[139] After the appropriate screw length has been determined, a 6.5-mm to 7.3-mm stainless steel cannulated screw is placed in a routine manner and advanced until approximately five threads engage the epiphysis (Figure 7). Carney and associates[140] reported progression of the SCFE greater than 10° in 9 of 22 hips (41%) when fewer than five threads engaged the epiphysis. When five or more threads engaged the epiphysis, no progression was reported. The screw should not be left protruding beyond the lateral aspect of the femoral shaft where it can be toggled by the soft tissues, leading to screw loosening.[141]

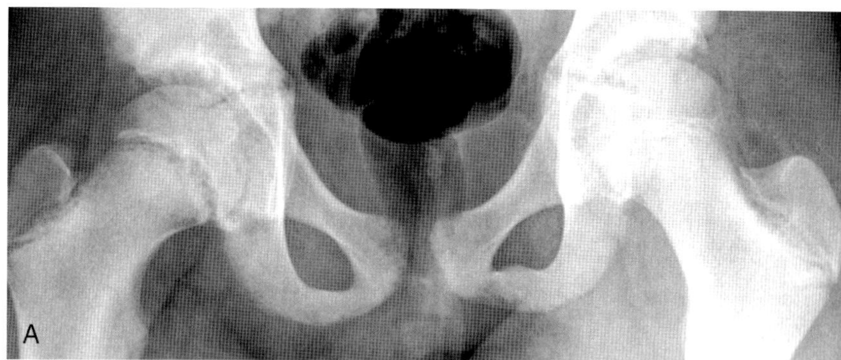

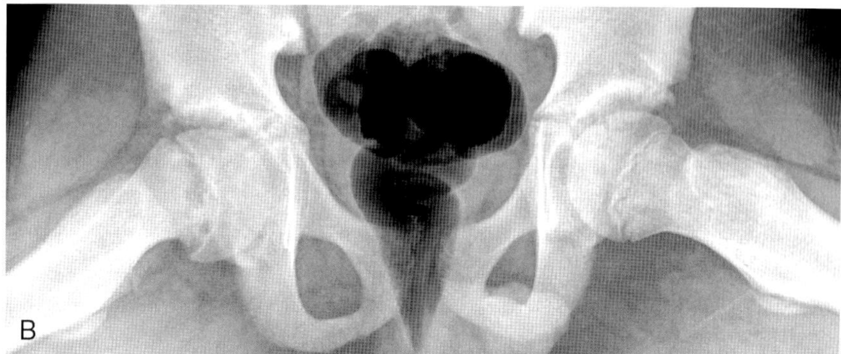

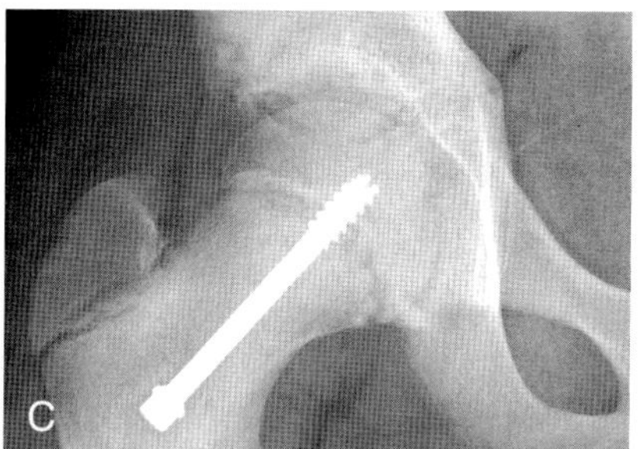

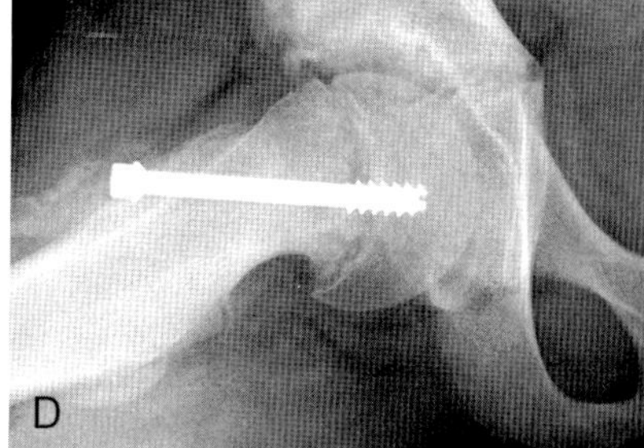

Figure 7 **A,** Initial AP radiograph of the pelvis of a boy age 11 years, 11 months with a stable right SCFE. **B,** Frog-lateral pelvic radiograph showing the right SCFE. **C,** Postoperative AP view of the pelvis shows screw placement perpendicular to the physis. **D,** Postoperative frog-lateral radiograph of the pelvis shows screw placement perpendicular to the physis.

At this point in the procedure, it must be confirmed that the screw tip is not in the joint space by using either variations on the "approach-withdraw" maneuver or arthrography.[142-146] The approach-withdraw maneuver indicates the position of the screw tip and helps avoid unrecognized screw penetration, which is associated with the blind spot that exists with individual views on the image intensifier. As the screw approaches the subchondral bone of the femoral head, and with the surgeon observing the image intensifier screen, the lower extremity is rotated from maximum internal rotation to maximum external rotation. During the first part of the rotation, the screw tip appears to move closer to the subchondral bone (approach), then moves away (withdraw). The instant of change from approach to withdrawal identifies the view in which the screw tip is shown in its true position. After surgery, the patient begins partial weight-bearing ambulation using crutches and gradually advances to full weight bearing after 4 to 6 weeks.

The results of single-screw fixation for patients with SCFE are good. Aronson and Carlson[47] reported excellent or good results in 36 of 38 mild slips (95%), in 10 of 11 moderate slips (91%), and in 8 of 9 severe slips (89%).[91] Osteonecrosis developed in only one patient (2%) with an unstable SCFE, and chondrolysis developed in none. Ward and associates[48] reported on 42 patients (53 hips) with a SCFE treated by single screw fixation. After an average follow-up of 32 months, 92% demonstrated physeal fusion and participated in full activities. No patient developed chondrolysis or osteonecrosis. The advantages of single-screw fixation for a patient with a stable SCFE include a high success rate, a low incidence of further slippage, and a low incidence of complications.[47,147,148] It is currently the most common treatment of SCFE in North America.

Bone Graft Epiphysiodesis With Iliac Crest or Allograft Bone Graft

In 1931, Ferguson and Howorth[28] first reported open epiphysiodesis with iliac crest bone graft to stabilize a SCFE. The surgical technique is characterized by an anterior iliofemoral exposure of the hip joint and removal of a rectangular window of bone from the anterior aspect of the femoral neck. A hollow mill is used to create a tunnel across the physis, and multiple corticocancellous strips of iliac crest bone graft are driven into the tunnel as bone pegs across the proximal femoral physis.

Epiphysiodesis avoids the complications associated with internal fixation including unrecognized pin protrusion, damage to the lateral epiphyseal vessels, and hardware failure. The graft is not inserted as deep as recommended for internal fixation; therefore, there is less risk of graft protrusion into the hip joint. However, the fixation provided by the iliac crest bone graft is not as secure as that achieved by internal fixation. Rao and associates[108] evaluated 43 patients (64 hips) treated by open bone peg epiphysiodesis. At the time of healing, further slippage developed in 27 hips (42%). Osteonecrosis developed in 4 hips (6%), chondrolysis in 3 (5%), and additional complications in 14 (22%). Adamczyk and associates[109] reported their 50-year experience with bone graft epiphysiodesis in 43 patients with 45 incidences of unstable SCFE, and 225 patients with 278 incidences of stable SCFE. Slip progression occurred in 6 of the patients (13%) with unstable SCFE and in 17 of the patients (6%) with stable SCFE. Other disadvantages of bone graft epiphysiodesis include increased blood loss, a longer duration of anesthesia, and a larger scar. As a result of these complications, open bone peg epiphysiodesis is no longer recommended as the initial treatment of SCFE.[108,109]

Adamczyk and associates[109] believe that the rate of reslippage with iliac crest bone graft is unacceptable and that the use of a fibular allograft should be considered for increased stability. Schmidt and associates[113] have recently developed a technique to percutaneously place a freeze-dried irradiated cortical strut allograft across the physis. The technique is similar to that used for the percutaneous insertion of a single screw, but instead of inserting a screw, a 10-mm cannulated reamer is placed over the guide pin to ream a channel to within 2 mm of the subchondral bone. A cortical strut allograft is then passed into the channel and advanced until at least 1 cm lay across the physis. Schmidt and associates[113] evaluated 33 patients (40 hips) after a mean follow-up of 3 years, 6 months and reported excellent Harris hip scores in 35 hips, good scores in 1, and fair in 2. Major complications developed in 6 hips (15%), including one each of osteonecrosis, chondrolysis, femoral neck fracture, subtrochanteric hip fracture, bilateral coxa vara deformity, and unilateral coxa vara deformity. Despite these complications, the authors recommend this technique, particularly for patients with severe SCFE.

Open Reduction With Corrective Osteotomy Through the Physis and Internal Fixation Using Multiple Pins

A cuneiform osteotomy through the physis is the ideal method to correct the retroversion deformity of the femoral neck, but the question of safety is relevant. The surgical technique is characterized by an anterior Smith-Peterson or anterolateral exposure of the hip.[114,115] A cuneiform-shaped wedge of bone is removed from the metaphysis of the femoral neck, which allows the epiphysis to be anatomically repositioned on the metaphysis without creating tension on the epiphyseal vasculature. After the femoral neck is sufficiently shortened, reduction and fixation of the epiphysis is accomplished internally using three pins. In one study, a cuneiform osteotomy was performed on 61 patients (66 hips) with 55 excellent results (83%), 6 good (9%), 2 fair (3%), and 3 poor (5%).[117] DeRosa and associates[114] evaluated 23 patients (27 hips) with a severe SCFE treated by cuneiform osteotomy. At an average follow-up of 8 years, 5 months, there were no excellent results, 19 good (70%), 4 fair (15%), and 4 poor (15%). Osteonecrosis developed in four hips (15%) and chondrolysis in eight (30%). Two patients (7%) lost fixation and required further surgery, a skin erosion over one of the pins developed in one patient and required pin removal, and a pressure sore developed in the buttock of another patient. Despite a 15% rate of osteonecrosis, DeRosa and associates[114] recommended cuneiform osteotomy for patients with severe SCFE.

Velasco and associates[115] evaluated 65 patients (66 hips) treated with open reduction of the SCFE. In 60 hips, the open reduction of the slip was combined with a cuneiform subcapital wedge resection of the femoral neck according to the technique described by Dunn and Angel.[149] At an average follow-up of 16 years, chondrolysis developed in 8 hips (12%), and osteonecrosis developed in 7 (11%). The results in 48 hips with a minimum follow-up of 10 years (average follow-up, 20.6 years) were good in 46%, moderate in 33%, and poor in 21%. Degenerative arthritis occurred in 19 of the 48 hips (40%). Because of the high risk of osteonecrosis and subsequent poor results in most studies, a physeal cuneiform osteotomy is not recommended as the initial treatment of SCFE.

Bilateral Hip Spica Cast

Hip spica cast immobilization provides prophylactic treatment of the opposite hip and avoids surgical complications. Hurley and associates[36] compared 169 patients treated with in situ fixation with 30 patients treated with a spica cast. In the in situ fixation group, a contralateral SCFE developed in 61 patients (36%) at a mean follow-up of 2.8 years. In the spica cast group, a contralateral SCFE developed in two patients (7%) at a mean follow-up of 3.6 years. Betz and associates[150] evaluated 32 patients (37 hips) treated with a hip spica cast without reduction. The cast was used until the metaphyseal lucency adjacent to the physis was no longer radiographically visible on the radiographs at an average follow-up of 12 weeks. Osteonecrosis did not develop in any of the patients, but progression of the slip occurred in two hips (5%), and chondrolysis in seven (19%). Meier and associates[107] evaluated 13 patients (17 hips) treated with a spica cast for an average of 12 weeks. Progression of the slip occurred in three hips (18%), chondrolysis in nine (53%), and full-thickness cast pressure sores in two (12%). There were a total of 14 complications in the 17 hips (82%). In addition to the high complication and slip progression rate, a hip spica cast is awkward and cumbersome for the wearer and family, particularly when the patient is obese. Spica cast treatment of SCFE is not recommended.

In Situ Fixation With Multiple Pins

Complications associated with multiple pins stemmed from a lack of understanding of the three-dimensional anatomy of SCFE and from poor intraoperative imaging techniques. As a result, fixation was often started on the lateral aspect of the femoral shaft, similar to the technique of treating a hip fracture in an adult. Because the proximal femur is retroverted in a patient with a SCFE, the fixation was often placed in the anterosuperior aspect of the epiphysis, achieving suboptimal fixation. To improve fixation, clinicians would angle the pin more posteriorly, often exiting the posterior aspect of the femoral neck and entering the epiphysis in the posterosuperior quadrant. This technique jeopardized the blood supply to the femoral head and also led to unrecognized pin protrusion with subsequent chondrolysis or osteonecrosis. Given the superior results of single central screw fixation, multiple pin fixation is now used infrequently in the treatment of a stable SCFE.

After the initial treatment of SCFE, the external rotational deformity of the lower extremity gradually improves as the inflammation resolves and the proximal femoral retroversion deformity remodels. The retroversion deformity may occasionally cause pain and loss of motion for the patient and may cause anterior femoroacetabular impingement, which can contribute to the early development of osteoarthritis.[123-127] When the retroversion deformity causes pain or loss of motion, the clinician may choose intertrochanteric osteotomy, basilar neck osteotomy, or open surgical dislocation with femoral neck osteoplasty as treatment.

Compensating Base-of-Neck Osteotomy With Stabilization In Situ of the SCFE Using Multiple Pin Fixation

Kramer and associates[119] described an anterosuperior-based wedge osteotomy at the base of the femoral neck with both the osteotomy and the SCFE stabilized with multiple pins. Barmada and associates[118] described an extracapsular basilar neck osteotomy implemented in an attempt to avoid osteonecrosis. The incidence of osteonecrosis is lower with basilar neck osteotomies compared with the cuneiform osteotomy; however, only 35° to 55° of correction is possible.[151] One benefit of the basilar neck osteotomy is improvement in hip motion; a disadvantage is that the procedure shortens the femoral neck, which may result in the greater trochanter impinging against the lateral aspect of the acetabulum during hip abduc-

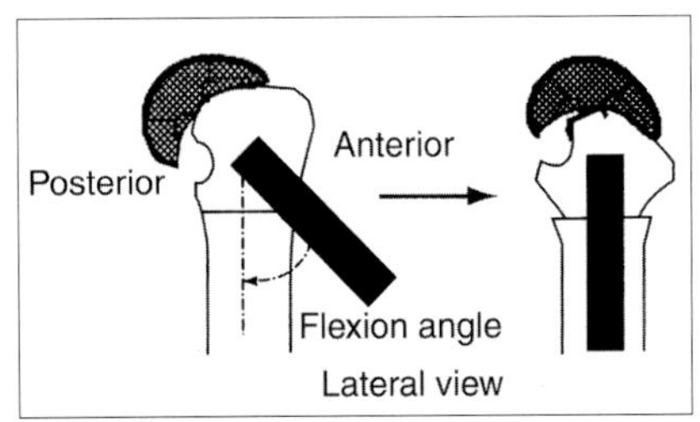

Figure 8 The Imhäuser flexion closing wedge intertrochanteric osteotomy for a SCFE. (Reproduced with permission from Kamegaya M, Saisu T, Ochiai N, Moriya H: Preoperative assessment for intertrochanteric femoral osteotomies in severe chronic slipped capital femoral epiphysis using computed tomography. *J Pediatr Orthop* 2005;14:71-78.)

tion. This femoral neck shortening may aggravate a limb-length discrepancy when there is premature closure of the proximal femoral physis, as is often seen in patients with SCFE.

Intertrochanteric Osteotomy With Internal Fixation

Southwick[65] described an intertrochanteric osteotomy through the lesser trochanter with flexion, abduction, and internal rotation of the distal fragment. This osteotomy improves hip motion and is not associated with osteonecrosis. The osteotomy is fixed with a compression hip screw and, if unstable, the SCFE is fixed with a cannulated screw. The intertrochanteric osteotomy is also a compensating osteotomy with correction limited to 45° on the AP radiograph and 60° on the lateral radiograph.[152] Because an anterolateral wedge of bone is removed, this osteotomy is also a shortening procedure. A risk of limb-length discrepancy exists when considerable correction is desired. Schai and associates[120] evaluated 51 patients with 30° to 60° slips treated with an intertrochanteric osteotomy at an average follow-up of 24 years. Moderate osteoarthritis developed in 14 patients (28%) and severe osteoarthritis in 9 patients (17%). In 35 patients (69%), the affected limb was shorter than the opposite side, and 2 patients (4%) underwent a limb-length equalization procedure. There was only one instance of osteonecrosis. The authors believed their results were superior to those treated with in situ fixation.[153] However, their results are at odds with the results of the long-term study of Carney and associates[53] in which those with realignment showed poorer results than those without realignment. In most studies, the results of intertrochanteric osteotomy using the Southwick technique are relatively poor compared with results using the current technique of in situ single-screw fixation; therefore, intertrochanteric osteotomy is not ideal for the initial treatment of SCFE.[65,120,152]

The Southwick osteotomy has now been replaced by the simpler Imhäuser flexion intertrochanteric osteotomy[63,121,122] (Figure 8). This osteotomy relies on the concept that the slip is essentially posterior, with secondary rotational deformity and minimal valgus or varus displacement.[55,69,154] The results of such an osteotomy are disparate. Kartenbender and associates[122] reviewed 39 severe SCFEs treated with an Imhäuser osteotomy at an average follow-up of 23.4 years. Three patients had severe degenerative disease and osteonecrosis developed in two patients. The number of excellent or good clinical results was 77%, whereas the excellent or good radiographic results using the Southwick classification were only 67%. Parsch and associates[121] noted one patient with osteonecrosis in stable SCFEs greater than 50°, yet concluded that they were unable to prove the advantage of osteotomy in late adult life.

Jerre and associates[155] evaluated the results of different realignment procedures in 36 patients (37 hips) at an average follow-up of 33.8 years (range, 26 to 42 years). Serious short-term complications developed in 7 of 22 hips (32%) treated with subcapital osteotomy, 3 of 11 hips (27%) with intertrochanteric osteotomy, and 3 of 4 hips (75%) treated with manipulative reduction. Long-term excellent or good results were reported in 9 of 22 hips (41%) treated with subcapital osteotomy, 4 of 11 (36%) treated with intertrochanteric osteotomy, and in none of the 4 hips (0%) treated with manipulative reduction.

Unstable SCFE

The treatment of an unstable SCFE is considerably more controversial than that of the stable SCFE. There is debate concerning an emergent or urgent reduction versus an elective reduction, an incidental reduction (improvement in the SCFE that occurs with positioning the patient on the operating table) versus a complete reduction, the magnitude of reduction, the role of joint decompression, and fixation with one or two screws. There is an increased risk of complications, particularly osteonecrosis, in patients with unstable SCFE.

This controversy regarding reduction was well documented by Mooney and associates[156] who surveyed the Pediatric Orthopaedic Society of North America membership about the treatment of unstable SCFE. Of the respondents; 57% favored urgent reduction (< 8 hours), 31% favored emergent reduction, and 12% favored elective treatment. An incidental reduction was favored by 84% of respondents, whereas 12% favored a formal (complete) manipulative reduction. Capsular decompression of the hematoma was not recommended by 65% of respondents, whereas 35% recommended decompression; 26% of those recommending decompression performed open decompression and 73% used a closed aspiration technique. Single-screw fixation was used by 57% of respondents, whereas 40% used double-screw fixation.

In the initial study that describes unstable SCFE and its increased risk for osteonecrosis, 25 acute stable SCFEs (24 patients) with 30 acute unstable SCFEs (30 patients) were compared.[56] There were 96% satisfactory results with no osteonecrosis in the 25 stable SCFEs, and 47% satisfactory results in the 30 unstable SCFEs. Osteonecrosis developed in 14 of 30 (47%) of the unstable SCFEs. Those with an acute slip were separated into two groups based on the time interval between the onset of symptoms and surgical stabilization. In the group that had surgical stabilization less than 48 hours after the onset of symptoms, the incidence of osteonecrosis was 88%. In the group that had surgical stabilization more than 48 hours after the onset of symptoms, the incidence of osteonecrosis was 32%. However, the data were inadequate to develop guidelines regarding the exact timing of surgical stabilization because the cause-effect relationship between the timing of surgical stabilization and the development of osteonecrosis could not be determined. It was possible that the more severe unstable SCFEs, which would likely have a higher risk of osteonecrosis, were stabilized sooner in an effort to reduce the child's discomfort as quickly as possible; the less severe unstable SCFEs, which theoretically had a lower risk of osteonecrosis, were stabilized later because the child was more comfortable.

Several authors have attempted to answer the questions regarding timing and surgical stabilization. The authors of one study evaluated 70 patients (81 hips) who had an unstable SCFE treated with gentle closed reduction and fixation using one or two screws or pins.[157] They reported complications in eight hips: three with chondrolysis (4%), three wound infections (4%), and two with osteonecrosis (2%). The authors concluded that a gentle reduction with percutaneous single-screw fixation is a stable, safe, and reliable method for treating patients with an unstable SCFE. Herman and associates[158] evaluated 15 unstable SCFEs (> 50% displacement) at an average follow-up of 2.8 years. Nine were treated by a gentle closed reduction and internal fixation, using either one or two screws. Five hips had a complete reduction of the SCFE, and osteonecrosis developed in three, whereas four hips had an incomplete reduction, and none developed osteonecrosis. The authors hypothesized that injury to the epiphyseal vasculature occurs at the time of the acute SCFE.

Peterson and associates[159] evaluated 91 patients with unstable SCFEs at an average follow-up of 44 months and especially evaluated the timing of the reduction and outcome regarding osteonecrosis. In 42 hips, a closed reduction was performed in less than 24 hours after presentation; osteonecrosis developed in 3 hips (7%). In 49 hips, a closed reduction was performed more than 24 hours after presentation, and osteonecrosis developed in 10 hips (20%). The authors hypothesized that the acute displacement of the femoral head may kink the posterior blood vessels, compromising the blood flow to the epiphysis. In this situation, a timely reduction of the SCFE may restore blood flow to the epiphysis. Gordon and associates[160] confirmed this concept with no occurrences of osteonecrosis in 10 unstable SCFEs treated within 24 hours with reduction, arthrotomy, and two-screw fixation.

Animal studies support the concept of early reduction and joint decompression. Beck and associates[161] evaluated the effects of increased intra-articular pressure on the blood flow to the femoral head. In 11 patients treated with open surgical dislocation for the femoroacetabular impingement, saline was injected into the intact intracapsular space while monitoring the blood flow to the femoral head with laser Doppler flowmetry. After an average intracapsular saline injection of 20 mL, loss of the pulsatile signal occurred with an average intra-articular pressure of 58 mm Hg. Aspiration of the joint caused a return of the pulsatile flow. These results support the recommendation to perform an urgent decompression of the intracapsular hematoma to optimize blood flow to the femoral head. Similarly, in the juvenile goat, Svalastoga and associates[162] showed that a joint pressure of 75 mm Hg resulted in a decrease in oxygen tension from 48 mm Hg to 29 mm Hg; traction in extension further decreased the oxygen tension. This study highlights the risks of treating a hip joint with an effusion by traction and indicates that aspiration should be strongly considered.

Several studies evaluated the question of how many screws should be used in the unstable SCFE; however, nearly all of the studies used in vitro animal models and were relatively far removed from the clinical situation. Karol and associates[136] compared one- and two-screw fixation in a calf model (testing a single load to failure) and found that single-screw fixation was 77% as stable as double-screw fixation. Kibiloski and associates[163] used the same model but studied the effects of physiologic shear loading, simulating slow walking and fast walking. The rates of creep were larger for the single-screw fixation group, particularly with fast walking, but the results were not statistically significant. The authors concluded that regardless of whether one or two screws are used, protected weight bearing is advisable in the postoperative period in the unstable SCFE. In an immature porcine model, Snyder and associates[164] studied torsional strength after removal of the perichondrium at the physeal level (analogous to the situation of the unstable SCFE in which the perichondrium at the physeal level has been compromised). This study differed from the studies done by both Karol and associates[136] and by Kibiloski and associates[163] who studied shear to failure, not torsion. Snyder and associates[164] found that two-screw fixation after removal of the perichondrium provided 43% of the stiffness and 74% of the strength of the intact physis in torsion. In an immature bovine model, Kishan and associates[165] evaluated one- and two-screw fixations in varying configurations at physiologically relevant loads and found no significant differences among three different screw configurations but did find that two-screw constructs were 66% stiffer and 66% stronger than single screw constructs.

Based on the literature to date, the authors recommend closed reduction, urgent hip joint aspiration/decompression, and single- or double-screw fixation for patients with unstable SCFE. One screw may not provide adequate fixation, but two screws may increase the risk of osteonecrosis and chondrolysis. In either situation, not bearing weight on the affected limb and the use of crutches for 6 to 8 weeks is recommended to prevent progression.

Prophylactic Fixation of the Contralateral Hip

The risk of a contralateral SCFE in a patient with unilateral SCFE is reported to be 2,335 times higher than the risk of an initial SCFE.[166] Schultz and associates[166] developed a decision analysis model with probabilities for the occurrence of a contralateral SCFE and concluded that prophylactic fixation of the contralateral hip was beneficial to the long-term outcome of that hip. The authors cautioned that the clinician must use sound judgment with respect to the age, gender, and endocrine status of the patient, including the preferences of the patient and family, before recommending prophylactic fixation of the contralateral hip. By contrast, Kocher and associates[167] also used a decision analysis model with probabilities for the occurrence of a contralateral SCFE but described a more limited group for whom the procedure would be beneficial. In their model, prophylactic fixation of the contralateral hip is favored for those in whom the probability of a contralateral SCFE is greater than 27% or in patients for whom reliable follow-up is not feasible. The difference in these studies is that Schultz and associates[166] used values from the literature for various incidences and probabilities of events (such as osteonecrosis, chondrolysis, severity of SCFE,), whereas Kocher and associates[167] used a questionnaire to determine patient preferences in a group of children without SCFE; the questionnaire posed scenarios for different outcomes and asked the children to rate preferences regarding prophylactic fixation from the context of the scenario.

Epidemiologic data also provide conflicting opinions regarding prophylactic fixation, with. prophylactic fixation recommended by some physicians and close observation recommended by others.[34,168-171] A Pediatric Orthopaedic Society of North America membership survey recommended prophylactic fixation of the contralateral hip only 12.2% of the time.[156]

Complications

Osteonecrosis

Osteonecrosis is a devastating complication, occurring infrequently in a stable SCFE but more frequently in an unstable SCFE[56] (Figure 9). Factors associated with osteonecrosis are an unstable SCFE, anterior physeal separation, overreduction of an unstable SCFE, attempted reduction of a stable SCFE, the placement of pins in the posterosuperior quadrant of the epiphysis, and cuneiform osteotomy.[53,56,131,132,172-175]

The patient with osteonecrosis typically reports pain in the groin or knee. On physical examination, a loss of range of motion of the hip (particularly internal rotation) exists, and the hip is irritable to passive internal and external rotation. The plain radiographs are unremarkable early in the course of the disorder, but changes diagnostic of osteonecrosis (collapse of the femoral head with cyst formation and sclerosis) develop after a few months. Osteonecrosis after SCFE will be radiographically apparent in all pa-

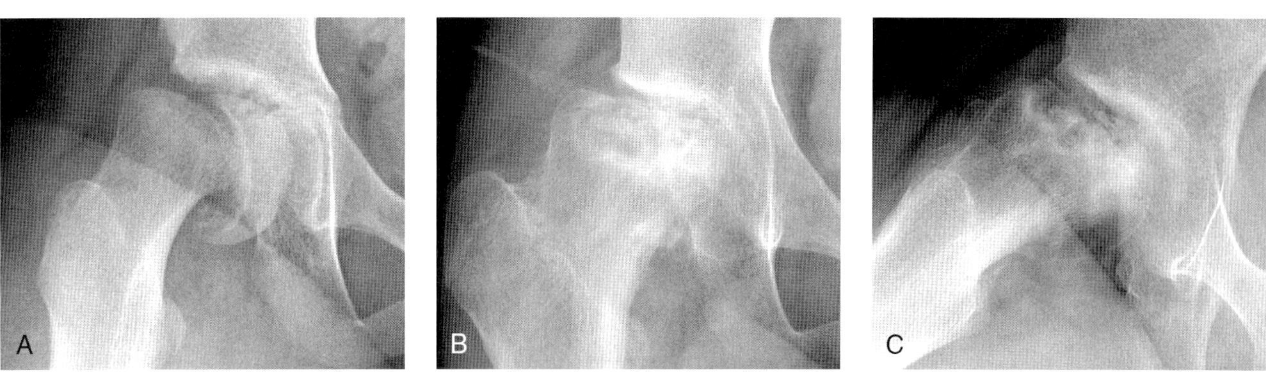

Figure 9 **A,** The AP radiograph of an unstable right SCFE in a girl age 11 years, 2 months. Emergent reduction and fixation was performed, but by the age of 12 years, 8 months, osteonecrosis was apparent on the AP **(B)** and lateral **(C)** radiographs.

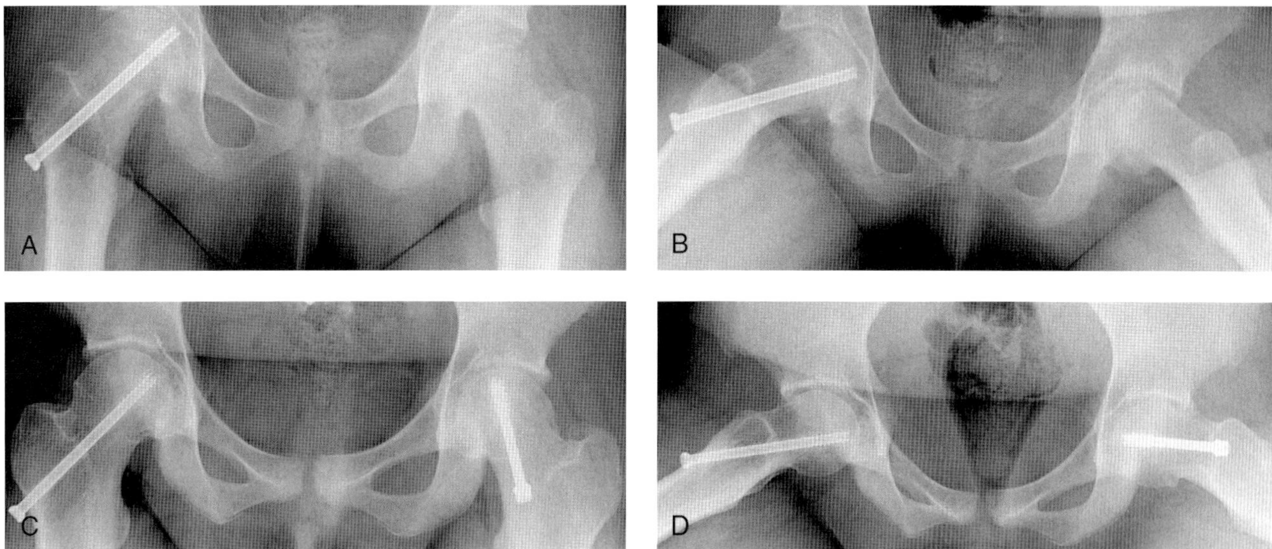

Figure 10 AP **(A)** and frog pelvis lateral **(B)** radiographs of a girl age 13 years, 6 months, who had previously undergone in situ fixation for a right SCFE. Note the protrusion of the screw into the joint space and the joint space narrowing, indicative of chondrolysis. Also note the opposite left SCFE. The right screw was slightly withdrawn along with in situ fixation of the left SCFE. At age 15 years, 5 months, the AP **(C)** and frog-lateral **(D)** radiographs show physeal closure of both hips and improvement in the joint space narrowing of the right hip.

tients within 1 year. An early bone scan or an MRI scan will often show asymmetry between the femoral heads, predicting the eventual development of osteonecrosis.[176] Krahn and associates[173] evaluated 22 patients with osteonecrosis after a mean follow-up of 31 years. Nine patients (41%) had reconstructive surgery, four during adolescence and five during adulthood. The remaining 13 patients had not yet had reconstructive surgery, but all had radiographic degenerative changes.

The treatment of osteonecrosis includes not bearing weight by using crutches, range-of-motion exercises, and anti-inflammatory medication. Internal fixation that protrudes into the joint should be repositioned in the epiphysis if the physis is open or removed if the physis is closed. Ten-year survivorship of the hip may approach 75% when an arthrogram and examination under anesthesia indicate that an osteotomy would result in a more congruous joint in a noninvolved portion of the femoral head.[177]

Chondrolysis

Chondrolysis is defined as a narrowing of the joint space by at least 50% compared with the opposite hip with unilateral chondrolysis, and less than 3 mm joint space with bilateral chondrolysis.[178-180] Chondrolysis may already be present when the patient first presents with

SCFE. However, in most patients with SCFE, the etiology of chondrolysis is secondary to unrecognized pin penetration of the femoral head at the time of surgery (Figure 10). In patients without pin penetration, an autoimmune phenomenon or some factor that interferes with cartilage nutrition may contribute to the chondrolysis. Factors associated with chondrolysis include unrecognized pin penetration, treatment in a hip spica cast, intertrochanteric osteotomy, severe SCFE, and prolonged symptoms before treatment.

The incidence of chondrolysis in patients with a SCFE was historically 5% to 7%, but many recent studies now support a far lower 1% to 2% incidence.[47,48] The patient usually reports pain in the groin or knee, and loss of hip motion, particularly internal rotation, is shown on physical examination. The diagnosis is confirmed by radiographs that show decreased joint width. An early bone scan that shows increased uptake in the hip with premature closure of the greater trochanter has been associated with an increased risk for the development of chondrolysis.[181] The incidence of chondrolysis increases with increasing severity of the SCFE. It is not increased in the black population as previously reported.[180,182-187] The frequency of chondrolysis is less with single-screw fixation than with fixation using multiple screws or pins.[188]

The treatment of chondrolysis, as with the treatment of osteonecrosis, is not particularly rewarding for the patient or the clinician. Non–weight-bearing ambulation with crutches, range-of-motion exercises, and anti-inflammatory medication may help alleviate symptoms. When there is screw protrusion, backing the screw out of the joint, or removing it if the physis is closed, will help minimize hip damage (Figure 10). Lengthening of the contracted muscle is recommended by some physicians for a hip with contracture, with arthrodesis required in severe situations.

Patients with chondrolysis have a better long-term prognosis than those with osteonecrosis. Tudisco and associates[189] evaluated nine patients with chondrolysis at a mean follow-up of 14 years and noted gradual regression of hip pain with restoration of the joint space after a mean of 10 months. At follow-up, five patients had mild pain after prolonged activity; all had some limitation of abduction and internal rotation.

Internal Fixation

The frequency of problems related to internal fixation (slip progression, implant breakage, and joint penetration) is decreasing with the use of fluoroscopically guided, cannulated single-screw fixation. The risk of fracture through an unused pinhole can be avoided by using fluoroscopy to position the guide pin correctly on the first attempt and by entering the bone proximal to the lesser trochanter.

Natural History Without Treatment

Two major issues arise with the untreated SCFE: the risk of further progression and the risk of degenerative joint disease in adult life. Unfortunately, there are few long-term studies of patients with SCFE and even fewer studies that also include untreated patients with SCFEs.[50,51,53,66,190-192]

Risk of Progression

The natural history of SCFE is unpredictable, and the risk of further progression is difficult to ascertain. Ordeberg and associates[193] reviewed studies of SCFEs without primary treatment 20 to 40 years after diagnosis. Although few patients had restrictions in their working capacity or social life, there was a risk of slip progression if the physis remained open.[194] Carney and associates[53] reported on 35 SCFEs that were initially observed; additional displacement occurred in 6 SCFEs (17%) after initial diagnosis, and 5 SCFEs became severe. Eleven of the 35 patients (31%) had an acute episode of SCFE superimposed on the chronic SCFE; these 11 slips all progressed to severe displacement and required surgical stabilization.

Risk of Degenerative Joint Disease

Howorth[195] stated that SCFE is likely the most frequent cause of degenerative joint disease of the hip in middle life and a common source of pain and disability. This conclusion is not necessarily supported by other studies. In reviewing a large study of patients with degenerative joint disease, the number of patients with known SCFE is low, averaging approximately 5%.[196-198] Murray[197] reported an association with SCFE in 80 of 200 patients (40%) believed to have primary degenerative joint disease. He described a tilt deformity caused by bone resorption laterally with new bone formation medially and believed this disorder to be compatible with an old SCFE. Stulberg and associates[199] also described a similar deformity, the pistol grip deformity, in 40% of patients without known prior hip disease undergoing total hip arthroplasty. This deformity was also believed to be compatible with an old SCFE. Resnick[200] refuted this theory in a pathologic study of 48 femoral heads of patients with a tilt deformity on radiographs that suggested the deformity was solely related to the remodeling changes of osteoarthritis. Whether subclinical forms of SCFE led to early osteoarthritis remains uncertain.

It is known that the severity of deformity in the untreated SCFE correlates with the long-term prognosis regarding degenerative joint disease.[53,66,153,191,192,201] Oram[191] reported on 22 untreated SCFEs, 11 of which were observed for more than 15 years. Those with moderate SCFEs retained good function for years, whereas degenerative joint disease with resultant poor function developed within 15 years in patients with severe SCFEs. Jerre[153,201] and Ross and associates[192] reported increasingly poor results with longer follow-up. Both groups reported many patients doing well early in the disease process; however, increasing symptoms and decreasing function developed with increasing age.

Carney and Weinstein[66] studied the natural history of the untreated, chronic SCFE in an evaluation of 31 hips in 28 patients at an average age of 55 years and at an average follow-up of 41 years. The average Iowa Hip Rating for the entire group was 89 points; the scores were: 92 in the 17 mild SCFEs, 87 in the 11 moderate SCFEs, and 75 in the 3 severe SCFEs. Although patients with mild SCFE appear to have a favorable prognosis, patients with moderate and severe SCFE have a high incidence of degenerative joint disease. At 41-year follow-up, an Iowa Hip Rating greater than 80 points was present in 100% of mild SCFEs and 64% of moderate and severe SCFEs. Degenerative changes were noted in 36% of the mild SCFEs and 100% of the moderate and severe SCFEs. However, poor results can occasionally occur even with minimal SCFEs.[50,53,66,192] The natural history of chronic (stable) SCFE is favorable, provided that displacement is mild and remains so.

There are few data on the natural history of untreated acute SCFEs. Progression begins with an acute episode, which is followed by a 2- to 3-week period of intolerance to weight bearing. As the pain and spasm subside, a degree of motion returns, although the hip remains moderately painful in a position of external rotation. Degenerative changes (joint space narrowing, subchondral bone cysts, epiphyseal collapse) develop within a few months, and the patient is left with residual flexion, adduction, and external rotation contractures.[51]

Long-Term Results of Treatment

Wilson and associates[38] reviewed 300 hips in 240 patients treated between 1936 and 1960; 187 were treated by fixation in situ with 81% good clinical results and 77% good radiographic results. Poorer results occurred in the 76 hips in which correction of the deformity had been attempted (60% good clinical results and 55% good radiographic results). Hall[190] reported on 138 patients, with the best results obtained with the use of multiple pins; 16 of 20 patients (80%) had excellent results. The worst results were seen after realignment had been attempted with manipulation or osteotomy; osteotomy of the femoral neck, in particular, led to poor results in 36% of the hips and osteonecrosis in 38%.

Patients with SCFE in southern Sweden were followed for more than 30 years.[193] Symptomatic treatment or fixation in situ resulted in high clinical ratings and few radiographic changes, with only 2% of the hips needing a secondary reconstructive procedure. When closed reduction and a spica cast were used, the combined rate of osteonecrosis and chondrolysis was 13%, and reconstructive procedures were needed in 35% of the hips. Femoral neck osteotomy was followed by a combined rate of osteonecrosis and chondrolysis of 30%, and reconstructive procedures were necessary in 15% of the hips.

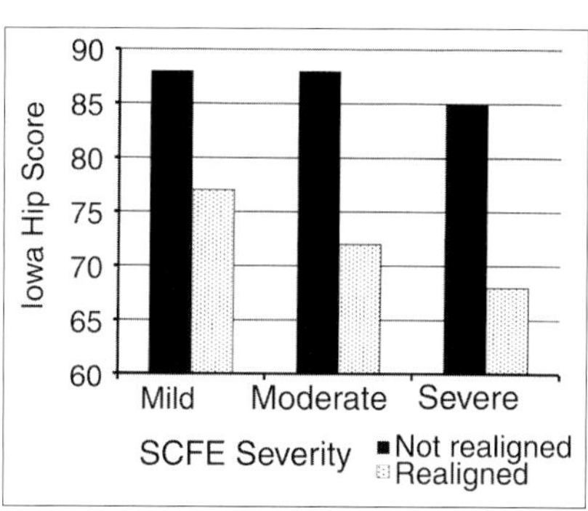

Figure 11 The graph shows worsening scores on the Iowa Hip Rating Scale for children with SCFE at 41-year average follow-up. Deterioration over time becomes more pronounced as slip severity increases.

Carney and associates[53] reported on 155 hips in 124 patients at a mean follow-up of 41 years using the Iowa Hip Rating and radiographic classification of degenerative joint disease (0 = no degenerative disease, 3 = severe degenerative disease). The SCFEs were mild in 42% of patients, moderate in 32%, and severe in 26%. Management of the chronic SCFEs involved symptomatic treatment in 25% of patients, a spica cast in 30%, fixation in situ in 24%, and osteotomy in 20%. Poorer results were associated with more severe slips and realignment (Figure 11). Osteonecrosis (12%) and chondrolysis (16%) were more common

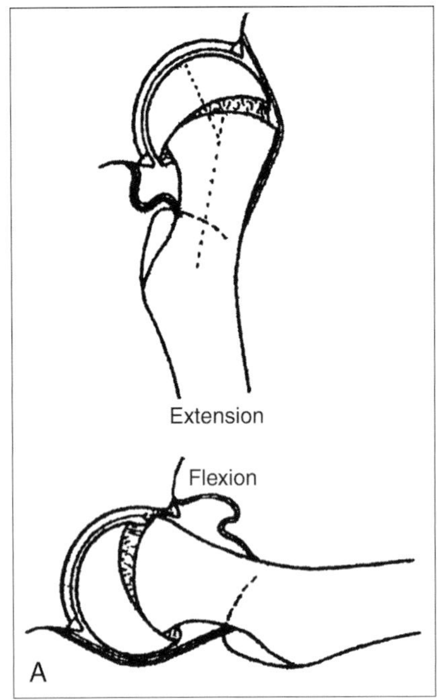

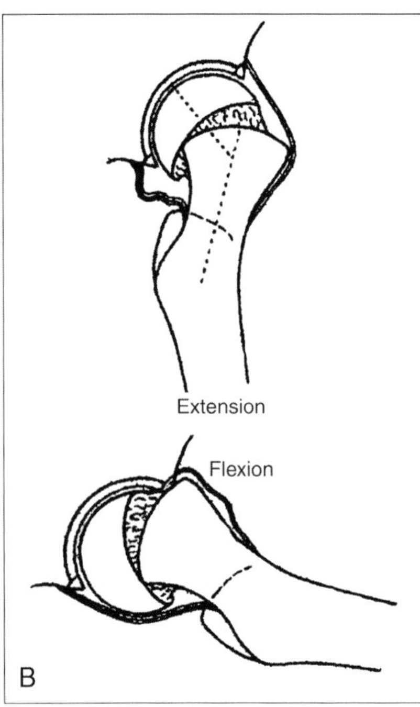

Figure 12 Schematic lateral drawings of varying types of degrees of SCFE in extension and flexion. **A,** Mild to moderate SCFE causes jamming of the femoral metaphysis against the acetabular cartilage in flexion. **B,** Severe SCFE with an impingement of the femoral neck against the acetabular rim in flexion. (Reproduced with permission from Leunig M. Casillas MM, Hamlet M, Hersche O, Nötzli H, Slongo T, Ganz R: Slipped capital femoral epiphysis: Early mechanical damage to the acetabular cartilage by a prominent femoral metaphysis. *Acta Orthop Scand* 2000;71:370-375.)

with increasing slip severity. Reduction was performed in 39 hips and realignment in 65 hips. For the 116 hips that had not been reduced, the mean Iowa Hip Rating was 85 points and the mean radiographic grade was 1.7. Osteonecrosis developed in 7 hips (6%) and chondrolysis in 14 (12%). For the 39 SCFEs that had been reduced, the mean Iowa Hip Rating was 72 points and the mean radiographic degenerative score was 2.4. Osteonecrosis developed in 12 hips (31%) and chondrolysis in 11 (28%). Twenty-seven hips with a chronic SCFE pinned in situ showed a mean hip rating of 90 points and a mean radiographic grade of 1.5. Osteonecrosis developed in one hip and chondrolysis in none.[53] These long-term study results support the use of in situ fixation as the treatment of choice for SCFE. Realignment was associated with appreciable complications and adversely affected the outcome. Regardless of slip severity, fixation in situ provided the best long-term function and delay of degenerative arthritis with the lowest risk of complications (Figure 11). Although limb-length discrepancy and motion in abduction and internal rotation were affected by the severity of the slip, function was not significantly impaired.

The conclusion from these studies is that regardless of the slip severity, fixation in situ provides the best long-term function, lowest complication risk, and most effective delay of degenerative arthritis. Many patients with SCFE do well with this treatment at long-term follow-up when the SCFE is of mild or moderate severity, good congruity between the femoral head and the acetabulum is maintained, and osteonecrosis and chondrolysis do not occur. In severe SCFEs or those with osteonecrosis or chondrolysis, a more rapid deterioration with degenerative changes occurs. SCFE differs from other pediatric hip disorders such as Legg-Calvé-Perthes disease and developmental hip dysplasia in that SCFE occurs at an age when most of the acetabular development is completed. Because of this acetabular maturity, adaptation to head deformity cannot occur.

Possible Future Directions

With newer technology that includes improved implants and intraoperative imaging, some surgeons are revisiting the role of transphyseal osteotomy, reduction, and fixation. This advancement has been brought about by the advent of surgical dislocation of the hip. As noted earlier, children treated with in situ fixation had better results than those treated with realignment. However, the realignment procedures used in those patients were either closed reductions in stable SCFEs, which should not be performed, or osteotomies done at a time when present-day improvements in intraoperative radiography and internal fixation did not exist. Therefore, will a realignment osteotomy performed today have a better outcome than those described in the long-term study of Carney and associates,[53] and, if so, will an osteotomy using current methods in a severe SCFE improve the natural history? This question is now being vigorously debated because of increasing evidence of potential mechanical damage that can occur from the prominent femoral metaphysis in a severe SCFE on the acetabular cartilage or femoracetabular impingement.[55,123,154,202]

In 14 adolescent hips with SCFE, Leunig and associates[123] noted labral and acetabular cartilage damage had occurred when the anterior femoral metaphysis was level with or extended past the epiphysis (Figures 12 and 13). This damage consisted of scars, tears, and erosions in the acetabular cartilage and ranged from partial to full-thickness loss. The femoral head cartilage was intact. These findings suggest that degenerative hip disease in children with SCFE can be triggered by early mechanical damage of the acetabular cartilage and that femoroacetabular impingement, which increases with SCFE severity, will result in significant long-term deterioration of the hip.

The technique of surgical dislocation of the hip with epiphyseal reorientation has been developed.[123,124] This technique involves a trochanteric osteotomy, gentle dislocation after a wide Z-capsulotomy, subperiosteal exposure of the posterior femoral neck, separation of the epiphysis through the physis, resection of the medial and posterior callus off the femoral neck, removal of the epiphyseal physis, reduction of the epiphysis without retinacular tension, and fixation of the epiphysis to the femoral neck.[124] The concept is that, with a properly and gently performed surgical dislocation of the hip, epiphyseal perfusion can be maintained during epiphyseal reorientation and avoid the high incidence of osteonecrosis that occurs when physeal resection with epiphyseal reduction is performed without surgical dislocation. Since 1996, Ganz has performed this procedure in 32 hips with a minimum follow-up of 18 months. Complications have included two fixation failures, the need for one varus/extension intertrochanteric osteotomy, and, most remarkably, no occurrence of osteonecrosis. (R. Ganz, MD, Chicago, IL, unpublished data, 2006.) This technique is demanding and should be performed by those appropriately trained. It still remains to be seen whether this new approach will result in improvement in long-term prognosis compared with results in a 41-year retrospective review by Carney and associates.[53]

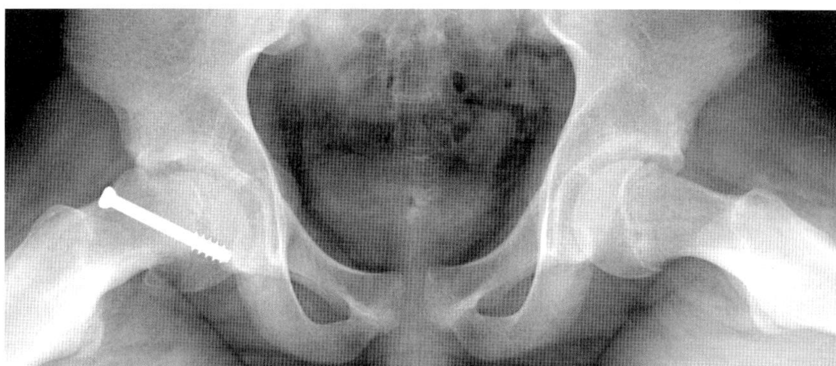

Figure 13 An example of impaction of the metaphysis on the acetabular rim when the hip is in the flexed position in a severe right SCFE in boy age 15 years, 5 months, after in situ single-screw central fixation. Note the early mild SCFE in the left hip.

Summary

The etiology of the idiopathic SCFE is a combination of both biomechanical and biochemical factors, whereas the role of genetics and heredity is variable. Naturally occurring SCFEs in animal models suggest that biochemical changes precede both physeal changes and subsequent SCFEs. Although pathologic changes of SCFE across species are the same, it appears that the etiology and pathophysiology are different. Several treatment modes, improved because of advances in imaging, exist for the stable SCFE, with single-screw fixation the most common treatment of SCFE currently used in North America. In the unstable SCFE, treatment is more controversial because of the increased risk of complications, especially osteonecrosis. Complications include osteonecrosis and chondrolysis, with better long-term prognosis for those with chondrolysis. Natural history without treatment entails the risk of progression and later degenerative joint disease of the hip. The conclusion drawn for long-term results of treatment is that regardless of severity, fixation in situ provides the best long-term function, lowest complication risk, and most effective delay of degenerative arthritis. Newer technologies include improved implants and intraoperative imaging, allowing surgeons to revisit the role of transphyseal osteotomy, reduction, and fixation. A current question is whether a realignment osteotomy performed today has a better outcome than that performed in the past. Finally, the technique of surgical dislocation of the hip with epiphyseal reorientation is considered; however, the long-term outcome is unknown.

References

1. Schein AJ: Acute severe slipped capital femoral epiphysis. *Clin Orthop Relat Res* 1967;51:151-166.

2. Segal LS, Weitzel PP, Davidson RS: Valgus slipped capital femoral epiphysis: Fact or fiction? *Clin Orthop Relat Res* 1996;322:91-98.
3. Loder RT, O'Donnell PW, Didelot WP, Kayes KJ: Valgus slipped capital femoral epiphysis. *J Pediatr Orthop* 2006;26:594-600.
4. Yngve DA, Moulton DL, Evans EB: Valgus slipped capital femoral epiphysis. *J Pediatr Orthop B* 2005;14:172-176.
5. Loder RT, Wittenberg B, DeSilva G: Slipped capital femoral epiphysis associated with endocrine disorders. *J Pediatr Orthop* 1995;15:349-356.
6. Wells D, King JD, Roe TF, Kaufman FR: Review of slipped capital femoral epiphysis associated with endocrine disease. *J Pediatr Orthop* 1993;13:610-614.
7. McAfee PC, Cady RB: Endocrinologic and metabolic factors in atypical presentations of slipped capital femoral epiphysis: Report of four cases and review of the literature. *Clin Orthop Relat Res* 1983;180:188-196.
8. Loder RT, Hensinger RN: Slipped capital femoral epiphysis associated with renal failure osteodystrophy. *J Pediatr Orthop* 1997;17:205-211.
9. Loder RT, Hensinger RN, Alburger PD, et al: Slipped capital femoral epiphysis associated with radiation therapy. *J Pediatr Orthop* 1998;18:630-636.
10. Liu S-C, Tsai C-C, Huang C-H: Atypical slipped capital femoral epiphysis after radiotherapy and chemotherapy. *Clin Orthop Relat Res* 2004;426:212-218.
11. Ninomiya S, Nagasaka Y, Tagawa H: Slipped capital femoral epiphysis: A study of 68 cases in the eastern half area of Japan. *Clin Orthop Relat Res* 1976;119:172-176.
12. Kelsey JL, Keggi KJ, Southwick WO: The incidence and distribution of slipped capital femoral epiphysis in Connecticut and southwestern United States. *J Bone Joint Surg Am* 1970;52:1203-1216.
13. Lehmann CL, Arons RP, Loder RT, Vitale MG: The epidemiology of slipped capital femoral epiphysis: An update. *J Pediatr Orthop* 2006;26:286-290.
14. Noguchi Y, Sakamaki T: Epidemiology and demographics of slipped capital femoral epiphysis in Japan: A multicenter study by the Japanese Paediatric Orthopaedic Association. *J Orthop Sci* 2002;7:610-617.
15. Hansson LI, Hägglund G, Ordeberg G: Slipped capital femoral epiphysis in southern Sweden 1910-1982. *Acta Orthop Scand Suppl* 1987;226:1-67.
16. Kocher MS, Bishop JA, Weed B, et al: Delay in diagnosis of slipped capital femoral epiphysis. *Pediatrics* 2004;113:e322-e325.
17. Loder RT, Starnes T, Dikos G, Aronsson DD: Demographic predictors of severity of stable slipped capital femoral epiphyses. *J Bone Joint Surg Am* 2006;88:97-105.
18. Loder RT: The demographics of slipped capital femoral epiphysis: An international multicenter study. *Clin Orthop Relat Res* 1996;322:8-27.
19. Kelsey JL, Acheson RM, Keggi KJ: The body build of patients with slipped capital femoral epiphysis. *Am J Dis Child* 1972;124:276-281.
20. KeepKidsHealty Website. Calculator BMI. Available at: http://www.keepkidshealthy.com/welcome/bmicalculator.html. Accessed September 10, 2007.
21. Centers for Disease Control and Prevention Website. Body Mass Index. www.cdc.gov/nccdphp/dnpa/bmi/bmi-for-age.html. Accessed September 10, 2007.
22. Bhatia NN, Pirpiris M, Otsuka NY: Body mass index in patients with slipped capital femoral epiphysis. *J Pediatr Orthop* 2006;26:197-199.
23. Manoff EM, Banffy MB, Winell JJ: Relationship between body mass index and slipped capital femoral epiphysis. *J Pediatr Orthop* 2005;25:744-746.
24. Poussa M, Schlenzka D, Yrjönen T: Body mass index and slipped capital femoral epiphysis. *J Pediatr Orthop B* 2003;12:369-371.
25. Loder RT, Farley FA, Herzenberg JE, Hensinger RN, Kuhn JL: Narrow window of bone age in children with slipped capital femoral epiphyses. *J Pediatr Orthop* 1993;13:290-293.
26. Loder RT, Starnes T, Dikos G: The narrow window of bone age in children with slipped capital femoral epiphysis: A reassessment one decade later. *J Pediatr Orthop* 2006;26:300-306.
27. Loder RT: A worldwide study on the seasonal variation of slipped capital femoral epiphysis. *Clin Orthop Relat Res* 1996;322:28-36.
28. Ferguson AB, Howorth MB: Slipping of the upper femoral epiphysis. *JAMA* 1931;97:1867-1872.
29. Morscher E: Strength and morphology of growth cartilage under hormonal influence of puberty: Animal experiments and clinical study on the etiology of local growth disorders during puberty. *Reconstr Surg Traumatol* 1968;10:3-104.
30. Hägglund G, Hansson LI, Ordeberg G: Epidemiology of slipped capital femoral epiphysis in southern Sweden. *Clin Orthop Relat Res* 1984;191:82-94.
31. Andrén L, Borgström KE: Seasonal variation of epiphysiolysis of the hip and possibility of causal factor. *Acta Orthop Scand* 1958;28:22-26.
32. Brown D: Seasonal variation of slipped capital femoral epiphysis in the United States. *J Pediatr Orthop* 2004;24:139-143.
33. Maffulli N, Douglas AS: Seasonal variation of slipped capital femoral epiphysis. *J Pediatr Orthop B* 2002;11:29-33.
34. Jerre R, Billing L, Hansson G, Wallin J: The contralateral hip in patients primarily treated for unilateral slipped upper femoral epiphysis. *J Bone Joint Surg Br* 1994;76:563-567.

35. Jerre R, Billing L, Hansson G, Karlsson J, Wallin J: Bilaterality in slipped capital femoral epiphysis: Importance of a reliable radiographic method. *J Pediatr Orthop B* 1996;5: 80-84.

36. Hurley JM, Betz RR, Loder RT, Davidson RS, Alburger PD, Steel HH: Slipped capital femoral epiphysis: The prevalence of late contralateral slip. *J Bone Joint Surg Am* 1996;78:226-230.

37. Stasikelis PJ, Sullivan CM, Phillips WA, Polard JA: Slipped capital femoral epiphysis: Prediction of contralateral involvement. *J Bone Joint Surg Am* 1996;78:1149-1155.

38. Wilson PD, Jacobs B, Schecter L: Slipped capital femoral epiphysis: An end-result study. *J Bone Joint Surg Am* 1965;47:1128-1145.

39. Sørensen KH: Slipped upper femoral epiphysis: Clinical study on aetiology. *Acta Orthop Scand* 1968;39:499-517.

40. Dreghorn CR, Knight D, Mainds CC, Blockey NJ: Slipped upper femoral epiphysis: A review of 12 years of experience in Glasgow (1972-1983). *J Pediatr Orthop* 1987;7:283-287.

41. Loder RT, Aronson DD, Greenfield ML: The epidemiology of bilateral slipped capital femoral epiphysis: A study of children in Michigan. *J Bone Joint Surg Am* 1993;75:1141-1147.

42. Segal LS, Davidson RS, Robertson WWJ, Drummond DS: Growth disturbance after pinning of juvenile slipped capital femoral epiphysis. *J Pediatr Orthop* 1991;11:631-637.

43. Stott S, Bidwell T: Epidemiology of slipped capital femoral epiphysis in a population with a high proportion of New Zealand Maori and Pacific children. *N Z Med J* 2003;116:U647.

44. Kitadai HK, Milani C, Nery CAS, Filho JL: Wiberg's center-edge angle in patients with slipped capital femoral epiphysis. *J Pediatr Orthop* 1999;19: 97-105.

45. Loder RT, Mehbod AA, Meyer CA, Meisterling M: Acetabular depth and race in young adults: A potential explanation of the differences in the prevalence of slipped capital femoral epiphysis (SCFE) between different racial groups? *J Pediatr Orthop* 2003; 23:699-702.

46. Fahey JJ, O'Brien ET: Acute slipped capital femoral epiphysis. *J Bone Joint Surg Am* 1965;47:1105-1127.

47. Aronson DD, Carlson WE: Slipped capital femoral epiphysis: A prospective study of fixation with a single screw. *J Bone Joint Surg Am* 1992;74: 810-819.

48. Ward WT, Stefko J, Wood KB, Stanitski CL: Fixation with a single screw for slipped capital femoral epiphysis. *J Bone Joint Surg Am* 1992;74:799-809.

49. Aadalen RJ, Weiner DS, Hoyt W, Herndon CH: Acute slipped capital femoral epiphysis. *J Bone Joint Surg Am* 1974;56:1473-1487.

50. Boyer DW, Mickelson MR, Ponseti IV: Slipped capital femoral epiphysis: Long-term follow-up of one hundred and twenty-one patients. *J Bone Joint Surg Am* 1981;63:85-95.

51. Ponseti I, Barta CK: Evaluation of treatment of slipping of the capital femoral epiphysis. *Surg Gynecol Obstet* 1948;86:87-97.

52. Casey BH, Hamilton HW, Bobechko WP: Reduction of acutely slipped capital femoral epiphysis. *J Bone Joint Surg Br* 1972;54:607-614.

53. Carney BT, Weinstein SW, Noble J: Long-term follow-up of slipped capital femoral epiphysis. *J Bone Joint Surg Am* 1991;73:667-674.

54. Jacobs B: Diagnosis and natural history of slipped capital femoral epiphysis. *Instr Course Lect* 1972;21:167-173.

55. Rab GT: The geometry of slipped capital femoral epiphysis: Implications for movement, impingement, and corrective osteotomy. *J Pediatr Orthop* 1999;19:419-424.

56. Loder RT, Richards BS, Shapiro PS, Reznick LR, Aronson DD: Acute slipped capital femoral epiphysis: The importance of physeal stability. *J Bone Joint Surg Am* 1993;75:1134-1140.

57. Kallio PE, Paterson DC, Foster BK, Lequesne GW: Classification in slipped capital femoral epiphysis: Sonographic assessment of stability and remodeling. *Clin Orthop Relat Res* 1993;294:196-203.

58. Kallio PE, Mah ET, Foster BK, Paterson DC, LeQuesne GW: Slipped capital femoral epiphysis: Incidence and assessment of physeal instability. *J Bone Joint Surg Br* 1995;77:752-755.

59. Aronsson DD, Loder RT: Treatment of the unstable (acute) slipped capital femoral epiphysis. *Clin Orthop Relat Res* 1996;322:99-110.

60. Rhoad RC, Davidson RS, Heyman S, Dormans JP, Drummond DS: Pretreatment bone scan in SCFE: A predictor of ischemia and avascular necrosis. *J Pediatr Orthop* 1999;19: 164-168.

61. Steel HH: The metaphyseal blanch sign of slipped capital femoral epiphysis. *J Bone Joint Surg Am* 1986;68: 920-922.

62. Klein A, Joplin RJ, Reidy JA, Hanelin J: Slipped capital femoral epiphysis: Early diagnosis and treatment facilitated by "normal" roentgenograms. *J Bone Joint Surg Am* 1952;34:233-239.

63. Kamegaya M, Saisu T, Ochiai N, Moriya H: Preoperative assessment for intertrochanteric femoral osteotomies in severe chronic slipped capital femoral epiphysis using computed tomography. *J Pediatr Orthop B* 2005;14: 71-78.

64. Loder RT, Blakemore LC, Farley FA, Laidlaw AT: Measurement variability of slipped capital femoral epiphysis. *J Orthop Surg (Hong Kong)* 2000;7: 33-42.

65. Southwick WO: Osteotomy through the lesser trochanter for slipped capital femoral epiphysis. *J Bone Joint Surg Am* 1967;49:807-835.

66. Carney BT, Weinstein SL: Natural history of untreated chronic slipped capital femoral epiphysis. *Clin Orthop Relat Res* 1996;322:43-47.

67. Weiner D: Pathogenesis of slipped capital femoral epiphysis: Current concepts. *J Pediatr Orthop B* 1996;5: 67-73.

68. Galbraith RT, Gelberman RH, Hajek PC, et al: Obesity and decreased femoral anteversion in adolescence. *J Orthop Res* 1987;5:523-528.

69. Gelberman RH, Cohen MS, Shaw BA, Kasser JR, Griffin PP, Wilkinson RH: The association of femoral retroversion with slipped capital femoral epiphysis. *J Bone Joint Surg Am* 1986; 68:1000-1007.

70. Pritchett JW, Perdue KD: Mechanical factors in slipped capital femoral epiphysis. *J Pediatr Orthop* 1988;8: 385-388.

71. Mirkopulos N, Weiner DS, Askew M: The evolving slope of the proximal femoral growth plate relationship to slipped capital femoral epiphysis. *J Pediatr Orthop* 1988;8:268-273.

72. Fishkin Z, Armstrong D, Shah H, Patra A, Mihaldo WM: Proximal femoral physis shear in slipped capital femoral epiphysis: A finite element study. *J Pediatr Orthop* 2006;26: 291-294.

73. Exner GU: Growth and pubertal development in slipped capital femoral epiphysis: A longitudinal study. *J Pediatr Orthop* 1986;6:403-409.

74. Speer DP: Experimental epiphysiolysis: Etiologic models of slipped capital femoral epiphysis, in Nelson JP (ed): *The Hip: Proceedings of the 12th Open Scientific Meeting of the Hip Society*. St. Louis, MO, CV Mosby, 1982, pp 68-88.

75. Harris WR: The endocrine basis for slipping of the upper femoral epiphysis. *J Bone Joint Surg Br* 1950;32:5-11.

76. Brenkel IJ, Dias JJ, Iqbal SJ, Gregg PJ: Thyroid hormone levels in patients with slipped capital femoral epiphysis. *J Pediatr Orthop* 1988;8:22-25.

77. Eisenstein A, Rothschild S: Biochemical abnormalities in patients with slipped capital femoral epiphysis and chondrolysis. *J Bone Joint Surg Am* 1976;58:459-467.

78. Mann DC, Weddington J, Richton S: Hormonal studies in patients with slipped capital femoral epiphysis without evidence of endocrinopathy. *J Pediatr Orthop* 1988;8:543-545.

79. Razzano CD, Nelson C, Eversman J: Growth hormone levels in slipped capital femoral epiphysis. *J Bone Joint Surg Am* 1972;54:1224-1226.

80. Wilcox PG, Weiner DS, Leighlye B: Maturation factors in slipped capital femoral epiphysis. *J Pediatr Orthop* 1988;8:196-200.

81. Nicolai RD, Grasemann H, Oberste-Berghaus C, Hövel M, Hauffa BP: Serum insulin-like growth factors IGF-1 and IGFBP-3 in children with slipped capital femoral epiphysis. *J Pediatr Orthop B* 1999;8:103-106.

82. Rennie AM: The inheritance of slipped upper femoral epiphysis. *J Bone Joint Surg Br* 1982;64:180-184.

83. Loder RT, Nechleba J, Sanders JO, Doyle P: Idiopathic slipped capital femoral epiphysis in Amish children. *J Bone Joint Surg Am* 2005;87:543-549.

84. Günal I, Ates E: The HLA phenotype in slipped capital femoral epiphysis. *J Pediatr Orthop* 1997;17:655-656.

85. Bednarz PA, Stanitski CL: Slipped capital femoral epiphysis in identical twins: HLA predisposition. *Orthopedics* 1998;21:1291-1293. Medline

86. Wong-Chung J, Al-Aali Y, Farid I, Al-Aradi A: A common HLA phenotype in slipped capital femoral epiphysis? *Int Orthop* 2000;24:158-159.

87. Flores M, Satish SG, Key T: Slipped capital femoral epiphysis in identical twins: Is there an HLA predisposition? *Bull Hosp Jt Dis* 2006;63:158-160. Medline

88. Agamanolis DP, Weiner DS, Lloyd JK: Slipped capital femoral epiphysis: A pathological study: I. A light microscopic and histochemical study of 21 cases. *J Pediatr Orthop* 1985;5: 40-46.

89. Ponseti IV, McClintock R: Pathology of slipping of the upper femoral epiphysis. *J Bone Joint Surg Am* 1956; 38:71-83.

90. Adamczyk MJ, Weiner DS, Nugent A, McBurney D, Horton WE Jr: Increased chondrocyte apoptosis in growth plates from children with slipped capital femoral epiphysis. *J Pediatr Orthop* 2005;25:440-444.

91. Agamanolis DP, Weiner DS, Lloyd JK: Slipped capital femoral epiphysis: A pathological study: II. An ultrastructural study of 23 cases. *J Pediatr Orthop* 1985;5:47-58.

92. McNicholas WT Jr, Wilkens BE, Blevins WE, et al: Spontaneous femoral capital physeal fractures in adult cats: 26 cases (1996-2001). *J Am Vet Med Assoc* 2002;221:1731-1736.

93. Craig LE: Physeal dysplasia with slipped capital femoral epiphysis in 13 cats. *Vet Pathol* 2001;38:92-97.

94. Queen J, Bennett D, Carmichael S: Femoral neck metaphyseal osteopathy in the cat. *Vet Rec* 1998;142: 159-162.

95. Root MV, Johnston SD, Olson PN: The effect of prepuberal and postpuberal gonadectomy on radial physeal closure in male and female domestic cats. *Vet Radiol Ultrasound* 1997;38: 42-47.

96. Stubbs WP, Bloomberg MS, Scruggs SL, Shille VM, Lane TJ: Effects of prepubertal gonadectomy on physical and behavioral development in cats. *J Am Vet Med Assoc* 1996;209:1864-1871.

97. Hill MA: Skeletal system and feet, in Leman AD, Straw BE, Mengeling WL, D'Allaire S, Taylor DJ, (eds): *Diseases of Swine*, ed 7. Ames, Iowa, Iowa State University Press, 1992, pp163-195.

98. Reiland S: Morphology of osteochondrosis and sequelae in pigs. *Acta Radiol Suppl* 1978;358:45-90.

99. Holmes RG: Separation of the upper femoral epiphysis in the coypu (*Myocastor coypus*). *Vet Rec* 1967;80:405-407.

100. Blenkinsopp WK, Blenkinsopp EC, Flack MB: Slipped femoral epiphysis in the coypu. *J Pathol Bacteriol* 1967; 93:690-693.

101. Dupuis J, Breton L, Drolet R: Bilateral epiphysiolysis of the femoral heads in two dogs. *J Am Vet Med Assoc* 1997;210:1162-1165.

102. Moores AP, Owen MR, Coe RJ, Brown PJ, Butterworth SJ: Slipped

capital femoral epiphysis in dogs. *J Small Anim Pract* 2004;45:602-608.

103. Lee R: Proximal femoral epiphyseal separation in the dog. *J Small Anim Pract* 1976;17:669-679.
104. Hamilton GF, Turner AS, Ferguson JG, Pharr JW: Slipped capital femoral epiphysis in calves. *J Am Vet Med Assoc* 1978;172:1318-1322.
105. Hull BL, Koenig GJ, Monke DR: Treatment of slipped capital femoral epiphysis in cattle: 11 cases (1974-1988). *J Am Vet Med Assoc* 1990;197: 1509-1512.
106. Rahme D, Comley A, Foster B, Cundy P: Consequences of diagnostic delays in slipped capital femoral epiphysis. *J Pediatr Orthop B* 2006;15: 93-97.
107. Meier MC, Meyer LC, Ferguson RL: Treatment of slipped capital femoral epiphysis with a spica cast. *J Bone Joint Surg Am* 1992;74:1522-1529.
108. Rao SB, Crawford AH, Burger RR, Roy DR: Open bone peg epiphyseodesis for slipped capital femoral epiphysis. *J Pediatr Orthop* 1996;16:37-48.
109. Adamczyk MJ, Weiner DS, Hawk D: A 50-year experience with bone graft epiphyseodesis in the treatment of slipped capital femoral epiphysis. *J Pediatr Orthop* 2003;23:578-583.
110. Aronson DD, Peterson DA, Miller DV: Slipped capital femoral epiphysis: The case for internal fixation in situ. *Clin Orthop Relat Res* 1992;281: 115-122.
111. Strong M, Lejman T, Michno P, Sulko J: Fixation of slipped capital femoral epiphyses with unthreaded 2-mm wires. *J Pediatr Orthop* 1996;16: 53-55.
112. Weiner DS, Weiner S, Melby A, Hoyt WH Jr: A 30-year experience with bone graft epiphysiodesis in the treatment of slipped capital femoral epiphysis. *J Pediatr Orthop* 1984;4:145-152.
113. Schmidt TL, Cimino WG, Seidel FG: Allograft epiphysiodesis for slipped capital femoral epiphysis. *Clin Orthop Relat Res* 1996;322:61-76.
114. DeRosa GP, Mullins RC, Kling TF Jr: Cuneiform osteotomy of the femoral neck in severe slipped capital femoral epiphysis. *Clin Orthop Relat Res* 1996;322:48-60.
115. Velasco R, Schai PA, Exner GU: Slipped capital femoral epiphysis: A long-term follow-up study after open reduction of the femoral head combined with subcapital wedge resection. *J Pediatr Orthop B* 1998;7:43-52.
116. Fish JB: Cuneiform osteotomy of the femoral neck in the treatment of slipped capital femoral epiphysis. *J Bone Joint Surg Am* 1984;66:1153-1168.
117. Fish JB: Cuneiform osteotomy of the femoral neck in the treatment of slipped capital femoral epiphysis. *J Bone Joint Surg Am* 1994;76:46-59.
118. Barmada R, Bruch RF, Gimbel JS, Ray RD: Base of the neck extracapsular osteotomy for correction of deformity in slipped capital femoral epiphysis. *Clin Orthop Relat Res* 1978;132: 98-101.
119. Kramer WG, Craig WA, Noel S: Compensating osteotomy at the base of the femoral neck for slipped capital femoral epiphysis. *J Bone Joint Surg Am* 1976;58:796-800.
120. Schai PA, Exner GU, Hansch O: Prevention of secondary coxarthrosis in slipped capital femoral epiphysis: A long-term follow-up study after corrective intertrochanteric osteotomy. *J Pediatr Orthop B* 1996;5:135-143.
121. Parsch K, Bühl T, Weller S: Intertrochanteric corrective osteotomy for moderate and severe chronic slipped capital femoral epiphysis. *J Pediatr Orthop B* 1999;8:223-230.
122. Kartenbender K, Cordier W, Katthagen B-D: Long-term follow-up study after corrective Imhäuser osteotomy for severe slipped capital femoral epiphysis. *J Pediatr Orthop* 2000;20: 749-756.
123. Leunig M, Casillas MM, Hamlet M, et al: Slipped capital femoral epiphysis: Early mechanical damage to the acetabular cartilage by a prominent femoral metaphysis. *Acta Orthop Scand* 2000;71:370-375.
124. Ganz R, Gill TJ, Gautier E, Ganz K, Krügel N, Berlemann U: Surgical dislocation of the adult hip: A technique with full access to the femoral head and acetabulum without the risk of avascular necrosis. *J Bone Joint Surg Br* 2001;83:1119-1124.
125. Spencer S, Millis MB, Kim Y-J: Early results of treatment for hip impingement syndrome in slipped capital femoral epiphysis and pistol grip deformity of the femoral head-neck junction using the surgical dislocation technique. *J Pediatr Orthop* 2006;26: 281-285.
126. Beck M, Leunig M, Parvizi J, Boutier V, Wyss D, Ganz R: Anterior femoroacetabular impingement: Part II. Midterm results of surgical treatment. *Clin Orthop Relat Res* 2004;418: 67-73.
127. Lavigne M, Parvizi J, Beck M, Siebenrock KA, Ganz R, Leunig M: Anterior femoroacetabular impingement: Part 1. Techniques of joint preserving surgery. *Clin Orthop Relat Res* 2004;418: 61-66.
128. O'Brien ET, Fahey JJ: Remodeling of the femoral neck after in-situ pinning for slipped capital femoral epiphysis. *J Bone Joint Surg Am* 1977;59:62-68.
129. Bellemans J, Fabry G, Molenaers G, Lammens J, Moens P: Slipped capital femoral epiphysis: A long-term follow-up, with special emphasis on the capacities for remodeling. *J Pediatr Orthop B* 1996;5:151-157.
130. Jerre R, Billing L, Karlsson J: Loss of hip motion in slipped capital femoral epiphysis: A calculation from the slipping angle. *J Pediatr Orthop B* 1996;5: 144-150.
131. Claffey TJ: Avascular necrosis of the femoral head: An anatomical study. *J Bone Joint Surg Br* 1960;42:802-809.
132. Brodetti A: The blood supply of the femoral neck and head in relation to the damaging effects of nails and screws. *J Bone Joint Surg Br* 1960;42: 794-801.

133. Walters R, Simon SR: Joint destruction: A sequel of unrecognized pin penetration in patients with slipped capital femoral epiphyses, in *The Hip: Proceedings of the Eighth Open Scientific Meeting of the Hip Society*. St. Louis, MO, CV Mosby, 1980, pp 145-164.

134. Blanco JS, Taylor B, Johnston CE II: Comparison of single pin vs multiple pin fixation in treatment of slipped capital femoral epiphysis. *J Pediatr Orthop* 1992;12:384-389.

135. Morrissy RT: Slipped capital femoral epiphysis: Technique of percutaneous in situ fixation. *J Pediatr Orthop* 1990;10:347-350.

136. Karol LA, Doane RM, Cornicelli SF, Zak PA, Haut RC, Manoli A II: Single versus double screw fixation for treatment of slipped capital femoral epiphysis: A biomechanical analysis. *J Pediatr Orthop* 1992;12:741-745.

137. Lee FY, Chapman CB: In situ pinning of hip for stable slipped capital femoral epiphysis on a radiolucent operating table. *J Pediatr Orthop* 2003;23:27-29.

138. Blasier RD, Ramsey JR, White RR: Comparison of radiolucent and fracture tables in the treatment of slipped capital femoral epiphysis. *J Pediatr Orthop* 2004;24:642-644.

139. Canale ST, Azar F, Young J, Beaty JH, Warner WC, Whitmer G: Subtrochanteric fracture fixation of slipped capital femoral epiphysis: A complication of unused drill holes. *J Pediatr Orthop* 1994;14:623-626.

140. Carney BT, Birnbaum P, Minter C: Slip progression after in situ single screw fixation for stable slipped capital femoral epiphysis. *J Pediatr Orthop* 2003;23:584-589.

141. Maletis GB, Bassett GS: Windshield-wiper loosening: A complication of in situ screw fixation of slipped capital femoral epiphysis. *J Pediatr Orthop* 1993;13:607-609.

142. Mosely C: The "approach-withdraw phenomenon" in the pinning of slipped capital femoral epiphysis. *Orthop Trans* 1985;9:947.

143. Burke JG, Sher JL: Intra-operative arthrography facilitates accurate screw fixation of a slipped capital femoral epiphysis. *J Bone Joint Surg Br* 2004;86:1197-1198.

144. Koval KJ, Lehman WB, Rose D, Koval RP, Grant A, Strongwater A: Treatment of slipped capital femoral epiphysis with a cannulated-screw technique. *J Bone Joint Surg Am* 1989;71:1370-1377.

145. Lehman WB, Grant A, Rose D, Pugh J, Norman A: A method of evaluating possible pin penetration in slipped capital femoral epiphysis using a cannulated internal fixation device. *Clin Orthop Relat Res* 1984;186:65-70.

146. Lehman WB, Menche D, Grant A, Norman A, Pugh J: The problem of evaluating in situ pinning of slipped capital femoral epiphysis: An experimental model and review of 63 consecutive cases. *J Pediatr Orthop* 1984;4:297-303.

147. Goodman WW, Johnson JT, Robertson WW Jr: Single screw fixation for acute and acute-on-chronic slipped capital femoral epiphysis. *Clin Orthop Relat Res* 1996;322:86-90.

148. Stevens DB, Short BA, Burch JM: In situ fixation of the slipped capital femoral epiphysis with a single screw. *J Pediatr Orthop B* 1996;5:85-89.

149. Dunn DM, Angel JC: Replacement of the femoral head by open operation in severe adolescent slipping of the upper femoral epiphysis. *J Bone Joint Surg Br* 1978;60-B:394-403.

150. Betz RR, Steel HH, Emper WD, Huss GK, Clancy M: Treatment of slipped capital femoral epiphysis: Spica cast immobilization. *J Bone Joint Surg Am* 1990;72:587-600.

151. Crawford AH: Role of osteotomy in the treatment of slipped capital femoral epiphysis. *J Pediatr Orthop B* 1996;5:102-109.

152. Southwick WO: Compression fixation after biplane intertrochanteric osteotomy for slipped capital femoral epiphysis. *J Bone Joint Surg Am* 1973;55:1218-1224.

153. Jerre T: A study in slipped upper femoral epiphysis with special reference to late functional and roentgenological results and the value of closed reduction. *Acta Orthop Scand* 1950;(suppl 6).

154. Cooperman DR, Charles LM, Pathria M, Latimer B, Thomspon GH: Postmortem description of slipped capital femoral epiphysis. *J Bone Joint Surg Br* 1992;74:595-599.

155. Jerne R, Hansson G, Wallin J, Karlsson J: Long-term results after realignment operations for slipped upper femoral epiphysis. *J Bone Joint Surg Br* 1996;78:745-750.

156. Mooney JF III, Sanders JO, Browne RH, et al: Management of unstable/acute slipped capital femoral epiphysis: Results of a survey of the POSNA membership. *J Pediatr Orthop* 2005;25:162-166.

157. de Sanctis N, Di Gennaro G, Pempinello C, Della Corte S, Carannante G: Is gentle manipulative reduction and percutaneous fixation with a single screw the best management of acute and acute-on-chronic slipped capital femoral epiphysis? *J Pediatr Orthop B* 1996;5:90-95.

158. Herman MJ, Dormans JP, Davidson RS, Drummond DS, Gregg JR: Screw fixation of grade III slipped capital femoral epiphysis. *Clin Orthop Relat Res* 1996;322:77-85.

159. Peterson MD, Weiner DS, Green NE, Terry CL: Acute slipped capital femoral epiphysis: The value and safety of urgent manipulative reduction. *J Pediatr Orthop* 1997;17:648-654.

160. Gordon JE, Abrahams MS, Dobbs MB, Luhmann SJ, Schoenecker PL: Early reduction, arthrotomy, and cannulated screw fixation in unstable slipped capital femoral epiphysis treatment. *J Pediatr Orthop* 2002;22:352-358.

161. Beck M, Siebenrock KA, Affolter B, Nützli H, Parvizi J, Ganz R: Increased intraarticular pressure reduces blood flow to the femoral head. *Clin Orthop Relat Res* 2004;424:149-152.

162. Svalastoga E, Kiær T, Jensen PE: The effect of intracapsular pressure and extension of the hip on oxygenation of the juvenile femoral epiphysis. *J Bone Joint Surg Br* 1989;71:222-226.

163. Kibiloski LJ, Doane RM, Karol LA, Haut RC, Loder RT: Biomechanical analysis of single- versus double-screw fixation in slipped capital femoral epiphysis at physiological load levels. *J Pediatr Orthop* 1994;14:627-630.

164. Snyder RR, Williams JL, Schmidt TL, Salsbury TL: Torsional strength of double- versus single-screw fixation in a pig model of unstable slipped capital femoral epiphysis. *J Pediatr Orthop* 2006;26:295-299.

165. Kishan S, Upasani V, Mahar A, et al: Biomechanical stability of single-screw versus two-screw fixation of an unstable slipped capital femoral epiphysis model: Effect of screw position in the femoral neck. *J Pediatr Orthop* 2006;26:601-605.

166. Schultz WR, Weinstein JN, Weinstein SL, Smith BG: Prophylactic pinning of the contralateral hip in slipped capital femoral epiphysis: Evaluation of long-term outcome for the contralateral hip with use of decision analysis. *J Bone Joint Surg Am* 2002;84-A:1305-1314.

167. Kocher MS, Bishop JA, Hresko MT, Millis MB, Kim Y-J, Kasser JR: Prophylactic pinning of the contralateral hip after unilateral slipped capital femoral epiphysis. *J Bone Joint Surg Am* 2004;86-A:2658-2665.

168. Hägglund G: The contralateral hip in slipped capital femoral epiphysis. *J Pediatr Orthop B* 1996;5:158-161.

169. MacLean JGB, Reddy SK: The contralateral slip. *J Bone Joint Surg Br* 2006;88:1497-1501.

170. Seller K, Raab P, Wild A, Krauspe R: Risk-benefit analysis of prophylactic pinning in slipped capital femoral epiphysis. *J Pediatr Orthop B* 2001;10: 192-196.

171. Castro FP Jr, Bennett JT, Doulens K: Epidemiological perspective on prophylactic pinning in patients with unilateral slipped capital femoral epiphysis. *J Pediatr Orthop* 2000;20: 745-748.

172. Dietz FR: Traction reduction of acute and acute-on-chronic slipped capital femoral epiphysis. *Clin Orthop Relat Res* 1994;302:101-110.

173. Krahn TH, Canale ST, Beaty JH, Warner WC, Lourenco P: Long-term follow-up of patients with avascular necrosis after treatment of slipped capital femoral epiphysis. *J Pediatr Orthop* 1993;13:154-158.

174. Tokmakova KP, Stanton RP, Mason DE: Factors influencing the development of osteonecrosis in patients treated for slipped capital femoral epiphysis. *J Bone Joint Surg Am* 2003; 85-A:798-801.

175. Ballard J, Cosgrove AP: Anterior physeal separation: A sign indicating a high risk for avascular necrosis after slipped capital femoral epiphysis. *J Bone Joint Surg Br* 2002;84:1176-1179.

176. Strange-Vognsen H, Wagner A, Dirksen K, et al: The value of scintigraphy in hips with slipped capital femoral epiphysis and the value of radiography and MRI after 10 years. *Acta Orthop Belg* 1999;65:33-38.

177. Mullins MM, Sood M, Hashemi-Nejad A, Catterall A: The management of avascular necrosis after slipped capital femoral epiphysis. *J Bone Joint Surg Br* 2005;87:1669-1674.

178. Maurer RC, Larsen IJ: Acute necrosis of cartilage in slipped capital femoral epiphysis. *J Bone Joint Surg Am* 1970; 52:39-50.

179. Vrettos BC, Hoffman EB: Chondrolysis in slipped upper femoral epiphysis. *J Bone Joint Surg Br* 1993;75:956-961.

180. Ingram AJ, Clarke MS, Clark CS Jr, Marshall WR: Chondrolysis complicating slipped capital femoral epiphysis. *Clin Orthop Relat Res* 1982;165:99-109.

181. Mandell GA, Keret D, Harcke HT, Bowen JR: Chondrolysis: Detection by bone scintigraphy. *J Pediatr Orthop* 1992;12:80-85.

182. Aronson DD, Loder RT: Slipped capital femoral epiphysis in Black children. *J Pediatr Orthop* 1992;12:74-79.

183. Bishop JO, Oley TJ, Stephenson CT, Hullos HS: Slipped capital femoral epiphysis: A study of 50 cases in Black children. *Clin Orthop Relat Res* 1978; 135:93-96.

184. Spero CR, Masciale JP, Tornetta P III, Star MJ, Tucci JJ: Slipped capital femoral epiphysis in Black children: Incidence of chondrolysis. *J Pediatr Orthop* 1992;12:444-448.

185. Kennedy JP, Weiner DS: Results of slipped capital femoral epiphysis in the Black population. *J Pediatr Orthop* 1990;10:224-227.

186. Orofino C, Innis JJ, Lowrey CW: Slipped capital femoral epiphysis in Negroes: A study of ninety-five cases. *J Bone Joint Surg Am* 1960;42:1079-1083.

187. Tillema DA, Golding JSR: Chondrolysis following slipped capital femoral epiphysis. *J Bone Joint Surg Am* 1971; 53:1528-1540.

188. Gonzalez-Moran G, Carsi B, Abril JC, Albinana J: Results after preoperative traction and pinning in slipped capital femoral epiphysis: K wires versus cannulated screws. *J Pediatr Orthop B* 1998;7:53-58.

189. Tudisco C, Caterini R, Farsetti P, Potenza V: Chondrolysis of the hip complicating slipped capital femoral epiphysis: Long-term follow-up of nine patients. *J Pediatr Orthop B* 1999; 8:107-111.

190. Hall JE: The results of treatment of slipped upper femoral epiphysis. *J Bone Joint Surg Br* 1957;39-B:659-673.

191. Oram V: Epiphysiolysis of the head of the femur: A follow-up examination with special reference to end results and the social prognosis. *Acta Orthop Scand* 1953;23:100-120.

192. Ross PM, Lyne ED, Morawa LG: Slipped capital femoral epiphysis: Long term results after 10-38 years.

Clin Orthop Relat Res 1979;141:176-180.

193. Ordeberg G, Hansson LI, Sandström S: Slipped capital femoral epiphysis in southern Sweden. *Clin Orthop Relat Res* 1987;220:148-154.

194. Jerre R, Hansson G, Wallin J, Karlsson J: Does a single device prevent further slipping of the epiphysis in children with slipped capital femoral epiphysis? *Arch Orthop Trauma Surg* 1997;116:348-351.

195. Howorth B: Slipping of the capital femoral epiphysis: History. *Clin Orthop Relat Res* 1966;48:11-32.

196. Johnston RC, Larson CB: Results of treatment of hip disorders with cup arthroplasty. *J Bone Joint Surg Am* 1969;51:1461.

197. Murray RO: The etiology of primary osteoarthritis of the hip. *Br J Radiol* 1965;38:810-824.

198. Solomon L: Patterns of osteoarthritis of the hip. *J Bone Joint Surg Br* 1976; 58:176-183.

199. Stulberg SD, Cordell LD, Harris WH: Unrecognized childhood hip disease: A major cause of idiopathic osteonecrosis of the hip, in *The Hip: Proceedings of the Third Open Scientific Meeting of The Hip Society*. St. Louis, MO, CV Mosby, 1975, pp 212-230.

200. Resnick D: The "tilt" deformity of the femoral head in osteoarthritis of the hip: A poor indicator of previous epiphysiolysis. *Clin Radiol* 1976;27: 355-363.

201. Jerre T: Early complications of osteosynthesis with a three flanged nail in situ for slipped epiphysis. *Acta Orthop Scand* 1958;27:126.

202. Richolt JA, Teschner M, Everett PC, Millis MB, Kikinis R: Impingement simulation of the hip in SCFE using 3D models. *Comput Aided Surg* 1999; 4:144-151.

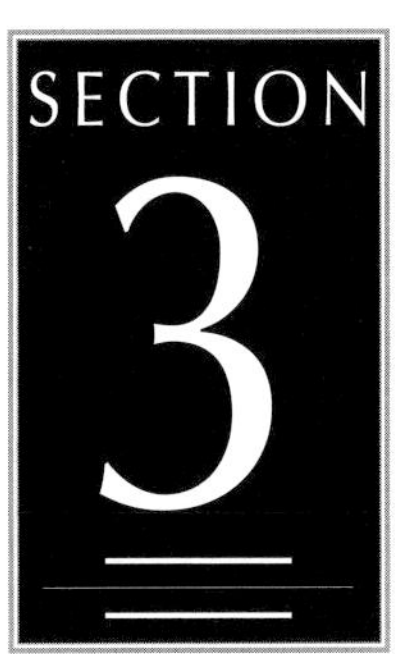

Bearing Surfaces in Total Hip Arthroplasty

Bearing Surfaces in Total Hip Arthroplasty

Total hip arthroplasty (THA) is a success story in the treatment of degenerative hip disease and a testament to the ingenuity and perseverance of innovators and designers who have contributed to its current incarnation. Paradigm shifts in the design of materials and manufacturing processes and improved biologic implant fixation and surgical techniques have transitioned this highly technical procedure from use by only a few highly experienced orthopaedic surgeons to a reliable and effective procedure used by many surgeons to treat millions of patients worldwide.

As the use of this technology has expanded, the demographics of patients treated with THA have mirrored this expansion. THA is no longer limited to low demand, elderly patients but is now offered to young, highly active patients whose demands for better implant performance have pushed the limits of current technology. Although many problems that arose in the early years of this procedure have been solved, a major cause of current implant failures is related to the bearing surfaces. The past two decades have seen quantum shifts in the understanding of tribology and the development of advanced bearing surfaces. The current challenge is to develop even longer-lasting bearing surfaces.

The understanding of the local biologic effects of polyethylene wear debris and its role in osteolysis has emerged as the single most important finding in implant survival and has led to the development of enhanced bearing surfaces. In the first chapter in this section, Catelas and Jacobs review findings that the biologic response to wear debris is related not only to the composition of the wear material but is also intimately related to the size, shape, and volume of the wear particles. A macrophage and cytokine-mediated response through the receptor activator of nuclear factor kappa-B (RANK)-RANK ligand pathway appears to be the key molecular and cellular path by which wear debris results in osteolysis. Phagocytosis of wear particles alters the normal homeostasis between osteoclasts and osteoblasts, resulting in a relative increase in osteoclast differentiation while detrimentally affecting mesenchymal stem cell osteoblast progenitors. Several studies showed that the smallest particles (submicron size) of polyethylene debris elicited the greatest bone resorption. Although larger particles can result in the same amount of resorption, larger volumes of particles are required. The shape of the particles is also important, with elongated particles upregulating this resorption pathway to a greater degree than globular particles.

Highly cross-linked polyethylene (HXPE) has been shown in simulators to have substantially less wear than conventional polyethylene. The widespread clinical use of this product has mirrored laboratory results. However, HXPE wear appears to generate particles that are both spheroid and oblong and smaller than those seen with conventional polyethylene. These particles seem to be more biologically active in terms of eliciting immune-mediated responses because of their smaller size and shape. A recent study comparing the rate of osteolysis measured by CT in young patients treated with THA with conventional polyethylene and HXPE reported very low rates of osteolysis in the group treated with HXPE.[1] Although the wear debris generated by HXPE may be more biologically active, it appears that the overall adverse biologic response may be mitigated because of the lower volume of debris compared with conventional polyethylene.

Ceramic-on-ceramic bearings offer several advantages—they are extremely hard materials, have exceptionally low wear rates, and the wear debris seems to be much less biologically active compared with other types of particles. The debris particles are generally uniformly round, with a size range that produces the least activation of the RANK pathway. When similar sizes and shapes of ceramic debris were directly compared with ultra-high–molecular-weight polyethylene debris, the ceramic particles resulted in a much lower cellular response. This study concluded that the likelihood of a significant osteolytic response was very low because of the extremely high concentration of ceramic particles that would be needed to reach that threshold. The widespread adoption of ceramic-on-ceramic bearings has been tempered by concerns about bearing fractures and audible squeaking during the gait cycle.

Second-generation metal-on-metal bearing surfaces (approved by the FDA in 1999) had, until recently, enjoyed an enthusiastic resurgence because of the improved designs, materials, and manufacturing tolerances. In the second chapter in this section, Beaulé and associates review the enhancements made in the second-generation metal-on-metal implant bearings. The newer designs include higher carbon levels, lower diametral clearance, and improved surface finishes. The higher carbon content in the materials used on the bearing surface appears to result in lower wear rates. Smoother surface finishes, which reduce asperities, also reduce wear rates. However, the most important factors in reducing wear rates in the second-generation metal-on-metal bearings are the roles of diametral clearance and head size. Extremely small differences between the femoral head diameter and the inner diameter of the acetabular component allow for better lubrication conditions. By trapping fluid in the relatively small space between the head and cup, the fluid layer can generate a physical separation between the metallic interfaces; this results in low or no contact and very low wear rates. Larger femoral heads also appear to enhance the effect of fluid-film separation.

Unfortunately, the promise of low wear rates and the use of large femoral heads have unfolded in an unexpected way. Reports of adverse local soft-tissue reactions in patients with metal-on-metal bearing surfaces began to appear in patients treated with THAs or hip resurfacing arthroplasties. Although these adverse reactions are relatively rare, they are unpredictable and can be catastrophic. A few correlations have been observed. It appears that smaller acetabular components (and thus smaller femoral heads) have higher failure rates. This may partly explain the higher failure rates observed in female patients. The malpositioning of components and the resultant edge-loading appear to result in higher failure rates. Acetabular designs with lower arc angles also perform poorly.

As described by Gonzalez and associates, implant failures have been correlated with the observations previously mentioned but fundamentally are related to wear particles (mainly cobalt and chromium ions), the diminished ability to systemically excrete locally generated particles, and susceptibility to adverse reactions to these particles. Metal wear particles, in contrast to polyethylene and ceramic particles, appear to be smaller (nanometer range) and contain not only round shapes but also needle-shaped debris. The inflammatory reaction is different and less prominent than that observed with polyethylene debris, suggesting a pathway other than the macrophage-mediated RANK pathway. The overall volume of wear particles observed in metal-on-metal bearings is much less than the volume seen with polyethylene bearings because the size of the particles is smaller by almost three orders of magnitude, but the absolute number of particles may be much greater. The cobalt and chromium ions that are detected locally as well as systemically are most accurately measured in the blood serum and are known to be high in number after the initial prosthesis implantation during the "run-in" period in which they are threefold to fivefold higher than after several years when a steady state is reached. Because these ions are excreted renally, concerns regarding the use of metal bearings in patients with renal insufficiency have long been recognized.

Chromosomal abnormalities also have been observed in patients with metal-on-metal bearings and in laboratory studies of human fibroblast, which showed increases in aneuploidy, translocation, and DNA damage after exposure to cobalt and chromium particles. The implications of this finding, if any, are not fully understood; however, there does not appear to be any substantial evidence that these chromosomal abnormalities lead to malignancy. Because there is concern that these ions can cross the placenta and damage fetal DNA, the use of metal-on-metal bearings in women of child-bearing age have been limited.

Initially believed to be a phenomenon observed only in hip resurfacing arthroplasty, pseudotumors (more recently referred to as adverse local tissue reactions) also occur in THAs with metal-on-metal bearing surfaces. Although these pseudotumors are not known to have malignant degeneration, they can cause substantial soft-tissue destruction. The sequelae of adverse local tissue reactions also extend to the bone; many observations of metal debris–induced osteolysis have been reported. The observation of higher failure rates in metal-on-metal THAs compared with hip resurfacing procedures may be a result of corrosion at the head-neck taper junction. Recent work has shown that this corrosion can lead to elevated metal ions in non–metal-on-metal hip bearing surfaces and raises speculation that the metal ion burden from the modular taper in addition to the ions generated at the bearing surface in a metal-on-metal THA may exceed threshold limits for failure.[2]

The dominant failure mode of metal-on-metal bearing appears to be aseptic loosening. Whether this loosening is related to metal ion release, pure mechanical failure, or a combination of the processes is still unknown and has definite ramifications on the choice of bearing surface at the time of revision hip arthroplasty, as described by Patel and associates in the last chapter in this section. These authors, while raising concerns similar to those of other works in this section, highlight the need for longer lasting bearing surfaces in revision THA, particularly in situations in which the etiology of failure is directly related to wear. Two of the most common reasons for failure after revision THA are instability and dislocation. These complications can be minimized through the use of larger head diameters at the time of revision surgery; however, the advantages of larger femoral heads must be weighed against potential problems with the bearing surface.

Metal-on-metal bearings have performed well in many patients. The current understanding of risk factors for failure, monitoring of symptomatic patients with metal-on-metal hip bearing surfaces, and recommended treatments are evolving. This technology should be used with caution until a thorough understanding emerges.

Hany Bedair, MD
Instructor, Orthopaedic Surgery
Massachusetts General Hospital
Harvard Medical School
Boston, Massachusetts

References

1. Mall NA, Nunley RM, Zhu JJ, Maloney WJ, Barrack RL, Clohisy JC: The incidence of acetabular osteolysis in young patients with conventional versus highly crosslinked polyethylene. *Clin Orthop Relat Res* 2011;469(2):372-381.
2. Cooper HJ, Della Valle CJ, Berger RA, et al: Corrosion at the head-neck taper as a cause for adverse local tissue reactions after total hip arthroplasty. *J Bone Joint Surg Am* 2012;94(18):1655-1661.

Dr. Bedair or an immediate family member is a member of a speakers' bureau or has made paid presentations on behalf of Cadence Pharmaceuticals and serves as a paid consultant to Zimmer.

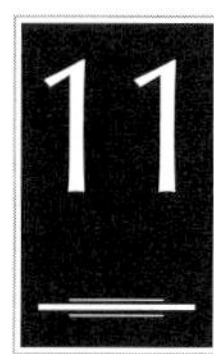

Biologic Activity of Wear Particles

Isabelle Catelas, PhD
Joshua J. Jacobs, MD

Abstract

Aseptic loosening resulting from periprosthetic osteolysis continues to be an important cause of hip implant failure. Wear particles from the bearing surfaces play a major role in initiating periprosthetic osteolysis, which is also potentiated by mechanical factors such as increased synovial fluid pressure. The precise mechanisms by which wear particles induce periprosthetic osteolysis have not been fully elucidated and remain an active subject of research. Particle characteristics such as composition, size, shape, and number (especially for particles in the most biologically active, submicrometer-size range) are recognized to significantly affect the overall cell and tissue response. The production of corrosion products, especially from metal-on-metal implants, also is a clinically significant issue, and individual variability in innate and adaptive immune responses is important but not yet completely defined. Because of the increasing need to implant hip prostheses in younger and more active patients, a better understanding of the biologic activity of wear particles from bearing couples is critical in the attempt to modulate the clinical effects of these particles and to develop materials with improved wear and corrosion resistance.

Metal-on-polyethylene bearing surfaces have been widely used in total hip replacements for the past 40 years. However, large numbers of polyethylene particles have been detected in the surrounding tissues, and they have been associated with bone resorption and implant failure caused by aseptic loosening.[1-4] The attempts to improve the wear characteristics of polyethylene over the years have included the use of carbon fiber additives, heat pressing, and, most recently, chemical cross-linking. There is strong research and clinical interest in highly cross-linked polyethylene (HXPE), but little is known about the biologic response to wear particles from this new generation of polyethylene. Metal-on-metal and ceramic-on-ceramic bearing surface combinations have been developed based on the concept that the use of harder materials can improve wear resistance.[5] Interest in metal-on-metal implants for total hip replacements has been revived within the past two decades with the introduction of new designs. Although the volumetric wear rate of metal-on-metal bearings is much lower than that of conventional metal-on-polyethylene bearings, the smaller size of the wear particles and the release of corrosion products have raised biologic concerns. Alumina and zirconia (Al_2O_3 and ZrO_2) ceramics are attractive as self-bearing materials because of their low coefficients of friction, high wettability and chemical stability, high hardness and excellent surface finish, and resistance to third-body scratching and wear. However, concerns exist about their extremely high modulus of elasticity compared

Dr. Catelas or an immediate family member is a member of a speakers' bureau or has made paid presentations on behalf of DePuy; and has stock or stock options held in Baxter Healthcare Corporation. Dr. Jacobs or an immediate family member serves as a board member, owner, officer, or committee member of the Bone and Joint Decade, U.S.A., the Hip Society, the Orthopaedic Research and Education Foundation, the Orthopaedic Research Society, InMotion, and NIAMS; serves as a paid consultant to or is an employee of Medtronic Sofamor Danek, the National Institutes of Health (NIAMS & NICHD), Wright Medical Technology, and Zimmer; has received research or institutional support from Arthrex, Biomet, DePuy, DJ Orthopaedics, Johnson & Johnson, Medtronic, Medtronic Sofamor Danek, the National Institutes of Health (NIAMS & NICHD), Nuvasive, Smith & Nephew, Stryker, Wright Medical Technology, Zimmer, Anesiva, Ctr Biom Adv Tech, Don Joy Orthopaedics, Pentax, Pioneer Labs – NUBAC, Spinal Kinetics, Omeros, and Anges; and has received nonincome support (such as equipment or services), commercially derived honoraria, or other non–research-related funding (such as paid travel) from Arthritis and Rheumatism and Taylor and Francis.

with bone, as well as their brittle material properties, which occasionally have caused component fracture.[6-8] This chapter will present a review of the literature that addresses the biologic activity of wear particles from these different types of bearing materials.

Characteristics of Wear Particles

Precise characterization of implant wear particles is important to understand their biologic effects. The composition, size, shape, and number of wear particles are known to play a role in the cell and tissue response.

The size of ultra-high molecular weight polyethylene (UHMWPE) particles isolated from in vitro hip simulators has been reported to be mainly between 0.1 and 1 μm.[9] The in vivo size and morphology of these particles has been demonstrated to be more variable. Most are globular spheroids between 0.1 and 0.4 μm in size, but some are platelet-shaped and are as large as 250 μm; others are fibrils or shreds.[10-13] Richards and associates[14] reported the presence of nanometer-size UHMWPE particles in vivo, but these particles accounted only for a small proportion of the total volume. Laurent and associates[15] studied HXPE particles and found that they were largely spheroidal or oblong and smaller than most UHMWPE particles. However, commercially available HXPE implants differ with respect to type of irradiation, radiation dose, method of thermal stabilization, machining, and final sterilization;[16] therefore, the resulting wear particles may differ in their characteristics.

A direct comparison of the available studies of wear particles from metal-on-metal implants is difficult because of the different implant designs and alloys from different manufacturers, as well as the different particle isolation and characterization techniques used in these studies. Doorn and associates[17] analyzed metal particles following enzymatic digestion of periprosthetic tissues. They found that most particles were round but that a small proportion were shard- or needle-shaped. When comparing different isolation protocols, Catelas and associates[18,19] found that a newly developed enzymatic protocol was less damaging to wear particles than the strong alkaline protocols used by earlier researchers to isolate metal particles. Using this new enzymatic protocol and particle embedding in resin to allow particle dispersion and facilitate morphology and elemental analysis, Catelas and associates[20-22] found that the wear particles produced by metal-on-metal implants in vitro and in vivo were in the nanometer size range and were mostly round or oval, but some were needle-shaped. The quantity of needle-shaped particles depended on the cycling period (for in vitro particles) or the implantation time (for in vivo particles). Most of the particles contained chromium (Cr) and oxygen (O) but no cobalt (Co) and therefore, were most likely chromium oxides. These findings corroborated those of Doorn and associates,[17] but differed to some extent from those reported by Brown and associates[23] who found only round and no needle-shaped cobalt-chromium particles in vitro. These discrepancies in shape and composition may be attributable to differences in the metallurgy of the prosthetic component alloys and the loading parameters; however, all of these researchers agreed that particles from metal-on-metal implants are in the nanometer-size range, have a high specific surface area (surface area/mass), and are subject to corrosion, which leads to the release of metal ions into the surrounding areas. Therefore, the effects of metal ions must be considered when analyzing the biologic response to these wear particles.

Lerouge and associates[24,25] analyzed alumina particles in tissue using scanning electron microscopy. They found uniform round particles with a size of 0.44 μm (± 0.25 μm). Yoon and associates[26] reported a similar size of 0.13 μm (± 7.21 μm). When using transmission electron microscopy in addition to scanning electron microscopy, some studies revealed a bimodal size range.[27,28] Transmission electron microscopic analysis of particles from tissues revealed the presence of 5- to 90-nm particles (24 nm ± 19 nm), whereas scanning electron microscopic analysis revealed particles in the size range of 0.05 μm to 3.2 μm.[27] By using microseparation of the prosthesis components with in vitro joint simulations, Tipper and associates[28] also found a bimodal distribution, with nanometer-size particles ranging from 1 to 35 nm and larger micrometer-size particles ranging from 0.021 to 10 μm.

Wear Particle-Induced Periprosthetic Osteolysis

The most common cause of implant failure is aseptic loosening resulting from periprosthetic osteolysis, which is primarily induced by the presence of wear particles and is potentiated by mechanical factors such as synovial fluid pressure. Periprosthetic osteolysis was first described as a cystic erosion of bone by Charnley in 1975.[29] Since then, it has been widely studied using in vitro, animal, and retrieval studies, and has been described as the cumulative result of biologic reactions that lead to increased bone resorption and decreased bone formation.

Many types of cells have been reported to be involved in wear particle-induced periprosthetic osteolysis, including macrophages, giant cells, osteoblasts, and fibroblasts.[30-32] Some studies also have described the recruitment and differentiation of osteoclast progenitors at the bone-implant interface as potentially early events in the pathogenesis of osteolysis.[33-35]

Periprosthetic tissues are characterized by the presence of granulation tissue rich in macrophages, wear particles, as well as inflammatory mediators including interleukin (IL)-1β, tumor necrosis factor (TNF)-α, prostaglandin E_2, and IL-6.[36-39] The cytokine pathways that modulate periprosthetic osteolysis have been extensively studied in recent years, and the importance of the pathway involving the receptor activator of nuclear factor kappa-B (RANK), the receptor activator of nuclear factor kappa-B ligand (RANKL), and osteoprotegerin (OPG) has emerged.[40-42] The RANK-RANKL-OPG pathway has been shown to be fundamental to the process of osteoclastogenesis because osteoclast precursors are unable to differentiate into mature osteoclasts in the absence of RANKL-RANK interaction. RANKL activates key pathways involved in osteoclast differentiation and function. It is a TNF-related cytokine produced by marrow stromal cells and osteoblasts. RANK, a member of the TNF-receptor superfamily, is present on osteoclasts and initiates osteoclastogenesis after binding with RANKL. OPG, a decoy receptor, also can bind to RANKL, thereby preventing its interaction with RANK and limiting its activity in osteoclastogenesis. Mandelin and associates[43] analyzed the particle-initiated inflammatory response in periprosthetic tissues from 11 patients with osteolysis to determine whether the response was associated with the upregulation of the RANK-RANKL-OPG system. They found that RANK and RANKL were upregulated and suggested that RANKL in the interface tissue could stimulate the differentiation of RANK-positive cells into osteoclasts capable of bone resorption.

Other mechanisms that may contribute to wear particle-induced periprosthetic osteolysis include the elevated production of reactive oxygen species by activated macrophages and osteoclasts, impaired periprosthetic bone formation secondary to disrupted osteogenesis, and compromised bone regeneration resulting from increased mesenchymal stem cell mortality caused by the wear particles.[44] The effects of wear particles on bone cells and their progenitors have only recently received attention.[45] Wang and associates[46,47] found that human mesenchymal stem cells exposed to commercially pure titanium (cpTi) particles demonstrated a lower viability and proliferation, reduced collagen type I and bone sialoprotein production, and suppression of bone sialoprotein but not osteocalcin, alkaline phosphatase, or collagen type I gene expression. When cells were exposed to zirconia particles, a decrease in cell proliferation and subsequent mineralization was measured, but there was no significant effect on osteoblastic gene markers. CpTi particles also were found to be more toxic than zirconia particles. These studies show that particle composition influences the viability, proliferation, as well as the gene and protein expression of osteoblast progenitors. Okafor and associates[48] also studied the effects of cpTi on human mesenchymal stem cells and found an increase in apoptosis, a decrease in cell proliferation, and the suppression of osteogenic differentiation after particle endocytosis. The addition of cytochalasin D (an inhibitor of phagocytosis) to the cpTi-stimulated human mesenchymal stem cell cultures inhibited these effects, demonstrating that phagocytosis was key to the adverse effects of cpTi particles on human mesenchymal stem cells. Chiu and associates[49] found that polymethylmethacrylate particles reduced murine bone marrow osteoprogenitor cell proliferation and differentiation when cells were exposed to the particles during the first 5 days of culture in osteogenic medium. Exposure of the bone marrow cells to polymethylmethacrylate particles after the fifth day of differentiation in osteogenic medium resulted in decreased cell proliferation but no reduction of alkaline phosphatase expression or mineralization, thus indicating that the cells were most sensitive to the particles during the first 5 days of differentiation.

In a very recent study, Caicedo and associates[50] examined the potential activation of the inflammasome pathway in human macrophages exposed to soluble metal ions and cobalt-chromium-molybdenum (Co-Cr-Mo) alloy particles. They found that these metal agents stimulate macrophage IL-1β secretion that is inflammasome-mediated. The authors concluded on a potential novel mechanism for implant particle reactivity in which contact with the particles would be sensed and transduced by macrophages into a proinflammatory response.

Biologic Response to Polyethylene Particles

Conventional metal-on-polyethylene total hip replacements produce relatively large quantities of polyethylene particles, and these particles have been the most important factor in initiating osteolysis. UHMWPE particles can be observed in histology sections using polarized light microscopy and have been identified in large numbers in tissues surrounding implants associated with bone resorption and failure caused by aseptic loosening.[1-4] These particles have been shown to elicit an inflammatory response due to macrophage and foreign body giant cell interaction and culminating in granuloma formation, osteolysis, and aseptic implant loosening. The influence of particle size and concentration was confirmed by in vivo studies that showed a direct relationship between polyethylene particles, macrophages, and osteolysis.[51-54] Green and associates[55] analyzed the in vitro bone resorption response of C3H murine peritoneal macrophages to grade GUR 1120 polyethylene particles of different sizes (0.24, 0.45, 1.71, and 7.62 μm) and at different doses (particle volume [μm^3] to macrophage ratios of 0.1:1, 1:1, 10:1, and 100:1). The smallest particles were the most active in stimulating bone-resorbing activity, at a ratio of 10 μm^3 per macrophage. Larger doses were necessary for the 0.45 and 1.71 μm particles, and the 7.62 μm particles were inactive at all tested doses. Cytokine amounts followed the same trend. Therefore, the size and dose of UHMWPE particles were important parameters influencing the osteolytic response of macrophages. Yang and associates[56] also analyzed the effects of UHMWPE particle shape, finding that different morphologies could elicit diverse cellular and apoptotic responses in a mouse air pouch model. Using the same model, Ren and associates[41] studied the gene expression of RANK and RANKL during the inflammatory response to globular or elongated UHMWPE particles. Elongated particles generated significantly higher RANK and RANKL gene expression than globular particles in pouch tissue, significantly higher IL-1β and TNF-α gene expression, and a higher cathepsin K gene expression. Histologic analysis revealed clusters of cells that were positive for tartrate-resistant acid phosphatase (TRAP) located in regions in contact with elongated particles. These data suggest that not only the size and dose but also the shape of UHMWPE particles critically influence the biologic response.

In vitro studies of cell response to polyethylene particles demonstrated that UHMWPE particles of different sizes stimulate macrophages to produce cytokines such as IL-1β, IL-6, TNF-α, and prostaglandin E_2.[57-59] However, there are discrepancies in the data, primarily because not all of the studies used the same cell lines, and some used particles that were not endotoxin free (leading to false positive results) or nonphysiologic. When comparing the macrophage response to UHMWPE particles with the macrophage response to other types of particles at similar sizes and concentrations, Petit and associates[60] found that UHMWPE particles induced faster and larger effects on TNF-α release than alumina particles.

The recent development of HXPE raised the question of the influence of cross-linking on the biologic activity of wear particles. Illgen and associates[61] compared the in vitro biologic activity of particles from Longevity HXPE (Zimmer, Warsaw, IN) and grade GUR 1050 conventional polyethylene (Zimmer), isolated from a hip simulator, and found no difference in the secretion of TNF-α and vascular endothelial growth factor (VEGF) at low and intermediate doses (0.1 and 0.75 surface area ratio, respectively). However, at the highest dose tested (2.5 surface area ratio), HXPE was significantly more inflammatory than conventional polyethylene. Both types of particles were predominantly round (granular), but the HXPE particles were somewhat smaller than the conventional polyethylene particles (0.111 μm versus 0.196 μm). Ingram and associates[62] also compared the inflammatory potential of HXPE and conventional polyethylene wear particles (all generated using a multidirectional pin-on-plate wear rig). The authors found that HXPE particles had a greater inflammatory potential than conventional polyethylene particles. Indeed, HXPE particles were able to stimulate cells to produce significantly elevated TNF-α levels at a concentration of only 0.1 μm^3 per cell; in contrast, a concentration of at least 10 μm^3 of the conventional polyethylene particles per cell was required to stimulate the cells. There was also a difference in particle sizes, with a higher percentage of HXPE particles than conventional polyethylene particles in the most biologically active submicrometer-size range. Ingram and associates[62] also reported the influence of the molecular weight and counterface roughness of the polyethylene and showed that higher levels of TNF-α were produced in the presence of particles of higher molecular weight polyethylene or relatively rough surfaces. All these studies show the importance of cross-linking, molecular weight, and

Table 1
Results of Immunohistochemical Staining and In Situ Hybridization Positive Cell Counts in Tissues Surrounding Metal-on-Metal Versus Metal-on-Polyethylene Hip Implants

Patient	CD 3	CD 68	Hybrid	IL-1β	IL-6	PDGF-α	TNF-α	TGF-β
Metal-on-metal								
1	35	36	0	220	1,982	551	1,324	725
2	10	28	0	1,945	3,822	2,900	1,807	662
3	19	33	0	1,627	2,429	2,450	1,719	1,382
4	17	13	0	827	1,064	1,195	889	314
5	7	9	0	1,079	1,301	1,360	632	832
Average	18	24	0	1,140	2,120	1,691	1,274	783
SD	11	12	0	677	1,095	961	511	387
SE	5	5	0	303	490	430	229	173
Metal-on-polyethylene								
1	10	77	0	1,189	2,237	1,206	1,941	1,637
2	5	77	0	2,739	3,572	2,478	3,063	2,284
3	4	36	0	479	798	372	1,239	963
4	5	91	0	2,792	4,284	2,763	3,665	4,003
5	11	97	0	2,125	2,843	1,470	2,623	2,853
Average	7	76	0	1,865	2,747	1,658	2,506	2,348
SD	3	24	0	1,009	1,333	973	948	1,164
SE	1	11	0	451	596	435	424	521
***P*-values**								
t-test	0.07	0.003		0.2	0.4	0.9	0.03	0.02
Mann-Whitney	0.06	0.01		0.2	0.5	0.9	0.05	0.02

CD 3 = CD 3 positive lymphocytes, CD 68 = CD 68 positive macrophages, IL = interleukin, PDGF-α = platelet-derived growth factor-α, TNF-α = tumor necrosis factor-α, TGF-β = transforming growth factor-β, SD = standard deviation, SE = standard error of mean.

(Adapted with permission from Campbell PA, Wang M, Amstutz HC, Goodman SB: Positive cytokine production in failed metal-on-metal total hip replacements. *Acta Orthop Scand* 2002;73:506-512.)

counterface roughness in determining the biologic activity of polyethylene particles. However, it is expected that the increase in particle biologic activity with higher molecular weight or higher cross-linking will probably be mitigated in vivo by lower wear volumes with HXPE.

Biologic Response to Metal Particles

Histiocytic and Specific Immunologic Responses

In a histologic study of periprosthetic tissues from different designs of metal-on-metal total hip replacements, Doorn and associates[17] found that the extent of the inflammatory reaction and the presence of foreign body-type giant cells were much less important in tissues surrounding metal-on-metal implants than in tissues surrounding metal-on-polyethylene implants. The authors postulated that the lower tissue reactivity resulted from the overall smaller size of wear particles from metal-on-metal bearings being an order of magnitude smaller than UHMWPE particles. In a comparison of the tissue response surrounding metal-on-metal and metal-on-polyethylene hip implants, Campbell and associates[63] reported fewer CD 68 positive macrophages and lower levels of transforming growth factor–β and TNF-α in the tissues surrounding metal-on-metal implants, but no difference in the quantities of CD 3 positive lymphocytes, IL-1β, IL-6, or platelet-derived growth factor-α (PDGF-α) (Table 1). Catelas and associates[64] analyzed the relationship between the production of cytokines and the quantity of metal wear particles in tissues and found that tissues surrounding failed metal-on-metal implants with low to moderate quantities of metal particles could induce the production of potentially osteolytic cytokines. However, the number of cells producing these cytokines tended to be lower than the number typically seen in tissues surrounding metal-on-polyethylene implants.

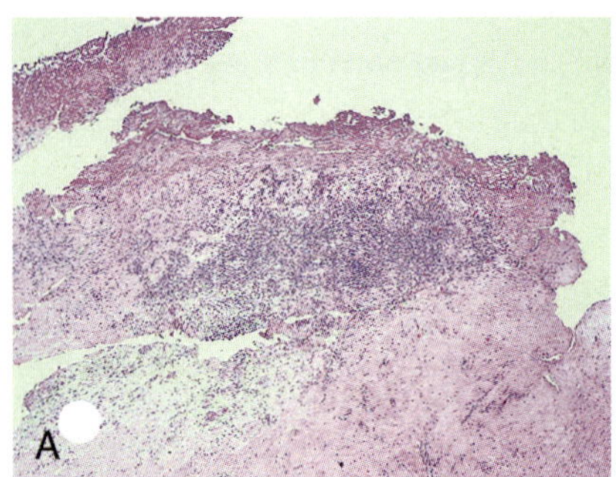

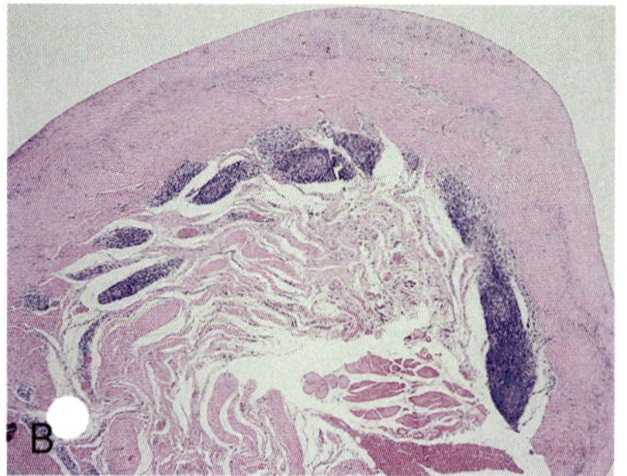

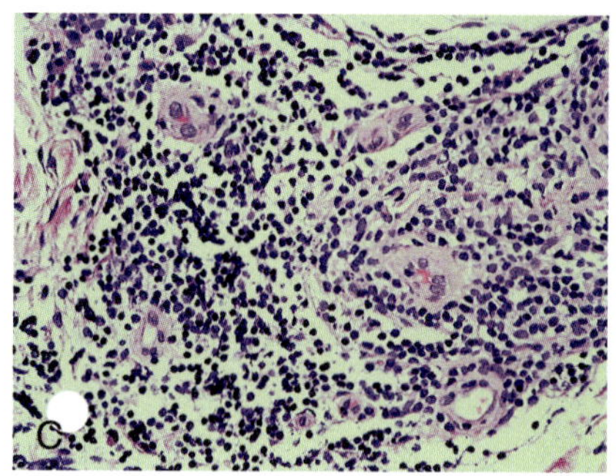

Figure 1 Histologic sections illustrating an ALVAL in tissues surrounding metal-on-metal implants. **A,** Inner capsular layer with infiltrates of diffusely distributed lymphocytes and fibrin exudates at the surface (×4). **B,** Perivascularity agglomerated lymphocytic infiltrates with secondary reaction centers in the intermediate vascular layer of a joint capsule (×20). **C,** High endothelial venules with marrow lumina and dense infiltrates of mononuclear cells in the capsular tissue (×40). (Reproduced with permission from Willert HG, Buchhorn GH, Fayyazi A, et al: Metal-on-metal bearings and hypersensitivity in patients with artificial hip joints: A clinical and histomorphological study. *J Bone Joint Surg Am* 2005;87:28-36.)

In addition to the potential of metal particles to induce osteolysis through macrophage activation, as observed in tissues surrounding conventional metal-on-polyethylene implants, concern has emerged regarding the possibility of specific immunologic responses to metal-on-metal implants. In their comparison study of tissues surrounding metal-on-metal and metal-on-polyethylene implants, Campbell and associates,[63] found a tendency toward more lymphocytes in tissues surrounding metal-on-metal implants. Similarly, Willert and associates[65] reported perivascular lymphocyte accumulations in tissues from 14 failed modern metal-on-metal implants and suggested that this reaction indicated a delayed hypersensitivity response to metal wear products. These immunologic responses could be caused by the release of metal ions that act as antigens and stimulate an allergic (hypersensitivity) reaction when they form an organometallic complex with proteins. However, it is still unclear whether implant loosening can be linked to an increased reactivity of the lymphocytes to metal particles or ions. Hallab and associates[66] investigated the incidence of lymphocyte reactivity to soluble cobalt, chromium, nickel (Ni), and titanium (Ti) using lymphocytes from patients with metal-on-metal implants compared to patients with metal-on-polyethylene implants and to patients with no implants (controls). Patients with metal-on-metal implants had significantly elevated serum cobalt and chromium concentrations (13- and 58-fold, respectively), which were correlated with elevated lymphocyte reactivity to cobalt and nickel, compared to patients having metal-on-polyethylene implants or patients in the control group. However, no etiologic link could be established between this lymphocyte reactivity and the poor performance of the implants. In a more recent study of failed modern metal-on-metal articulations, Willert and associates[67] also reported the presence of lymphocytic infiltrates, plasma cells and sometimes eosinophilic granulocytes, high endothelial venules, localized bleeding, fibrin exudation, necrosis, and macrophages with drop-like inclusions (Figure 1). This response was described as an aseptic, lymphocyte-dominated, vasculitis-associated lesion (ALVAL) or a lymphocyte-dominated immunological answer (LYDIA). Other authors also reported individual cases of lymphocytic infiltration around failed modern metal-on-metal implants.[68-70] In another study, Pandit and associates[71] recently reported the presence of pseudotumors surrounding metal-on-metal surface replacements. These pseudotumors were characterized by an extensive necrosis of dense connective tissue, a focally heavy macrophage and lymphocytic infiltration, and, in some patients, the presence of plasma cells and eosinophils. The observed reaction was somewhat similar to the ALVAL reaction reported by Willert and associates;[67] however, there was a more diffuse lymphocyte infiltrate as well as extensive connective tissue necrosis. The causes of these pseudotumors were not fully elucidated, but the potential effects of wear particles and a possible hypersensitivity reaction were mentioned. All patients in this study were female, and therefore preoperative sensitization to metal might have been a factor. Also, all revisions were done within 5 years of implantation (rather short implantation times). Unfortunately,

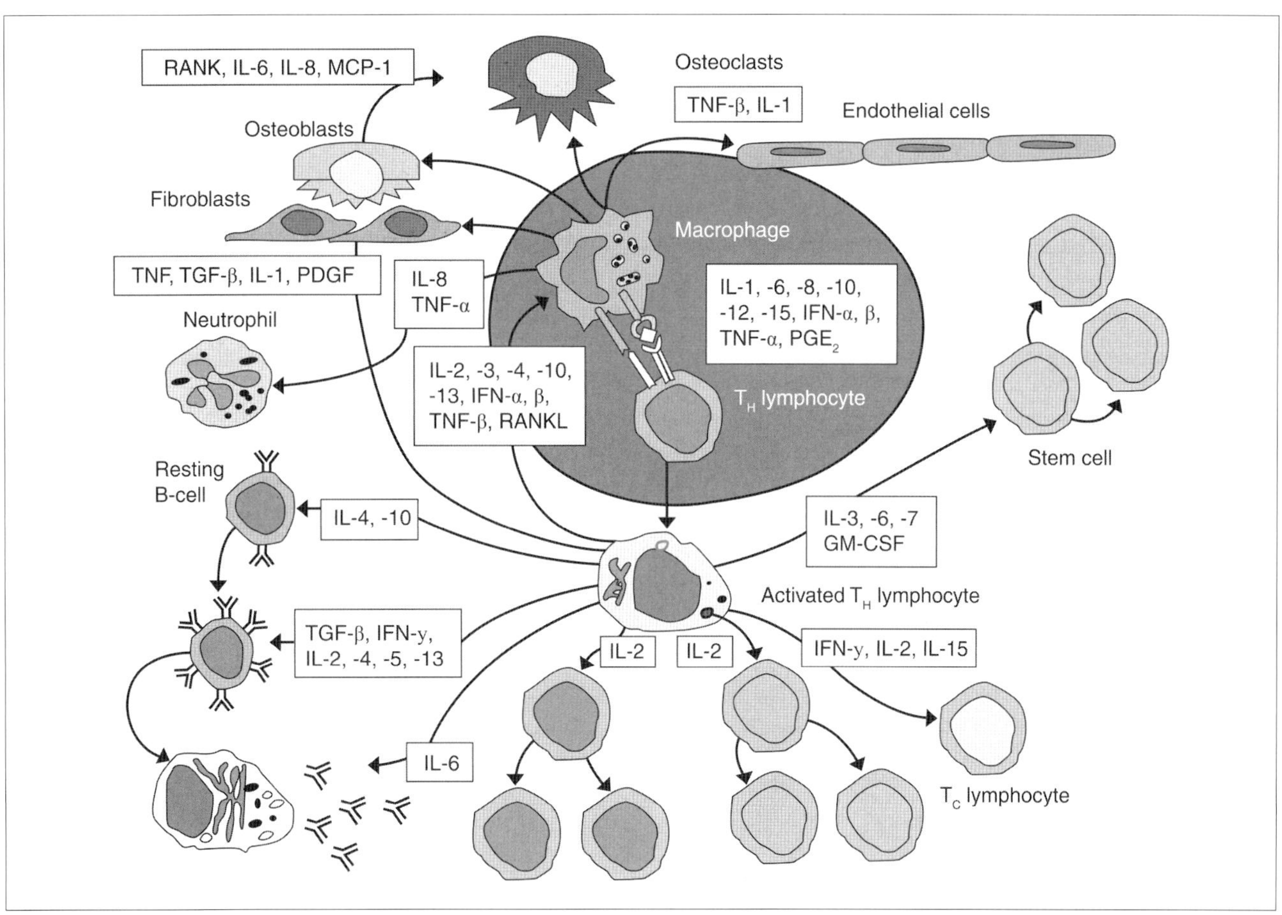

Figure 2 Illustration showing the complex interrelationship between wear products and cells of the innate and adaptive immune systems. GM-CSF = granulocyte monocyte-colony stimulating factor, IFN = interferon, MCP = monocyte chemoattractant protein, PDGF = platelet-derived growth factor, PGE_2 = prostaglandin E_2, T_c = cytotoxic T lymphocyte, TGF = transforming growth factor, T_H = T helper lymphocyte. (Reproduced with permission from Jacobs JJ, Campbell PA, Konttinen YT: Implant Wear Symposium 2007 Biologic Work Group: How has the biologic reaction to wear particles changed with newer bearing surfaces? *J Am Acad Orthop Surg* 2008;16(suppl 1):S49-S55.)

no gold standard test currently exists for the clinical diagnosis of implant-associated metal allergy because cutaneous patch testing to assess metal hypersensitivity may not relate to allergic response in the deep periprosthetic environment.[72] Although the link between aseptic loosening and hypersensitivity reactions remains to be clearly established,[73] there is increasing evidence that hypersensitivity plays a role in the pathogenesis of osteolysis.[74] The incidence of premature failure of metal-on-metal joint arthroplasty caused by a specific immunologic response is probably low but is currently unknown. Figure 2 shows the complex interrelationship between the wear products and cells of the innate and adaptive immune systems.

There are also concerns that the metal wear particles generated by a metal-on-metal hip implants may have cytotoxic effects as they disperse throughout the body. The systemic dissemination of soluble and particulate corrosion products includes the presence of metallic particles in the liver and spleen,[75] raising questions about potential genotoxicity.

Metal Ions and Genotoxic Potential

Ion levels have been measured in whole blood, serum, erythrocytes, and urine. Because of complex issues associated with the analysis of metal ions (including sample collection and statistical methodologies) there has been significant variability in the techniques used by different investigators, and this lack of uniformity makes the comparison of results difficult.[76]

In a randomized clinical trial, MacDonald and associates[77] reported significantly higher levels of metal ions in the urine and erythrocytes of patients with metal-on-metal implants than in patients with metal-on-polyethylene implants. Also, the levels of cobalt, chromium, and titanium ions measured in urine were higher than those measured in erythrocytes. Walter and associates[78] found higher levels of cobalt and chromium ions in serum or plasma than in red blood cells of patients with metal-on-metal implants. Engh and associates[79] also recently found higher levels of chromium and titanium in serum than in erythrocytes. Overall, these studies suggest that serum may better reflect the true ion levels when blood is used to assess systemic ion levels.[78] Brodner and associates[80] specifically studied serum cobalt concentrations in patients during the first 5 years after a total hip arthroplasty with a metal-on-metal articulation and found moderate concentrations of 1 μg/L at 1 year and 0.7 μg/L at 5 years. These results led to the conclusion that the serum cobalt concentrations did not reflect the higher run-in wear of metal-on-metal implants. In a study of modern metal-on-metal surface arthroplasties, Skipor and associates[81] reported that serum chromium levels were 22, 23, and 21 times higher at 3, 6, and 12 months after surgery, respectively, than before surgery; the corresponding serum cobalt levels were eight, seven, and six times higher after surgery. The authors reported that serum chromium and cobalt values found with the current generation of surface arthroplasties were in the same range as those found with conventional metal-on-metal total hip replacements.[81] In contrast, when comparing the levels of serum cobalt and chromium in patients with metal-on-metal resurfacings or metal-on-metal total hip implants, Clarke and associates[82] found median serum levels of 38 nmol/L for cobalt and 53 nmol/L for chromium in patients with metal-on-metal resurfacings compared with 22 nmol/L for cobalt and 19 nmol/L for chromium in patients with metal-on-metal total hip implants. However, this study was a retrospective analysis in which two different metal-on-metal implant designs and shorter follow-up periods were used for patients treated with resurfacing implants compared with patients treated with metal-on-metal total hip implants. In a very recent study, Antoniou and associates[83] compared the blood ion levels of patients after hip resurfacings with the ASR System (DePuy, Warsaw, IN) or metal-on-metal total hip implants using a 28- or 36-mm femoral head. After 1 year, the patients with hip resurfacings had blood metal ion levels similar to those of the patients with total hip implants. Langton and associates[84] analyzed the effects of the femoral head component size and the orientation of the acetabular component and found that both parameters could influence the overall concentration of metal ions in the whole blood of patients with metal-on-metal resurfacings. The authors reported higher ion concentrations in patients with smaller components and when the inclination angle was greater than 45° and the anteversion angle exceeded 20°.[84]

When present in high concentrations, both Co^{2+} and Cr^{3+} ions have been reported to be capable of inducing macrophage necrosis in vitro.[85] However, Co^{2+} appeared to be more toxic than Cr^{3+} considering that 40 to 50 times more Cr^{3+} was needed to induce a similar level of macrophage mortality and TNF-α release.[86,87] In theory, carcinogenic and other biologic risks, including mutagenesis, also can be associated with these metal ions. Although cobalt and chromium ions are most stable as Co^{2+} and Cr^{3+} at neutral pH, soluble Cr^{6+} ions can freely pass through the cell membrane, in comparison with Cr^{3+} ions, which cannot freely move across the lipid membrane and therefore do not easily enter the cells. After Cr^{6+} ions traverse the cell membrane, they are reductively metabolized within the cells, where they can cause a diverse range of genetic lesions. Some of these lesions can present a physical barrier to DNA replication or transcription and can promote apoptosis or terminal growth arrest. Other lesions, such as ternary DNA adducts, may be premutagenic. For example, Cr^{6+} ion exposure has been shown to elicit a classic DNA damage response in cells, including activation of the p53 signaling pathway and cell cycle arrest or apoptosis.[88] Quievryn and associates[89] reported that the reduction of Cr^{6+} led to dose-dependent formation of both mutagenic and replication-blocking DNA lesions in human fibroblasts. Similarly, Papageorgiou and associates[90] found an increase in aneuploidy, chromosome translocations, and DNA damage in human fibroblasts exposed to cobalt-chromium particles. Ladon and associates,[91] investigating changes in metal levels and chromosome aberrations in patients with metal-on-metal Metasul (Zimmer) implants for less than 2 years, showed a statistically significant increase in both chromosome translocations and aneuploidy in peripheral blood lymphocytes at 6, 12, and 24 months after surgery. However, secondary analyses did not show any statistically significant correlations between chromosome translocation indices and cobalt or chromium concentrations in whole blood. Massè and associates[92] also found that the incidence of markers of chromosomal damage in lymphocytes did not correlate with any of the ion levels (cobalt, chromium, nickel, molybdenum) measured in the blood and urine of patients who had received a Metasul component.

Biologic Response to Ceramic Particles

The alumina-on-alumina total hip implants have been in clinical use for more than 30 years, primarily in Europe. Ceramics in bulk form do not undergo oxidative environmental degradation and have been considered inert. However, in particulate form, they have been reported to be capable of eliciting a macrophage response.[93-95] Catelas and associates[95] found an increase in macrophage mortality and TNF-α release with increasing alumina or zirconia particle size and concentration in vitro. There was no significant difference between the cell response to alumina or zirconia but the overall cell response was lower than that observed with high-density polyethylene particles at similar sizes and concentrations. Petit and associates[60] also reported lower levels of TNF-α after macrophage exposure to alumina particles compared with UHMWPE polyethylene particles. Using chemiluminescence assay for reactive oxygen species, Nagase and associates[96] found that the most biologically active size of alumina particles was 1 to 7 μm. Catelas and associates[94] found that both alumina and zirconia induced macrophage apoptotic cell death. The induction of apoptosis was size- and concentration-dependent, and reached a plateau above 150 particles per macrophage with a particle size of 1.3 μm. Hatton and associates[97] compared the effects of two types of ceramic wear particles on TNF-α production by human peripheral blood mononuclear cells (PBMNC) from six donors. When wear particles obtained by microseparation (bimodal size of particles, 5 to 20 nm and 0.2 to 10 μm) were used, a greater volume was required to activate the PBMNC than when alumina powder particles (0.5 μm) were used. PBMNC from all donors produced significantly elevated levels of TNF-α when stimulated with 100 μm^3 of alumina powder per cell, but as much as 500 μm^3 of the microseparation particles per cell were necessary to have PBMNC from some donors produce similar levels of TNF-α. The authors attributed the differences in cell response to the variations in particle size, as there were fewer particles in the critical size range (0.1 to 1 μm) among the microseparation wear particles. In a comparison of the biologic activity of ceramic particles (both alumina and zirconia) and high-density polyethylene particles on murine calvarial bone, Warashina and associates[98] found that the ceramic particles induced a much lower inflammatory response and much less bone resorption than the polyethylene particles. Considering the high volumetric concentration of ceramic particles needed to generate a significant level of cytokine production, it is unlikely that the concentration threshold would ever be reached in vivo.[97] Overall, these studies suggest that ceramic particles can activate a macrophage response in a fashion similar to the response of the other types of particles, although to a lesser extent.

Lerouge and associates[25] compared the histology of pseudomembranes from ceramic-on-ceramic and metal-on-polyethylene total hip implants in a semiquantitative in vivo study, finding no significant difference in cellular reaction. However, the characterization of the particles from ceramic-on-ceramic hip implants revealed that 76% of these particles consisted of zirconia particles used to opacify the cement used for fixation and only 12% were alumina particles originating from the articulation. The authors concluded that the cellular reaction was caused by the zirconia particles in the cement rather than the alumina particles from the bearing and that the aseptic loosening of the ceramic cups resulted from the cement fragmentation caused by mechanical factors.[25] Nevertheless, osteolysis has been reported in association with ceramic wear particles. Yoon and associates[26] found osteolysis of the femur in 23 hips and osteolysis of the pelvis in 49 hips in a study of 103 noncemented Mittelmeir with a Biolox femoral head (Osteo AG, Selzach, Switzerland) ceramic-on-ceramic total hip implants at a mean 92-month follow-up. Histologic and electron microscopy analysis of the periprosthetic membranes revealed abundant ceramic wear particles with a mean size of 0.71 μm (range, 0.13 to 7.2 μm). The interface tissue consisted of rather vascular fibrous connective tissue rich in macrophages containing electron-dense material within phagosomes. Ten patients had revision surgery for loosening and migration of the acetabular component. The authors concluded that ceramic wear particles could stimulate a foreign body reaction leading to periprosthetic osteolysis.[26] However, Yoo and associates,[99] in a more recent study, reported encouraging results with respect to fracture, osteolysis, and wear at a 5-year minimum follow-up after total hip arthroplasty using a modern cementless-stem, alumina-on-alumina implant. They found radiographic evidence of bone ingrowth, no implant loosening, and no detectable wear. D'Antonio and associates[100] also reported encouraging results at a 62-month follow-up after implantation of a newer alumina-on-alumina cementless design with 99.7% of the cups stable, only 1.4% osteolysis, and no fractures. However, longer follow-up is required before conclusions can be drawn regarding the long-term outcome of using cementless ceramic-on-ceramic implants. A recent study by Yoon and associates[101] analyzed the long-term results of a newer cementless implant design with a tapered, fully porous-coated cobalt-chromium stem (Autophor 900-S; Osteo AG). At an average 17-year follow-up of 127 hip replacements (43 ceramic-on-polyethylene and 84 ceramic-on-ceramic), the femoral component survival rate was 94.5%. In a recent long-term study of ceramic acetabular components with alumina ceramic femoral heads, Hannouche and associates[102] found 85% survival of cemented cups and 61.2% survival of cementless cups in 118 hips after 20 years. Only three hips had osteolysis, and none had detectable wear.

Summary

It is clear that implant wear and corrosion can lead to the production of degradation products, a highly inflammatory biologic response, periprosthetic bone loss, and aseptic loosening. The biologic activity is highly dependent on particle characteristics and the quantity of wear particles in the most biologically active submicrometer-size range. The local and systemic effects of the wear particles and corrosion products also remain clinically significant issues. To minimize the clinical impact of implant wear, efforts should continue to focus not only on developing and studying newer materials with improved wear, corrosion resistance, and less biologic reactivity, but also on elucidating the cellular and molecular mechanisms leading to periprosthetic osteolysis in order to identify new approaches for therapeutic intervention. Several investigations already have been conducted in an attempt to reverse or even suppress the biologic response to wear particles. These approaches include the use of corticosteroids and nonsteroidal anti-inflammatory drugs, antiosteolytic agents (such as bisphosphonates), antioxidants, RANKL inhibitors, gene therapy for the delivery of anti-inflammatory agents (such as anti–TNF-α agents), and osteogenic growth factors to stimulate periprosthetic bone formation. To date, however, there is no approved drug therapy to prevent or inhibit periprosthetic osteolysis.

References

1. Willert HG, Bertram H, Buchhorn GH: Osteolysis in alloarthroplasty of the hip: The role of ultra-high molecular weight polyethylene wear particles. *Clin Orthop Relat Res* 1990;258: 95-107.
2. Amstutz HC, Campbell P, Kossovsky N, Clarke IC: Mechanism and clinical significance of wear debris-induced osteolysis. *Clin Orthop Relat Res* 1992;276:7-18.
3. Cooper RA, McAllister CM, Borden LS, Bauer TW: Polyethylene debris-induced osteolysis and loosening in uncemented total hip arthroplasty: A cause of late failure. *J Arthroplasty* 1992;7:285-290.
4. Schmalzried TP, Jasty M, Harris WH: Periprosthetic bone loss in total hip arthroplasty: Polyethylene wear debris and the concept of the effective joint space. *J Bone Joint Surg Am* 1992; 74:849-863.
5. Schey JA: Systems view of optimizing metal on metal bearings. *Clin Orthop Relat Res* 1996;329:S115-S127.
6. Dorlot JM: Wear patterns of alumina-alumina ceramic hip implants. *Clin Orthop Relat Res* 1991;272:88-93.
7. Nizard RS, Sedel L, Christel P, Meunier A, Soudry M, Witvoet J: Ten-year survivorship of cemented ceramic-ceramic total hip prosthesis. *Clin Orthop Relat Res* 1992;282:53-63.
8. Sedel L: Clinical follow-up of alumina-alumina ceramic bearings in total hip arthroplasty. *Clin Orthop Relat Res* 1994;298:62-69.
9. Endo M, Tipper JL, Barton DC, Stone MH, Ingham E, Fisher J: Comparison of wear, wear debris and functional biological activity of moderately crosslinked and non-crosslinked polyethylene in hip prostheses. *Proc Inst Mech Eng H* 2002;216: 111-122.
10. Campbell P, Ma S, Yeom B, McKellop H, Schmalzried TP, Amstutz HC: Isolation of predominantly sub-micron sized UHMWPE wear particles from periprosthetic tissues. *J Biomed Mater Res* 1995;29:127-131.
11. Margevicius KJ, Bauer TW, McMahon JT, Brown SA, Merritt K: Isolation and characterization of debris from around total joint prostheses. *J Bone Joint Surg Am* 1994;76: 1664-1675.
12. Shanbhag AS, Jacobs JJ, Glant TT, Gilbert JL, Black J, Galante JO: Composition and morphology of wear debris in failed uncemented total hip replacement. *J Bone Joint Surg Br* 1994; 76:60-67.
13. Visentin M, Stea S, Squarzoni S, Antonietti B, Reggiani M, Toni A: A new method for isolation of polyethylene wear debris from tissue and synovial fluid. *Biomaterials* 2004;25:5531-5537.

14. Richards L, Brown C, Stone MH, Fisher J, Ingham E, Tipper JL: Identification of nanometre-sized ultra-high molecular weight polyethylene wear particles in samples retrieved in vivo. *J Bone Joint Surg Br* 2008;90: 1106-1113.
15. Laurent MP, Johnson TS, Crowninshield RD, Blanchard CR, Bhambri SK, Yao JQ: Characterization of a highly cross-linked ultrahigh molecular-weight polyethylene in clinical use in total hip arthroplasty. *J Arthroplasty* 2008;23:751-761.
16. Atienza C Jr, Maloney WJ: Highly cross-linked polyethylene bearing surfaces in total hip arthroplasty. *J Surg Orthop Adv* 2008;17:27-33.
17. Doorn PF, Mirra JM, Campbell PA, Amstutz HC: Tissue reaction to metal on metal total hip prostheses. *Clin Orthop Relat Res* 1996;329:S187-S205.
18. Catelas I, Bobyn JD, Medley JB, et al: Effects of digestion protocols on the isolation and characterization of metal-metal wear particles: I. Analysis of particle size and shape. *J Biomed Mater Res* 2001;55:320-329.
19. Catelas I, Bobyn JD, Medley JJ, Zukor DJ, Petit A, Huk OL: Effects of digestion protocols on the isolation and characterization of metal-metal wear particles: Part II. Analysis of ion release and particle composition. *J Biomed Mater Res* 2001;55:330-337.
20. Catelas I, Bobyn JD, Medley JB, Krygier JJ, Zukor DJ, Huk OL: Size, shape, and composition of wear particles from metal-metal hip simulator testing: Effects of alloy and number of loading cycles. *J Biomed Mater Res A* 2003;67:312-327.
21. Catelas I, Medley JB, Campbell PA, Huk OL, Bobyn JD: Comparison of in vitro with in vivo characteristics of wear particles from metal-metal hip implants. *J Biomed Mater Res B Appl Biomater* 2004;70:167-178.
22. Catelas I, Campbell PA, Bobyn JD, Medley JB, Huk OL: Wear particles from metal-on-metal total hip replacements: Effects of implant design and implantation time. *Proc Inst Mech Eng H* 2006;220:195-208.
23. Brown C, Fisher J, Ingham E: Biological effects of clinically relevant wear particles from metal-on-metal hip prostheses. *Proc Inst Mech Eng H* 2006; 220:355-369.
24. Lerouge S, Huk O, Yahia LH, Sedel L: Characterization of in vivo wear debris from ceramic-ceramic total hip arthroplasties. *J Biomed Mater Res* 1996;32:627-633.
25. Lerouge S, Huk O, Yahia LH, Witovet J, Sedel L: Ceramic-ceramic and metal-polyethylene total hip replacements: Comparison of pseudomembranes after loosening. *J Bone Joint Surg Br* 1997;79:135-139.
26. Yoon TR, Rowe SM, Jung ST, Seon KJ, Maloney WJ: Osteolysis in association with a total hip arthroplasty with ceramic bearing surfaces. *J Bone Joint Surg Am* 1998;80:1459-1468.
27. Hatton A, Nevelos JE, Nevelos AA, Banks RE, Fisher J, Ingham E: Alumina-alumina artificial hip joints: Part I. A histological analysis and characterization of wear debris by laser capture microdissection of tissues retrieved at revision. *Biomaterials* 2002;23:3429-3440.
28. Tipper JL, Hatton A, Nevelos JE, et al: Alumina-alumina artificial hip joints: Part II. Characterization of the wear debris from in vitro hip joint simulations. *Biomaterials* 2002;23: 3441-3448.
29. Charnley J: Fracture of femoral prostheses in total hip replacement: A clinical study. *Clin Orthop Relat Res* 1975;111:105-120.
30. Rubash HE, Sinha RK, Shanbhag AS, Kim SY: Pathogenesis of bone loss after total hip arthroplasty. *Orthop Clin North Am* 1998;29:173-186.
31. Neale SD, Athanasou NA: Cytokine receptor profile of arthroplasty macrophages, foreign body giant cells and mature osteoclasts. *Acta Orthop Scand* 1999;70:452-458.
32. Jacobs JJ, Roebuck KA, Archibeck M, Hallab NJ, Glant TT: Osteolysis: Basic science. *Clin Orthop Relat Res* 2001; 393:71-77.
33. Neale SD, Fujikawa Y, Sabokbar A, et al: Human bone-derived cells support formation of human osteoclasts from arthroplasty-derived cells in vitro. *J Bone Joint Surg Br* 2000;82: 892-900.
34. Hirashima Y, Ishiguro N, Kondo S, Iwata H: Osteoclast induction from bone marrow cells is due to pro-inflammatory mediators from macrophages exposed to polyethylene particles: A possible mechanism of osteolysis in failed THA. *J Biomed Mater Res* 2001;56:177-183.
35. Greenfield EM, Bi Y, Ragab AA, Goldberg VM, Van De Motter RR: The role of osteoclast differentiation in aseptic loosening. *J Orthop Res* 2002;20:1-8.
36. Kim KJ, Rubash HE, Wilson SC, D'Antonio JA, McClain EJ: A histologic and biochemical comparison of the interface tissues in cementless and cemented hip prostheses. *Clin Orthop Relat Res* 1993;287:142-152.
37. Xu JW, Konttinen YT, Lassus J, et al: Tumor necrosis factor-alpha (TNF-alpha) in loosening of total hip replacement (THR). *Clin Exp Rheumatol* 1996;14:643-648.
38. Goodman SB, Chin RC, Chiou SS, Schurman DJ, Woolson ST, Masada MP: A clinical-pathologic-biochemical study of the membrane surrounding loosened and non-loosened total hip arthroplasties. *Clin Orthop Relat Res* 1989;244:182-187.
39. Ingham E, Fisher J: The role of macrophages in osteolysis of total joint replacement. *Biomaterials* 2005;26:1271-1286.
40. Haynes DR, Crotti TN, Potter AE, et al: The osteoclastogenic molecules RANKL and RANK are associated with periprosthetic osteolysis. *J Bone Joint Surg Br* 2001;83:902-911.
41. Ren W, Yang SY, Fang HW, Hsu S, Wooley PH: Distinct gene expression of receptor activator of nuclear factor-kappaB and rank ligand in the inflammatory response to variant morphol-

ogies of UHMWPE particles. *Biomaterials* 2003;24:4819-4826.

42. Granchi D, Amato I, Battistelli L, et al: Molecular basis of osteoclastogenesis induced by osteoblasts exposed to wear particles. *Biomaterials* 2005;26: 2371-2379.

43. Mandelin J, Li TF, Liljeström M, et al: Imbalance of RANKL/RANK/OPG system in interface tissue in loosening of total hip replacement. *J Bone Joint Surg Br* 2003;85:1196-1201.

44. Wang ML, Sharkey PF, Tuan RS: Particle bioreactivity and wear-mediated osteolysis. *J Arthroplasty* 2004;19:1028-1038.

45. Goodman SB, Ma T, Chiu R, Ramachandran R, Smith RL: Effects of orthopaedic wear particles on osteoprogenitor cells. *Biomaterials* 2006;27: 6096-6101.

46. Wang ML, Nesti LJ, Tuli R, et al: Titanium particles suppress expression of osteoblastic phenotype in human mesenchymal stem cells. *J Orthop Res* 2002;20:1175-1184.

47. Wang ML, Tuli R, Manner PA, Sharkey PF, Hall DJ, Tuan RS: Direct and indirect induction of apoptosis in human mesenchymal stem cells in response to titanium particles. *J Orthop Res* 2003;21:697-707.

48. Okafor CC, Haleem-Smith H, Laqueriere P, Manner PA, Tuan RS: Particulate endocytosis mediates biological responses of human mesenchymal stem cells to titanium wear debris. *J Orthop Res* 2006;24:461-473.

49. Chiu R, Ma T, Smith RL, Goodman SB: Polymethylmethacrylate particles inhibit osteoblastic differentiation of bone marrow osteoprogenitor cells. *J Biomed Mater Res A* 2006;77:850-856.

50. Caicedo MS, Desai R, McAllister K, Reddy A, Jacobs JJ, Hallab NJ. Soluble and particulate Co-Cr-Mo alloy implant metals activate the inflammasome danger signaling pathway in human macrophages: A novel mechanism for implant debris reactivity. *J Orthop Res* 2009;27:847-854.

51. Goodman SB, Fornasier VL, Lee J, Kei J: The histological effects of the implantation of different sizes of polyethylene particles in the rabbit tibia. *J Biomed Mater Res* 1990;24:517-524.

52. Goodman S, Aspenberg P, Song Y, et al: Tissue ingrowth and differentiation in the bone-harvest chamber in the presence of cobalt-chromium-alloy and high-density-polyethylene particles. *J Bone Joint Surg Am* 1995; 77:1025-1035.

53. Trindade MC, Song Y, Aspenberg P, Smith RL, Goodman SB: Proinflammatory mediator release in response to particle challenge: Studies using the bone harvest chamber. *J Biomed Mater Res* 1999;48:434-439.

54. Brooks RA, Sharpe JR, Wimhurst JA, Myer BJ, Dawes EN, Rushton N: The effects of the concentration of high density polyethylene particles on the bone implant interface. *J Bone Joint Surg Br* 2000;82:595-600.

55. Green TR, Fisher J, Matthews JB, Stone MH, Ingham E: Effect of size and dose on bone resorption activity of macrophages by in vitro clinically relevant ultra high molecular weight polyethylene particles. *J Biomed Mater Res* 2000;53:490-497.

56. Yang SY, Ren WP, Park YS, et al: Diverse cellular and apoptotic responses to variant shapes of UHMWPE particles in a murine model of inflammation. *Biomaterials* 2002;23:3535-3543.

57. Shanbhag AS, Jacobs JJ, Black J, Galante JO, Glant TT: Human monocyte response to particulate biomaterials generated in vivo and in vitro. *J Orthop Res* 1995;13:792-801.

58. Horowitz SM, Gonzales JB: Effects of polyethylene on macrophages. *J Orthop Res* 1997;15:50-56.

59. Voronov I, Santerre JP, Hinek A, Callahan JW, Sandhu J, Boynton EL: Macrophage phagocytosis of polyethylene particles in vitro. *J Biomed Mater Res* 1998;39:40-51.

60. Petit A, Catelas I, Antoniou J, Zukor DJ, Huk OL: Differential apoptotic response of J774 macrophages to alumina and ultra-high-molecular-weight polyethylene particles. *J Orthop Res* 2002;20:9-15.

61. Illgen RL II , Forsythe TM, Pike JW, Laurent MP, Blanchard CR: Highly crosslinked vs conventional polyethylene particles: An in vitro comparison of biologic activities. *J Arthroplasty* 2008;23:721-731.

62. Ingram JH, Stone M, Fisher J, Ingham E: The influence of molecular weight, crosslinking and counterface roughness on TNF-alpha production by macrophages in response to ultra high molecular weight polyethylene particles. *Biomaterials* 2004;25:3511-3522.

63. Campbell PA, Wang M, Amstutz HC, Goodman SB: Positive cytokine production in failed metal-on-metal total hip replacements. *Acta Orthop Scand* 2002;73:506-512.

64. Catelas I, Campbell PA, Dorey F, Frausto A, Mills BG, Amstutz HC: Semi-quantitative analysis of cytokines in MM THR tissues and their relationship to metal particles. *Biomaterials* 2003;24:4785-4797.

65. Willert H, Buchhorn G, Fayyazi A, Lohmann C: Histopathological changes around metal/metal joints indicate delayed type hypersensitivity: Preliminary results of 14 cases. *Osteologie* 2000;9:2-16.

66. Hallab NJ, Anderson S, Caicedo M, Skipor A, Campbell P, Jacobs JJ: Immune responses correlate with serum-metal in metal-on-metal hip arthroplasty. *J Arthroplasty* 2004;19:88-93.

67. Willert HG, Buchhorn GH, Fayyazi A, et al: Metal-on-metal bearings and hypersensitivity in patients with artificial hip joints: A clinical and histomorphological study. *J Bone Joint Surg Am* 2005;87:28-36.

68. Al-Saffar N: Early clinical failure of total joint replacement in association with follicular proliferation of B-lymphocytes: A report of two cases. *J Bone Joint Surg Am* 2002;84:2270-2273.

69. Böhler M, Kanz F, Schwarz B, et al: Adverse tissue reactions to wear parti-

cles from Co-alloy articulations, increased by alumina-blasting particle contamination from cementless Ti-based total hip implants: A report of seven revisions with early failure. *J Bone Joint Surg Br* 2002;84:128-136.

70. Davies AP, Willert HG, Campbell PA, Learmonth ID, Case CP: An unusual lymphocytic perivascular infiltration in tissues around contemporary metal-on-metal joint replacements. *J Bone Joint Surg Am* 2005;87:18-27.

71. Pandit H, Glyn-Jones S, McLardy-Smith P, et al: Pseudotumours associated with metal-on-metal hip resurfacings. *J Bone Joint Surg Br* 2008;90: 847-851.

72. Jacobs JJ, Campbell PA, T Konttinen YT: How has the biologic reaction to wear particles changed with newer bearing surfaces? *J Am Acad Orthop Surg* 2008;16:S49-S55.

73. Jacobs JJ, Hallab NJ: Loosening and osteolysis associated with metal-on-metal bearings: A local effect of metal hypersensitivity? *J Bone Joint Surg Am* 2006;88:1171-1172.

74. Hallab NJ, Anderson S, Stafford T, Glant T, Jacobs JJ: Lymphocyte responses in patients with total hip arthroplasty. *J Orthop Res* 2005;23:384-391.

75. Urban RM, Tomlinson MJ, Hall DJ, Jacobs JJ: Accumulation in liver and spleen of metal particles generated at nonbearing surfaces in hip arthroplasty. *J Arthroplasty* 2004;19:94-101.

76. MacDonald SJ, Brodner W, Jacobs JJ: A consensus paper on metal ions in metal-on-metal hip arthroplasties. *J Arthroplasty* 2004;19:12-16.

77. MacDonald SJ, McCalden RW, Chess DG, et al: Metal-on-metal versus polyethylene in hip arthroplasty: A randomized clinical trial. *Clin Orthop Relat Res* 2003,406:282-296.

78. Walter LR, Marel E, Harbury R, Wearne J: Distribution of chromium and cobalt ions in various blood fractions after resurfacing hip arthroplasty. *J Arthroplasty* 2008;23:814-821.

79. Engh CA Jr, MacDonald SJ, Sritulanondha S, Thompson A, Naudie D, Engh CA: Metal ion levels after metal-on-metal total hip arthroplasty: A randomized trial [2008 John Charnley Award]. *Clin Orthop Relat Res* 2009;467:101-111.

80. Brodner W, Bitzan P, Meisinger V, Kaider A, Gottsauner-Wolf F, Kotz R: Serum cobalt levels after metal-on-metal total hip arthroplasty. *J Bone Joint Surg Am* 2003;85:2168-2173.

81. Skipor AK, Campbell PA, Patterson LM, Amstutz HC, Schmalzried TP, Jacobs JJ: Serum and urine metal levels in patients with metal-on-metal surface arthroplasty. *J Mater Sci Mater Med* 2002;13:1227-1234.

82. Clarke MT, Lee PT, Arora A, Villar RN: Levels of metal ions after small- and large-diameter metal-on-metal hip arthroplasty. *J Bone Joint Surg Br* 2003;85:913-917.

83. Antoniou J, Zukor DJ, Mwale F, Minarik W, Petit A, Huk OL: Metal ion levels in the blood of patients after hip resurfacing: A comparison between twenty-eight and thirty-six-millimeter-head metal-on-metal prostheses. *J Bone Joint Surg Am* 2008; 90:142-148.

84. Langton DJ, Jameson SS, Joyce TJ, Webb J, Nargol AV: The effect of component size and orientation on the concentrations of metal ions after resurfacing arthroplasty of the hip. *J Bone Joint Surg Br* 2008;90:1143-1151.

85. Catelas I, Petit A, Vali H, et al: Quantitative analysis of macrophage apoptosis vs. necrosis induced by cobalt and chromium ions in vitro. *Biomaterials* 2005;26:2441-2453.

86. Catelas I, Petit A, Zukor DJ, Huk OL: Cytotoxic and apoptotic effects of cobalt and chromium ions on J774 macrophages: Implication of caspase-3 in the apoptotic pathway. *J Mater Sci Mater Med* 2001;12:949-953.

87. Catelas I, Petit A, Zukor DJ, Antoniou J, Huk OL: TNF-alpha secretion and macrophage mortality induced by cobalt and chromium ions in vitro: Qualitative analysis of apoptosis. *Biomaterials* 2003;24:383-391.

88. O'Brien TJ, Ceryak S, Patierno SR: Complexities of chromium carcinogenesis: Role of cellular response, repair and recovery mechanisms. *Mutat Res* 2003;533:3-36.

89. Quievryn G, Peterson E, Messer J, Zhitkovich A: Genotoxicity and mutagenicity of chromium (VI)/ ascorbate-generated DNA adducts in human and bacterial cells. *Biochemistry* 2003;42:1062-1070.

90. Papageorgiou I, Yin Z, Ladon D, et al: Genotoxic effects of particles of surgical cobalt chrome alloy on human cells of different age in vitro. *Mutat Res* 2007;619:45-58.

91. Ladon D, Doherty A, Newson R, Turner J, Bhamra M, Case CP: Changes in metal levels and chromosome aberrations in the peripheral blood of patients after metal-on-metal hip arthroplasty. *J Arthroplasty* 2004;19:78-83.

92. Massè A, Bosetti M, Buratti C, Visentin O, Bergadano D, Cannas M: Ion release and chromosomal damage from total hip prostheses with metal-on-metal articulation. *J Biomed Mater Res B Appl Biomater* 2003;67:750-757.

93. Catelas I, Huk OL, Petit A, Zukor DJ, Marchand R, Yahia L: Flow cytometric analysis of macrophage response to ceramic and polyethylene particles: Effects of size, concentration, and composition. *J Biomed Mater Res* 1998; 41:600-607.

94. Catelas I, Petit A, Zukor DJ, Marchand R, Yahia L, Huk OL: Induction of macrophage apoptosis by ceramic and polyethylene particles in vitro. *Biomaterials* 1999;20:625-630.

95. Catelas I, Petit A, Marchand R, Zukor DJ, Yahia L, Huk OL: Cytotoxicity and macrophage cytokine release induced by ceramic and polyethylene particles in vitro. *J Bone Joint Surg Br* 1999;81:516-521.

96. Nagase M, Nishiya H, Takeuchi H: Effect of particle size on alumina-induced production of reactive oxygen metabolites by human leukocytes. *Scand J Rheumatol* 1995;24:102-107.

97. Hatton A, Nevelos JE, Matthews JB, Fisher J, Ingham E: Effects of clinically relevant alumina ceramic wear particles on TNF-alpha production by human peripheral blood mononuclear phagocytes. *Biomaterials* 2003;24: 1193-1204.

98. Warashina H, Sakano S, Kitamura S, et al: Biological reaction to alumina, zirconia, titanium and polyethylene particles implanted onto murine calvaria. *Biomaterials* 2003;24:3655-3661.

99. Yoo JJ, Kim YM, Yoon KS, Koo KH, Song WS, Kim HJ: Alumina-on-alumina total hip arthroplasty: A five-year minimum follow-up study. *J Bone Joint Surg Am* 2005;87:530-535.

100. D'Antonio J, Capello W, Manley M, Naughton M, Sutton K: Alumina ceramic bearings for total hip arthroplasty: Five-year results of a prospective randomized study. *Clin Orthop Relat Res* 2005;436:164-171.

101. Yoon TR, Rowe SM, Kim MS, Cho SG, Seon JK: Fifteen- to 20-year results of uncemented tapered fully porous-coated cobalt-chrome stems. *Int Orthop* 2008;32:317-323.

102. Hannouche D, Hamadouche M, Nizard R, Bizot P, Meunier A, Sedel L: Ceramics in total hip replacement. *Clin Orthop Relat Res* 2005;430:62-71.

Metal-on-Metal Bearings in Total Hip Arthroplasty

Paul E. Beaulé, MD, FRCSC
Steven A. Mussett, MBChB, FRCSC
John B. Medley, PhD, PEng

Abstract

The demand for total hip arthroplasty is increasing, as are patients' expectations to return to high activity levels. Metal-on-metal bearings are being used in an effort to maximize the longevity of primary hip replacements. Acetabular component inclination has been a recognized aspect of surgical technique for more than 20 years; it now is considered critical, especially in hip resurfacing or implantation of a stem-type device with a larger diameter femoral head and a monoblock acetabular component. It is important to understand the indications for using metal-on-metal bearings as well as the key clinical factors for avoiding early implant failure.

Metal-on-metal implant articulation bearings were introduced during the 1960s but fell out of favor after poor bearing and implant designs led to disappointing clinical results.[1-4] Metal-on-polyethylene bearings had better clinical results and became the preferred articulation bearing.[5] However, some early metal-on-metal prostheses had satisfactory outcomes, and improved understanding of bearing design eventually led to a renewal of interest in the use of metal-on-metal bearings.[6] A second generation of metal-on-metal bearings with improved design and manufacturing was approved in 1999 for clinical use by the US Food and Drug Administration. The current generation of metal-on-metal bearings has been in use longer than bearings composed of metal on highly cross-linked polyethylene, oxonium on highly cross-linked polyethylene, or delta ceramic on delta ceramic.[7] The advantages of metal on metal compared with other bearing materials include better wear properties and, consequently, potentially greater longevity of the prosthesis; use of a larger femoral head diameter, which permits a greater range of motion and thereby reduces the risk of dislocation after primary or revision surgery; and preservation of acetabular bone stock (when a large-diameter femoral head is used).

Wear Characteristics

Second-generation metal-on-metal bearings have better wear characteristics than first-generation bearings. Decreased wear reduces the risk of wear particle–induced osteolysis[8] or a hypersensitivity reaction.[9,10] Laboratory studies[11-13] comparing different types of cobalt-chromium-molybdenum alloys found that the important factors determining wear resistance are carbon levels, diametral clearance, and surface finish. One study[14] specifically found that the amount of carbon dissolved in the matrix is very important. Cobalt-chromium-molybdenum metal-on-metal bearing alloys are manufactured using either a wrought or cast process. Wrought material has a small grain size with a fine, homogenous distribution of

Dr. Beaulé or an immediate family member is a member of a speakers' bureau or has made paid presentations on behalf of Wright Medical Technology; serves as a paid consultant to or is an employee of Brainlab and Wright Medical Technology; serves as an unpaid consultant to Getinge USA; and has received research or institutional support from Stryker, Wright Medical Technology, and Zimmer. Dr. Medley or an immediate family member has received nonincome support (such as equipment or services), commercially derived honoraria, or other non–research-realted funding (such as paid travel) from Medtronic Spinal & Biologics. Neither Dr. Mussett nor an immediate family member has received anything of value from or owns stock in a commercial company or institution related directly or indirectly to the subject of this chapter.

carbides (a carbide is a compound of carbon with a less electronegative element). Cast material has large grains with blocky carbides; it can be subjected to heat treatment to produce a more uniform distribution of carbides along grain boundaries and in the matrix.[5] Dowson and associates[12] compared wrought and cast cobalt-chromium-molybdenum alloy metal-on-metal hip bearings with a low (less than 0.05%) or high (more than 0.20%) carbon content and found higher wear rates in the bearings with low carbon content. The study did not distinguish between the amount of carbon in carbides compared with the amount dissolved in the alloy matrix. There was no significant difference between the wrought and cast materials in the absence of other factors, and heat treatment did not have a significant effect on wear. This finding was confirmed by other studies.[5]

Rieker and associates[6] found a positive correlation between wear rate and clearance in the laboratory setting. Diametral clearance may be the most important parameter influencing the wear of a metal-on-metal bearing.[9,10] The clearance must be adequate to allow polar (rather than equatorial) articulation of the contact zone that remains polar under the mechanical deformation occurring when the prosthesis is loaded. Polar articulation refers to the femoral head and inner acetabular component surface making contact at the dome, whereas equatorial articulation refers to contact at the widest part of the femoral head. Polar bearing contact patterns result in less wear, probably because fluid ingress optimizes surface-protective, elastohydrodynamic lubrication, which creates beneficial surface deformation in the contact zone, and the subsequent egress of wear-generated particles.[9,10] If the clearance is too small, equatorial bearing occurs and fluid entrainment cannot take place; the resulting high frictional torque leads to seizing and subsequent loosening. McKee[15] recognized inadequate clearance as the mechanism for early failures of the McKee-Farrar prosthesis; as a result, in 1968 the femoral head component was slightly downsized. Seizure also frequently occurred with use of the equatorial-bearing Stanmore metal-on-metal hip implant.[16] Excessive wear also can occur if the diametral clearance is too great; one study reported a wear rate 16 times greater than average.[17] Many manufacturers make metal-on-metal bearings with a diametral clearance of 100 to 200 μm to maximize fluid entrapment and ensure polar bearing.

The influence of diametral clearance recently was considered in more detail. Metal-on-metal implant wear in a hip simulator was found to be related to the film thickness of the lubricant fluid, as determined using Dowson's explanation of elastohydrodynamic theory.[9,10] Efforts were made to relate the thickness of the lubricant fluid film to surface roughness using the λ parameter (the ratio of the thickness of the fluid film to the composite root-mean-square surface roughness). The fluid film thickness and the λ parameter for a specific surface roughness are closely correlated with the effective radius of the bearing.[9,10] The effective radius is a geometric parameter that contains both radial clearance and femoral component head size; it can be expressed by the formula $R = R_H (R_H + C)/C$, where R is the effective radius, R_H is the radius of the head, and C is the radial clearance (the difference between femoral head and acetabular cup radii or, more simply, one half of the diametral clearance). The concept of decreased wear with increasing effective radius was supported by in vitro simulator data and some in vivo clinical data.[18] Effective radius increases with lubricant fluid film thickness and the λ parameter, and wear decreases when the radius of the femoral head is as large as possible and the radial clearance is as small as possible.[9,10] The effective radius can be controlled by the device manufacturer.

A hip bearing with a large effective radius has a larger contact zone and thus a lower contact stress than a bearing with a smaller effective radius. Provided the contact area remains polar and has a small peripheral inlet region, lubricant can be more easily entrained and thus develop into a thicker, more protective fluid film. In addition, a large-diameter head, which often contributes to a large effective radius, has a higher surface velocity during activities and thus creates a higher entrainment velocity for the lubricant, further increasing lubricant film thickness. When activity levels are low, fluid films slowly decrease in thickness and eventually break down; thus, fluid films are not initially available to protect the surface when activity levels subsequently increase. When activity begins, the surfaces are likely to be in direct contact, and other conditions at the surface influence wear.

The manufacturer has some control over the alloy microstructure, particularly over the amount of dissolved carbon. Varano and associates[14] proposed that higher levels of dissolved carbon make the surface microstructure resistant to a strain-induced transformation, which is associated with higher wear. Thus, a higher level of dissolved carbon was considered beneficial. Varano and

Table 1
The Advantages and Disadvantages of Metal-on-Metal Bearings

Advantages
Low wear rate
Reduced risk of osteolysis
Improved longevity
Larger diameter femoral head
Improved range of motion
Reduced risk of dislocation
Preserved acetabular bone stock (compared with a metal-on-polyethylene bearing surface)
Disadvantages
Metal ion release
Risk of carcinogenicity
Risk of chromosomal damage
Pregnancy risk (teratogenic, mutagenic)
Metal hypersensitivity

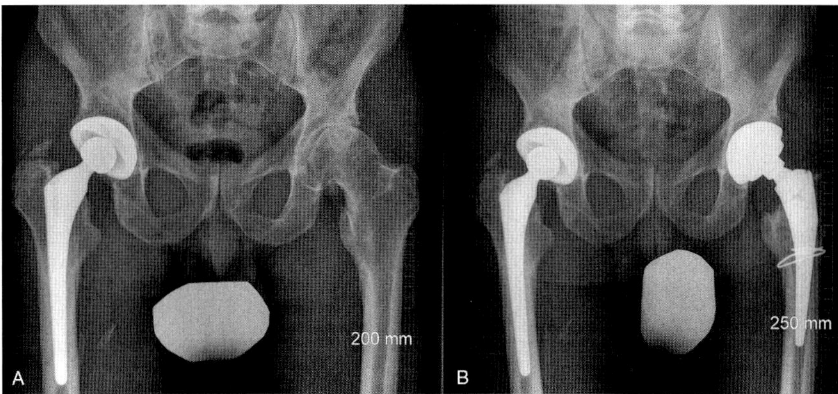

Figure 1 **A,** AP radiograph of the pelvis in a 43-year-old patient showing a right total hip replacement with a cementless metal-on-polyethylene implant and advanced arthritis in the left hip. **B,** AP radiograph of the left total hip replacement using a large metal-on-metal bearing with a modular, large-head femoral component (ProFemur TL Total Hip System, Wright Medical Technology, Memphis, TN).

associates[14] noted that a large effective radius also would reduce contact stress and thus surface strain, thereby reducing strain-induced transformation. Although the effectiveness of higher levels of dissolved carbon in reducing in vivo wear has not been determined, it is interesting to note that a high effective radius might help reduce wear by reducing contact stress during surface contact. A cobalt-chromium-molybdenum alloy with a high level of carbon tends to have a higher level of dissolved carbon; a metal-on-metal hip implant that was made from an alloy with a high carbon content (perhaps having more dissolved carbon) and that has a low clearance and a large diameter (thus, a high effective radius) is likely to have a lower wear rate.

Clinical Indications and Advantages

The use of metal-on-metal implants is associated with several advantages (Table 1). Multiple studies have reported a significant reduction in bearing wear and subsequent osteolysis.[8,19,20] Retrieval analyses of second-generation metal-on-metal implants found a 20-fold reduction in linear wear rate and a more than 60-fold reduction in volumetric wear rate, compared with traditional, not intentionally cross-linked polyethylene implants.[20] This factor may lead to increased implant longevity and a need for fewer revision surgeries, which would be of immense value for young, active patients.

A second advantage of using a metal-on-metal implant is the ability to use a larger diameter femoral head (Figure 1), which has better wear characteristics than a smaller diameter femoral head. In addition, using a larger femoral head component can be important in treating a patient with instability, because increasing the head size reduces the risk of dislocation.[21,22] The increased head size allows for a greater head-to-neck ratio, which increases the primary arc of motion by reducing the risk of the femoral neck impinging on the edge of the cup at opposite ends of the range of motion.[23] Increasing the femoral head size increases the excursion distance from the point the neck impinges to the point the hip dislocates.

The reported incidence of hip instability after revision surgery ranges from 8% to 14%.[24-26] Very large femoral heads (having a diameter greater than 40 mm) with a polyethylene liner have been used with some success in revision procedures necessitated by instability, but the demands on the polyethylene are great.[27,28] The advantage of using a metal-on-metal bearing in revision procedures for instability is that the wall of the acetabular component can be relatively thin (4 mm), permitting the size of the femoral head to be maximized without compromising the acetabular bone stock. A metal-on-metal bearing also can be useful when a liner must be cemented into a well-fixed acetabular shell because the locking mechanism is damaged. Cementing an all-metal liner allows access to a wider range of large femoral heads[29,30] (Figure 2).

Both first- and second-generation metal-on-metal prostheses are associated with good rates of clinical survivorship and low rates of osteol-

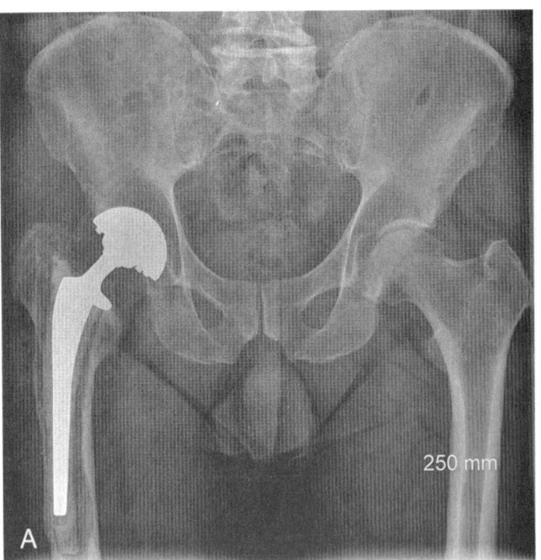

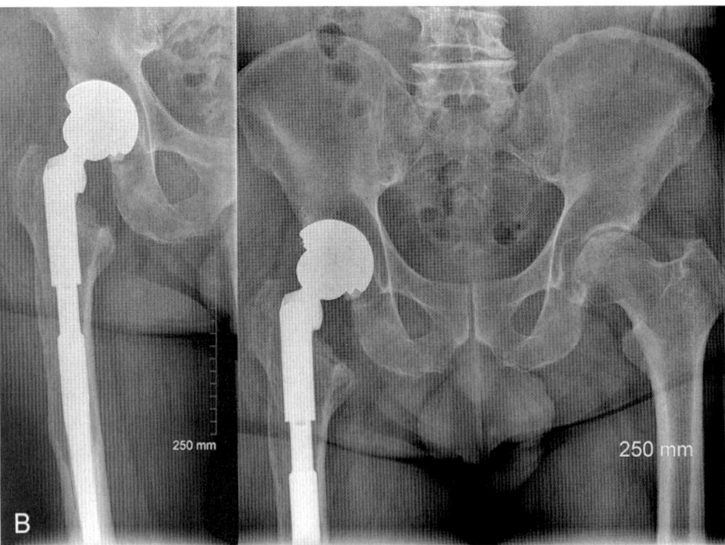

Figure 2 **A,** AP radiograph showing aseptic loosening of a right total hip replacement in a 73-year-old man. **B,** AP hip (left) and AP pelvic (right) radiographs showing revision to a modular femoral stem (Link, Hamburg, Germany) with a large-head metal-on-metal bearing (BFH, Wright Medical Technology), which was achieved by cementing the liner into the well-fixed existing cementless shell.

ysis. Long and associates[31] found good results at 5- to 11-year follow-up after 161 hip replacements using a Metasul hip implant (Zimmer, Warsaw, IN) with a 28-mm femoral head component. Six revision surgeries were needed, including one for aseptic loosening and one for instability. A focal radiolucency, identified as calcar resorption, was identified in nine patients. Saito and associates[32] reported excellent mid-term results at average 6.4-year follow-up after hip replacements using the Metasul implant. The survival rate was 99.1%, and no patients had osteolysis or loosening. Grübl and associates[33] reviewed the 10-year results of 105 hips with a second-generation metal-on-metal total hip replacement. The survival rate was 98.6%, and osteolysis was rarely reported. At a minimum 5-year follow-up, Migaud and associates[34] compared 39 patients treated with a metal-on-metal total hip replacement with a 28-mm femoral head component with 39 matched patients treated with a ceramic-on-polyethylene total hip replacement with a 28-mm femoral head component. The metal-on-metal hip implants fared better than the ceramic-on-polyethylene implants. Nine of the patients with a ceramic-on-polyethylene implant had osteolysis, and seven required revision; neither osteolysis nor revision was found in the patients with a metal-on-metal implant. The 5-year survival rate was 100% for the metal-on-metal implants and 97.2% for the ceramic-on-polyethylene implants.

Cuckler and associates[35] compared the results of using a 28-mm or 38-mm femoral head in metal-on-metal hip replacements. The dislocation rate was 2.5% with the 28-mm head; there were no dislocations with the 38-mm head. Peters and associates[36] found no dislocations in 136 patients with a 38-mm head, compared with a 2.5% rate (four dislocations) in 160 patients with a 28-mm head. The 38-mm heads were inserted using a posterior approach, and the 28-mm heads were inserted using a Hardinge approach. Subsequently, 469 metal-on-metal hip replacements with a 38-mm head were inserted using a posterior approach; only two dislocations occurred.

The use of large-head metal-on-metal hip implants reduces the likelihood of dislocation and therefore leads to fewer postoperative restrictions and a higher postoperative activity level.[35] This factor is especially relevant because returning to recreational activities is an important patient expectation after total hip replacement.[37] Improved activity levels after hip replacement are associated with higher patient satisfaction rates.[38,39] In high-activity patients, a metal-on-metal hip implant has the benefit of being able to withstand impact loading; no implant fractures have been recorded.

The use of metal-on-metal articulations has facilitated the reintroduction of hip resurfacing, with excellent short-term results.[40-42] On the acetabular side, the relatively thin wall of the metal cup and the lack of keyholes means that less bone stock is taken than with the first generation of cemented metal-on-polyethylene hip resurfacing sockets.[43] Although the rate of wear debris–induced failures after hip resurfacing has been significantly reduced with the introduction of metal-on-metal bearings, patient selection and proper surgical technique remain the key determinants of clinical success.[44]

Table 2
The Relationship Between Acetabular Cup Inclination and Metal Ion Concentration in Whole Blood

	Ion Concentration	
Cup Inclination	Cobalt	Chromium
More than 55° (steep)	9.8 μg/L (range, 0.6 to 111.3 μg/L)	9.7 μg/L (range, 0.6 to 94.6 μg/L)
55° or less	2.4 μg/L (range, 0.4 to 31.5 μg/L)	3.6 μg/L (range, 0.2 to 32.2 μg/L)

(Adapted with permission from De Haan R, Pattyn C, Gill HS, Murray DW, Campbell PA, De Smet KA: Correlation between inclination of the acetabular component and metal ion levels in metal-on-metal hip resurfacing replacement. *J Bone Joint Surg Br* 2008;90:1291-1297.)

Clinical Contraindications and Disadvantages

Metal Ion Release

Multiple clinical studies have documented an elevation in patients with a metal-on-metal implant of cobalt and chromium ions in blood, serum, erythrocytes, and urine, as well as an accumulation in the abdominal lymph nodes, liver, and spleen.[45-48] In a randomized, controlled comparison study of metal-on-metal and metal-on-polyethylene total hip replacements, MacDonald and associates[47] reported a 7.9-fold increase in erythrocyte cobalt and a 2.3-fold increase in erythrocyte chromium, as well as a 35-fold increase in urinary cobalt and a 17-fold increase in urinary chromium. Metal-on-metal implants have a biphasic wear pattern. The wear rates are highest during an initial bedding-in phase, with peak levels occurring 6 to 12 months after surgery. The wear rate steadily decreases during the subsequent 12 months to a continuing state of slow, steady wear; however, metal ion levels appear to remain elevated over time.[33] Increased ion concentration has been reported after exercise, but this finding is controversial; the concentration may be related to a decrease in urinary ion excretion rather than an increase in ion production during exercise.[49]

Most metal ions are excreted in the urine and therefore are of most concern in patients with impaired renal function.[50] The value of monitoring metal ion levels is unclear. Jacobs and associates[51] concluded that, although metal ion concentration may be routinely monitored in the future, presently it is primarily useful as a research tool. Nonetheless, assessment of ion levels can be used to identify a malfunctioning or malpositioned total hip replacement.[52] The importance of proper acetabular component orientation (a cup abduction angle of less than 50°) for wear properties and metal ion release was recently discussed[53-55] (Table 2). Langton and associates[53] looked at the influence of acetabular component abduction on metal ion levels, finding that smaller femoral head components (less than 51 mm) were associated with higher levels of metal ion release. It remains unclear how implant design (diametral clearance and inner bearing diameter) influences wear properties in relation to acetabular component position. The inner bearing surface design of monoblock acetabular shells is different from that of modular acetabular metal liners; for example, some monoblock acetabular shells are less than 180° (a hemisphere) and may be only 164°.[56] In addition, some acetabular components have a relatively thick central pole, which lateralizes the hip's center of rotation and decreases the overall surface area for bearing contact. These types of shell designs may have a narrower range of acceptable cup abduction and may be more susceptible to edge-loading wear because of the smaller area of surface contact[54,55] (Table 3). This factor is extremely important because substantial wear of metal-on-metal bearings is associated with significant soft tissue reactions.[57] De Haan and associates[55] recently reported that hip resurfacings with a cup placed at more than 55° of abduction had significantly higher cobalt and chromium ion levels (Table 2) and that smaller femoral component sizes were outliers in terms of ion release. Acetabular component designs with a lower arc of cover (164° compared with an average arc of cover of 170°) had significantly higher concentrations of cobalt and chromium ions when they were placed at more than 55° of abduction (Table 3).

Adverse Tissue Reaction

Metal-on-metal hip replacements may be associated with higher rates of malignancy secondary to metal ion release. However, a review of cancer incidence in all patients on the Finnish registry who underwent

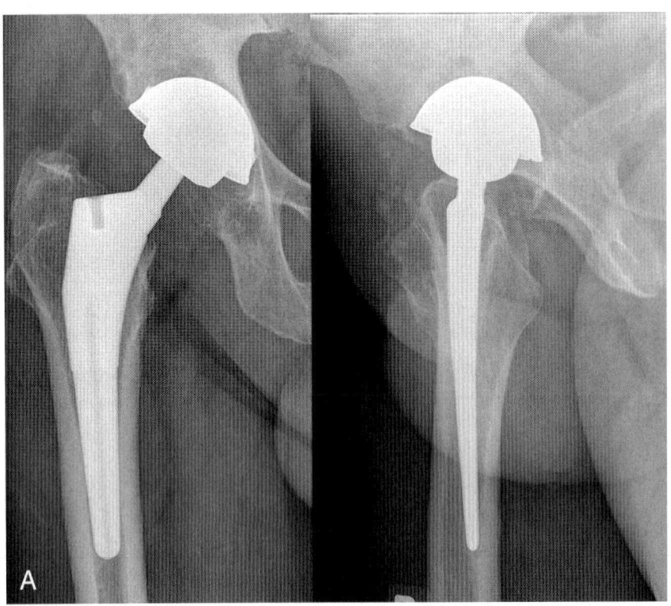

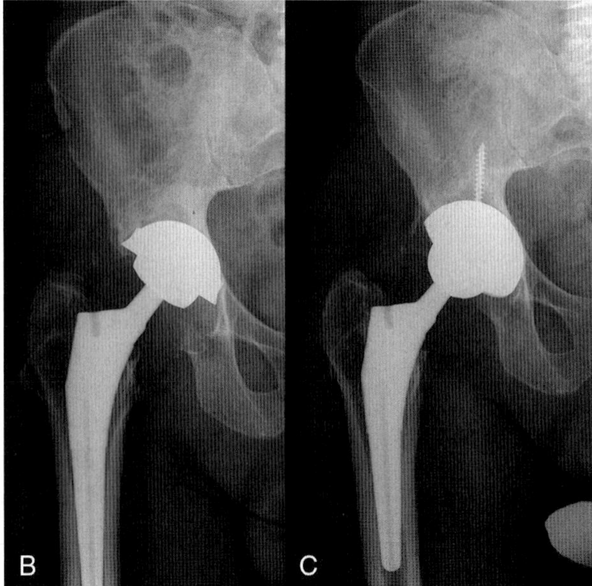

Figure 3 **A,** AP (left) and lateral (right) radiographs of the right hip in a 70-year-old man 14 months after a metal-on-metal total hip replacement and 6 months after the onset of thigh and groin pain. There is evidence of osteolysis at the dome of the acetabular component; the septic workup was negative. **B,** AP radiograph of the right hip (taken 6 months after the radiographs shown in part A) showing migration of the acetabular component. **C,** AP radiograph taken 1 year after isolated revision of the acetabular component with conversion to a metal-on-polyethylene bearing (Trabecular Metal Revision Shell with Longevity liner; Zimmer, Warsaw, IN).

Table 3
The Relationship Between Acetabular Arc of Cover With a Steep Cup Inclination (> 55°) and Metal Ion Concentration in Whole Blood

	Ion Concentration	
Arc of Cover	Cobalt	Chromium
164°	10.2 μg/L (range, 0.8 to 111.3 μg/L)	10.4 μg/L (range, 0.6 to 94.6 μg/L)
170°	2.1 μg/L (range, 0.6 to 6.4 μg/L)	3.0 μg/L (range, 0.9 to 7.6 μg/L)

(Adapted with permission from De Haan R, Pattyn C, Gill HS, Murray DW, Campbell PA, De Smet KA: Correlation between inclination of the acetabular component and metal ion levels in metal-on-metal hip resurfacing replacement. *J Bone Joint Surg Br* 2008;90:1291-1297.)

total hip replacement between 1980 and 1999 found no increased risk among those who had a metal-on-metal implant compared with the general population.[58] Although this study reported an increased incidence of prostate cancer and melanoma after hip arthroplasty, the current evidence does not confirm that the risk is increased. Large epidemiologic studies with longer follow-up periods and an adjustment for comorbidities are necessary to obtain an accurate estimate of the risk.[59] Chromosomal abnormalities (translocations and aneuploidy) were found to be increased in patients with metal-on-metal or metal-on-polyethylene bearings.[60,61]

Willert and associates[62] described an aseptic, lymphocyte-dominated, vasculitis-associated lesion that appears as persistent hip pain in patients with a metal-on-metal hip implant and in some patients is associated with osteolysis (Figure 3). The incidence of this hypersensitivity reaction was low (less than 0.3%), and it may have been linked to wear of the prosthesis. Although the overall volume of wear particles released from a metal-on-metal implant is less than the volume of polyethylene debris from a metal-on-polyethylene implant, the total number of particles released from a metal-on-metal implant may be greater.[63] Milosev and associates[64] found high levels of osteolysis in low carbon, metal-on-metal alloy articulations, and this clinical experience was confirmed by other studies of low carbon alloy implants.[65] In a retrieval analysis, Reinisch and associates[66] found higher wear rates in low carbon alloy implants, compared with high carbon alloy implants.

Pseudotumors were reported in 17 female patients with metal-on-metal hip resurfacing.[57] These patients had pain or a malfunctioning prosthesis at a mean of 17 months after surgery. A cystic mass was found in

8 of the 13 patients who underwent imaging studies. Fourteen of the 17 patients underwent further surgery; the cup abduction was found to be significantly higher in those with a soft-tissue mass. This study had several limitations—the severity of the soft-tissue reaction was not graded and cystic lesions and masses were not differentiated. Griffiths and associates[67] found that these types of masses, which they called granulomatous pseudotumors, also occurred in female patients with metal-on-polyethylene bearings, with similar destructive processes. Symptoms appeared more rapidly in patients with metal-on-metal bearings than in patients with metal-on-polyethylene bearings, but development of the pseudotumor was related to excessive particulate wear debris in all patients. Additional longitudinal research is required to determine the incidence of pseudotumors and whether they are limited to female patients or to patients with a smaller femoral component.

There has been concern about the use of metal-on-metal bearings in women of childbearing age because the effects of metal ions on a fetus are unknown. Although Brodner and associates[68] did not find that ions cross the placenta, a more recent study by Ziaee and associates,[69] using more sensitive measurement techniques, did find that ions cross the placenta. Because of the theoretic mutagenic and teratogenic risk, women are advised to delay metal-on-metal hip replacement until after childbearing or to delay childbearing for 1 to 2 years after receiving a metal-on-metal hip replacement.

Summary

Improvements in design and manufacturing as well as an improved understanding of in vivo biomechanics and wear have led to renewed interest in the use of metal-on-metal hip bearings. Metal-on-metal bearing surfaces offer several advantages over metal-on-polyethylene, ceramic-on-polyethylene, or ceramic-on-ceramic surfaces. Metal-on-metal bearings have very low wear rates, and osteolysis is infrequent. Metal on metal allows the use of a larger diameter femoral head; the result is a greater range of motion, increased stability, and resistance to fracture. Patients are less restricted and more satisfied. These advantages are important not only for young, high-demand patients but also for patients at risk of dislocation. In revision surgery, the use of a larger femoral head component reduces the risk of dislocation and can successfully treat instability. There are concerns about elevated levels of metal ions and their theoretic consequences, as well as the possibility of metal hypersensitivity; longer term studies are required to resolve the clinical implications of these concerns. With careful patient selection, attention to surgical technique, and vigilant clinical follow-up, metal-on-metal total joint arthroplasty can provide predictable results with excellent long-term survival rates.

References

1. McKee GK, Watson-Farrar J: Replacement of arthritic hips by the McKee-Farrar prosthesis. *J Bone Joint Surg Br* 1966;48:245-259.
2. McKee GK, Chen SC: The statistics of the McKee-Farrar method of total hip replacement. *Clin Orthop Relat Res* 1973;95:26-33.
3. Ring PA: Total replacement of the hip joint: A review of a thousand operations. *J Bone Joint Surg Br* 1974;56:44-58.
4. Amstutz HC, Grigoris P: Metal on metal bearings in hip arthroplasty. *Clin Orthop Relat Res* 1996;329:S11-S34.
5. Nevelos J, Shelton JC, Fisher J: Metallurgical considerations in the wear of metal-on-metal hip bearings. *Hip Int* 2004;14:1-10.
6. Rieker CB, Schön R, Konrad R, et al: Influence of the clearance on in-vitro tribology of large diameter metal-on-metal articulations pertaining to resurfacing hip implants. *Orthop Clin North Am* 2005;36:135-142.
7. Fisher J, Jin Z, Tipper J, Stone M, Ingham E: Tribology of alternative bearings. *Clin Orthop Relat Res* 2006;453:25-34.
8. Jacobsson SA, Djerf K, Wahlström O: Twenty-year results of McKee-Farrar versus Charnley prosthesis. *Clin Orthop Relat Res* 1996;139:S60-S68.
9. Dowson D: Tribological principles in metal-on-metal hip joint design. *Proc Inst Mech Eng H* 2006;220:161-171.
10. Rieker CB, Schön R, Köttig P: Development and validation of second-generation metal-on-metal bearing: Laboratory studies and analysis of retrievals. *J Arthroplasty* 2004;19:5-11.
11. Chan FW, Bobyn JD, Medley JB, Krygier JT, Tanzer M: Wear and lubrication of metal-on-metal hip implants. *Clin Orthop Relat Res* 1999;369:10-24.
12. Dowson D, Hardaker C, Flett M, Isaac GH: A hip joint simulator study of the performance of metal-on-metal joints: Part I. The role of materials. *J Arthroplasty* 2004;19:118-123.
13. Streicher RM, Semlitsch M, Schön R, Weber H, Rieker C: Metal-on-metal articulation for artificial hip joints: Laboratory study and clinical results. *Proc Inst Mech Eng H* 1996;210:223-232.
14. Varano R, Bobyn JD, Medley JB, Yue S: The effect of microstructure on the wear of cobalt-based alloys used in metal-on-metal hip implants. *Proc Inst Mech Eng H* 2006;220:145-159.
15. McKee GK: Development of total prosthetic replacement of the hip. *Clin Orthop Relat Res* 1970;72:85-103.
16. Wilson JN, Scales JT: Loosening of total hip replacements with cement

fixation: Clinical findings and laboratory studies. *Clin Orthop Relat Res* 1970;72:145-160.

17. McKellop H, Park S, Chiesa R, et al: In vivo wear of three types of metal on metal hip prostheses during two decades of use. *Clin Orthop Relat Res* 1996;329:S128-S140.
18. Medley JB: Tribology of bearing materials, in Amstutz HC, ed: *Hip Resurfacing: Principles, Indications, Technique and Results*. Philadelphia, PA, Elsevier, 2008, pp 33-44.
19. Schmalzried TP, Peters PC, Maurer BT, Bragdon CR, Harris WH: Long duration metal-on-metal total hip replacements with low wear of the articulating surfaces. *J Arthroplasty* 1996; 11:322-331.
20. Sieber HP, Rieker CB, Köttig P: Analysis of 118 second-generation metal-on-metal retrieved hip implants. *J Bone and Joint Surg Br* 1999; 81:46-50.
21. Berry DJ, von Knoch M, Schleck CD, Harmsen WS: Effect of femoral head diameter and operative approach on risk of dislocation after primary total hip arthroplasty. *J Bone Joint Surg Am* 2005;87:2456-2463.
22. Amstutz HC, Le Duff MJ, Beaulé PE: Prevention and treatment of dislocation after total hip replacement using large diameter balls. *Clin Orthop Relat Res* 2004;429:108-116.
23. Chandler DR, Glousman R, Hull D, et al: Prosthetic hip range of motion and impingement: The effects of head and neck geometry. *Clin Orthop Relat Res* 1982;166:284-291.
24. Alberton GM, High WA, Morrey BF: Dislocation after revision total hip arthroplasty: An analysis of risk factors and treatment options. *J Bone Joint Surg Am* 2002;84:1788-1792.
25. Phillips CB, Barrett JA, Losina E, et al: Incidence rates of dislocation, pulmonary embolism, and deep infection during the first six months after elective total hip replacement. *J Bone Joint Surg Am* 2003;85:20-26.
26. Mahomed NN, Barrett JA, Katz JN, et al: Rates and outcomes of primary and revision total hip replacement in the United States Medicare population. *J Bone Joint Surg Am* 2003;85: 27-32.
27. Beaulé PE, Schmalzried TP, Udomkiat P, Amstutz HC: Jumbo femoral head for the treatment of recurrent dislocation following total hip replacement. *J Bone Joint Surg Am* 2002; 84:256-263.
28. Halley D, Glassman AH, Crowninshield RD: Recurrent dislocation after revision total hip replacement with a large prosthetic femoral head: A case report. *J Bone Joint Surg Am* 2004;86:827-830.
29. Ebramzadeh E, Beaulé PE, Culwell JL, Amstutz HC: Fixation strength of an all-metal acetabular component cemented into an acetabular shell: A biomechanical analysis. *J Arthroplasty* 2004;19:45-49.
30. Beaulé PE, Ebramzadeh E, LeDuff MJ, Prasad R, Amstutz HC: Cementing a liner into a stable cementless acetabular shell in revision hip surgery: The double-socket technique. *J Bone Joint Surg Am* 2004;86:929-934.
31. Long WT, Dorr LD, Gendelman V: An American experience with metal-on-metal total hip arthroplasties: A 7-year follow-up study. *J Arthroplasty* 2004;19:29-34.
32. Saito S, Ryu J, Watanabe T, Ishii K, Saigo K: Midterm results of Metasul metal-on-metal total hip arthroplasty. *J Arthroplasty* 2006;21:1105-1110.
33. Grübl A, Marker M, Brodner W, et al: Long-term follow-up of metal-on-metal total hip replacement. *J Orthop Res* 2007;25:841-848.
34. Migaud H, Jobin A, Chantelot C, Giraud F, Laffargue P, Duquennoy A: Cementless metal-on-metal hip arthroplasty in patients less than 50 years of age: Comparison with a matched control group using ceramic-on-polyethylene after a minimum 5-year follow-up. *J Arthroplasty* 2004;19:23-28.
35. Cuckler JM, Moore KD, Lombardi AV Jr, McPherson E, Emerson R: Large versus small femoral heads in metal-on-metal total hip arthroplasty. *J Arthroplasty* 2004;19:41-44.
36. Peters CL, McPherson E, Jackson JD, Erickson JA: Reduction in early dislocation rate with large-diameter femoral heads in primary total hip arthroplasty. *J Arthroplasty* 2007;22:140-144.
37. Wright JG, Rudicel S, Feinstein AR: Ask patients what they want: Evaluation of individual complaints before total hip replacement. *J Bone Joint Surg Br* 1994;76:229-234.
38. Lieberman JR, Dorey FJ, Shekelle P, et al: Outcome after total hip arthroplasty: Comparison of a traditional disease-specific and a quality-of-life measurement of outcome. *J Arthroplasty* 1997;12:639-645.
39. Beaulé PE, Dorey FJ, Hoke R, Le Duff MJ, Amstutz HC: The value of patient activity level in clinical outcome of total hip arthroplasty. *J Arthroplasty* 2006;21:547-552.
40. Amstutz HC, Beaulé PE, Dorey FJ, Le Duff MJ, Campbell PA, Gruen TA: Metal-on-metal hybrid surface arthroplasty: Two to six-year follow-up. *J Bone Joint Surg Am* 2004;86: 28-39.
41. Daniel J, Pynsent PB, McMinn DJ: Metal-on-metal resurfacing of the hip in patients under the age of 55 years with osteoarthritis. *J Bone Joint Surg Br* 2004;86:177-184.
42. Treacy RB, McBryde CW, Pynsent PB: Birmingham hip resurfacing arthroplasty: A minimum follow-up of five years. *J Bone Joint Surg Br* 2005;87: 167-170.
43. Vendittoli PA, Lavigne M, Girard J, Roy AG: A randomised study comparing resection of acetabular bone at resurfacing and total hip replacement. *J Bone Joint Surg Br* 2006;88:997-1002.
44. Beaulé PE: Surface arthroplasty of the hip: A review and current indications. *Semin Arthroplasty* 2005;16:70-76.
45. Brodner W, Bitzan P, Meisinger V, Kaider A, Gottsauner-Wolf F, Kotz R: Serum cobalt levels after metal-on-metal total hip arthroplasty. *J Bone Joint Surg Am* 2003;85:2168-2173.

46. Schaffer AW, Pilger A, Engelhardt C, Zweymuller K, Ruediger HW: Increased blood cobalt and chromium after total hip replacement. *J Toxicol Clin Toxicol* 1999;37:839-844.

47. MacDonald SJ, McCalden RW, Chess DG, et al: Metal-on-metal versus polyethylene in hip arthroplasty: A randomized clinical trial. *Clin Orthop Relat Res* 2003;406:282-296.

48. Urban RM, Tomlinson MJ, Hall DJ, Jacobs JJ: Accumulation in liver and spleen of metal particles generated at nonbearing surfaces in hip arthroplasty. *J Arthroplasty* 2004;19:94-101.

49. Bitsch RG, Zamorano M, Loidolt T, Heisel C, Jacobs JJ, Schmalzreid TP: Ion production and excretion in a patient with a metal-on-metal bearing hip prosthesis: A case report. *J Bone Joint Surg Am* 2007;89:2758-2763.

50. Brodner W, Grohs JG, Bitzan P, Meisinger V, Kovarik J, Kotz R: Serum cobalt and serum chromium level in 2 patients with chronic renal failure after total hip prosthesis implantation with metal-metal gliding contact. *Z Orthop Ihre Grenzgeb* 2000; 138:425-429.

51. Jacobs JJ, Skipor AK, Campbell PA, Hallab NJ, Urban RM, Amstutz HC: Can metal levels be used to monitor metal-on-metal hip arthroplasties? *J Arthroplasty* 2004;19:59-65.

52. Brodner W, Grübl A, Jankovsky R, Meisinger V, Lehr S, Gottsauner-Wolf F: Cup inclination and serum concentration of cobalt and chromium after metal-on-metal total hip arthroplasty. *J Arthroplasty* 2004;19: 66-70.

53. Langton DJ, Jameson SS, Joyce TJ, Webb J, Nargol AV: The effect of component size and orientation on the concentrations of metal ions after resurfacing arthroplasty of the hip. *J Bone Joint Surg Br* 2008;90:1143-1151.

54. Williams S, Leslie I, Isaac G, Jin Z, Ingham E, Fisher J: Tribology and wear of metal-on-metal hip prostheses: Influence of cup angle and head position. *J Bone Joint Surg Am* 2008;90: 111-117.

55. De Haan R, Pattyn C, Gill HS, Murray DW, Campbell PA, De Smet KA: Correlation between inclination of the acetabular component and metal ion levels in metal-on-metal hip resurfacing replacement. *J Bone Joint Surg Br* 2008;90:1291-1297.

56. Shimmin A, Beaulé PE, Campbell P: Metal-on-metal hip resurfacing arthroplasty. *J Bone Joint Surg Am* 2008; 90:637-654.

57. Pandit H, Glyn-Jones S, McLardy-Smith P, et al: Pseudotumors associated with metal-on-metal hip resurfacings. *J Bone Joint Surg Br* 2008;90: 847-851.

58. Visuri TI, Pukkala E, Pulkkinen P, Paavolainen P: Cancer incidence and causes of death among total hip replacement patients: A review based on Nordic cohorts with a special emphasis on metal-on-metal bearings. *Proc Inst Mech Mech Eng H* 2006;220: 399-407.

59. Tharani R, Dorey FJ, Schmalzreid TP: The risk of cancer following total hip or knee arthroplasty. *J Bone Joint Surg Am* 2001;83:774-780.

60. Ladon D, Doherty A, Newson R, Turner J, Bhamra M, Case CP: Changes in metal levels and chromosome aberrations in the peripheral blood of patients after metal-on-metal hip arthroplasty. *J Arthroplasty* 2004;19:78-83.

61. Daley B, Doherty AT, Fairman B, Case CP: Wear debris from hip or knee replacements causes chromosomal damage in human cells in tissue culture. *J Bone Joint Surg* 2004;86: 598-606.

62. Willert HG, Buchorn G, Fayaayazi A, Lohmann C: Histopathological changes around metal/metal joints indicate delayed type hypersensitivity: Preliminary results of 14 cases. *Osteologie* 2000;9:2.

63. Campbell P, Shen FW, McKellop H: Biologic and tribologic considerations of alternative bearing surfaces. *Clin Orthop Relat Res* 2004;418:98-111.

64. Milosev I, Trebse R, Kovac S, Cör A, Pisot V: Survivorship and retrieval analysis of Sikomet metal-on-metal total hip replacements at a mean of seven years. *J Bone Joint Surg Am* 2006; 88:1173-1182.

65. Park YS, Moon YW, Lim SL, Yang YM, Ahn G, Choi YL: Early osteolysis following second-generation metal-on-metal hip replacement. *J Bone Joint Surg Am* 2005;87:1515-1521.

66. Reinisch G, Judmann KP, Lhotke C, Lintner F, Zweymüller KA: Retrieval study of uncemented metal-metal hip prostheses revised for early loosening. *Biomaterials* 2003;24:1081-1091.

67. Griffiths HJ, Burke J, Bonfiglio TA: Granulomatous pseudotumors in total joint replacement. *Skeletal Radiol* 1987;16:146-152.

68. Brodner W, Grohs JG, Bancher-Todesca D, et al: Does the placenta inhibit the passage of chromium and cobalt after metal-on-metal total hip arthroplasty? *J Arthroplasty* 2004;19: 102-106.

69. Ziaee H, Daniel J, Datta AK, Blunt S, McMinn DJ: Transplacental transfer of cobalt and chromium in patients with metal-on-metal hip arthroplasty: A controlled study. *J Bone Joint Surg Br* 2007;89:301-305.

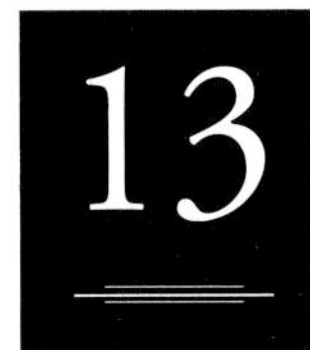

The Evolution and Modern Use of Metal-on-Metal Bearings in Total Hip Arthroplasty

Mark H. Gonzalez, MD, MEng
Ryan Carr, MD
Sharon Walton, MD
William M. Mihalko, MD, PhD

Abstract

Metal-on-metal bearings have been used in total hip arthroplasty for decades. Because younger patients with higher physical demands are now being treated with hip arthroplasty, the popularity and use of metal-on-metal bearings has increased over the past 10 years. New concerns, however, have emerged regarding the percentage of patients with a hypersensitivity reaction or pseudotumor formation after arthroplasty with these bearings. These concerns have raised questions concerning long-term outcomes for patients treated with metal-on-metal bearings. It is important for orthopaedic surgeons to review these issues so that better educated decisions can be made in treating their patients.

First-generation metal-on-metal hip implants were introduced in the late 1930s. Despite long-term survival, many implants showed significant radiographic loosening.[1] Poor manufacturing techniques, crude designs, and the lack of adequate fixation were some of the problems encountered with the early designs.[1-4] Additional concerns over metal sensitivity and the early success of the metal-on-polyethylene Charnley prosthesis eventually led to a decline in the use of metal-on-metal hip implants.[2] In 1984, there was renewed interest in the metal-on-metal hip prosthesis because of evolving evidence of very low volumetric wear rates and a lack of periprosthetic inflammatory changes, unlike those seen in the polyethylene designs. The growing interest in metal-on-metal bearings used in implants for total hip arthroplasty (THA) has heightened concerns over the effects of the metal ions released from the degradation of these implants. This fact, coupled with recent Australian and US experience of increased revision rates with the ASR Hip System (DePuy, Warsaw, IN; device recently recalled in the United States) and the British medical alert concerning hip resurfacing devices has made surgeons aware of the possible reaction to particulate metal debris that patients may experience and that may increase the risk for an early revision.[5,6] Monitoring recommendations from the British medical device alert for patients with metal-on-metal bearings are summarized in **Table 1**.[5] This chapter will discuss the literature regarding the local and systemic effects of metal-on-metal implants as well as hypersensitivity and carcinogenic effects.

Dr. Gonzalez or an immediate family member has received royalties from Johnson & Johnson; serves as a paid consultant to or is an employee of Smith & Nephew and owns stock or stock options in Ortho Sensing Technology. Dr. Mihalko or an immediate family member has received royalties from Aesculap/B. Braun; is a member of a speakers' bureau or has made paid presentations on behalf of Aesculap/B. Braun; serves as a paid consultant to or is an employee of Aesculap/B. Braun; has received research or institutional support from Aesculap/B. Braun, Smith & Nephew, Stryker, and Corin USA; and has received nonincome support (such as equipment or services), commercially derived honoraria, nor other non–research-related funding (such as paid travel) from Aesculap/B. Braun. Neither of the following authors or any immediate family member has received anything of value from or owns stock in a commercial company or institution related directly or indirectly to the subject of this chapter: Dr. Carr and Dr. Walton.

Table 1
Monitoring Recommendation From the British Medical Device Alert for Patients With Metal-on-Metal Bearings

Patient follow-up should be done at least annually for 5 years postoperatively and more frequently in the presence of symptoms. Beyond 5 years, follow up in accordance with locally agreed protocols.

Evaluate patients with painful metal-on-metal hip replacements. Specific tests should include an evaluation of cobalt and chromium ion levels in the patient's blood and cross-sectional imaging, including MRI or ultrasound scanning.

Consider measuring cobalt and chromium ion levels in the blood and/or cross-sectional imaging for the following patient groups:
- Patients with radiologic features associated with adverse outcomes, including component position
- Patients with small component size (hip resurfacing arthroplasty only)
- If the patient or surgeon is concerned about a metal-on-metal hip replacement
- Cohorts of patients in which there is concern about higher than expected rates of failure

If either cobalt or chromium ion levels are elevated above seven parts per billion, a second test should be performed 3 months after the first to identify patients who require closer surveillance, which may include cross-sectional imaging.

If imaging shows soft-tissue reactions, fluid collections, or tissue masses, revision surgery should be considered

Wear Characteristics of Metal, Polyethylene, and Ceramic Prostheses

An analysis of second-generation metal-on-metal hip prostheses showed a biphasic wear distribution comparable to first-generation prostheses. The initial volumetric run-in wear rate is threefold to fivefold that of the steady-state wear rate.[4] This is believed to result from the opposing surface asperities that are polished away during initial use. Steady-state wear is believed to occur after one million cycles (mc) and produces a volumetric wear rate of 0.43 mm^3/y (range, 0.02 to 1.63 mm^3/y) for the low carbon Sikomet prosthesis (Endoprothetik AG, Modling, Austria) and 1.0 ± 1.64 mm^3/mc for the high carbon Metasul prosthesis (Zimmer, Warsaw, IN).[7,8] Particle analysis demonstrates mean particle size in the range of 25 to 36 nm and generates 4×10^{12} to 6×10^{13} particles per million cycles as shown in high and low carbon pairings.[9]

This pattern differs from polyethylene prostheses that produce a monophasic wear pattern and a volumetric wear rate of 16.6 ± 0.4 mm^3/mc to 20.0 ± 2.6 mm^3/mc.[10] Particle analysis showed particles in the range of 0.1 to 10 μm and generation of 5×10^{11} particles per million cycles.[9] Polyethylene prostheses produce larger particles and greater volumetric wear than metallic prostheses.

Ceramic prostheses also have a monophasic wear pattern. The volumetric wear rates are 0.05 to 1.6 mm^3/mc.[11,12] Particle analysis demonstrates mean particle size of 0.39 μm (range, 0.13 to 78.4 μm).[3] Ceramic prostheses produce lower volumetric wear rates compared to metallic and polyethylene prostheses.

Volumetric wear is now understood to comprise tribology (the science related to the mechanisms of friction, lubrication, and wear of surfaces that are in relative motion with each other), as well as the composition of the prostheses. Low carbon pairings of a femoral head and an acetabular cup were shown to have significantly higher bedding-in and steady-state wear rates than mixed and high carbon pairings.[9] Mixed evidence also has led to the belief that larger femoral heads (of approximately 36 mm) produce fluid film lubrication conditions that allow more of the load to be carried by the fluid film as opposed to asperity contact seen in smaller femoral heads and in those with mixed lubrication conditions. Lubrication films within the bearing are important because the thicker the film, the lower the number of wear particles produced by the bearing. Analysis showed that 16- and 22.25-mm femoral heads produce no surface separation, and volumetric wear rates of 4.85 mm^3/mc and 6.3 mm^3/mc, respectively.[13] Larger femoral heads of 28 mm and 36 mm produce mixed and fluid film lubrications and volumetric wear rates of 0.54 mm^3/mc and 0.07mm^3/mc, respectively.[13]

Clearance is also clinically significant. The clearance of a bearing relates to the difference between the convex and concave curvatures of the opposite sides of the bearing. In the metal-on-metal hip, if the ball is slightly smaller (for example, 30 μm), then the bearing allows fluid film to form and decreases bearing wear. Evidence reveals that an increase in clearance results in greater volumetric wear,[14] whereas a decrease in clearance results in increased fluid film thickness and decreased contact pressure. However, there is a fine balance between having a low clearance, which optimizes the fluid film condition, and a clearance that is too low and increases the contact pressure. Critically low clearance rates cause concern for the reemergence of locking, increased friction, and increased wear rates.[15] Equatorial contact resulting from decreased clearance has shown greater wear rates and a higher release of particulate debris.

Metal-on-Polyethylene Versus Metal-on-Metal

It is now widely accepted that the larger polyethylene particles seen in metal-on-polyethylene bearing surfaces stimulate the activation of multinucleated giant cells, causing bone reabsorption and aseptic loosening. An examination of tissue adjacent to the prostheses during revisions has revealed inflamed periarticular tissue.[16] Histologic examination of the joint capsule showed polyethylene particles within macrophages.[16] Aseptic loosening is now understood to result from a biologically induced reaction stimulated by polyethylene particles. Twenty-year survival rates in metal-on-polyethylene THA prostheses with no reoperation were 81.3%, and 89.4% with no component removal or revision for aseptic loosening; however, implant survivorship has been reported as low as 73%.[17] Because of the high incidence of aseptic failure, alternate materials (including metal-on-metal prostheses) are being studied.

Although metallic particles seen in metal-on-metal hip prostheses did not produce the aseptic loosening response of polyethylene particles, there is convincing evidence that the greater number of metallic particles stimulates an immunologic reaction similar to type IV hypersensitivity,[8] which is discussed in greater detail later in this chapter. Histologic examination reveals diffuse and perivascular lymphocytic aggregates in the presence of moderate metallic wear debris.[8] Further evaluation shows persistently high levels of chromium and cobalt in serum and urine. The deleterious effects of metallic particles on levels of CD4 and CD8 T lymphocytes also have been reported.[18] Although the clinical significance has not yet been determined, there are concerns regarding the carcinogenic and mutagenic effects of metal particles. Despite a lower incidence of osteolysis in metal-on-metal THAs, aseptic loosening remained the dominant feature at the time of revision.[8]

Nickel, cobalt, and chromium are the most common metal allergens. Currently, it is unclear if early osteolysis seen in metal-on-metal hip implants is caused by preexisting metal sensitivity or if patients later develop sensitivity as a result of the failed THA and exposure to a large amount of particulate metal debris. In a study by Park et al,[19] 165 patients treated with metal-on-metal hip implants were evaluated. Within 24 months of surgery, nine patients had radiographic evidence of osteolysis. Skin-patch testing determined that eight of the nine patients had a higher sensitivity to cobalt chloride in comparison with a control group. The authors concluded that patients who had radiographic findings of osteolysis had significantly higher rates of sensitivity to metals in comparison to control groups.[19] Willert et al[20] evaluated the first 19 consecutive revisions of metal-on-metal hip implants performed at a single institution for patients with hip pain and osteolysis. At 1- to 7-year follow-ups, three of five patients treated with revision to a metal-on-metal hip prosthesis had persistent pain in the hip and thigh. The 14 patients treated with revision to alumina-on-polyethylene or metal-on-polyethylene prostheses had symptom relief. It was believed that the patients treated with revision to metal-on-metal hip implants had become sensitized to the metal particles, and an immunologic reaction led to the persistent painful symptoms.[20] However, the overall incidence of tissue reaction to metal-on-metal hip implants remains low. Engh et al[21] evaluated 828 patients (945 hips) treated with large head (36 mm) metal-on-metal hip prostheses and determined that 3 patients had a local tissue reaction that was likely attributed to the metal-on-metal implant (0.3%). The authors continued to use metal-on-metal implants but considered a sensitivity reaction to the metal as a possible factor in all failed implants.[21]

The incidence of hypersensitivity is markedly increased in metal-on-metal hip prostheses compared with metal-on-polyethylene prostheses. Although metallic ions induce an immunologic reaction, it is not clear if this response contributes to the development of osteolysis.

A recent analysis of surface engineered metal-on-metal prostheses containing titanium niobium, chromium nitrogen, chromium-carbon-nitrogen, and diamond-like carbon produced a volumetric wear rate 36 times lower and a metallic ion concentration rate 20 times lower than traditional metal-on-metal prostheses.[22] In prosthetic designs using metals, the possibility remains for producing extremely low volumetric wear rates and low metallic ion concentrations, which has the potential to reduce the incidence of hypersensitivity, minimize osteolysis, and prolong prostheses survival rates.

Metal-on-metal implants remain a viable alternative, especially in younger and more active patients in whom implant longevity is an issue, although the problem of hypersensitivity must be considered. An alternative to traditional THA is hip resurfacing with metal-on-metal designs, but this approach has recently been questioned by the British National Health Service.[6]

Hip Resurfacing

Several different metal-on-metal hip resurfacing designs exist, including the Conserve Plus (Wright Medical Technology, Arlington, TN), the McMinn prosthesis (Corin Medical, Cirencester, England), the Cormet (Corin, Tampa, FL), and the Birmingham (Smith & Nephew, Memphis, TN). Each design consists of a high carbon chromium-cobalt alloy with a press-fit acetabular cup and cemented femoral stem. The differences among the prostheses result from the manufacturing process of the alloy. Wrought alloy is harder than cast alloy and can be highly polished, thus producing more wear resistance and decreased surface roughness compared with cast alloy.[23] Additional processing can include postcast heat treatments, such as solution heat treatment or hot isostatic processing. This process can cause depletion of surface carbides, which are a mix of carbon and the surrounding metal.[23] These carbides are significantly harder than the surrounding metal and provide a higher resistance to wear. Although processing was originally believed to produce different wear characteristics, recent analysis has not shown a significant difference.[24,25] Instead, wear is considered to be a function of radial clearance, lubrication conditions, carbon content, and surface roughness.[23,26]

McKellop et al[27] reported similar wear rates between hip resurfacing and THA. The development of pseudotumors is a unique characteristic of the metallic wear particles in hip resurfacing.[28] Although the etiology of pseudotumors is likely multifactorial, it is believed that toxic levels of metallic ions contribute to their development.[28] Among 1,300 metal-on-metal hip resurfacing prostheses, 12 were found to contain a soft-tissue mass.[28] Histologic examination showed metallic wear particles within necrotic connective tissue surrounded by macrophages and lymphocytes.[28] Although rare occurrences of cysts with lymphocytic infiltration have been seen in THA, this response is considered to be more extensive and suggestive of a new complication unique to hip resurfacing. The predilection to women is not well understood but may suggest a prior sensitivity to metallic ions.[28] Recently, reports have linked smaller size femoral heads with a higher likelihood of metal reactivity about these implants.[29] The smaller femoral head seems to be susceptible to higher wear rates because of the smaller contact area in an acetabular component that is aligned with greater inclination and or anterversion.[29,30] The higher wear rate of a smaller femoral head needs to be considered when an orthopaedic surgeon is weighing the pros and cons of a metal-on-metal bearing. If templating suggests the need for small head and acetabular component sizes, then hard-on-hard bearings, such as ceramic bearings, should be considered.

Radiographic analysis of resurfaced hips has shown a 77% incidence of femoral neck narrowing.[31] Hing et al[31] identified narrowing greater than 10% in 28% of patients, although there has been no indication that this finding is of clinical significance.[32] The etiology of femoral neck narrowing is largely unknown but may be related to stress shielding or a decreased blood supply to the femoral head and neck, as seen in the posterior approach to hip resurfacing.

Femoral neck fracture is identified as the most common and significant complication associated with hip resurfacing, with an overall incidence ranging from 1.46% to 7.2%. A learning curve for surgeons is also related to the hip resurfacing procedure.[32-35] In a study by Shimmin and Back,[32] femoral neck notching and varus placement of more than 5° was seen in 46.6% and 71.1% of patients, respectively. No case of femoral neck fracture was identified in prostheses placed in valgus position in relationship to the preoperative neck-shaft angle;[32] however, prostheses placed in excessive valgus position were associated with notching along the superior lateral border of the femoral neck.[34] Marker et al[33] reported that 12 of 14 femoral neck fractures (86%) occurred in the first 69 hip resurfacing procedures performed by a single surgeon, after which time the incidence decreased to 0.4%, thereby suggesting a learning curve. However, Shimmin and Back[32] did not find any association between the surgeon's experience and the incidence of femoral neck fractures. To help identify patients at risk for this complication, Beaulé and Antoniades[26] developed the surface arthroplasty risk index. Evidence shows that resurfaced hips with higher surface arthroplasty risk index numbers were more likely to fail. When surgeons implemented stricter patient selection criteria (body mass index < 35, no osteopenia, no femoral cysts > 1 cm), the overall complication rate decreased from 13.4% to 2.1%, and femoral neck fractures decreased from 7.2% to 0.8%.[35]

Early analyses of hip resurfacing procedures seemed to indicate higher rates of revision among females when compared with males. This difference is now attributed to the smaller femoral heads used in female patients and the decreased area of contact that can result from excessive inclination and/or anteversion of the acetabulum.[29,30,36] McBryde et al[36] reported a similar risk of revision in both sexes when the same size component was used. It was concluded that revision rates were more significantly related to femoral head size than to sex.

Resurfacing Versus Total Hip Arthroplasty

Although THA has traditionally produced excellent results in older patients, significantly higher failure rates have occurred in younger patients.[37-39] Although the transition to cementless prostheses did not show any early significant differences in implant survival rates compared with cemented prostheses, a recent analysis by Lombardi et al[40] showed excellent long-term survival rates for uncemented proximal porous-coated titanium tapered stems. Kaplan-Meier analysis showed a 95.5% cumulative survival rate for any stem revision at 20 years.[40] Although uncemented prostheses have excellent long-term survival rates, hip resurfacing helps maintain bone stock and offers a relatively easy transition to THA. Recent studies indicate similar survival rates in patients younger than 55 years treated with hip resurfacing compared with THA.[41] The larger femoral heads used in hip resurfacing are believed to provide greater stability, fewer dislocations, and greater range of motion. Proponents also believe that hip resurfacing produces a more physiologic load transfer than stemmed prostheses, thereby minimizing stress shielding, bone remodeling, and bone loss.[42] Although some surgeons believe this load transfer enables patients to resume higher levels of activity, gait studies do not indicate superiority. Gait characteristics between patients treated with hip resurfacing and large femoral head THAs were not found to be statistically different; however, Lavigne et al[43] reported significant differences in gait characteristics in patients treated with THAs with smaller femoral heads. Although hip resurfacing offers several advantages to THA, hip resurfacing remains more technically challenging. For this reason, some orthopaedic surgeons believe that hip resurfacing should not replace THA but should serve as a viable alternative.

Wear Particle Consideration in Metal-on-Metal Prostheses

Local Toxicity

Tissue samples obtained from hips with metal-on-metal prostheses were markedly more ulcerated than those obtained from hips with metal-on-polyethylene implants, particularly in the area adjacent to areas of perivascular lymphocytic infiltration.[44] This type of reaction is consistent with an aseptic lymphocytic vasculitis-associated lesion (type IV hypersensitivity reaction) because there was no histologic evidence of acute infection.[44,45] The characteristic histologic features of tissue from patients with metal-on-metal implants were perivascular infiltrates of T and B lymphocytes, plasma cells, high endothelial venules, massive fibrin exudation, the accumulation of macrophages, and infiltrates of eosinophilic granulocytes and necrosis. There was no such immune response in the tissues of patients with nonmetal implants.[44]

Mikhael et al[45] described two patients with metal-on-metal implant failure who presented with signs that mimicked a hip infection. The etiology of symptoms differed between the two patients. The first patient had a local hypersensitivity type IV reaction to the metal-on-metal implant. Previously reported clinical presentations have included pain within 10 months to 5 years following THA surgery or early radiographic signs of loosening. In this study, the patient also had constitutional symptoms and elevated serum levels of inflammatory biomarkers. Tissue specimens from the patient showed perivascular lymphocytic infiltrates and was positive for B and T lymphocytes, similar to the results in studies by Hallab et al[46,47] involving human lymphocytes and metal alloy degradation. The second patient had a mismatch between the sizes of the femoral head and the acetabular socket that led to a rapid increase in the production of local metal debris and tissue hyperreactivity to the metal. In contrast to the chronic inflammation identified in the first patient, the samples from the second patient revealed acellular necrotic tissue. The large amount of metal debris caused an inflammatory reaction leading to elevated inflammatory markers, which were probably exacerbated by some form of metal hypersensitivity. The inappropriate pairing of the acetabular and femoral components also may have caused elevated inflammatory markers. Both patients had complete resolution of symptoms following exchange of the metal liner for a polyethylene component.[45]

Systemic Toxicity

Multiple studies have shown elevated metal ions in the serum and urine of patients with metal-on-metal implants (particularly in those with long-term implants).[48-51] In a 4-year prospective study assessing serum levels of metal ions in patients with THAs, cobalt levels were shown to steadily decrease over a 4-year period compared with chromium levels.[52] Furthermore, metal-on-metal bearings with a large diameter resulted in a greater systemic exposure of metal ions than bearings with a small diameter.[53]

The number of chromosomal aberrations found in patients with metal-on-metal bearings was greater than those in a control group. Structural aberrations were not seen in the control group, and this difference was highly significant ($P = 0.003$).[54] Also, the number of chromosomal aberrations in the metal-on-metal group was greater than in patients who had revision surgery from metal-on-metal to metal-on-polyethylene implants.[54,55] The clinical consequences of the chromosomal changes seen in this study are unknown, and it is unknown if the changes are present in other cells in the body. Decreased levels of CD8(+) T cells and an increase in the number of debris particles in the liver and spleen were found in patients with metal-on-metal THAs compared with a control group.[56,57] In one rare instance, granulomas had formed in the liver, spleen, and abdominal lymph nodes in response to the heavy accumulation of wear debris from a hip prosthesis.[57] Cobalt and chromium have also been shown to cross the placenta in women with metal-on-metal THAs.[58] Although the pathologic importance of these results have not been elucidated, they emphasize the need for additional investigations into the effect of chronic exposure to elevated levels of metal ions produced by orthopaedic implants.

Hypersensitivity Responses

Components of metal alloys, such as benzoyl peroxide, have been shown to be potential allergens in patients treated with THAs.[45] It is clear that some patients have excessive immune reactions directly associated with implanted metallic materials leading to an aseptic lymphocytic vasculitis-associated lesion.[44,45] However, these reactions are rare, with reported estimated prevalences of 1% to 2% and up to 5% for certain alloys such as cobalt and chromium.[59] In one study, blood samples were taken from patients with no known prior metal allergies or exposures having a primary THA. Repeat blood samples were taken 3 months to 1 year later. Sensitivity to at least one of the antigens developed in 32% of the patients, but a severe reaction developed in only 5%.[59] In a histologic analysis of patients with metal-on-metal THAs at a mean follow-up of 77 months postoperatively, it was concluded that periprosthetic osteolysis and aseptic loosening in the hips were possibly associated with hypersensitivity to metal debris.[20] The lymphocyte response to serum protein complexed with metal from implant degradation was investigated using human lymphocytes from healthy volunteers. Even in healthy patients, there is a lymphocyte proliferative response to both cobalt-chromium-molybdenum and titanium alloy metalloprotein degradation products. Histologic samples were taken from patients who had hip revision surgery with ceramic, metal-on-polyethylene, or metal-on-metal implants. The induction of T cell activation by metal particles suggests that lymphocytes may contribute to the inflammation that mediates osteolysis in patients with particle debris.[60]

Carcinogenic Effects

Animal studies have documented the carcinogenic potential of orthopaedic implant materials. Small increases in rat sarcoma rates were correlated with metal implants; however, lymphomas were more common in rats with metallic implants.[61] The occurrence of tumor-like reactions at the site of metallic implants in humans also has been reported.[62] The most common lesion was a malignant fibrous histiocytoma.[63] Slight increases in the risk of lymphoma and leukemia were observed in patients with metal-on-metal THAs.[64] In contrast, studies have shown a decreased incidence of certain tumors, including breast carcinoma, sarcoma, and stomach cancer in patients with metal-on-metal THAs. In a 1988 Swedish study of 154 patients treated with THA and followed for 20 years, the overall relative risk of cancer increased by 3%, with most cancers originating from connective tissue.[64] A 1996 Finnish study evaluated the incidence of cancer in patients with metal-on-metal THAs compared with patients with polyethylene implants. There was a 4% and 4.5% increase in the incidence of cancer in the metal-on-metal and polyethylene groups, respectively. Also, there was a threefold to fourfold risk for tumors of the lymphatic and hematopoietic systems after THA compared with a control group.[65] Neither study separated patients with degenerative and inflammatory joint disease, suggesting that there could be factors other than THA that play a major role in the origin of cancer.

Practice Recommendations

This chapter's authors avoid the use of metal-on-metal endbearing hip replacements in patients requiring a cup size smaller than 50 to 52 mm. A full radius (180°) cup should be used with high carbon content. Surgical technique is paramount, especially in properly placing the acetabular cup. Excessive anteversion or lateral opening can produce end loading and increased metallic wear.

Patients are followed with an examination and radiographic evaluation every 12 months. Patients with pain or radiologic signs of early implant failure are evaluated for cobalt-chromium ion levels and with MRI. Patients with elevated ion levels alone are reevaluated in 3 to 6 months with repeat ion level testing and imaging. Revision is advised if there is a soft-tissue reaction or abnormal fluid collection noted on imaging studies.

Summary

Clearly, there seems to be a subset of patients that may be more susceptible to complications caused by metallic debris from metal-on-metal bearing articulations. Whether this susceptibility is related to implant size, implant contact area, a combination of patient genetic factors, or patient predisposition is not yet clear. Long-term epidemiologic studies are needed to fully address the issues of metal implant-associated local and remote toxicity, as well as hypersensitivity reactions and carcinogenesis. Advances in science and patient screening procedures will increase the understanding of host compatibility to metal implants. However, it should be remembered that modern metal-on-metal bearings have achieved good results in most patients.

References

1. Dumbleton JH, Manley MT: Metal-on-metal total hip replace-

ment: What does the literature say? *J Arthroplasty* 2005;20(2): 174-188.

2. Amstutz HC, Grigoris P: Metal on metal bearings in hip arthroplasty. *Clin Orthop Relat Res* 1996; 329(Suppl):S11-S34.
3. Santavirta S, Böhler M, Harris WH, et al: Alternative materials to improve total hip replacement tribology. *Acta Orthop Scand* 2003;74(4):380-388.
4. Amstutz HC, Campbell P, McKellop H, et al: Metal on metal total hip replacement workshop consensus document. *Clin Orthop Relat Res* 1996;329(Suppl): S297-S303.
5. Meier B: With warning, a hip device is withdrawn. *New York Times*, March 9, 2010.
6. Medical Device Alert: All metal-on-metal (MoM) hip replacements. Ref: MDA/2010/033. Issued: April 22, 2010. http://www.mhra.gov.uk/Publications/Safetywarnings/MedicalDeviceAlerts/CON079157. Accessed September 3, 2010.
7. Anissian HL, Stark A, Good V, Dahlstrand H, Clarke IC: The wear pattern in metal-on-metal hip prostheses. *J Biomed Mater Res* 2001;58(6):673-678.
8. Milosev I, Trebse R, Kovac S, Cör A, Pisot V: Survivorship and retrieval analysis of Sikomet metal-on-metal total hip replacements at a mean of seven years. *J Bone Joint Surg Am* 2006;88(6): 1173-1182.
9. Firkins PJ, Tipper JL, Saadatzadeh MR, et al: Quantitative analysis of wear and wear debris from metal-on-metal hip prostheses tested in a physiological hip joint simulator. *Biomed Mater Eng* 2001;11(2):143-157.
10. St John KR, Zardiackas LD, Poggie RA: Wear evaluation of cobalt-chromium alloy for use in a metal-on-metal hip prosthesis. *J Biomed Mater Res B Appl Biomater* 2004;68(1):1-14.
11. Fisher J, Jin ZM, Tipper JL, Stone MH, Ingham E: Tribology of alternative bearings. *Clin Orthop Relat Res* 2006;453:25-34.
12. Stewart T, Tipper J, Streicher R, Ingham E, Fisher J: Long-term wear of HIPed alumina on alumina bearings for THR under microseparation conditions. *J Mater Sci Mater Med* 2001; 12(10-12):1053-1056.
13. Smith SL, Dowson D, Goldsmith AA: The effect of femoral head diameter upon lubrication and wear of metal-on-metal total hip replacements. *Proc Inst Mech Eng H* 2001;215(2):161-170.
14. Udoifa IJ, Yew A, Jin ZM: Contact mechanics analysis of metal-on-metal hip resurfacing prostheses. *Proc Inst Mech Eng H* 2004; 218(5):293-305.
15. Goldsmith AA, Dowson D, Isaac GH, Lancaster JG: A comparative joint simulator study of the wear of metal-on-metal and alternative material combinations in hip replacements. *Proc Inst Mech Eng H* 2000;214(1):39-47.
16. Müller ME: The benefits of metal-on-metal total hip replacements. *Clin Orthop Relat Res* 1995;311:54-59.
17. Berry DJ, Harmsen WS, Cabanela ME, Morrey BF: Twenty-five-year survivorship of two thousand consecutive primary Charnley total hip replacements: Factors affecting survivorship of acetabular and femoral components. *J Bone Joint Surg Am* 2002;84-A(2):171-177.
18. Hart AJ, Skinner JA, Winship P, et al: Circulating levels of cobalt and chromium from metal-on-metal hip replacement are associated with CD8+ T-cell lymphopenia. *J Bone Joint Surg Br* 2009; 91(6):835-842.
19. Park YS, Moon YW, Lim SJ, Yang JM, Ahn G, Choi YL: Early osteolysis following second-generation metal-on-metal hip replacement. *J Bone Joint Surg Am* 2005;87(7):1515-1521.
20. Willert HG, Buchhorn GH, Fayyazi A, et al: Metal-on-metal bearings and hypersensitivity in patients with artificial hip joints: A clinical and histomorphological study. *J Bone Joint Surg Am* 2005; 87(1):28-36.
21. Engh CA Jr, Ho H, Engh CA: Metal-on-metal hip arthroplasty: Does early clinical outcome justify the chance of an adverse local tissue reaction? *Clin Orthop Relat Res* 2010;468(2):406-412.
22. Fisher J, Hu XQ, Stewart TD, et al: Wear of surface engineered metal-on-metal hip prostheses. *J Mater Sci Mater Med* 2004; 15(3):225-235.
23. Grigoris P, Roberts P, Panousis K, Bosch H: The evolution of hip resurfacing arthroplasty. *Orthop Clin North Am* 2005;36(2): 125-134.
24. Nevelos J, Shelton JC, Fisher J: Metallurgical considerations in the wear of metal-on-metal hip bearings. *Hip Int* 2004;14(1): 1-10.
25. Dowson D, Hardaker C, Flett M, Isaac GH: A hip joint simulator study of the performance of metal-on-metal joints: Part I. The role of materials. *J Arthroplasty* 2004;19(8, Suppl 3):118-123.
26. Beaulé PE, Antoniades J: Patient selection and surgical technique for surface arthroplasty of the hip. *Orthop Clin North Am* 2005; 36(2):177-185.
27. McKellop H, Amstutz H, Lu B, Timmerman I,Carroll M: A hip simulator study of the wear of large diameter, metal-on-metal hip surface replacements, in *Society for Biomaterials 27th Annual Meeting Transactions*. Mt Laurel, NJ, Society for Biomaterials, 2001, p 339.

28. Pandit H, Glyn-Jones S, McLardy-Smith P, et al: Pseudotumours associated with metal-on-metal hip resurfacings. *J Bone Joint Surg Br* 2008;90(7): 847-851.
29. Langton DJ, Jameson SS, Joyce TJ, Hallab NJ, Natu S, Nargol AV: Early failure of metal-on-metal bearings in hip resurfacing and large-diameter total hip replacement: A consequence of excess wear. *J Bone Joint Surg Br* 2010;92(1):38-46.
30. Langton DJ, Jameson SS, Joyce TJ, Webb J, Nargol AV: The effect of component size and orientation on the concentrations of metal ions after resurfacing arthroplasty of the hip. *J Bone Joint Surg Br* 2008;90(9): 1143-1151.
31. Hing CB, Young DA, Dalziel RE, Bailey M, Back DL, Shimmin AJ: Narrowing of the neck in resurfacing arthroplasty of the hip: A radiological study. *J Bone Joint Surg Br* 2007;89(8):1019-1024.
32. Shimmin AJ, Back D: Femoral neck fractures following Birmingham hip resurfacing: A national review of 50 cases. *J Bone Joint Surg Br* 2005;87(4):463-464.
33. Marker DR, Seyler TM, Jinnah RH, Delanois RE, Ulrich SD, Mont MA: Femoral neck fractures after metal-on-metal total hip resurfacing: A prospective cohort study. *J Arthroplasty* 2007;22 (7, Suppl 3):66-71.
34. Mont MA, Schmalzried TP: Modern metal-on-metal hip resurfacing: Important observations from the first ten years. *J Bone Joint Surg Am* 2008;90(Suppl 3): 3-11.
35. Mont MA, Seyler TM, Ulrich SD, et al: Effect of changing indications and techniques on total hip resurfacing. *Clin Orthop Relat Res* 2007;465:63-70.
36. McBryde CW, Theivendran K, Thomas AM, Treacy RB, Pynsent PB: The influence of head size and sex on the outcome of Birmingham hip resurfacing. *J Bone Joint Surg Am* 2010;92(1): 105-112.
37. Beaulé PE, Dorey FJ, LeDuff M, Gruen T, Amstutz HC: Risk factors affecting outcome of metal-on-metal surface arthroplasty of the hip. *Clin Orthop Relat Res* 2004;418:87-93.
38. Duffy GP, Berry DJ, Rowland C, Cabanela ME: Primary uncemented total hip arthroplasty in patients < 40 years old: 10- to 14-year results using first-generation proximally porous-coated implants. *J Arthroplasty* 2001;16(8, Suppl 1):140-144.
39. Ortiguera CJ, Pulliam IT, Cabanela ME: Total hip arthroplasty for osteonecrosis: Matched-pair analysis of 188 hips with long-term follow-up. *J Arthroplasty* 1999;14(1):21-28.
40. Lombardi AV Jr, Berend KR, Mallory TH, Skeels MD, Adams JB: Survivorship of 2000 tapered titanium porous plasma-sprayed femoral components. *Clin Orthop Relat Res* 2009;467(1): 146-154.
41. Buergi ML, Walter WL: Hip resurfacing arthroplasty: The Australian experience. *J Arthroplasty* 2007;22(7 Suppl 3):61-65.
42. Daniel J, Pynsent PB, McMinn DJ: Metal-on-metal resurfacing of the hip in patients under the age of 55 years with osteoarthritis. *J Bone Joint Surg Br* 2004; 86(2):177-184.
43. Lavigne M, Vendittoli P-A, Nantel J, Prince F: Abstract: Gait analysis in three types of hip replacement. *75th Annual Meeting Procedings*. Rosemont, IL, American Academy of Orthopaedic Surgeons, 2008, p 431.
44. Davies AP, Willert HG, Campbell PA, Learmonth ID, Case CP: An unusual lymphocytic perivascular infiltration in tissues around contemporary metal-on-metal joint replacements. *J Bone Joint Surg Am* 2005;87(1):18-27.
45. Mikhael MM, Hanssen AD, Sierra RJ: Failure of metal-on-metal total hip arthroplasty mimicking hip infection: A report of two cases. *J Bone Joint Surg Am* 2009; 91(2):443-446.
46. Hallab NJ, Anderson S, Stafford T, Glant T, Jacobs JJ: Lymphocyte responses in patients with total hip arthroplasty. *J Orthop Res* 2005;23(2):384-391.
47. Hallab NJ, Mikecz K, Vermes C, Skipor A, Jacobs JJ: Orthopaedic implant related metal toxicity in terms of human lymphocyte reactivity to metal-protein complexes produced from cobalt-base and titanium-base implant alloy degradation. *Mol Cell Biochem* 2001; 222(1-2):127-136.
48. Back DL, Young DA, Shimmin AJ: How do serum cobalt and chromium levels change after metal-on-metal hip resurfacing? *Clin Orthop Relat Res* 2005;438: 177-181.
49. Brodner W, Bitzan P, Meisinger V, Kaider A, Gottsauner-Wolf F, Kotz R: Serum cobalt levels after metal-on-metal total hip arthroplasty. *J Bone Joint Surg Am* 2003;85-A(11):2168-2173.
50. Schaffer AW, Pilger A, Engelhardt C, Zweymueller K, Ruediger HW: Increased blood cobalt and chromium after total hip replacement. *J Toxicol Clin Toxicol* 1999;37(7):839-844.
51. Sauvé P, Mountney J, Khan T, De Beer J, Higgins B, Grover M: Metal ion levels after metal-on-metal ring total hip replacement: A 30-year follow-up study. *J Bone Joint Surg Br* 2007;89(5): 586-590.
52. Daniel J, Ziaee H, Pradhan C, Pynsent PB, McMinn DJ: Blood and urine metal ion levels in young and active patients after Birmingham hip resurfacing ar-

throplasty: Four-year results of a prospective longitudinal study. *J Bone Joint Surg Br* 2007;89(2):169-173.

53. Clarke MT, Lee PT, Arora A, Villar RN: Levels of metal ions after small- and large-diameter metal-on-metal hip arthroplasty. *J Bone Joint Surg Br* 2003;85(6):913-917.

54. Dunstan E, Ladon D, Whittingham-Jones P, Carrington R, Briggs TW: Chromosomal aberrations in the peripheral blood of patients with metal-on-metal hip bearings. *J Bone Joint Surg Am* 2008;90(3):517-522.

55. Ladon D, Doherty A, Newson R, Turner J, Bhamra M, Case CP: Changes in metal levels and chromosome aberrations in the peripheral blood of patients after metal-on-metal hip arthroplasty. *J Arthroplasty* 2004;19(8, Suppl 3):78-83.

56. Hart AJ, Hester T, Sinclair K, et al: The association between metal ions from hip resurfacing and reduced T-cell counts. *J Bone Joint Surg Br* 2006;88(4):449-454.

57. Urban RM, Jacobs JJ, Tomlinson MJ, Gavrilovic J, Black J, Peoc'h M: Dissemination of wear particles to the liver, spleen, and abdominal lymph nodes of patients with hip or knee replacement. *J Bone Joint Surg Am* 2000;82(4):457-476.

58. Ziaee H, Daniel J, Datta AK, Blunt S, McMinn DJ: Transplacental transfer of cobalt and chromium in patients with metal-on-metal hip arthroplasty: A controlled study. *J Bone Joint Surg Br* 2007;89(3):301-305.

59. Merritt K, Rodrigo JJ: Immune response to synthetic materials: Sensitization of patients receiving orthopaedic implants. *Clin Orthop Relat Res* 1996;326:71-79.

60. Hallab NJ, Mikecz K, Vermes C, Skipor A, Jacobs JJ: Differential lymphocyte reactivity to serum-derived metal-protein complexes produced from cobalt-based and titanium-based implant alloy degradation. *J Biomed Mater Res* 2001;56(3):427-436.

61. Memoli VA, Urban RM, Alroy J, Galante JO: Malignant neoplasms associated with orthopedic implant materials in rats. *J Orthop Res* 1986;4(3):346-355.

62. Jacobs JJ, Urban RM, Wall J, Black J, Reid JD, Veneman L: Unusual foreign-body reaction to a failed total knee replacement: Simulation of a sarcoma clinically and a sarcoid histologically. A case report. *J Bone Joint Surg Am* 1995;77(3):444-451.

63. Tait NP, Hacking PM, Malcolm AJ: Malignant fibrous histiocytoma occurring at the site of a previous total hip replacement. *Br J Radiol* 1988;61(721):73-76.

64. Visuri T, Pukkala E, Paavolainen P, Pulkkinen P, Riska EB: Cancer risk after metal on metal and polyethylene on metal total hip arthroplasty. *Clin Orthop Relat Res* 1996;329(Suppl):S280-S289.

65. Paavolainen P, Pukkala E, Pulkkinen P, Visuri T: Cancer incidence in Finnish hip replacement patients from 1980 to 1995: A nationwide cohort study involving 31,651 patients. *J Arthroplasty* 1999;14(3):272-280.

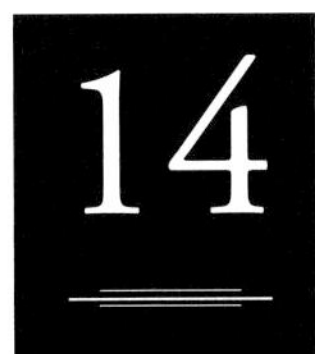

Alternative Bearing Surface Options for Revision Total Hip Arthroplasty

Deepan Patel, MD
Javad Parvizi, MD, FRCS
Peter F. Sharkey, MD

Abstract

Despite the overall success of total hip arthroplasty (THA), there has been an increase in the rate of revision hip surgeries performed each year in the United States. These revision surgeries result in several billion dollars in health care costs. Bearing surface wear can result in the need for revision surgery through a variety of mechanisms. Many implant failures necessitating the need for revision surgeries occur secondary to dislocations, which are often related to prothesis wear and eventual loosening of the components. Wear also can lead to osteolysis and may play a role in aseptic loosening. Specific concerns regarding the wear rates of metal-on-polyethylene (the most common bearing surface) have encouraged the manufacture of newer polyethylene implants with improved wear properties, as well as alternative bearing surfaces. The goal is to improve the durability of revision implants and/or reduce the incidence of revision THAs. Revision arthroplasty involves using alternative surfaces, such as replacing the metal femoral head with a ceramic component or changing the entire prosthesis to a metal-on-metal or ceramic-on-ceramic articulation. It is important to review the characteristics of these alternative bearing surface options and their contributions to improved THA tribology and prolonged prosthesis longevity.

The choice of a bearing surface for a revision THA should consider factors such as the patient's age and activity level, the cost of the implant, and both the surgeons' and patients' preferences. Although laboratory studies and small clinical trials have generated optimistic results for these alternative implants in vitro and in vivo, much still needs to be learned about the long-term performance of these materials in patients after total hip revision surgery.

Total hip arthroplasty (THA) is a treatment option for patients with advanced stages of degenerative joint disease. For these patients, joint surgery improves the quality of life and provides relief from the chronic, persistent pain that interferes with daily activities and is refractory to conservative therapy. More than 200,000 artificial hips were implanted last year in the United States. The success of this surgery is attributed to advances in prosthetic devices and surgical techniques, which have ultimately led to reduced risks and an increase in immediate and long-term benefits. However, despite the success of THA, there has been an annual increase in the rate (approximately 7% to 8%) of revision hip surgeries performed in the United States, which translates to several billion dollars in health care costs.[1,2]

Many implant failures requiring revision surgery occur secondary to dislocations that are often related to wear of the prostheses. Bearing surface wear can cause osteolysis and eventual loosening of the components.[1,3,4] Other less common causes of failure include joint infection, limb-length inequality, and gradual bone loss around the implant. Specific concerns exist over the wear rates of the most common bearing surface—the metal-on-polyethylene implant—in younger, more active patients who are at an increased risk for prosthesis wear and future revision surgery. The relative motion between the two bearing surfaces contributes to the generation of most of the in vivo, wear-related, particulate debris.[4] This debris leads to macrophage accumulation and a subsequent inflammatory response. The presence of lytic enzymes, proinflammatory cytokines, and bone-resorbing mediators in the area of the prosthesis have been documented.[4] This process results in osteolysis that can cause aseptic loosening and fixation failure.[5,6]

Revision THA is considered by many surgeons to be a more technically complicated procedure with inferior outcomes compared with primary THA. Problems arise because of the diminished quality of bone and the inability to adequately secure the components of the revision hip replacement. In addition, removing the original hip implant can necessitate more extensive surgery and bone loss. These factors, coupled with the discovery of periprosthetic wear debris, has encouraged the development and manufacture of newer polyethylene implants with improved wear properties as well as alternative bearing surfaces. The ultimate goals are to improve the durability of revision implants and reduce the incidence of re-revision THAs. Revision surgery may include replacing the metal femoral head with a ceramic component or changing the entire prosthesis to a metal-on-metal or ceramic-on-ceramic articulation. The characteristics of these alternative bearing surface options and their contribution to improved THA tribology and component longevity are discussed in this chapter.

Tribology

Before any formal discussion of alternative bearing surfaces, it is important to first review the principles of tribology and how it relates to implant design. Tribology refers to the science of surfaces (for example, bearings) interacting under an applied load and in relative motion. Broadly defined, tribology encompasses three aspects of science and technology—wear, lubrication, and friction.

Wear refers to the removal of material and the resultant generation of particles caused by the relative motion between two opposing surfaces under loading. There are three known mechanisms of wear: adhesion, abrasion, and fatigue.[7] Adhesive wear is caused by the bonding between two surfaces in close contact and the matter that is subsequently pulled off the weaker surface.[8] Abrasive wear involves the removal of material from the softer surface secondary to microcutting from hard surface asperities that have rooted themselves into the opposing soft surface.[8] Fatigue refers to the progressive and localized structural damage that occurs when a material is subjected to repetitive loading cycles, such as exists in an artificial hip joint.[8]

Lubrication occurs when two opposing surfaces are separated by a lubricant film that carries the force of the applied load as a fluid pressure and removes the load from the opposing surface materials.[9] Boundary lubrication arises when the two bodies are not completely separated; thus, occasional abrasion from hard surface asperities will occur.[7,9] The gamma (λ) ratio compares fluid-film thickness to surface roughness. A higher λ value translates into reduced friction and wear.[7] A λ value greater than 3 indicates fluid-film or hydrodynamic lubrication in which complete separation of the bearing surfaces is achieved, and abrasive wear is minimal (if present at all).[7]

Friction is the force that opposes the relative motion or tendency toward such motion of two surfaces in contact.[10] Ideally, when prostheses are designed, bearing surfaces are manufactured to be smoother to reduce the coefficient of friction and yield lower frictional forces across the joint. The coefficient of friction of a normal hip joint is 0.008 to 0.02; most artificial hip joints are designed with a coefficient at or below those values.[11]

Metal-on-Polyethylene Prostheses

Much of the current success of THA is attributed to the work of Charnley, whose implant design became the foremost model for arthroplasty by the 1970s. Charnley's design consisted of three parts: the stainless steel femoral component, a polyethylene acetabular component, and cement to fix the component to bone. The Charnley implant used a small 22-mm femoral head to decrease the wear rate of the joint; however, it was later recognized that smaller femoral heads could increase the rate of hip dislocation.[7]

Currently, the most common bearing surface used in hip replacement is a cobalt alloy femoral head that

---

Dr. Parvizi or an immediate family member serves as a board member, owner, officer, or committee member of the American Association of Hip and Knee Surgeons, the American Board of Orthopaedic Surgery, the British Orthopaedic Association, the Hip Society, the Orthopaedic Research and Education Foundation, the Orthopaedic Research Society, and SmartTech; serves as a paid consultant to or is an employee of Stryker; and has received research or institutional support from 3M, the Musculoskeletal Transplant Foundation, Smith & Nephew, and Stryker. Dr. Sharkey or an immediate family member serves as a board member, owner, officer, or committee member of Physician Recommended Nutriceuticals and the American Association of Hip and Knee Surgeons; has received royalties from Stryker and Stelkast; serves as a paid consultant to or is an employee of Stryker; has received research or institutional support from Stryker and Stelkast; and owns stock or stock options in Cross Current, Physician Recommended Nutriceuticals, CardoMedical, and Knee Creations. Neither Dr. Patel nor any immediate family member has received anything of value from or owns stock in a commercial company or institution related directly or indirectly to the subject of this chapter.

articulates with an ultra-high–molecular weight polyethylene (UHMWPE) acetabular cup. The advantages of this design are that it is a proven product, which has demonstrated excellent results in clinical studies; is nontoxic to patients; is cost effective; and allows the surgeon some flexibility with implantation because of multiple polyethylene liner options.[6] However, one major disadvantage of this bearing couple is that the longevity of this prosthesis can be compromised by eventual wearing of the UHMWPE cup, resulting in subsequent osteolysis and failure of the joint.[3,12] Given these concerns, when revising a THA, this chapter's authors prefer to reserve the use of metal-on-polyethylene implants for elderly and/or less active patients who have a reduced risk for component wear. Nonetheless, if a well-fixed, cemented, all-polyethylene socket or a nonmodular liner with minimal wear is present, the risk-to-benefit ratio of removing this device must be carefully considered.

UHMWPE is manufactured by either extrusion, bulk compression molding, or net-shape molding, and its wear properties can be enhanced by irradiating the material to induce cross-linking.[13] Cross-linked UHMWPE has more than 95% improved wear resistance compared with non–cross-linked polyethylene.[14] Non–cross-linked polyethylene can generate approximately 0.1 mm/y microparticulate debris, with a mean particle size of 0.4 μm.[11] Oxidative degradation secondary to sterilization of polyethylene by gamma radiation has been cited as an important cause of polyethylene deformation, accelerated wear, and, ultimately, liner fracture.[6] Additionally, laboratory studies have shown a tradeoff, with gamma radiation resulting in increased wear resistance at the cost of lower yield strength, ultimate tensile strength, and percentage of strain on the polyethylene before it fails.[14] To counter these detrimental effects, the manufacturing process has been modified and improved to incorporate sterilization in an inert atmosphere, such as nitrogen or argon gas, to prevent oxidation of free radicals, which reduce the mechanical properties of components.[14] When planning for a revision THA, the surgeon should try to determine the type of polyethylene currently implanted and should assess the risk for future failure if the component is not revised.

In an effort to further improve the wear properties of the polyethylene cup, highly cross-linked UHMWPE was developed in the late 1990s.[15,16] The theory behind this new composite material suggests that cross-linking improves wear resistance by decreasing adhesive and abrasive wear.[17] However, radiation alone generates free radicals only, and these free radicals can couple with other free radicals and cross-link only if the polymeric chains are given mobility. This can be achieved through annealing or remelting the polyethylene. In the annealing process, the polyethylene is heated to a temperature below its melting point.[18] Annealing preserves mechanical and fatigue properties of the material, but it still contains free radicals because there is not enough mobility for all free radicals to cross-link.[18] In the remelting process, the polyethylene is heated to a temperature beyond its melting point, which results in lower mechanical and fatigue properties; however, there are no detectable residual free radicals after the process.[18]

In vitro studies have reported that highly cross-linked UHMWPE offers the additional advantage of having wear properties that are independent of the femoral head size.[3,15,19] This is a major advantage compared with conventional UHMWPE components, which exhibits increased wear in proportion to an increasing femoral head size. Using larger femoral heads is particularly important in revision surgery where the risk of postoperative dislocation is increased. Using larger heads translates into increased hip range of motion, reduced dislocation rates, and a lack of component-to-component impingement.[19-21] In a study by Muratoglu et al,[22] significant improvements in the wear resistance characteristics of UHMWPE were reported with up to 10 Mrads of gamma radiation. With more than 10 mrads of gamma radiation, the mechanical properties of the polyethylene exponentially decline, and the rate of improved wear resistance begins to drastically diminish. Caution must be taken when introducing more cross-linking into the polyethylene because studies have reported an indirect relationship of more cross-linking with loss of material fatigue strength, ultimate strength, and the percentage of ultimate elongation, leading to polyethylene fracture and long-term component failure.[14,22-24]

Metallic alloys used for hip implants should have a high level of corrosion resistance as well as mechanical properties that can withstand the demanding requirements of the replaced hip. The three materials used for artificial femoral heads are titanium, stainless steel, and cobalt-chromium alloys. All three metallic alloys have a modulus of elasticity significantly higher than that of bone, which causes the implant to be stiffer than natural bone.[25] Titanium femoral heads have great biocompatibility and low levels of corrosion in vivo, along with the lowest modulus of elasticity compared to cobalt-based alloys or surgical stainless steel.[25] However, because titanium has significant vulnerability to abrasion, it is no longer used as a femoral head bearing.[13] Concerns have been expressed about in vivo corrosion in surgical stainless steel alloys used for hip implants.[16] The low carbon in 316 L stainless steel reduces corrosion rates and is still used for some hip replacements, predominantly outside the United States.[16] Cast or forged cobalt-chromium components offer more resistance to corrosion compared with stainless steel. Forged components have a smaller grain size and greater hardness compared with cast alloys.[13] Currently, cobalt-chromium, which is well suited for long-term weight bearing, is the most common metallic surface used for femoral head replacements. Although surgeons are unlikely to encounter a titanium or stainless steel femoral head during revision THA, this contingency should be considered if the primary surgery was done before the early 1990s or outside the United States.

Ceramic-on-Polyethylene Implants

An alternative bearing option available for revision THA is the replacement of metallic femoral heads with ceramic components, mainly alumina or zirconium. Both materials offer improved biocompatibility and durability compared with their metallic counterparts. Alumina bearings have high hardness, wettability (lower friction), lower surface roughness, and high tensile strength.[26] These properties may translate to a fivefold to tenfold reduction in polyethylene wear and a higher resistance to femoral head surface abrasion.[26,27] The zirconium femoral head has even higher hardness and burst strength compared with the alumina head; however, in vivo studies have shown that it is not as thermostable as alumina.[28] Practically speaking, this makes it dangerous to sterilize zirconium components in an autoclave. In a case study by Haraguchi et al,[28] deterioration and an increase in the surface roughness of two zirconia ceramic femoral head implants was associated with in vivo phase transformation of the ceramics after implantation. Therefore, despite its high mechanical durability, many surgeons and implant designers believe that zirconia is not stable enough to be considered an optimal bearing surface for femoral head replacement. Nonetheless, the product is still available and is an option for revision THA.

Oxidized zirconium alloy implants, made from a zirconium base that is heated and infused with oxygen so that the outer coating of the metal transforms into a ceramic shell, have recently been introduced. These implants retain the light yet strong characteristics of the zirconium metal while also adopting the smooth, tough properties inherent in ceramic implants. Specifically, the ceramic coating reduces friction between the oxidized zirconium femoral head and the polyethylene cup leading to potentially diminished wear compared with standard metal-on-polyethylene devices.[29,30] Oxidized zirconium also is harder and more than 4,900 times more resistant to scratching compared with cobalt-chromium and has a minimum fatigue load equivalent to its metal counterparts.[29] However, with oxidized zirconium, the ceramic coating is thin and can be easily scratched, greatly diminishing its wear properties. When revising an oxidized zirconium head, it should be carefully inspected and revised if scratched. Interestingly, oxidized zirconium contains no detectable level of nickel, which some investigators suspect causes allergic reactions in patients following the implantation of metal bearings.[29] It is hoped that clinical trials will confirm the superior qualities of oxidized zirconium. Replacing a metal head with a ceramic head during revision surgery is generally discouraged. If any damage of the femoral trunion is present, the risk of catastrophic head fracture is increased. An oxidized zirconium head could potentially provide enhanced wear protection without the risk of fracture.

Metal-on-Metal Implants

Metal-on-metal hip implants were first introduced in the 1950s with limited success.[31] Many surgeons and implant manufacturers believed that the initial problems associated with metal-on-metal components resulted from poor manufacturing practices for the first generation of this type of prosthesis (specifically, poor alloy quality and mismatched articulating surfaces) rather than from design flaws.[32] However, despite poor manufacturing practices, some first-generation metal-on-metal implants lasted more than 20 years in vivo.[33,34] This fact, combined with the potential for 100 times less wear debris versus polyethylene components (because of increased hardness) and resistance to dislocation, has led to a renewed interest in second-generation metal-on-metal implants.[27,35,36] The particles generated by metal-on-metal implants are smaller than those generated by polyethylene and are less likely to result in macrophage stimulation.[27] Also, it is now understood that there is an early spike in the level of metal debris during the "breaking in" period; after this period, there is a large decrease in the number of particles produced.[37] Hip simulator studies and laboratory measurements of friction and wear in metal-on-metal joints have identified wear rates of approximately 0.01 mm/y with a mean particle debris size of 0.05 μm.[11,38] Metal-on-metal implants also allow for a larger femoral head, which leads to increases in sliding velocity and pulls more fluid into the articulation.[7,38] This ultimately results in greater joint stability and fewer postoperative dislocations.[7] When performing revision THA for chronic instability, the use of a metal-on-metal articulation should be considered.

Second-generation metal-on-metal designs developed in the late 1980s, such as the Metasul Hip (Zimmer Orthopaedics, Warsaw, IN) featured lower steady-state wear rates, optimal clearance, and improved tribology versus earlier devices. The conventional plastic polyethylene insert in the Metasul Hip implant has a cobalt-chromium metal inlay that articulates with the cobalt-chromium-molybdenum metallic alloy of the femoral head.[39] In a 5-year follow-up study of 78 patients with metal-on-metal uncemented THAs, Wagner and Wagner[39] reported no metallosis at the time of revision, a reduction in wear properties, and no evidence that the metal-on-metal articulation led to additional complications in vivo. Newer cobalt-chromium-molybdenum bearings also have an intrinsic capacity to smooth surface scratches caused by third-body particles.[40] In a small, randomized controlled study, Pabinger et al[41] reported that the metal-on-metal implants showed lower migration rates at 6 and 12 months (0.13 mm and 0.27 mm, respectively) compared with ceramic-on-polyethylene prostheses (0.63 mm and 0.82 mm, respectively). There were no significant differences reported between the two surfaces in terms of radiolucency, activity limitations, degree of pain, or range of motion.[41] A prospective, randomized, clinical trial of 171 patients, which compared 95 patients with a metal-on-metal prosthesis with a control group of 76 patients with a metal-on-polyethylene prosthesis, reported no statistically significant differences in the average Harris hip scores, degree of pain, presence of a limp, range of motion, and radiolucencies.[42] A 7-year follow-up study on the clinical performance of 161 THAs with Metasul metal-on-metal hip prostheses reported no complications from failed cup fixation, no evidence of large amounts of particulate debris, and no other unusual complications.[43]

Despite the advantages of metal-on-metal prostheses, concerns exist over the long-term biologic effect of metal particulate wear debris released into body tissues and fluids. Studies have reported an association between wear and metal sensitivity in patients. Metallosis results in the potential for mutagenic and carcinogenic effects, as well as a possible delayed-type hypersensitivity response to the metal ions.[7,44,45] The term "metallosis" has been used to describe the intraoperative findings of gross metallic debris and blackening of periprosthetic tissue.[45] The quantity of metal debris generated annually from a metal-on-metal prosthesis can be up to 500 times the number of polyethylene particles produced from a traditional metal-on-polyethylene implant.[46] Many studies have reported the release of cytokines and inflammatory mediators secondary to low to moderate doses of metallic particulate debris, which in theory may lead to cell destruction and subsequent periprosthetic osteolysis and aseptic loosening.[44,47-50] In contrast, other studies have suggested that metallic debris is too small to induce an inflammatory cascade and is not associated with loosening of the prosthesis.[51,52] Various clinical trials and laboratory studies have shown higher levels (up to 50 to 100 times higher) of cobalt and chromium in the blood and urine of patients with metal-on-metal implants compared with normal human levels.[7,44,53,54] Consequently, the use of metal-on-metal bearings is precluded in patients with chronic renal failure because of the risk of reduced urine clearance of metallic ions and in women of childbearing age because of the possibility of metal particles crossing the placenta.[55,56] A Finnish study compared the incidence of cancer after metal-on-metal total THA versus metal-on-polyethylene implantation.[57] Results showed an increased ratio for all cancers in the metal-on-metal group (0.95) over the polyethylene group (0.76), which translated into an overall risk of cancer in the metal-on-metal group of 1.23-fold compared with the risk in patients who had metal-on-polyethylene THAs.[57] Despite the suggestion that metallic implants may lead to carcinogenic and other adverse effects, other factors may also be contributing to the overall risks; therefore, more studies are needed to fully explore this issue.[57] Revising a metal-on-metal THA creates numerous issues. Metal-on-metal acetabular components are often nonmodular. If a surgeon decides not to use a metal-on-metal articulation, equipment should be available to revise the entire acetabular component. Alternatively, a dual mobility polyethylene insert (for example, Mobile Bearing Hip; Stryker Orthopaedics, Mahwah, NJ) can be inserted into the existing acetabular shell.

Ceramic-on-Ceramic Implants

The appeal of a ceramic-on-ceramic hip implant is the inherent properties of improved hardness and durability compared with a metal implant, as well as its biologic inertness in the body. Ceramic is regarded as the hardest bearing material used in THA, and it is the bearing surface that is most resistant to wear.[58] In vivo, ceramic implant debris usually produces no inflammatory response or osteolysis. Ceramic implants are often used in a younger, more active patient who is at risk of wearing out the bearing in his or her lifetime.[58] Hip simulator studies and laboratory measurements of friction and wear in ceramic-on-ceramic joint implants have identified wear rates of approximately 0.0001 mm/y with a mean particle debris size of 0.02 μm.[59] As was the case with first-generation metal-on-metal total hip prostheses, early ceramic prostheses had design flaws and material inequalities that commonly led to catastrophic fractures, impingement, implant loosening, and higher than predicted wear rates.[60-62] Improvements in implant design and the material grain structure of ceramic devices have produced a bearing surface with improved hardness, fracture toughness, and burst strength compared with early designs.[7] These properties are attributed to smaller average grain size and lower porosity of the ceramic material and its higher density and purity.[63] In a study comparing the results of ceramic-on-ceramic with metal-on-polyethylene bearings, D'Antonio et al[64] reported that revisions were necessary in 2.7% of patients with ceramic (alumina) bearings compared with 7.5% of the control group with metal-on-polyethylene bearings. Osteolysis was reported in 1.4% of the patients with an alumina bearing compared with 14.0% of the control group.[64]

Ceramics also are hydrophilic, which allows for improved wettability of the joint articulation.[7] This attribute, combined with the ability to polish a ceramic bearing to a low surface roughness, allows for a higher λ ratio compared with its metal counterpart and less friction and overall wear.[7,65] Because laboratory trials have demonstrated no ion release from the wear of ceramic bearings, in theory these bearings are more biologically compatible; however, these same studies have reported some ceramic particle-induced inflammatory reaction, but it is much less than seen with metal debris.[66] In the revision setting, even with copious irrigation, residual debris (such as bone, metal, and polymethylmethacrylate cement) may be present. Because ceramic-on-ceramic bearings are highly resistant to third body wear caused by debris, a ceramic-on-ceramic bearing should be considered for a young patient undergoing revision of all hip components.

Ceramic-on-ceramic implants also have disadvantages. Early alumina-on-alumina models, plagued with faulty designs and poor manufacturing, experienced excessive wear rates of 5 to 9 μm/y to 90 μm over 3 years.[67] The most common concerns surrounding ceramic bearings are the heightened fracture risk because of brittleness, the potential for acetabular liner chipping over time, the limited availability in femoral neck lengths, and postoperative squeaking with joint movement. The fracture rate of newer ceramic models is reported at 0.012%, and the incidence of acetabular liner chipping occurs in approximately 1% to 2% of all implants.[68] Squeaking has been reported in metal-on-metal bearings but is more common with ceramic articulations. In metal-on-polyethylene implants, squeaking may be attributed to femoral head wear through the polyethylene liner and the resulting articulation with the metal cup underneath.[69] Squeaking of a metal-on-polyethylene bearing requires urgent evaluation and treatment. In ceramic-on-ceramic implants, malpositioning of the cup can lead to component impingement and squeaking.[70] A relatively low incidence of squeaking (1 in 700 patients) has been reported with newer models of ceramic-on-ceramic implants.[69] Revision surgeries secondary to the failure of ceramic implants, most notably ceramic fracture, is complicated by the presence of highly abrasive ceramic particulate debris.[71] Nevertheless, an approach using total synovectomy, cup exchange, and the insertion of a new ceramic femoral ball minimizes the chance of accelerated bearing wear and the need for additional revision surgeries.[72] The limited choices of head, neck, and liner sizes available with ceramic components creates an added challenge when they are used in revision surgery.

Despite concerns, the outlook for ceramic implants appears positive. In a 5-year minimum follow-up study of alumina-on-alumina THAs in 79 patients younger than 65 years (93 hips), postoperative imaging and examination results showed no hip dislocations, component loosening, wear, or osteolysis.[73] In addition, ceramic fractures did not occur in any of the patients under ordinary circumstances.[73] A prospective, randomized, multicenter study with 495 patients and 514 hips compared patients with an alumina-on-alumina ceramic bearing to a control group with cobalt chromium-on-polyethylene bearings.[74] No significant differences in clinical outcomes were observed after a mean follow-up of 4 years.[74] No fractures of the ceramic head or liner were reported nor were any revisions needed because of liner-related complications.[74] These encouraging results with newer ceramic bearings may provide a safe option for younger and more active patients in need of primary or revision THAs.

Ceramic-on-Metal Implants

The most recent combination of bearing surfaces introduced for joint reconstruction is the ceramic-on-metal implant. Early studies reported lower friction, wear, and ion levels (specifically, cobalt and chromium) in ceramic-on-metal bearings compared with metal-on-metal implants and nearly equivalent tribologic properties as ceramic-on-ceramic implants.[75,76] These results are further supported by in vitro studies that evaluated the tribology of various bearing surfaces. The differential hardness of ceramic-on-metal bearings and ceramic-like coatings on metal reduce wear and metallic ion levels by up to 50% compared with metal-on-metal articulations.[77] In a study by Firkins et al,[78] the differential hardness of the ceramic-on-metal bearings contributed to the approximately 100-fold lower wear rates of these implants compared with metal-on-metal implants. Although early investigative clinical trials have reported optimistic results for ceramic-on-metal hip replacements, further long-term studies are needed before surgeons can confidently choose these bearing surfaces for treating their patients.

Discussion of Bearing Surface Options

Each of the previously discussed bearing surface options may be suitable for patients undergoing revision THA because of their favorable wear rates and low incidence of osteolysis (**Table 1**). A metal-on-polyethylene hip bearing is the workhorse of revision THA because of its very good wear resistance, multiple liner options, and lower cost versus other bearing surfaces. Polyethylene is not associated with in vivo toxicity, and osteolysis usually occurs only with significant wear. However, these benefits come at the cost of increased wear rates compared with other bearing surfaces. Metal-on-metal implants offer higher wear resistance and long-term in vivo durability and easily support larger diameter femoral heads, which reduce the risk of dislocation. However, concerns about the biotoxicity of wear particles should be considered before making this type of bearing a routine choice in THA. Because ceramic-on-ceramic implants have the highest wear resistance, have good long-term in vivo results, and show minimal evidence of particle toxicity, these implants are often used in younger, more active patients. The disadvantages of ceramic-on-ceramic implants include the risk of acetabular liner chipping, catastrophic fracturing of the implant, and squeaking. However, these concerns may be subjugated when considering ceramic bearings for younger patients because of the need to avoid future revision surgery that may occur secondary to implant wear (**Table 2**).

Table 1
Comparison of Hip Implant Materials

Properties	Metal-on-Polyethylene	Metal-on-Metal	Ceramic-on-Ceramic
Hardness (MPa)	Low	350	2,300
Fracture risk	Yes	No	Yes
Run-in wear	100 µm	25 µm	1 µm
Steady-state wear	10-20 µm	5 µm	0-3 µm
Metal ion level in body fluids	N/A	Yes	N/A
Cell toxicity	N/A	Yes	N/A
Allergic component	Yes, minor	Yes, major	No
Squeaking	No	Yes	Yes
Clicking	No	Yes	Yes

N/A = not available

Table 2
Advantages and Disadvantages of Hip Implant Materials

	Metal-on-Polyethylene	Metal-on-Metal	Ceramic-on-Ceramic
Advantages	High wear resistance No toxicity Low cost Multiple liner options Proven product	Very high wear resistance Larger head diameters Long in vivo experience	Highest wear resistance Bioinert Long in vivo experience Wettability Decreased surface roughness Resistant to oxidative wear
Disadvantages	Reduced material properties Material failure Increased bioactivity Particles/osteolysis	Increased ion levels Delayed-type hypersensitivity response Carcinogenic Corrosion at metal junctions Precise machining required	Acetabular liner chipping Fracture risk Squeaking Increased cost Limited neck lengths

Summary

Over the years, impressive advances in the design and durability of bearing surfaces for THA have occurred. The choice of a bearing surface for revision THA should take into account factors such as the patient's age and activity level, the cost of the implant, and both the surgeon's and patient's preference and experience with various bearing options. Currently, most revision THAs are performed using a metal-on-polyethylene articulation. However, as the revision burden increases and the average age of patients undergoing revision surgery decreases, the use of more durable bearing surfaces should be considered. Although laboratory studies and small clinical trials have reported optimistic in vivo results for alternative bearing surface options, much has to be learned about the long-term performance of these materials in patients treated with revision THA. Although long-term clinical studies confirming the better wear performance of newer bearing surfaces are needed, a decline in the incidence of wear-induced osteolysis and loosening with these new bearing surface options for revision THA is likely based on optimistic and extensive in vitro evaluation.

References

1. Furnes O, Havelin LI, Espehaug B, Engesaeter LB, Lie SA, Vollset SE: The Norwegian registry of joint prostheses: 15 beneficial years for both the patients and the health care. *Tidsskr Nor Laegeforen* 2003;123(10): 1367-1369.
2. Kurtz S, Mowat F, Ong K, Chan N, Lau E, Halpern M: Prevalence of primary and revision total hip and knee arthroplasty in the United States from 1990 through 2002. *J Bone Joint Surg Am* 2005;87(7):1487-1497.
3. Harris WH: The problem is osteolysis. *Clin Orthop Relat Res* 1995;311:46-53.
4. Jazrawi LM, Kummer FJ, Di-Cesare PE: Alternative bearing surfaces for total joint arthroplasty. *J Am Acad Orthop Surg* 1998;6(4):198-203.
5. Schmalzried TP, Kwong LM, Jasty M, et al: The mechanism of loosening of cemented acetabular components in total hip arthroplasty: Analysis of specimens retrieved at autopsy. *Clin Orthop Relat Res* 1992;274:60-78.
6. Harris WH, Muratoglu OK: A review of current cross-linked polyethylenes used in total joint arthroplasty. *Clin Orthop Relat Res* 2005;430:46-52.
7. Heisel C, Silva M, Schmalzried TP: Bearing surface options for total hip replacement in young patients. *Instr Course Lect* 2004; 53:49-65.
8. Garvey R: Wear rates impact maintenance priorities. Machinery Lubrication Website. 2003. http://www.machinerylubrication.com/Read/468/wear-rate-maintenance. Accessed November 16, 2010.
9. Jacobson B: Thin film lubrication of real surfaces. *Tribology Intl* 2000;33:205-210.
10. Czichos H: *Tribology: A Systems Approach to the Science and Technology of Friction, Lubrication, and Wear*. Amsterdam, The Netherlands, Elsevier Scientific Publishing, 1978, p 414.
11. Dumbleton JH, Manley MT, Edidin AA: A literature review of the association between wear rate and osteolysis in total hip arthroplasty. *J Arthroplasty* 2002;17(5): 649-661.
12. Sochart DH: Relationship of acetabular wear to osteolysis and loosening in total hip arthroplasty. *Clin Orthop Relat Res* 1999;363: 135-150.
13. McKellop HA: Bearing surfaces in total hip replacements: State of the art and future developments. *Instr Course Lect* 2001;50: 165-179.
14. McKellop H, Shen FW, Lu B, Campbell P, Salovey R: Effect of sterilization method and other modifications on the wear resistance of acetabular cups made of ultra-high molecular weight polyethylene: A hip-simulator study. *J Bone Joint Surg Am* 2000; 82-A(12):1708-1725.
15. Muratoglu OK, Bragdon CR, O'Connor DO, Jasty M, Harris WH: A novel method of cross-linking ultra-high-molecular-weight polyethylene to improve wear, reduce oxidation, and retain mechanical properties: Recipient of the 1999 HAP Paul Award. *J Arthroplasty* 2001;16(2): 149-160.
16. Sharkey PF, Hozack WJ, Dorr LD, Maloney WJ, Berry D: The bearing surface in total hip arthroplasty: Evolution or revolution. *Instr Course Lect* 2000; 49:41-56.
17. Kurtz SM, Manley M, Wang A, Taylor S, Dumbleton J: Comparison of the properties of annealed crosslinked (Crossfire) and conventional polyethylene as hip bearing materials. *Bull Hosp Jt Dis* 2002-2003;61(1-2):17-26.
18. Wannomae KK, Christensen SD, Freiberg AA, Bhattacharyya S, Harris WH, Muratoglu OK: The effect of real-time aging on the oxidation and wear of highly cross-linked UHMWPE acetabular liners. *Biomaterials* 2006;27(9): 1980-1987.
19. Burroughs BR, Rubash HE, Harris WH: Femoral head sizes larger than 32 mm against highly cross-linked polyethylene. *Clin Orthop Relat Res* 2002;405:150-157.
20. Livermore J, Ilstrup D, Morrey B: Effect of femoral head size on wear of the polyethylene acetabu-

lar component. *J Bone Joint Surg Am* 1990;72(4):518-528.

21. Burroughs BR, Golladay GJ, Hallstrom B, Harris WH: A novel constrained acetabular liner design with increased range of motion. *J Arthroplasty* 2001;16(8, Suppl 1):31-36.
22. Muratoglu OK, Bragdon CR, O'Connor DO, et al: Unified wear model for highly crosslinked ultra-high molecular weight polyethylenes (UHMWPE). *Biomaterials* 1999;20(16):1463-1470.
23. McKellop HA, Shen FW, Campbell P, Ota T: Effect of molecular weight, calcium stearate, and sterilization methods on the wear of ultra high molecular weight polyethylene acetabular cups in a hip joint simulator. *J Orthop Res* 1999;17(3):329-339.
24. Colwell CW, et al: Effect of head size and crosslinking on wear in polyethylene acetabular components. *Trans AAHKS* 2001;11:46.
25. Leventhal GS: Titanium: A metal for surgery. *J Bone Joint Surg Am* 1951;33-A(2):473-474.
26. Clarke IC, Manaka M, Green DD, et al: Current status of zirconia used in total hip implants. *J Bone Joint Surg Am* 2003; 85-A(Suppl 4):73-84.
27. Manley MT, Dumbleton J: Bearing surfaces, in Barrack RL, Booth RE Jr, Lonner JH, eds: *Orthopaedic Knowledge Update: Hip and Knee Reconstruction*, ed 3. Rosemont, IL, American Academy of Orthopaedic Surgeons, 2006, pp 333-344.
28. Haraguchi K, Sugano N, Nishii T, Miki H, Oka K, Yoshikawa H: Phase transformation of a zirconia ceramic head after total hip arthroplasty. *J Bone Joint Surg Br* 2001;83(7): 996-1000.
29. Smith & Nephew: Welcome to Oxinium Hip and Knee Placements. 2003-2005. http://www.oxinium.co.uk/index.php. Accessed September 22, 2010.
30. Bourne RB, Barrack R, Rorabeck CH, Salehi A, Good V: Arthroplasty options for the young patient: Oxinium on cross-linked polyethylene. *Clin Orthop Relat Res* 2005;441:159-167.
31. Amstutz HC, Le Duff MJ: Background of metal-on-metal resurfacing. *Proc Inst Mech Eng H* 2006;220(2):85-94.
32. Willert HG, Buchhorn GH, Göbel D, et al: Wear behavior and histopathology of classic cemented metal on metal hip endoprostheses. *Clin Orthop Relat Res* 1996; 329(Suppl):S160-S186.
33. Jacobsson SA, Djerf K, Wahlström O: Twenty-year results of McKee-Farrar versus Charnley prosthesis. *Clin Orthop Relat Res* 1996;329(Suppl):S60-S68.
34. Jacobsson SA, Djerf K, Wahlström O: A comparative study between McKee-Farrar and Charnley arthroplasty with long-term follow-up periods. *J Arthroplasty* 1990;5(1):9-14.
35. MacDonald SJ, McCalden RW, Chess DG, et al: Metal-on-metal versus polyethylene in hip arthroplasty: A randomized clinical trial. *Clin Orthop Relat Res* 2003;406: 282-296.
36. Dorr LD, Wan Z, Longjohn DB, Dubois B, Murken R: Total hip arthroplasty with the use of the Metasul metal-on-metal articulation: Four to seven-year results. *J Bone Joint Surg Am* 2000;82(6): 789-798.
37. Archibeck MJ, Jacobs JJ, Black J: Alternate bearing surfaces in total joint arthroplasty: Biologic considerations. *Clin Orthop Relat Res* 2000;379:12-21.
38. Dowson D, Jin ZM: Metal-on-metal hip joint tribology. *Proc Inst Mech Eng H* 2006;220(2): 107-118.
39. Wagner M, Wagner H: Medium-term results of a modern metal-on-metal system in total hip replacement. *Clin Orthop Relat Res* 2000;379:123-133.
40. McKellop H, Park SH, Chiesa R, et al: In vivo wear of three types of metal on metal hip prostheses during two decades of use. *Clin Orthop Relat Res* 1996;329 (Suppl):S128-S140.
41. Pabinger C, Biedermann R, Stöckl B, Fischer M, Krismer M: Migration of metal-on-metal versus ceramic-on-polyethylene hip prostheses. *Clin Orthop Relat Res* 2003;412:103-110.
42. Jacobs M, Gorab R, Mattingly D, Trick L, Southworth C: Three- to six-year results with the Ultima metal-on-metal hip articulation for primary total hip arthroplasty. *J Arthroplasty* 2004;19(7, Suppl 2):48-53.
43. Long WT, Dorr LD, Gendelman V: An American experience with metal-on-metal total hip arthroplasties: A 7-year follow-up study. *J Arthroplasty* 2004;19 (8, Suppl 3):29-34.
44. Lhotka C, Szekeres T, Steffan I, Zhuber K, Zweymüller K: Four-year study of cobalt and chromium blood levels in patients managed with two different metal-on-metal total hip replacements. *J Orthop Res* 2003;21(2): 189-195.
45. McGovern TF, Moskal JT: Radiographic evaluation of periprosthetic metallosis after total knee arthroplasty. *J South Orthop Assoc* 2002;11(1):18-24.
46. Silva M, Heisel C, Schmalzried TP: Metal-on-metal total hip replacement. *Clin Orthop Relat Res* 2005;430:53-61.
47. Lee SH, Brennan FR, Jacobs JJ, Urban RM, Ragasa DR, Glant TT: Human monocyte/macrophage response to cobalt-chromium corrosion products and titanium particles in patients with total joint replacements. *J Orthop Res* 1997;15(1):40-49.

48. Shanbhag AS, Jacobs JJ, Black J, Galante JO, Glant TT: Human monocyte response to particulate biomaterials generated in vivo and in vitro. *J Orthop Res* 1995;13(5): 792-801.

49. Korovessis P, Petsinis G, Repanti M: Zweymueller with metal-on-metal articulation: Clinical, radiological and histological analysis of short-term results. *Arch Orthop Trauma Surg* 2003; 123(1):5-11.

50. Park YS, Moon YW, Lim SJ, Yang JM, Ahn G, Choi YL: Early osteolysis following second-generation metal-on-metal hip replacement. *J Bone Joint Surg Am* 2005;87(7):1515-1521.

51. Green TR, Fisher J, Stone M, Wroblewski BM, Ingham E: Polyethylene particles of a "critical size" are necessary for the induction of cytokines by macrophages in vitro. *Biomaterials* 1998; 19(24):2297-2302.

52. Willert HG, Semlitsch M: Tissue reactions to plastic and metallic wear products of joint endoprostheses. *Clin Orthop Relat Res* 1996;333:4-14.

53. Grübl A, Weissinger M, Brodner W, et al: Serum aluminium and cobalt levels after ceramic-on-ceramic and metal-on-metal total hip replacement. *J Bone Joint Surg Br* 2006;88(8):1003-1005.

54. Savarino L, Greco M, Cenni E, et al: Differences in ion release after ceramic-on-ceramic and metal-on-metal total hip replacement: Medium-term follow-up. *J Bone Joint Surg Br* 2006;88(4): 472-476.

55. Santavirta S, Böhler M, Harris WH, et al: Alternative materials to improve total hip replacement tribology. *Acta Orthop Scand* 2003;74(4):380-388.

56. Jacobs JJ, Skipor AK, Doorn PF, et al: Cobalt and chromium concentrations in patients with metal on metal total hip replacements. *Clin Orthop Relat Res* 1996;329 (Suppl):S256-S263.

57. Visuri T, Pukkala E, Paavolainen P, Pulkkinen P, Riska EB: Cancer risk after metal on metal and polyethylene on metal total hip arthroplasty. *Clin Orthop Relat Res* 1996;329(Suppl):S280-S289.

58. Hannouche D, Hamadouche M, Nizard R, Bizot P, Meunier A, Sedel L: Ceramics in total hip replacement. *Clin Orthop Relat Res* 2005;430:62-71.

59. Tipper JL, Hatton A, Nevelos JE, et al: Alumina-alumina artificial hip joints: Part II. Characterisation of the wear debris from in vitro hip joint simulations. *Biomaterials* 2002;23(16):3441-3448.

60. Mittelmeier H, Heisel J: Sixteen-years' experience with ceramic hip prostheses. *Clin Orthop Relat Res* 1992;282:64-72.

61. Walter A: On the material and the tribology of alumina-alumina couplings for hip joint prostheses. *Clin Orthop Relat Res* 1992;282: 31-46.

62. Mahoney OM, Dimon JH III: Unsatisfactory results with a ceramic total hip prosthesis. *J Bone Joint Surg Am* 1990;72(5): 663-671.

63. D'Antonio J, Capello W, Manley M: Alumina ceramic bearings for total hip arthroplasty. *Orthopedics* 2003;26(1):39-46.

64. D'Antonio J, Capello W, Manley M, Naughton M, Sutton K: Alumina ceramic bearings for total hip arthroplasty: Five-year results of a prospective randomized study. *Clin Orthop Relat Res* 2005;436:164-171.

65. Prudhommeaux F, Hamadouche M, Nevelos J, Doyle C, Meunier A, Sedel L: Wear of alumina-on-alumina total hip arthroplasties at a mean 11-year followup. *Clin Orthop Relat Res* 2000;379:113-122.

66. Germain MA, Hatton A, Williams S, et al: Comparison of the cytotoxicity of clinically relevant cobalt-chromium and alumina ceramic wear particles in vitro. *Biomaterials* 2003;24(3):469-479.

67. Boutin P, Christel P, Dorlot JM, et al: The use of dense alumina-alumina ceramic combination in total hip replacement. *J Biomed Mater Res* 1988;22(12):1203-1232.

68. Garino JP: Ceramic component fracture: Trends and recommendations with modern components based on improved reporting methods, in D'Antonio JA, Dietrich M, eds: *Bioceramics and Alternative Bearings in Joint Arthroplasty: 10th Biolox Symposium Proceedings*. Darmstadt, Germany, Steinkopff Verlag, 2005, pp 157-168.

69. Walter WL, Insley GM, Walter WK, Tuke MA: Edge loading in third generation alumina ceramic-on-ceramic bearings: Stripe wear. *J Arthroplasty* 2004; 19(4):402-413.

70. Eickmann T, Masakazu M, et al: Squeaking and neck-socket impingement in a ceramic total hip arthroplasty. *Key Eng Mater* 2003; 240-242:849-852.

71. Barrack RL, Burak C, Skinner HB: Concerns about ceramics in THA. *Clin Orthop Relat Res* 2004;429:73-79.

72. Allain J, Roudot-Thoraval F, Delecrin J, Anract P, Migaud H, Goutallier D: Revision total hip arthroplasty performed after fracture of a ceramic femoral head: A multicenter survivorship study. *J Bone Joint Surg Am* 2003; 85-A(5):825-830.

73. Yoo JJ, Kim YM, Yoon KS, Koo KH, Song WS, Kim HJ: Alumina-on-alumina total hip arthroplasty: A five-year minimum follow-up study. *J Bone Joint Surg Am* 2005;87(3):530-535.

74. Capello WN, Dantonio JA, Feinberg JR, Manley MT: Alternative bearing surfaces: Alumina ceramic

bearings for total hip arthroplasty. *Instr Course Lect* 2005;54: 171-176.

75. Williams S, Schepers A, Isaac G, et al: Ceramic-on-metal hip arthroplasties: A comparative in vitro and in vivo study. *Clin Orthop Relat Res* 2007;465:23-32.

76. Brockett C, Williams S, Jin Z, Isaac G, Fisher J: Friction of total hip replacements with different bearings and loading conditions. *J Biomed Mater Res B Appl Biomater* 2007;81(2):508-515.

77. Fisher J, Jin Z, Tipper J, Stone M, Ingham E: Tribology of alternative bearings. *Clin Orthop Relat Res* 2006;453:25-34.

78. Firkins PJ, Tipper JL, Ingham E, Stone MH, Farrar R, Fisher J: A novel low wearing differential hardness, ceramic-on-metal hip joint prosthesis. *J Biomech* 2001; 34(10):1291-1298.

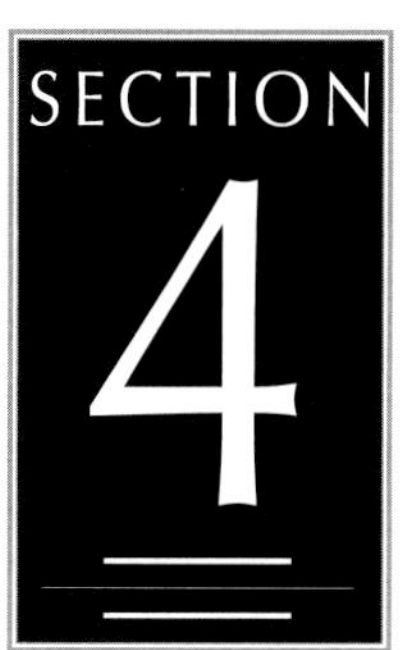

Primary Total Hip Arthroplasty

Primary Total Hip Arthroplasty

Primary total hip arthroplasty (THA) is one of the most successful surgical procedures ever devised, as measured by patient satisfaction and quality-of-life improvements. THAs are currently performed at a rate of approximately 300,000 per year in the United States and are projected to increase to more than 500,000 per year by 2030. Major advances have been made since the inception of this procedure by Sir John Charnley more than 50 years ago; many of these developments have focused on more reliable implant fixation and material improvements. In the past decade, orthopaedic surgeons have seen an emphasis on accelerating patient recovery from THA through the use of multimodal approaches such as enhanced pain management, reduced surgical trauma, and accelerated postoperative rehabilitation. Continued efforts have been made to find the ideal bearing surface to minimize wear debris and increase implant longevity. Despite the successes and improvements in primary THA, complications continue to occur. The five chapters in this section present topics that are relevant to any orthopaedic surgeon performing primary THA.

The first chapter by Dennis and associates is a wonderful overview of the basics of hip arthroplasty and covers topics ranging from the selection of implant materials to the management of postoperative complications. The second chapter, also by Dennis and associates, and the third chapter, by Berend and associates, discuss intraoperative decision making during primary THA. The fourth chapter, by Dutton and Rubash, presents a discussion of cementless fixation in elderly patients—a growing demographic of primary THA. The fifth chapter, by Parvizi and associates, describes the advances made in postoperative pain management that have allowed patients to recover more quickly from primary THA.

Dennis and associates discuss the suggested thought process for every surgeon who has a patient being considered for primary THA. This includes planning for fixation and choosing the bearing surface and surgical approach. The authors provide an excellent review of bearing materials used in THA, including highly cross-linked polyethylene and metal-on-metal and ceramic-on-ceramic components. The pros and cons of all the bearing couples are discussed, along with the balance that must be struck between reducing wear and decreasing the risks of complications such as fracture, squeaking, and allergic response to metal debris. The chapter also covers the common complications of dislocation and venous thromboembolism, with tips on avoidance and management. The authors also provide an excellent review of the risk factors for instability.

In the first of two chapters dealing with intraoperative considerations, Dennis and associates provide an overview of various surgical approaches for primary THA and the pros and cons of each surgical approach relative to exposure, ease of recovery, and risks for dislocation. The preoperative and intraoperative methods of assessing limb-length discrepancy are reviewed, along with tips on the anatomic landmarks for intraoperative assessment. Guidance for acetabular component positioning is provided regarding inclination and anteversion, and excellent advice is offered on how the body habitus and the position on the surgical table can affect acetabular positioning. This chapter is a "must read" for the hip surgeon. In the other chapter dealing with intraoperative considerations, Berend and associates examine the issues involved in achieving joint stability and equal limb lengths in primary THA. Factors associated with stability and limb length, the effect and role of various surgical approaches and techniques, and the management of instability with and without limb-length inequality are discussed. Overall, the authors provide a comprehensive review of instability and limb-length inequality in primary THA, with tips for avoiding and managing these complications. The techniques and results of revision surgery for instability are also presented, ranging from-soft-tissue augmentation to modular head/liner exchange to constrained liner usage.

Dutton and Rubash discuss a formerly controversial topic—the use of cementless femoral fixation in elderly patients. Over the past decade, many surgeons have adopted this technique. The number of elderly patients treated with primary THA is increasing because of increasing life expectancy. The advantages of cementless implants include the promises of improved implant survival and femoral bone preservation, decreased surgical time, and reduced cardiopulmonary compromise. Dutton and Rubash provide a comprehensive literature review of the outcomes of cementless fixation in older patients.

In the fifth chapter in this section, postoperative pain management techniques after primary THA are discussed by Parvizi and associates. Two critical elements of contemporary pain management are mentioned—preemptive analgesia and preventive multimodal techniques. The authors discuss the theoretic and practical applications of these two techniques with regard to primary THA. Techniques of anesthesia, such as spinal and epidural analgesia, can influence blood loss, postoperative nausea, and the speed of recovery. Multimodal analgesics, including nonsteroidal anti-inflammatory drugs, cyclooxygenase-2 inhibitors, gabapentin, pregabalin, and ketamine may assist in preemptive pain control. Postoperative use of intravenous patient-controlled analgesia, transdermal patient-controlled analgesia, and capsaicin are also discussed.

These five chapters remain relevant to primary THA because of their broad topics and comprehensive coverage. However, in the past few years, increasing attention has been focused on problems arising from the hard-on-hard bearing surface couples. Numerous articles have cited the incidence of squeaking in ceramic-on-ceramic bearings and the possibility that this portends an increased rate of wear.[1-4] Studies on metal-on-metal bearings describe the phenomenon of edge loading and the excessive production of metallic debris.[5,6] Hypersensitivity to metallic debris also has been described and often can lead to massive soft-tissue destruction.[7] In current THA procedures, orthopaedic surgeons are most likely to choose a highly cross-linked polyethylene liner as the primary bearing surface. There is also an increased interest in the direct anterior approach. Proponents of this surgical exposure espouse its less invasive and intermuscular nature and believe there is less tissue trauma as demonstrated by circulating enzymes[8] and postoperative imaging.[9] Numerous studies have shown that primary THA, performed via a variety of surgical approaches, can have excellent results.

Edwin P. Su, MD
Associate Professor of Clinical Orthopedics
Weill Cornell University Medical Center
Hospital for Special Surgery
New York, New York

References

1. Porat M, Parvizi J, Sharkey PF, Berend KR, Lombardi AV Jr, Barrack RL: Causes of failure of ceramic-on-ceramic and metal-on-metal hip arthroplasties. *Clin Orthop Relat Res* 2012;470(2):382-387.
2. Ki SC, Kim BH, Ryu JH, Yoon DH, Chung YY: Squeaking sound in total hip arthroplasty using ceramic-on-ceramic bearing surfaces. *J Orthop Sci* 2011;16(1):21-25.
3. Schroder D, Bornstein L, Bostrom MP, Nestor BJ, Padgett DE, Westrich GH: Ceramic-on-ceramic total hip arthroplasty: Incidence of instability and noise. *Clin Orthop Relat Res* 2011;469(2):437-442.
4. Choi IY, Kim YS, Hwang KT, Kim YH: Incidence and factors associated with squeaking in alumina-on-alumina THA. *Clin Orthop Relat Res* 2010;468(12):3234-3239.
5. Glyn-Jones S, Pandit H, Kwon YM, Doll H, Gill HS, Murray DW: Risk factors for inflammatory pseudotumour formation following hip resurfacing. *J Bone Joint Surg Br* 2009;91(12):1566-1574.
6. Mahendra G, Pandit H, Kliskey K, Murray D, Gill HS, Athanasou N: Necrotic and inflammatory changes in metal-on-metal resurfacing hip arthroplasties. *Acta Orthop* 2009;80(6):653-659.
7. Kwon YM, Thomas P, Summer B, et al: Lymphocyte proliferation responses in patients with pseudotumors following metal-on-metal hip resurfacing arthroplasty. *J Orthop Res* 2010;28(4):444-450.
8. Bergin PF, Doppelt JD, Kephart CJ, et al: Comparison of minimally invasive direct anterior versus posterior total hip arthroplasty based on inflammation and muscle damage markers. *J Bone Joint Surg Am* 2011;93(15):1392-1398.
9. Bremer AK, Kalberer F, Pfirrmann CW, Dora C: Soft-tissue changes in hip abductor muscles and tendons after total hip replacement: comparison between the direct anterior and the transgluteal approaches. *J Bone Joint Surg Br* 2011;93(7):886-889.

Dr. Su or an immediate family member serves as a paid consultant to Smith & Nephew and has received research or institutional support from Smith & Nephew.

Basics of Primary Total Hip Arthroplasty: Preoperative and Postoperative Decisions

Douglas A. Dennis, MD
Raymond H. Kim, MD
Thomas S. Thornhill, MD
Robert T. Trousdale, MD

Abstract

Preoperative planning, choice of implant-bearing surface materials to reduce wear, factors to minimize the incidence of postoperative dislocation, and the critical postoperative care issues to facilitate a rapid recovery are important considerations in patients undergoing total hip arthroplasty.

The decision to perform a total hip arthroplasty (THA) is based on clinical, functional, and radiographic criteria. Plain radiographs should show destructive arthropathy of the involved hip. Moreover, the surgeon must evaluate other possible sources of pain that could either mask, intensify, or complicate the pain pattern produced by the hip arthrosis. The clinical criteria should determine that the patient's symptoms can be corrected only with a THA. The patient should have undergone an adequate trial of medical therapy, physical therapy, and adjustment of functional activity. The functional criterion should be limitation or failure of the patient to perform reasonable physical activities because of the arthrosis.

Preoperative Planning

It is essential that the surgeon and patient align their goals and incentives. Informed consent is critical, but a more accurate description of the process would be "informed decision making." This indicates that the patient and family have actively participated in the decision-making process. The patient must understand that surgery is the only remaining option to improve function. At this point, the surgeon must discuss and document the known complications of the procedure and anesthesia, as well as any additional complications that may occur due to the patient's associated medical conditions.

The surgeon must determine the best choice of implant and discuss the risks and benefits of a THA and alternative treatment options with the patient. Is it best that the implant be cemented or cementless? Should the bearing surface be metal on cross-linked polyethylene, ceramic on ceramic, or metal on metal? Should resurfacing arthroplasty be considered? Should a large femoral head diameter be chosen to improve the head-neck ratio? What is the best surgical approach for the patient? Is it best to use a small posterolateral muscle-sparing approach or should an anterolateral approach be selected, particularly if the patient is at increased risk of postoperative dislocation? Is it best to perform the surgical procedure with a minimally invasive or standard incision? The advantages and disadvantages of the numerous issues that must be shared with the patient are discussed later in this chapter.

As patients are generally admitted the day of surgery, their medical history, including anesthesia risks, must be evaluated and known before the surgical procedure. The demographics of patients undergoing THAs are similar to those who have multiple medical comorbidities such as cardiovascular and respiratory disease. Moreover, the limited function caused by the arthritis may prevent the patient from exercising sufficiently to unmask silent coronary artery disease. To minimize perioperative risks, the patient must have a complete medical evaluation prior to surgery, typically performed by the patient's internist. In recent years the use of a beta-blocker in many patients has proved

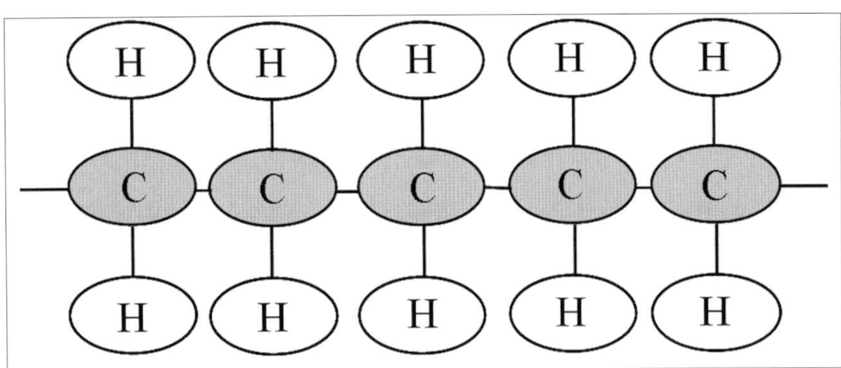

Figure 1 The chemical structure of polyethylene, showing long chains of carbon (C) with attached hydrogen (H) atoms.

to lower perioperative risk.[1-5] There are also data indicating that the pleiotropic effects of statins may reduce perioperative morbidity following noncardiac surgery.[6] This discussion should be held in concert with the patient's internist.

The emerging use of drug-eluting cardiac stents has created a large pool of patients who are on long-term anticoagulation medication. Recent studies of thrombosis in drug-eluting stents has led to the recommendation that the patient be maintained on clopidogrel for at least 1 year following stent insertion,[7-9] which substantially increases the risk of bleeding. Preoperative discussion with the patient's cardiologist is wise to determine the best treatment methodology, such as delaying the surgical procedure until this medication can be discontinued or considering perioperative platelet transfusion.

The surgeon must also preoperatively review the radiographs to be certain that the chosen implant can be sized to the patient's bone. This can be done either with plain or digital radiographs as long as a sizing marker is used to determine the percentage of magnification. Because most implanted femoral components are now cementless, it is imperative to be certain that the implant will reproduce femoral offset and leg length while being able to accommodate any anatomic variances. For example, in developmental dysplasia of the hip, the femur is often excessively anteverted, so a modular femoral component to correct the anteversion is desirable. In these patients, there is frequently acetabular deficiency that may require either a bone graft or prosthetic augmentation to obtain proper fixation.

Bearing Surface Materials

The failure of a THA secondary to particle-induced osteolysis, often associated with polyethylene wear rates greater than 0.2 mm/year,[10] has resulted in the development of various alternative bearing materials, including highly cross-linked polyethylene (HXLPE), metal-on-metal, and ceramic-on-ceramic designs.

Highly Cross-Linked Polyethylene

Polyethylene consists of long chains of carbon with attached hydrogen atoms (Figure 1). The production of HXLPE initially requires the production of free radicals, in which hydrogen atoms are removed from the carbon chains. Creation of free radicals can be accomplished by exposure of polyethylene to either gamma or electron beam irradiation or chemically by the use of peroxides. Most currently available HXLPE products are exposed to an irradiation dose of 5 to 10 Mrad. Exposure to higher doses offers limited improvements in wear properties and reduces mechanical properties (such as fatigue strength and fracture toughness), risking premature material failure. HXLPE is then created by the formation of covalent carbon-carbon bonds between adjacent free radicals, creating an interconnected, three-dimensional material with improved wear characteristics[11] (Figure 2). Avoiding of oxygen exposure during this process is critical because oxygen can combine with free radicals, resulting in chain scission, reduced molecular weight, and inferior wear properties due to oxidation.[11] The material is then treated with a thermal stabilization process (remelting or annealing), which frees the free radicals trapped within the crystalline region, allowing them to combine with each other and further reducing the potential for polyethylene oxidation.

Recent clinical reports with the use of various HXLPE materials have demonstrated substantial reductions in both wear and the incidence of osteolysis when compared with traditional polyethylene.[12-14] Triclot and associates[14] performed a prospectively randomized review of 102 THA patients implanted with either highly cross-linked Durasul (Zimmer, Warsaw, IN; 9.5-Mrad electron beam irradiation) or contemporary Sulene (Zimmer; 2.5- to 4.0-Mrad gamma irradiation in nitrogen) polyethylene inserts. At a mean follow-up of 4.9 years, the mean femoral head penetration rate was 0.025 mm/year in the Durasul group versus 0.106 mm/year in the

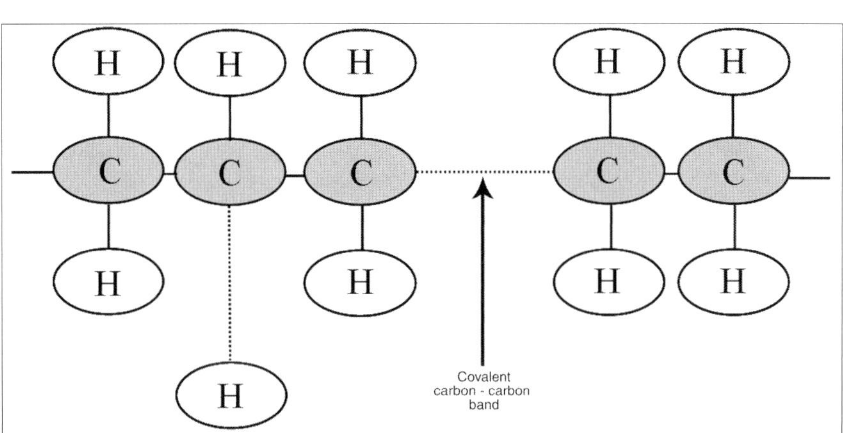

Figure 2 The chemical structure of HXLPE, created by the formation of covalent carbon-carbon bonds between adjacent free radicals, creating an interconnected, three-dimensional material.

Sulene group (P = 0.0027). The mean volumetric wear was 55% less in the Durasul group (P = 0.0058). Leung and associates[13] performed another randomized study of THA subjects implanted with either a Marathon (DePuy, Warsaw, IN) moderately cross-linked polyethylene liner (5 Mrad) or a conventional Enduron (DePuy) liner. Seventy-six participants (36 Marathon, 40 Enduron) were evaluated using CT scans at a mean follow-up of 6.1 years to determine the presence of osteolysis. Twelve of the Enduron participants (30%) and 6 Marathon patients (16.7%) demonstrated osteolytic lesions of 1 cm or larger (P = 0.19). The average lesion volume was significantly larger for Enduron patients (7.0 ± 6.7 cm^3) than those with Marathon acetabular liners (1.2 ± 0.7 cm^3; P = 0.001).

Although midterm clinical analyses have demonstrated substantial improvements in wear resistance, longer follow-up is needed to establish the long-term safety of HXLPE materials.[15] As previously mentioned, mechanical properties are reduced as the irradiation dose used to cross-link polyethylene is increased.[11,14,16] Fatigue cracking of retrieved HXLPE acetabular liners prepared with higher dose (9- to 10-Mrad) irradiation methods has been reported, often associated with thin polyethylene and vertical cup placement.[17,18] Continued clinical analyses are required to further evaluate the wear resistance benefits and ideal irradiation dose for HXLPE.

Metal-on-Metal

Metal-on-metal THA designs have been used for more than three decades. Premature failures encountered in the early years of use were often related to inferior materials and manufacturing processes. Substantial design improvements ensued to improve the durability of these devices. Critical design factors in the manufacture of metal-on-metal implants include the choice of metal material, equatorial versus polar contact patterns, boundary versus fluid-film lubrication, diametral clearance, and surface roughness.

Forged, high-carbon cobalt-chromium-molybdenum material is currently favored by most manufacturers due to its excellent hardness, wear resistance, and "self-healing" capacity to polish out surface scratches that may occur.[19] Equatorial contact between the femoral head and acetabular component was typical in first-generation metal-on-metal THA designs and often resulted in increased frictional torque, boundary lubrication, and an increased risk of failure due to implant seizing and premature loosening. Polar bearing contact patterns have been shown to reduce wear, believed secondary to the allowance of fluid ingress for lubrication as well as egress of wear debris particles[20] (Figure 3).

With boundary lubrication, transmitted loads are carried by asperity contacts between the two surface layers. With fluid-film lubrication, loads are carried by a fluid film that separates the bearing surfaces, reducing wear. Factors favoring fluid-film lubrication include polar contact patterns, reduced surface roughness, reduced diametral clearance dimension between the femoral head and acetabular liner, and increased femoral head diameter.[21-23]

The reported advantages of metal-on-metal THA implants include very low wear and subsequent osteolysis, increased range of motion to impingement secondary to the availability of larger femoral head diameters, and the potential to monitor implant performance by serial assessment of metal ion levels.[24-29] Sieber and associates[25] performed a wear analysis of 118 retrieved second-generation metal-on-metal implants and observed a linear wear rate (after initial wear-in phase) of 5 μm/year, which is at least 20 times less than linear wear rates with traditional polyethylene, and a volumetric wear rate of 0.3 mm^3/year, which is at least 60 times lower than with use of traditional polyethylene.

Reported concerns with metal-

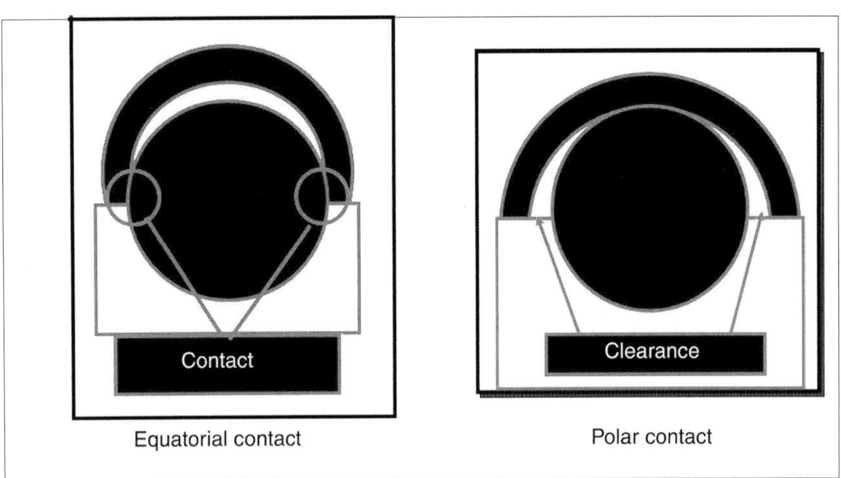

Figure 3 Equatorial versus polar bearing contact patterns.

on-metal THA implants are the elevation in serum and urine metal ion levels typically observed in subjects implanted with these devices and the subsequent risk of carcinogenicity or teratogenic effects.[30-32] Sauvé and associates[30] analyzed metal ion levels in a 30-year follow-up study of subjects implanted with the Ring metal-on-metal THA implant and found levels of cobalt and chromium were elevated by five and three times, respectively. Another report analyzing different metal-on-metal THA designs observed cobalt ion levels 50 times higher and chromium ion levels 100 times higher than controls.[31] Because of these ion elevations, many recommend avoiding metal-on-metal THA implants in patients with renal insufficiency or in females of childbearing age. Because of the potential carcinogenic effects of the associated metal ions, numerous investigations have been performed that have shown no increase in overall cancer risk in patients implanted with metal-on-metal THA designs versus the general population.[33-35]

An additional concern with metal-on-metal THA designs is the risk of metal-induced hypersensitivity reactions.[36,37] Willert and associates[36] analyzed periprosthetic tissue from 19 failed metal-on-metal THA implants and observed perivascular infiltration of both lymphocytes and plasma cells consistent with a hypersensitivity reaction. Associated joint effusions and tissue necrosis were commonly seen. Although the prevalence of this phenomenon appears low, close follow-up of metal-on-metal THA patients is merited to analyze the incidence and clinical significance of hypersensitivity reactions.

Clinical results of both first- and second-generation metal-on-metal THA implants have been favorable, with a low incidence of osteolysis and good survivorship.[26,27] Jacobsson and associates[26] compared the results of 107 McKee-Farrar (metal-on-metal) and 70 Charnley (metal-on-polyethylene) THA implants at an average follow-up of 20 years and observed a 20-year aseptic probability of survival of 77% and 73%, respectively, with minimal osteolysis in the metal-on-metal group. Grübl and associates[27] analyzed 105 second-generation metal-on-metal implants at a minimum follow-up of 10 years and observed a 98.6% probability of survival, with rare osteolysis and no renal insufficiency.

Ceramic-on-Ceramic

Ceramic-on-ceramic prostheses were first implanted by Boutin in 1970.[38] Many first-generation failures, including ceramic fracture rates as high as 7.5%,[38] were attributed to inferior ceramic material (large grain size, low density, increased porosity) and poor manufacturing processes (sphericity deviations, diametral clearance mismatches, large taper tolerances).[39,40] Early failures resulted in multiple mechanical property improvements, including clean-room processing, improved sintering techniques to reduce grain size and increase material strength, hot isostatic pressing to increase density and improve surface finish, proof testing, and laser marking to reduce stress raisers within the ceramic.[39,41-43] These changes have resulted in substantial increases in material strength and hardness, as well as a reduction in grain size and the incidence of ceramic fracture.

Alumina ceramic (Al_2O_3) was initially used because of its excellent hardness, biocompatibility, wettability, fluid-film lubrication, and low coefficient of friction.[44] Zirconia ceramic was introduced in the 1980s to address alumina fracture. Pure zirconia is unstable, exhibiting three crystalline phases (monoclinic, cubic, and tetragonal).[44] Stability is provided with the addition of oxides (yttrium) to maintain zirconia in the tetragonal phase. Yttrium-stabilized zirconia has a small grain size (0.2 μm) and exhibits nearly double the fracture toughness of alumina ceramic.[45] Zirconia, however, may undergo phase transformation from the tetragonal to monoclinic phase over time.[44,46] Phase transformation to the monoclinic phase results in increased surface roughness and may account for the inferior wear characteristics of zirconia as compared with alumina ceramic.[46]

More recently, alumina matrix composite (AMC) ceramics have been developed that combine the hardness and excellent wear characteristics of alumina with the fracture resistance of zirconia ceramic.[47,48] Testing of AMC composites of alumina and zirconia (Biolox delta; CeramTec AG, Plochingen, Germany) has demonstrated a nearly twofold increase in fracture toughness when compared with alumina ceramic, with maintenance of excellent wear resistance. AMC ceramic composites are currently approved by the US Food and Drug Administration (FDA) for use only as femoral head components. AMC-on-AMC ceramic couples currently remain under FDA study, although they are clinically implanted internationally. Major advantages reported for the use of ceramic THA designs are extremely low wear rates (attributed to material hardness), low surface roughness (Ra = 0.02 μm), and increased wettability that favors a fluid-film lubrication regimen.[44] In vivo retrieval linear wear rates as low as 0.016 to 0.025 mm/year have been observed,[49-51] which is approximately 4,000 times less than with historical metal-on-polyethylene devices. Bohler and associates[52] found that the concentration of debris in periprosthetic membranes of loosened implants was 2 to 22 times lower with alumina-on-alumina than with metal-on-polyethylene wear couples. Higher wear rates can be observed, particularly in association with loose or vertically positioned sockets, femoral neck-acetabular rim impingement, and with the use of poor quality alumina ceramic.[39] Stripe wear has been observed in retrievals due to intragranular ceramic loss believed to be secondary to impingement and femoral head microseparation.[48]

An additional advantage of ceramic bearings is the relative bioinertness of ceramic microparticulate debris. Analyses of periprosthetic membranes of failed alumina-on-alumina implants typically demonstrate a fibrocytic response with limited inflammatory cells. In a study by Sedel and associates,[53] prostaglandin E_2 levels in retrieved membranes surrounding loosened prostheses were 69 ± 56 fmol/mg in failed alumina ceramic implants versus 202 ± 156 fmol/mg in failed metal-on-polyethylene implants. Petit and associates[54] compared the macrophage response to alumina and polyethylene microparticulate debris of identical size and volume by measuring the production of tumor necrosis factor-α, a cytokine known to induce osteolysis. They observed 8 to 10 times higher levels of tumor necrosis factor-α release in the presence of polyethylene than with exposure to alumina microparticulate. These data are supported by numerous long-term clinical studies that show a very limited incidence of osteolysis associated with ceramic THA designs.[44,51,55-57]

Disadvantages associated with ceramic THA bearing materials include the risk of fracture or squeaking, a risk of premature bearing wear in ceramic components revised because of fracture due to remaining third-body microparticulate debris, increased cost, and a reduced range of error during component implantation.[38,44,57-63] Willmann[59] reported a fracture rate of 0.02% based on implantation of more than 1.5 million ceramic femoral heads since 1974. Hannouche and associates[58] observed 13 fractures (0.23%) in a group of 5,500 patients with ceramic THA implants. Fracture rates of ceramic implants are affected by material quality, manufacturing techniques, component malposition resulting in ceramic impingement, and patient factors. Squeaking following implantation of ceramic THA materials historically has been rare. Lusty and associates,[57] in a recent analysis of a third-generation alumina-on-alumina ceramic THA implant, observed this phenomenon in 0.3% (1 of 301 cases). However, Jarrett and associates (unpublished data presented at the American Association of Hip and Knee Surgeons annual meeting, 2006) observed an incidence of squeaking of 7% (10 of 159) in a group of subjects implanted with a modular design in which the ceramic liner is positioned within a titanium encasement that has an extended rim designed to prevent metal-on-ceramic impingement. The exact etiology of squeaking remains unclear but is theorized to be related to factors that enhance femoral head microseparation and femoral neck-acetabular component impingement such as component malposition,[62] patient factors (younger, heavier, taller),[60,62] and implant designs with elevated acetabular component rims.[60]

The results of using alumina-on-alumina in THA have been favorable, with minimal failures related to the ceramic material and absent or minimal incidence of periprosthetic osteolysis.[51,57,64] In the recent analysis by Lusty and associates,[57] a rate of survival based on revision for either aseptic loosening or osteolysis was 99% at 7-year follow-up.

Avoiding Instability

Dislocation after THA is a frustrating complication, with a reported incidence of 0 to 10%.[65-74] It may

Table 1
Risk Factors for Dislocation After a THA

Preoperative	Intraoperative	Postoperative
Previous hip surgery	Intraoperative patient positioning	Incorrect limb positioning
Gender	Surgical approach	Trochanteric nonunion/ migration
Mental health disorders	Capsular repair	Retained foreign debris
Neuromuscular disorders	Component malposition	Entrapped soft tissues
Alcohol abuse	Decreased prosthetic offset	
Older age (octogenarians)	Decreased soft-tissue tension	
	Femoral head-neck ratio	
	Femoral head diameter	
	Acetabular liner geometry	
	Retained periacetabular osteophytes/cementophytes	

occur in either a posterior, anterior, or superior direction. Posterior dislocations result from lower extremity positioning in excessive flexion, adduction, and internal rotation. Limb placement in extension, adduction, and external rotation risks anterior dislocation.

Most initial dislocations occur early, with 60% to 70% reported within the first 6 weeks following the surgical procedure.[75,76] The risk of recurrent dislocation is variable, with two large series reporting an incidence of approximately 33%.[77,78] The risk of recurrent dislocation is greater in patients suffering their initial dislocation late, after primary healing has occurred.[76] von Knoch and associates[79] reviewed 19,680 patients following THA and observed that 165 (0.8%) suffered their initial dislocation more than 5 years postoperatively (mean, 11.3 years), and 55% of those with late dislocation suffered a recurrent dislocation. Risk factors observed for late dislocation included female gender, younger age, trauma, polyethylene wear greater than 2 mm, and cognitive or motor neurologic impairment.[79-81]

Risk Factors

Risk factors can be classified into preoperative, intraoperative, and postoperative categories (Table 1). A predominant preoperative risk factor for dislocation is previous hip surgery.[66,75,76,78] Woo and Morrey[78] found a twofold increase in dislocation in those with previous hip surgery (158 of 3,259; 4.8%) versus those without previous hip surgery (171 of 7,241; 2.4%; $P < 0.001$). Dislocation occurs twice as frequently in females and three times as often in females who suffer a late dislocation.[66,75,76,78,80] Additional preoperative risk factors for dislocation include mental health disorders, neuromuscular disease, alcoholism, and advanced age.[75,76,82-84]

Intraoperative patient positioning can affect the incidence of dislocation by enhancing the probability of acetabular component malpositioning.[78,85] The normal lumbar lordosis is decreased from the standing position to the lateral decubitus position by as much as 20° to 35°, resulting in pelvic flexion and increasing the risk of acetabular component retroversion when the patient is in an erect position.[85] Placement in the lateral decubitus position often results in pelvis adduction (10°-15°), increasing the risk of vertical cup placement. Anterior tilt of the patient positioned in the lateral decubitus position is fairly common, enhancing the chance of acetabular component placement in less anteversion than desired.[78]

The risk of dislocation is highest when a posterolateral surgical approach is used.[70,78,85-87] Berry and associates[87] analyzed the 10-year dislocation rates in more than 21,000 THAs and observed dislocation rates with a 28-mm femoral head of 3% with the anterolateral approach, 3.5% with the transtrochanteric approach, and 6.9% with the posterolateral surgical approach. Dislocation rates using a posterolateral approach can be reduced with posterior capsular repair. Robinson and associates[70] reported a 7.5% rate of dislocation using this approach without capsular or external rotator musculature repair versus less than 1% when the capsule was repaired.

Component malposition, particularly of the acetabular component, is a critical factor in dislocation.[66,78,82] Lewinnek and associates[69] determined that the "safe zone" of acetabular component position was 40° ± 10° of abduction and 15° ± 10° of anteversion. Patients with acetabular components positioned within this safe zone had an incidence of dislocation of 1.5% versus 6% in those in whom the acetabular component was oriented outside this range ($P < 0.05$).

Failure to restore both vertical and horizontal soft-tissue length risks dislocation. Vertical length is determined by the level of femoral neck resection, prosthetic neck length, and axial acetabular component position. Horizontal soft-tissue tension is determined by the level of neck resection, the length of femoral neck selected, and the femoral component offset. Horizontal length (offset) may be increased by a more distal femoral neck resection and selection of a longer femoral neck or with the use of femoral components with increased offset built into the component.

Additional prosthetic risk factors for hip dislocation include the femoral head-neck ratio, the femoral head diameter, and acetabular liner geometry. Larger femoral head-neck ratios are favored because they increase the range of motion to impingement. This ratio can be increased both with the use of larger femoral head diameters and the selection of femoral components with narrower neck diameters, particularly in the coronal plane.[88] Many have reported reduced dislocation with larger femoral head diameters, particularly greater than 36 mm.[87,89-91] Crowninshield and associates[91] demonstrated that the use of larger femoral head diameters results in increased displacement (drop height and lateral displacement) required for dislocation as long as the acetabular component is not vertically positioned. Impingement can still occur with large diameter femoral heads, but it typically involves osseous impingement (proximal femur against the pelvis), in contrast to component-component impingement with lesser diameter femoral heads.[92,93]

The use of modular extended lip acetabular liners theoretically improves hip stability by providing additional support in regions of compromised hip stability.[94] Cobb and associates[94] reviewed patients treated with a 10° extended lip versus a standard, nonelevated liner. The incidence of dislocation in those with an extended lip liner was 1.43% (25 of 1,949) versus 2.35% (50 of 1,068) when a nonelevated rim liner was used ($P = 0.04$). The use of elevated-lip liners risks premature polyethylene wear and component loosening due to earlier neck-liner impingement, particularly when used in combination with a long femoral neck with a femoral-neck skirt.[94,95] Modular lateralized liners increase horizontal soft-tissue tension, theoretically reducing the risk of dislocation; however, clinical data are lacking with the use of these devices.

Noncompliance with postoperative instructions regarding limb positioning is the most frequent cause of early postoperative THA dislocation. Perioperative education, emphasizing the need to avoid lower limb positioning in excessive flexion, adduction, and internal rotation (posterior dislocation) or placement of the extended limb in marked external rotation (anterior dislocation), is imperative to minimize dislocation. Other postoperative risk factors include trochanteric nonunion associated with proximal migration of the trochanteric fragment greater than 2 cm and entrapment of either soft tissue or foreign debris postoperatively.[67,78,96-98]

Dislocation Management

Postoperative THA dislocations can be managed by either nonsurgical or surgical methods. The best nonsurgical management of THA dislocation is prevention, by using good surgical technique and educating the patient on the mechanisms of dislocation and the importance of avoiding high-risk limb positions. Should dislocation occur, most can be treated with closed reduction (longitudinal traction plus hip rotation) with appropriate anesthesia. Additional external devices, such as hip abduction braces, knee immobilization splints, or a hip spica cast, can be used after reduction to lessen the risk of recurrent dislocation.[99-102] The success of nonsurgical treatment is variable, with 10% to 44% eventually requiring surgical treatment.[78,80]

Surgical treatment is considered when a concentric reduction is not obtainable by closed methods or when nonsurgical treatment of recurrent dislocation is unsuccessful. Multiple surgical procedures may be used (Table 2). The choice of surgical procedure is based on the etiology of the dislocation. A determination of the accuracy of component position is critical. If substantial malposition is found, reorientation of the acetabular component is often required, particularly if retroversion is present. Daly and Morrey[103] reviewed 95 patients reoperated for chronic THA instability and observed that correction of retroversion of the acetabular component was the procedure most likely to produce a stable hip. If acetabular component malposition is limited, insertion of a modular, elevated-lip liner can reorient the peripheral boundaries of the acetabular component, providing additional support in regions of compromised hip stability.[94] If component placement is satisfactory but soft-tissue tension is inadequate, distal advancement of the greater trochanter can be used to increase abductor muscle tension and function. Kaplan and associates[104] used this technique to treat 21 recurrent dislocations, obtaining hip stability in 76% (16 of 21). The soft-tissue tension can also be increased by increasing femoral neck length or by using lateralized modular acetabular component liners.

Table 2
Surgical Options for Recurrent Hip Instability

Component revision
Extended-lip acetabular liner
Acetabular augmentation
Trochanteric reattachment/advancement
Constrained acetabular component
Bipolar/tripolar acetabular component
Increased femoral head diameter
Increased femoral neck length
Impingement correction

As previously discussed, larger femoral head diameters can lessen dislocation secondary to increased hip motion until component impingement occurs. The use of jumbo femoral head diameters in surgical treatment of the unstable THA is therefore logical, although long-term clinical data supporting this concept are not yet available other than when a bipolar or tripolar acetabular prosthesis is selected. These devices offer additional hip stability because motion can occur at multiple bearing surfaces, thus allowing increased motion before the femoral head dislodges from the acetabular component. Beaulé and associates[105] reported on 12 cases of recurrent dislocation revised with a jumbo femoral head (11 of 12 with a tripolar construct) at mean follow-up duration of 6.5 years. No further hip instability was observed in 11 of 12 cases (91.7%). When the previous treatment modalities have failed, the use of constrained acetabular components is considered. Indications for these devices include extremity shortening, excessive weakening or loss of the hip musculature, an elderly and disoriented patient, and a multiply revised THA that continues to dislocate. Disadvantages of these components include reduced motion until impingement, premature polyethylene wear, and component loosening, as well as mechanical breakdown of the constraining mechanism with recurrent dislocation. Results of the use of constrained acetabular components are variable, with failure rates ranging from 0 to 42% with follow-up durations up to 10 years.[106-108]

Results of revision for hip instability are variable and often related to the type and extent of the surgical procedure. Correction of hip instability with surgical treatment has been reported to occur in 60% to 70% of patients treated with surgery.[78,81] Failure to correct all factors contributing to dislocation intraoperatively was often associated with failure of the revision. Many of the surgical methods described can be used in combination to achieve THA stability (Figure 4).

Patient Management: Start to Finish

In addition to performing a technically sound operation, a successful THA requires comprehensive management of the patient from the preoperative visit in the office to postoperative care after discharge from the hospital.

Preoperative Patient Education

Patients commonly approach their hip replacement with significant anxiety. The fear of the unknown can be minimized with preoperative education for the patient as well as the patient's family or caregivers. Educational material in the form of handbooks, videotapes, and patient education classes can provide useful information and has been shown to have beneficial effects on the outcome of total joint arthroplasty patients.[109-111] It is important for the surgeon to be attentive to the patient's specific fears and to provide appropriate reassurance. The surgeon should understand the patient's preoperative expectations to ensure that the patient has realistic goals for the postoperative recovery and acceptable activities after a THA. Patient satisfaction postoperatively is influenced by whether the patient's preoperative goals and expectations are achieved.[112] Length of hospital stay should also be discussed with patients preoperatively so that they can anticipate the timing of postoperative discharge from the hospital.[111]

Anesthesia Optimization

Anesthesia for total joint arthroplasty has dramatically evolved over the past decade. In addition to reducing postoperative pain, anesthesia techniques have been developed with the goal of minimizing the use of parenteral narcotics to prevent medication side effects such as nausea, vomiting, oversedation, bowel and urinary retention, and pruritus, while allowing patients to participate in their physical therapy rehabilitation. Multimodal anesthesia, incorporating preemptive analgesics and regional nerve blocks, is an effective means of achieving pain control and avoiding prolonged hospitalization due to inadequate pain control or complications resulting from medication side effects.[113-118] The use of preemptive analgesics (long-acting oral narcotics and nonsteroidal anti-inflammatory medications) that are administered before surgery has been demonstrated to effectively reduce postoperative pain.[114,117,119-122] Advancements in techniques for peripheral nerve blockade, using lumbar plexus or sciatic nerve blocks, now provide improved regional pain control postoperatively.[114-116,120]

Weight-Bearing Status After THA

Postoperative instructions on the amount of allowed weight bearing should be provided to both the patient and the physical therapists involved in mobilizing the patient after surgery. It is reasonable to permit weight bearing as tolerated when good implant fixation is achieved and the surgical exposure avoids violation of the abductor mechanism. Historically, patients with cementless femoral stems were required to ambulate with protected weight bearing or even no weight bearing for up to 12 weeks, out of concern for stem subsidence. Multiple recent studies, however, demonstrate excellent results using cementless THAs, even with unrestricted weight bearing.[123-126] Rapid mobilization beginning the day of surgery or the following morning is recommended to avoid complications associated with immobilization (such as thrombosis, ileus, or pneumonia).

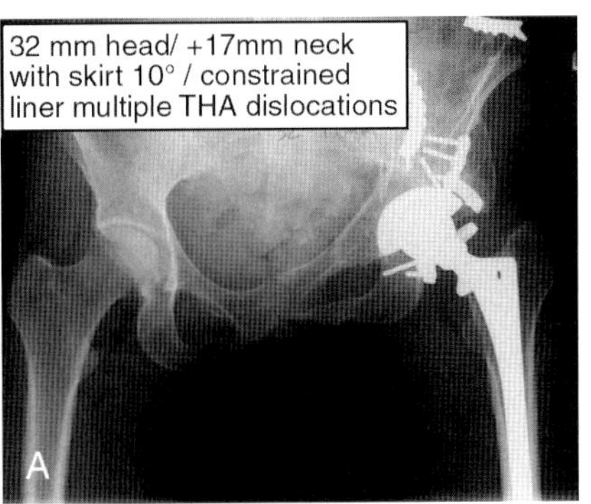

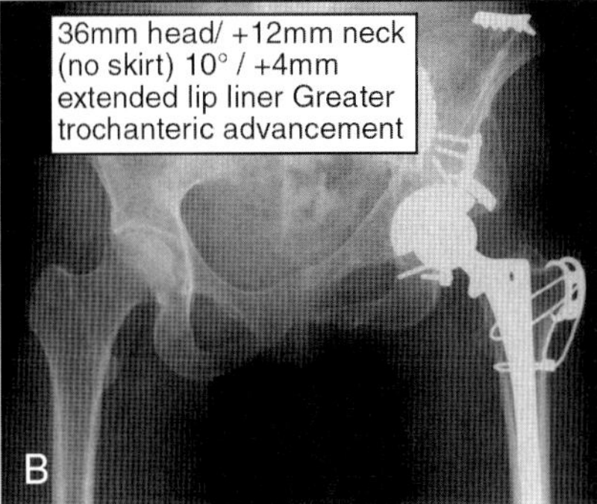

Figure 4 **A,** Preoperative radiograph of the pelvis of a patient who sustained multiple THA dislocations despite the presence of a constrained liner. Note the wide femoral neck skirt resulting in a reduced femoral head-neck ratio. **B,** AP pelvic radiograph following revision THA involving femoral head (larger diameter/no femoral neck skirt) and liner (nonconstrained) exchange, greater trochanteric advancement, and subsequent resolution of hip instability.

Dislocation Precautions

Some controversy exists regarding the need to adhere to postoperative restrictions designed to limit postoperative dislocation, such as avoiding certain limb positions. Although two studies question the role of patient restrictions in preventing dislocation, these studies examined patients who underwent a THA using an anterolateral approach.[127,128] Most believe patients should receive instructions on avoiding certain ranges of motion and limb positions that increase the risk of postoperative dislocation.[129,130]

Deep Vein Thrombosis Prophylaxis

Patients undergoing THA are at increased risk for venous thromboembolism. Katz and associates[131] reported a 0.93% nonfatal pulmonary embolism rate in 58,521 Medicare patients undergoing THA at 90 days postoperatively. From the Scottish morbidity record, Howie and associates[132] reported a 0.22% fatal pulmonary embolism (90-day) rate in 44,785 patients undergoing THA. The American College of Chest Physicians provided their most recent evidence-based guidelines for thromboembolic prophylaxis in 2004.[133] The grade 1A guidelines are recommendations based on clear evidence of benefit and are supported by consistent results from randomized clinical trials. The grade 1A recommendations for postoperative pharmacologic thromboembolic prophylactic agents include warfarin with a target international normalized ratio of 2.5, low-molecular-weight heparin, or fondaparinux. They recommended at least 10 days of postoperative prophylaxis and 28 to 35 days of prophylaxis for high-risk patients (history of deep vein thrombosis or pulmonary embolism, cancer, obesity, and advanced age).

Recognizing that the benefits of preventing symptomatic pulmonary emboli should be balanced by the risks of bleeding complications, the American Academy of Orthopaedic Surgeons has preoperative, intraoperative, and postoperative guidelines based on a systematic review and meta-analysis of the literature.[134] Preoperatively, patients should be assessed for elevated risk for pulmonary embolism and bleeding. Intraoperatively, the use of regional anesthesia and mechanical prophylaxis should be considered. Postoperatively, acceptable chemoprophylactic agents for patients at standard risk of both pulmonary embolism and major bleeding include aspirin, low-molecular-weight heparin, synthetic pentasaccharides, or warfarin.

Summary

Before THA is performed, the goals of the surgeon and patient should be in alignment. The surgeon must select the best choice of implant and discuss possible risks and benefits with the patient. Preoperative patient education, optimization of anesthesia, providing instructions on weight-bearing status and hip precautions, and administration of thromboembolic prophylactic measures are some of the important details that should be carefully managed by the surgeon to ensure a successful THA.

References

1. Daumerie G, Fleisher LA: Perioperative beta-blocker and statin therapy. *Curr Opin Anaesthesiol* 2008;21:60-65.

2. Biccard BM, Sear JW, Foëx P: Meta-analysis of the effect of heart rate achieved by perioperative beta-adrenergic blockade on cardiovascular outcomes. *Br J Anaesth* 2008;100:23-28.

3. Berg C, Berger DH, Makia A, et al: Perioperative beta-blocker therapy

and heart rate control during noncardiac surgery. *Am J Surg* 2007;194: 189-191.

4. Noordzij PG, Poldermans D, Schouten O, et al: Beta-blockers and statins are individually associated with reduced mortality in patients undergoing noncardiac, nonvascular surgery. *Coron Artery Dis* 2007;18:67-72.
5. Wiesbauer F, Schlager O, Domanovits H, Wildner B, Maurer G, Muellner M: Perioperative beta-blockers for preventing surgery-related mortality and morbidity: A systematic review and meta-analysis. *Anesth Analg* 2007;104:27-41.
6. Perler BA: The effect of statin medications on perioperative and long-term outcomes following carotid endarterectomy or stenting. *Semin Vasc Surg* 2007;20:252-258.
7. Pfisterer M, Brunner-La Rocca HP, Buser PT, et al: Late clinical events after clopidogrel discontinuation may limit the benefit of drug-eluting stents: An observational study of drug-eluting versus bare-metal stents. *J Am Coll Cardiol* 2006;48:2584-2591.
8. Eisenstein EL, Anstrom KJ, Kong DF, et al: Clopidogrel use and long-term clinical outcomes after drug-eluting stent implantation. *JAMA* 2007;297: 159-168.
9. Spertus JA, Kettelkamp R, Vance C, et al: Prevalence, predictors, and outcomes of premature discontinuation of thienopyridine therapy after drug-eluting stent placement: Results from the PREMIER registry. *Circulation* 2006;113:2803-2809.
10. Wan Z, Dorr LD: Natural history of femoral focal osteolysis with proximal ingrowth smooth stem implant. *J Arthroplasty* 1996;11:718-725.
11. McKellop H, Shen FW, Lu B, Campbell P, Salovey R: Development of an extremely wear-resistant ultra high molecular weight polyethylene for total hip replacements. *J Orthop Res* 1999;17:157-167.
12. Digas G, Kärrholm J, Thanner J, Malchau H, Herberts P: Highly cross-linked polyethylene in total hip arthroplasty: Randomized evaluation of penetration rate in cemented and uncemented sockets using radiostereometric analysis. *Clin Orthop Relat Res* 2004;429 :6-16.
13. Leung SB, Egawa G, Stepniewski A, Beykirch S , Engh CA Jr, Engh CA Sr: Incidence and volume of pelvic osteolysis at early follow-up with highly cross-linked and noncross-linked polyethylene. *J Arthroplasty* 2007;22(6, suppl 2):134-139.
14. Triclot P, Grosjean G, El Masri F, Courpied JP, Hamadouche M: A comparison of the penetration rate of two polyethylene acetabular liners of different levels of cross-linking: A prospective randomised trial. *J Bone Joint Surg Br* 2007;89:1439-1445.
15. Jacobs CA, Christensen CP, Greenwald AS, McKellop H: Clinical performance of highly cross-linked polyethylenes in total hip arthroplasty. *J Bone Joint Surg Am* 2007;89:2779-2786.
16. Baker DA, Bellare A, Pruitt L: The effects of degree of crosslinking on the fatigue crack initiation and propagation resistance of orthopedic-grade polyethylene. *J Biomed Mater Res A* 2003;66:146-154.
17. Tower SS, Currier JH, Currier BH, Lyford KA, Van Citters DW, Mayor MB: Rim cracking of the cross-linked longevity polyethylene acetabular liner after total hip arthroplasty. *J Bone Joint Surg Am* 2007;89:2212-2217.
18. Kurtz SM, Hozack W, Turner J , et al: Mechanical properties of retrieved highly cross-linked crossfire liners after short-term implantation. *J Arthroplasty* 2005;20:840-849.
19. Schey JA: Systems view of optimizing metal on metal bearings. *Clin Orthop Relat Res* 1996;329:S115-S127.
20. Chan FW, Bobyn JD, Medley JB, Krygier JJ, Tanzer M: The Otto Aufranc Award: Wear and lubrication of metal-on-metal hip implants. *Clin Orthop Relat Res* 1999;369:10-24.
21. Brockett CL, Harper P, Williams S, et al: The influence of clearance on friction, lubrication and squeaking in large diameter metal-on-metal hip replacements. *J Mater Sci Mater Med* 2007;19:1575-1579.
22. Isaac GH, Thompson J, Williams S, Fisher J: Metal-on-metal bearings surfaces: Materials, manufacture, design, optimization, and alternatives. *Proc Inst Mech Eng H* 2006;220: 119-133.
23. Dowson D, Hardaker C, Flett M, Isaac GH: A hip joint simulator study of the performance of metal-on-metal joints: Part II. Design. *J Arthroplasty* 2004;19:124-130.
24. Schmalzried TP, Peters PC, Maurer BT, Bragdon CR, Harris WH: Long-duration metal-on-metal total hip arthroplasties with low wear of the articulating surfaces. *J Arthroplasty* 1996; 11:322-331.
25. Sieber HP, Rieker CB, Kottig P: Analysis of 118 second-generation metal-on-metal retrieved hip implants. *J Bone Joint Surg Br* 1999;81: 46-50.
26. Jacobsson SA, Djerf K, Wahlström O: Twenty-year results of McKee-Farrar versus Charnley prosthesis. *Clin Orthop Relat Res* 1996;329:S60-S68.
27. Grübl A, Marker M, Brodner W, et al: Long-term follow-up of metal-on-metal total hip replacement. *J Orthop Res* 2007;25:841-848.
28. Burroughs BR, Hallstrom B, Golladay GJ, Hoeffel D, Harris WH: Range of motion and stability in total hip arthroplasty with 28-, 32-, 38-, and 44-mm femoral head sizes. *J Arthroplasty* 2005;20:11-19.
29. Jacobs JJ, Skipor AK, Patterson LM, et al: Metal release in patients who have had a primary total hip arthroplasty: A prospective, controlled, longitudinal study. *J Bone Joint Surg Am* 1998;80:1447-1458.
30. Sauvé P, Mountney J, Khan T, De Beer J, Higgins B, Grover M: Metal ion levels after metal-on-metal Ring total hip replacement: A 30-year follow-up study. *J Bone Joint Surg Br* 2007;89:586-590.

31. Lhotka C, Szekeres T, Steffan I, Zhuber K, Zweymüller K: Four-year study of cobalt and chromium blood levels in patients managed with two different metal-on-metal total hip replacements. *J Orthop Res* 2003;21:189-195.

32. Brodner W, Bitzan P, Meisinger V, Kaider A, Gottsauner-Wolf F, Kotz R: Serum cobalt levels after metal-on-metal total hip arthroplasty. *J Bone Joint Surg Am* 2003;85-A:2168-2173.

33. Nyrén O, McLaughlin JK, Gridley G, et al: Cancer risk after hip replacement with metal implants: A population-based cohort study in Sweden. *J Natl Cancer Inst* 1995;87: 28-33.

34. Paavolainen P, Pukkala E, Pulkkinen P, Visuri T: Cancer incidence in Finnish hip replacement patients from 1980 to 1995: A nationwide cohort study involving 31,651 patients. *J Arthroplasty* 1999;14:272-280.

35. Visuri TI, Pukkala E, Pulkkinen P, Paavolainen P: Cancer incidence and causes of death among total hip replacement patients: A review based on Nordic cohorts with a special emphasis on metal-on-metal bearings. *Proc Inst Mech Eng H* 2006;220: 399-407.

36. Willert HG, Buchhorn GH, Fayyazi A, et al: Metal-on-metal bearings and hypersensitivity in patients with artificial hip joints: A clinical and histomorphological study. *J Bone Joint Surg Am* 2005;87:28-36.

37. Davies AP, Willert HG, Campbell PA, Learmonth ID, Case CP: An unusual lymphocytic perivascular infiltration in tissues around contemporary metal-on-metal joint replacements. *J Bone Joint Surg Am* 2005;87:18-27.

38. Boutin P: Arthroplastie totale de la hanche par prothèse en alumine frittée: Etude expérimentale et premières applications cliniques. *Rev Chir Orthop Reparatrice Appar Mot* 1972;58: 229-246.

39. Walter A: On the material and the tribology of alumina-alumina couplings for hip joint prostheses. *Clin Orthop Relat Res* 1992;282:31-46.

40. Winter M, Griss P, Scheller G, Moser T: Ten-to 14-year results of a ceramic hip prosthesis. *Clin Orthop Relat Res* 1992;282:73-80.

41. Wu C, Rice RW, Johnson D, Platt BA: Grain size dependence of wear in ceramics. *Ceram Eng Sci Proc* 1985;6: 995-1011.

42. Heros HJ, Willmann G: Ceramics in total hip arthroplasty: History, mechanical properties, clinical results, and current manufacturing state of the art. *Semin Arthroplasty* 1998;9: 123-134.

43. Sedel L: The tribology of hip replacement, in Kenwright J, Duparc J, Fulford P (eds): *European Instructional Course Lectures.* London, England, British Editorial Society of Bone and Joint Surgery, 1997, pp 25-33.

44. Hannouche D, Hamadouche M, Nizard R, Bizot P, Meunier A, Sedel L: Ceramics in total hip replacement. *Clin Orthop Relat Res* 2005;430:62-71.

45. Cales B: Zirconia as a sliding material: Histologic, laboratory, and clinical data. *Clin Orthop Relat Res* 2000;379: 94-112.

46. Haraguchi K, Sugano N, Nishii T, Miki H, Oka K, Yoshikawa H: Phase transformation of a zirconia ceramic head after total hip arthroplasty. *J Bone Joint Surg Br* 2001;83:996-1000.

47. Masson B: Emergence of the alumina matrix composite in total hip arthroplasty. *Int Orthop* 2007 [Epub ahead of print].

48. Stewart TD, Tipper JL, Insley G, Streicher RM, Ingham E, Fisher J: Long-term wear of ceramic matrix composite materials for hip prostheses under severe swing phase microseparation. *J Biomed Mater Res B Appl Biomater* 2003;66:567-573.

49. Dorlot JM, Christel P, Meunier A: Wear analysis of retrieved alumina heads and sockets of hip prostheses. *J Biomed Mater Res* 1989;23:299-310.

50. Jazrawi LM, Bogner E, Della Valle CJ, et al: Wear rates of ceramic-on-ceramic bearing surfaces in total hip implants. *J Arthroplasty* 1999;14: 781-786.

51. Hamadouche M, Boutin P, Daussange J, Bolander ME, Sedel L: Alumina-on-alumina total hip arthroplasty: A minimum 18.5-year follow-up study. *J Bone Joint Surg Am* 2002;84-A:69-77.

52. Bohler M, Mochida Y, Bauer TW, Plenk H Jr, Salzer M: Wear debris from two different alumina-on-alumina total hip arthroplasties. *J Bone Joint Surg Br* 2000;82:901-909.

53. Sedel L, Simeon J, Meunier A, Villette JM, Launay SM: Prostaglandin E2 level in tissue surrounding aseptic failed total hips: Effects of materials. *Arch Orthop Trauma Surg* 1992;111: 255-258.

54. Petit A, Catelas I, Antoniou J, Zukor DJ, Huk OL: Differential apoptotic response of J774 macrophages to alumina and ultra-high-molecular-weight polyethylene particles. *J Orthop Res* 2002;20:9-15.

55. Bizot P, Nizard R, Hamadouche M, Hannouche D, Sedel L: Prevention of wear and osteolysis: Alumina-on-alumina bearing. *Clin Orthop Relat Res* 2001;393 :85-93.

56. Nizard R, Pourreyron D, Raould A, Hannouche D, Sedel L: Alumina-on-alumina hip arthroplasty in patients younger than 30 years old. *Clin Orthop Relat Res* 2008;466:317-323.

57. Lusty PJ, Tai CC, Sew-Hoy RP, Walter WL, Walter WK, Zicat BA: Third-generation alumina-on-alumina ceramic bearings in cementless total hip arthroplasty. *J Bone Joint Surg Am* 2007;89:2676-2683.

58. Hannouche D, Nich C, Bizot P, Meunier A, Nizard R, Sedel L: Fractures of ceramic bearings: History and present status. *Clin Orthop Relat Res* 2003;417:19-26.

59. Willmann G: Ceramics for total hip replacement: What a surgeon should know. *Orthopedics* 1998;21:173-177.

60. Yang CC, Kim RH, Dennis DA : The squeaking hip: A cause for concern-disagrees. *Orthopedics* 2007;30: 739-742.

61. Ranawat AS, Ranawat CS: The squeaking hip: A cause for concern-

agrees [Comment]. *Orthopedics* 2007; 30:738, 743.

62. Walter WL, O'Toole GC, Walter WK, Ellis A, Zicat BA: Squeaking in ceramic-on-ceramic hips: The importance of acetabular component orientation. *J Arthroplasty* 2007;22: 496-503.
63. Allain J, Roudot-Thoraval F, Delecrin J, Anract P, Migaud H, Goutallier D: Revision total hip arthroplasty performed after fracture of a ceramic femoral head: A multicenter survivorship study. *J Bone Joint Surg Am* 2003;85:825-830.
64. Bizot P, Banallec L, Sedel L, Nizard R: Alumina-on-alumina total hip prostheses in patients 40 years of age or younger. *Clin Orthop Relat Res* 2000;379:68-76.
65. Eftekhar NS: Dislocation and instability complicating low friction arthroplasty of the hip joint. *Clin Orthop Relat Res* 1976;121:120-125.
66. Morrey BF: Instability after total hip arthroplasty. *Orthop Clin North Am* 1992;23:237-248.
67. Ritter MA: Dislocation and subluxation of the total hip replacement. *Clin Orthop Relat Res* 1976;121:92-94.
68. Lachiewicz PF, Paterno SA: Dislocation of total hip replacements: Causes, prevention, and outcome of treatment. *Complications Orthop* 1996; 3:14-18.
69. Lewinnek GE, Lewis JL, Tarr R, Compere C, Zimmerman J: Dislocations after total hip replacement arthroplasties. *J Bone Joint Surg Am* 1978;60:217-220.
70. Robinson RP, Robinson HJ Jr, Salvati EA: Comparison of the transtrochanteric and posterior approaches for total hip replacement. *Clin Orthop Relat Res* 1980;147:143-147.
71. Khatod M, Barber T, Paxton E, Namba R, Rithian D: An analysis of the risk of hip dislocation with a contemporary total joint registry. *Clin Orthop Relat Res* 2006;447:19-23.
72. Meek RM, Allan DB, McPhillips G, Kerr L, Howie CR: Epidemiology of dislocation after total hip arthroplasty. *Clin Orthop Relat Res* 2006;447:9-18.
73. Morrey BF: Results of reoperation for hip dislocation: The big picture. *Clin Orthop Relat Res* 2004;429:94-101.
74. Phillips CB, Barrett JA, Losina E, et al: Incidence rates of dislocation, pulmonary embolism, and deep infection during the first six months after elective total hip replacement. *J Bone Joint Surg Am* 2003;85:20-26.
75. Ali Khan MA, Brakenbury PH, Reynolds IS: Dislocation following total hip replacement. *J Bone Joint Surg Br* 1981;63:214-218.
76. Lindberg HO, Carlsson AS, Gentz CF, Pettersson H: Recurrent and non-recurrent dislocation following total hip arthroplasty. *Acta Orthop Scand* 1982;53:947-952.
77. Kristiansen B, Jorgensen L, Holmich P: Dislocation following total hip arthroplasty. *Arch Orthop Trauma Surg* 1985;103:375-377.
78. Woo RYG, Morrey BF: Dislocations after total hip arthroplasty. *J Bone Joint Surg Am* 1982;64:1295-1306.
79. von Knoch M, Berry DJ, Harmsen WS, et al: Late dislocation after total hip arthroplasty. *J Bone Joint Surg Am* 2002;84:1949-1953.
80. Coventry MB: Late dislocations in patients with Charnley total hip arthroplasty. *J Bone Joint Surg Am* 1985; 67:832-841.
81. Daly PJ, Morrey BF: Operative correction of an unstable total hip arthroplasty. *J Bone Joint Surg Am* 1992;74: 1334-1343.
82. Fackler CD, Poss R: Dislocation in total hip arthroplasties. *Clin Orthop Relat Res* 1980;151:169-178.
83. Ekelund A, Rydell N, Nilsson OS: Total hip arthroplasty in patients 80 years of age and older. *Clin Orthop Relat Res* 1992;281:101-106.
84. Newington DP, Bannister GC, Fordyce M: Primary total hip replacement in patients over 80 years of age. *J Bone Joint Surg Br* 1990;72:450-452.
85. McCollum DE, Gray WJ: Dislocation after total hip arthroplasty: Causes and prevention. *Clin Orthop Relat Res* 1990;261:159-170.
86. Vicar AJ, Coleman CR: A comparison of the anterolateral, transtrochanteric, and posterior surgical approaches in primary total hip arthroplasty. *Clin Orthop Relat Res* 1984;188:152-159.
87. Berry DJ, von Knoch M, Schleck CD, Harmsen WS: Effect of femoral head diameter and operative approach on risk of dislocation after primary total hip arthroplasty. *J Bone Joint Surg Am* 2005;87:2456-2463.
88. Krushell RJ, Burke DW, Harris WH: Range of motion in contemporary total hip arthroplasty: The impact of modular head-neck component. *J Arthroplasty* 1991;6:97-101.
89. Peters CL, McPherson E, Jackson JD, Erickson JA: Reduction in early dislocation rate with large-diameter femoral heads in primary total hip arthroplasty. *J Arthroplasty* 2007;22(6 , suppl 2):140-144.
90. Amstutz HC, Le Duff MJ, Beaulé PE: Prevention and treatment of dislocation after total hip replacement using large diameter balls. *Clin Orthop Relat Res* 2004;429 :108-116.
91. Crowninshield RD, Maloney WJ, Wentz DH, et al: Biomechanics of large femoral heads: What they do and don't do. *Clin Orthop Relat Res* 2004;429 :102-107.
92. Burroughs BR, Hallstrom B, Golladay GJ, et al: Range of motion and stability in total hip arthroplasty with 28-, 32-, 38-, and 44-mm femoral head sizes. *J Arthroplasty* 2005;20: 11-19.
93. Bartz RL, Nobel PC, Kadakia NR, Tullos HS: The effect of femoral component head size on posterior dislocation of the artificial hip joint. *J Bone Joint Surg Am* 2000;82: 1300-1307.
94. Cobb TK, Morrey BF, Ilstrup DM: The elevated-rim acetabular liner in total hip arthroplasty: Relationship to postoperative dislocation. *J Bone Joint Surg Am* 1996;78:80-86.
95. Lawton RL, Morrey BF: Dislocation after long-necked total hip arthro-

plasty. *Clin Orthop Relat Res* 2004;422: 164-166.

96. Turner RS: Postoperative total hip prosthetic femoral head dislocations: Incidence, etiologic factors, and management. *Clin Orthop Relat Res* 1994; 301:196-204.

97. Grigoris P, Grecula MJ, Amstutz HC: Dislocation of a total hip arthroplasty caused by iliopsoas tendon displacement. *Clin Orthop Relat Res* 1994;306: 132-135.

98. Vakili F, Salvati EA, Warren RF: Entrapped foreign body within the acetabular cup in total hip replacement. *Clin Orthop Relat Res* 1980;150: 159-162.

99. Clayton ML, Thirupathi RG: Dislocation following total hip arthroplasty: Management by special brace in selected patients. *Clin Orthop Relat Res* 1983;177:154-159.

100. Mallory TH, Vaughn BK, Lombardi AV Jr, et al: Prophylactic use of a hip cast-brace following primary and revision total hip arthroplasty. *Orthop Rev* 1988;17:178-183.

101. Dewal H, Maurer SL, Tsai P, Su E, Hiebert R, Di Cesare PE: Efficacy of abduction bracing in the management of total hip arthroplasty dislocation. *J Arthroplasty* 2004;19:733-738.

102. Williams JF, Gottesman MJ, Mallory TH: Dislocation after total hip arthroplasty: Treatment with an above-knee hip spica cast. *Clin Orthop Relat Res* 1982;171:53-58.

103. Daly PJ, Morrey BF: Operative correction of an unstable total hip arthroplasty. *J Bone Joint Surg Am* 1992;74: 1334-1343.

104. Kaplan SJ, Thomas WH, Poss R: Trochanteric advancement for recurrent dislocation after total hip arthroplasty. *J Arthroplasty* 1987;2:119-124.

105. Beaulé PE, Schmalzried TP, Udomkiat P, et al: Jumbo femoral head for the treatment of recurrent dislocation following total hip replacement. *J Bone Joint Surg Am* 2002;84:256-263.

106. Berend KR, Lombardi AV Jr , Mallory TH, et al: The long-term outcome of 755 consecutive constrained acetabular components in total hip arthroplasty examining the successes and failures. *J Arthroplasty* 2005;20(7, suppl 3):93-102.

107. Su EP, Pellicci PM: The role of constrained liners in total hip arthroplasty. *Clin Orthop Relat Res* 2004;420: 122-129.

108. Bremner BR, Goetz DD, Callaghan JJ , et al: Use of constrained acetabular components for hip instability: An average 10-year follow-up study. *J Arthroplasty* 2003;18(7, suppl 1):131-137.

109. Daltroy LH, Morlino CI, Eaton HM, Poss R, Liang MH: Preoperative education for total hip and knee replacement patients. *Arthritis Care Res* 1998; 11:469-478.

110. Lin PC, Lin LC, Lin JJ : Comparing the effectiveness of different educational programs for patients with total knee arthroplasty. *Orthop Nurs* 1997; 16:43-49.

111. Pour AE, Parvizi J, Sharkey PF, Hozack WJ, Rothman RH: Minimally invasive hip arthroplasty: What role does patient preconditioning play? *J Bone Joint Surg Am* 2007;89:1920-1927.

112. Dorr LD, Thomas D, Long WT, Polatin PB, Sirianni LE: Psychologic reasons for patients preferring minimally invasive total hip arthroplasty. *Clin Orthop Relat Res* 2007;458: 94-100.

113. Buckenmaier CC III, Xenos JS, Nilsen SM: Lumbar plexus block with perineural catheter and sciatic nerve block for total hip arthroplasty. *J Arthroplasty* 2002;17:499-502.

114. Hebl JR, Kopp SL, Ali MH, et al: A comprehensive anesthesia protocol that emphasizes peripheral nerve blockade for total knee and total hip arthroplasty. *J Bone Joint Surg Am* 2005;87:63-70.

115. Horlocker TT, Kopp SL, Pagnano MW, Hebl JR: Analgesia for total hip and knee arthroplasty: A multimodal pathway featuring peripheral nerve block. *J Am Acad Orthop Surg* 2006;14: 126-135.

116. Pagnano MW, Hebl J, Horlocker T: Assuring a painless total hip arthroplasty: A multimodal approach emphasizing peripheral nerve blocks. *J Arthroplasty* 2006;21:80-84.

117. Skinner HB, Shitani EY: Results of a multimodal analgesic trial involving patients with total hip or total knee arthroplasty. *Am J Orthop* 2004;33: 85-92.

118. Viscusi ER, Parvizi J, Tarity TD : Developments in spinal and epidural anesthesia and nerve blocks for total joint arthroplasty: What is new and exciting in pain management. *Instr Course Lect* 2007;56:139-145.

119. Aida S, Fujihara H, Taga K, Fukuda S, Shimoji K: Involvement of presurgical pain in preemptive analgesia for orthopedic surgery: A randomized double blind study. *Pain* 2000;84: 169-173.

120. Buvanendran A, Kroin JS, Tuman KJ, et al: Effects of perioperative administration of a selective cyclooxygenase 2 inhibitor on pain management and recovery of function after knee replacement: A randomized controlled trial. *JAMA* 2003;290:2411-2418.

121. Mallory TH, Lombardi AV Jr, Fada RA, Dodds KL, Adams JB: Pain management for joint arthroplasty: Preemptive analgesia. *J Arthroplasty* 2002; 17(4, suppl 1):129-133.

122. Wall PD: The prevention of postoperative pain. *Pain* 1988;33:289-290.

123. Bottner F, Zawadsky M, Su EP, et al: Implant migration after early weight bearing in cementless hip replacement. *Clin Orthop Relat Res* 2005;436: 132-137.

124. Rao RR, Sharkey PF, Hozack WJ, Eng K, Rothman RH: Immediate weightbearing after uncemented total hip arthroplasty. *Clin Orthop Relat Res* 1998;349:156-162.

125. Strom H, Nilsson O, Milbrink J, Mallmin H, Larsson S: Early migration pattern of the uncemented CLS stem in total hip arthroplasties. *Clin Orthop Relat Res* 2007;454:127-132.

126. Woolson ST, Adler NS: The effect of partial or full weight bearing ambulation after cementless total hip arthroplasty. *J Arthroplasty* 2002;17:820-825.

127. Peak EL, Parvizi J, Ciminiello M, et al: The role of patient restrictions in reducing the prevalence of early dislocation following total hip arthroplasty: A randomized, prospective study. *J Bone Joint Surg Am* 2005;87: 247-253.

128. Talbot NJ, Brown JH, Treble NJ: Early dislocation after total hip arthroplasty: Are postoperative restrictions necessary? *J Arthroplasty* 2002;17: 1006-1008.

129. Paterno SA, Lachiewicz PF, Kelley SS: The influence of patient-related factors and the position of the acetabular component on the rate of dislocation after total hip replacement. *J Bone Joint Surg Am* 1997;79: 1202-1210.

130. Morrey BF: Difficult complications after hip joint replacement. *Clin Orthop Relat Res* 1997;344:179-187.

131. Katz JN, Losina E, Barrett J, et al: Association between hospital and surgeon procedure volume and outcomes of total hip replacement in the United States Medicare population. *J Bone Joint Surg Am* 2001;83: 1622-1629.

132. Howie C, Hughes H, Watts AC: Venous thomboembolism associated with hip and knee replacement over a ten-year period: A population-based study. *J Bone Joint Surg Br* 2005;87: 1675-1680.

133. Geerts WH, Pineo GF, Heit JA , et al: Prevention of venous thromboembolism: The Seventh ACCP Conference on Antithrombotic and Thrombolytic Therapy. *Chest* 2004;126: 338S-400S.

134. American Academy of Orthopaedic Surgeons: Clinical Guideline on Prevention of Symptomatic Pulmonary Embolism in Patients Undergoing Total Hip or Knee Arthroplasty. http://www.aaos.org/Research/guidelines/PE_guideline.pdf. Accessed October 29, 2008.

Primary Total Hip Arthroplasty: Intraoperative Decisions and Surgical Techniques

*Douglas A. Dennis, MD
Raymond H. Kim, MD
*Thomas S. Thornhill, MD
*Robert T. Trousdale, MD

Abstract

Intraoperative decisions and surgical techniques are important factors in the success of a total hip arthroplasty. Each of the available surgical exposures has advantages and disadvantages. Reproducing accurate leg length and precisely implanting the acetabular and femoral components also are critical.

Several surgical approaches can be used for primary total hip arthroplasty (THA), and surgeons should be familiar with the technique for each exposure as well as its advantages and disadvantages.

Anterolateral Approach

The anterolateral approach is commonly used for primary or revision THA. The acetabular exposure is excellent, and the sciatic nerve can be avoided.[1-4] In addition, the anterolateral exposure offers a lower risk of postoperative dislocation than a posterior approach. However, the abductor musculature must be violated, and proximal abductor muscle splitting carries a risk of superior gluteal nerve injury. The incidence of heterotopic ossification is greater than with a posterior approach.[5,6]

The skin incision is centered over the greater trochanter, extending distally in line with the femur and proximally either in a straight line or slightly curved posteriorly. The tensor fascia lata is divided along the length of the incision. The gluteus medius is identified, and the anterior third of the muscle is elevated anteriorly, leaving a tendinous cuff for later repair (Figure 1). The proximal split of the gluteus medius should not extend beyond 5 cm to avoid superior gluteal nerve injury. The gluteus minimus is identified, released, and preserved for later repair. An anterior capsulotomy can then be performed to allow access to the hip joint.

After implantation of the components, the abductor mechanism should be repaired, either tendon to tendon (if a cuff of abductor tendon was preserved) or tendon to bone (using nonabsorbable suture through drill holes in the greater trochanter).

Direct Lateral Approach

The direct lateral approach is a variant of the anterolateral approach. The incision is made into the anterior portion of the gluteus medius. The anterior aspect of the vastus lateralis is elevated distally while maintaining fascial continuity.[7] The advantages of the direct lateral approach are similar to those of the anterolateral approach: excellent acetabular exposure, avoidance of the sciatic nerve, and a decreased risk of postoperative dislocation. The

Douglas A. Dennis, MD or the department with which he is affiliated has received research or institutional support from DePuy, Zimmer, and Ceramtec, has received royalties from DePuy, and is a consultant for or an employee of DePuy. Thomas S. Thornhill, MD or the department with which he is affiliated has received research or institutional support from DePuy, Biomet, and Smith & Nephew and royalties from DePuy. Robert T. Trousdale, MD or the department with which he is affiliated has received royalties from DePuy and Wright Medical.

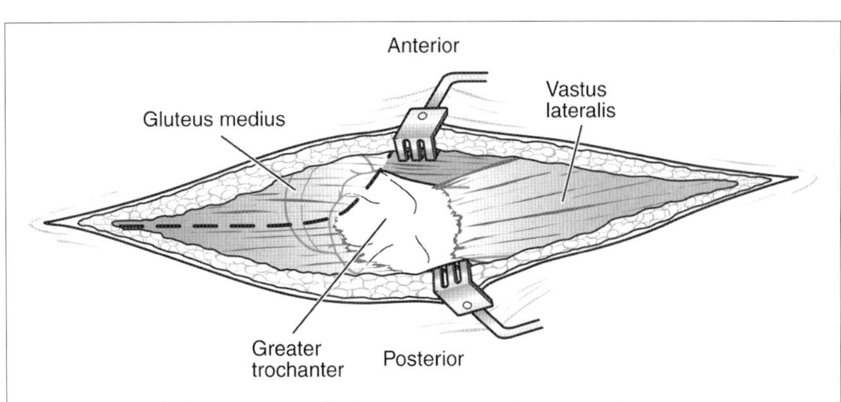

Figure 1 Schematic diagram of the anterolateral approach showing the gluteal muscle incision and the elevation required to expose the hip capsule.

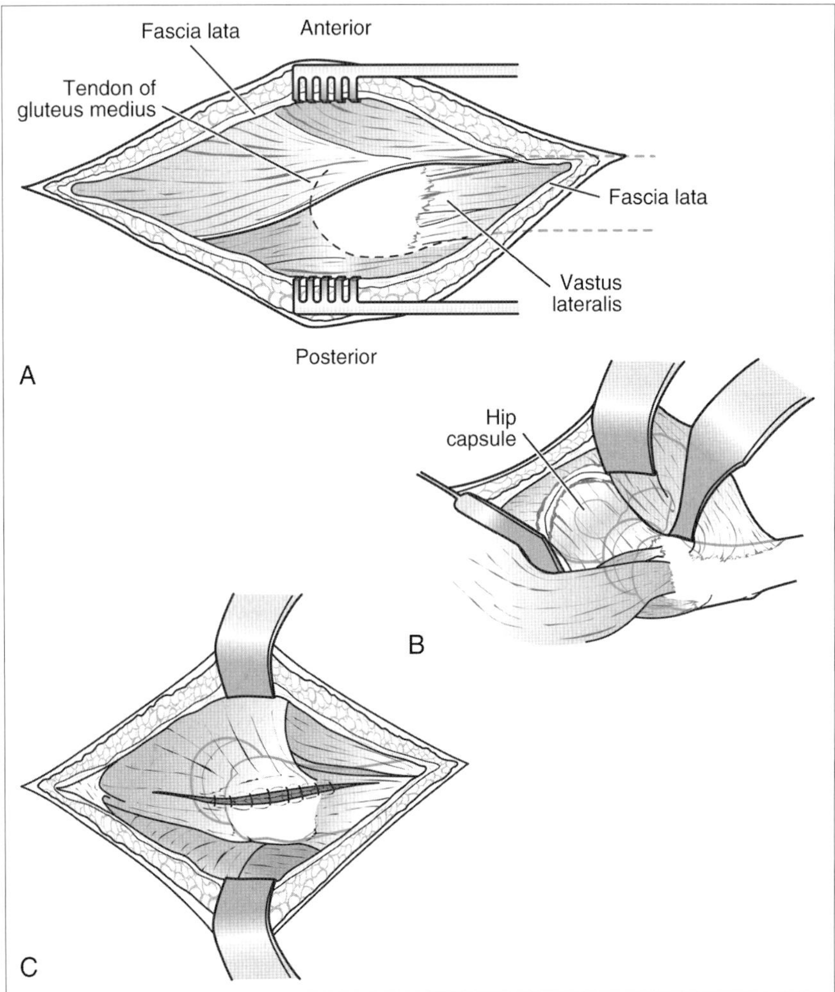

Figure 2 Schematic diagram of the direct lateral approach. **A,** Elevation of the anterior third of the gluteus medius and anterior aspect of the vastus lateralis. **B,** Exposure of the hip joint. **C**, Abductor repair.

disadvantages include the need for incision of the abductor musculature, the risk of superior gluteal nerve injury with proximal muscle splitting, and the risk of postoperative heterotopic ossification.[2,8,9]

The skin incision is centered over the greater trochanter, as in the anterolateral approach. The tensor fascia lata is divided along the length of the incision. The gluteus medius is identified, and the anterior third of the muscle is dissected from the greater trochanter anteriorly, leaving a tendinous cuff for later repair (Figure 2, *A*). The exposure continues distally with elevation of the anterior aspect of the vastus lateralis distal to the trochanter (Figure 2, *B*). The fascial continuity of the abductor musculature and vastus lateralis is maintained. An anterior capsulotomy can be done to allow access into the hip joint. The abductor is repaired to the cuff of tendon preserved during the exposure (Figure 2, *C*).

Posterolateral Approach

The posterolateral approach also is commonly used for primary and revision THA.[10] Its advantages, in comparison with the anterolateral and direct lateral approaches, include less abductor muscle damage, less severe early postoperative limping, and a lower incidence of heterotopic ossification. The disadvantages include a greater risk of dislocation.[2] The rate of dislocation was 4% to 9.5% when a posterior approach was used without repair of the posterior capsule and external rotators; however, rates as low as 0.4% have been reported when the posterior capsule and external rotators were repaired.[2,11-14] In contrast, the reported rates of dislocation are 0.7% to 2.2% when an anterolateral approach was used and 0.4% to 2.2%

when a direct lateral approach was used.[4,11]

The skin incision is made longitudinally and centered over the greater trochanter. The proximal portion of the incision can be gently curved posteriorly. The tensor fascia lata and gluteus maximus muscle are then divided along the length of the incision. With the hip internally rotated, the short external rotator muscles can be identified and released at their insertion onto the greater trochanter; they are preserved for later repair (Figure 3, *A*). The posterior capsule is identified, and a capsulotomy is done from the posterosuperior acetabulum toward the greater trochanter and distally along the posterior aspect of the greater trochanter (Figure 3, *B*). The capsule should be preserved for later repair. The hip can then be dislocated posteriorly for access to the joint (Figure 3, *C*). After the prosthesis is implanted, the posterior capsule and short external rotators are repaired through drill holes into the greater trochanter, using nonabsorbable suture.

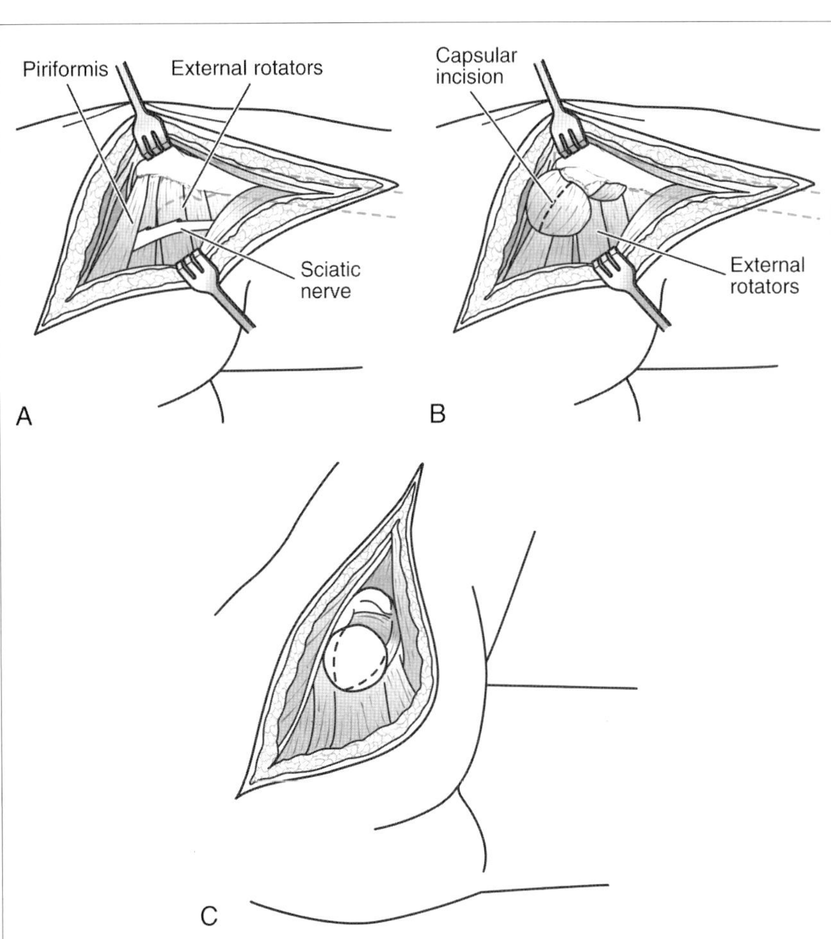

Figure 3 Schematic diagram of the posterolateral approach. **A,** Exposure of the piriformis and external rotators. **B,** Capsular incision. **C,** The exposed hip joint after dislocation.

Other Surgical Approaches

Anterior, transtrochanteric, and various minimally invasive approaches have been described for primary THA. The anterior approach also has been used for several other hip procedures.[15-21] Its advantages include preservation of the abductor mechanism and a low rate of postoperative dislocation (0.61%).[19] The disadvantages include an increased risk of femoral cutaneous nerve injury and difficulty in obtaining access to the proximal femur for implantation of the femoral component; the use of a specialized operating table often is required. Matta and associates[19] described the use of an anterior approach with the patient positioned supine on a PROfx table (Orthopaedic Systems, Union City, CA). A longitudinal skin incision is made 2 cm posterior and 1 cm distal to the anterosuperior iliac spine to a point 2 cm anterior to the greater trochanter. The tensor fascia lata is divided along the length of the incision. Deep to the fascial layer, the interval between the tensor and sartorius muscles is bluntly created to protect the lateral femoral cutaneous nerve. Medial and lateral retractors can be placed to expose the hip capsule, and the reflected head of the rectus femoris can be elevated to facilitate exposure. A capsulotomy is performed to allow access to the hip joint. Using traction and external rotation, the hip is dislocated anteriorly; if the bone is osteoporotic, undue force must be avoided to minimize the risk of fracture. The femoral exposure for stem preparation is accomplished by hyperextension, adduction, and external rotation of the hip (Figure 4).

Although the transtrochanteric approach is used primarily for revision procedures, it can be valuable for a primary THA if the patient has severe acetabuli protrusio, an anatomic distortion of the proximal femur or acetabulum, or an unstable hip in which

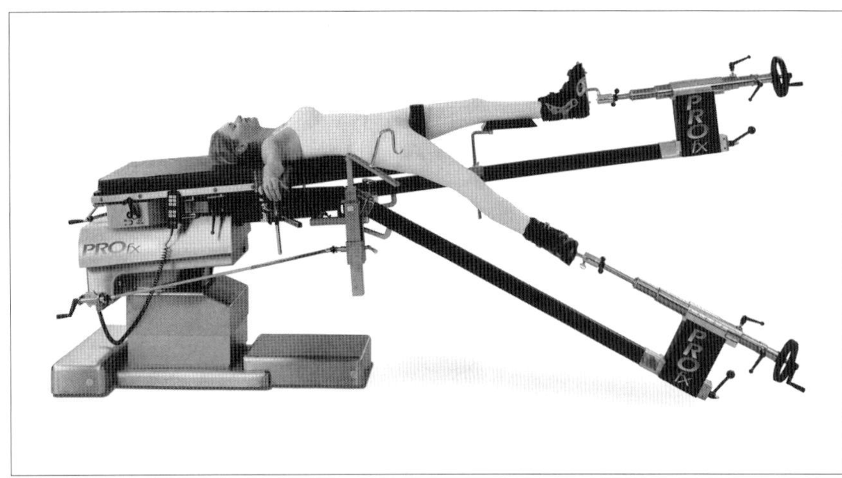

Figure 4 Photograph showing the placement of a patient on the operating table when the anterior approach is used, with the hip hyperextended and externally rotated for implantation of the femoral component.

the trochanter can be advanced to enhance stability. The advantage is extensile exposure of both the acetabulum and femur. The primary disadvantage is the risk of trochanteric nonunion. Several methods of trochanteric reattachment have been described, typically using wire, cables, or trochanteric clamps.

Several minimally invasive surgical approaches have been described, including a two-incision anterior approach and small-incision variants of the anterior, anterolateral, direct lateral, and posterolateral exposures.[22,23] Early studies of the two-incision approach reported rapid rehabilitation and excellent outcomes.[24-26] More recent studies criticized the two-incision technique because of the significant learning curve required and early complications, including fracture and component malposition.[27-30] Anatomic studies found that the two-incision approach caused greater damage to the abductor muscle than the miniposterior approach.[31] A study of patients who underwent a miniposterior THA on one hip and a two-incision THA on the other hip found that the patients were more satisfied with the miniposterior procedure.[32] Minimally invasive surgical techniques typically are more difficult than standard, more extensile exposures. A minimally invasive technique should be used only if an adequate exposure can be created without unnecessary soft-tissue damage, the fixation will be equivalent to that achieved using a standard exposure, and complications such as component malpositioning or fracture can be avoided.

Leg Length Assessment

After THA, patients frequently report that the surgical leg is longer than the contralateral leg. Many factors affect both true and perceived leg length, and it is essential that the surgeon evaluate leg length both preoperatively and intraoperatively. The surgical leg frequently is shorter than the contralateral leg because of arthritic degeneration of the hip joint. A discrepancy in the relative length of the legs also may be the result of an earlier fracture, a varus or valgus knee deformity, a history of growth arrest, or another condition. The legs may appear to differ in length because of scoliosis or a long-standing pelvic obliquity in compensation for a shortened arthritic extremity. A false limb-length discrepancy also can exist if fixed soft-tissue contractures are present about the hip; a fixed abduction contracture typically causes the leg to appear longer than it actually is, and a fixed adduction contracture creates the appearance of a shorter leg. Preoperative templating of hip radiographs is essential in determining true leg length; the surgeon must choose a component that reproduces the offset and has sufficient femoral neck length to accommodate soft-tissue tension.

Leg length is related to hip stability. Lengthening the surgical leg can decrease impingement, increase soft-tissue tension, and increase stability; however, overlengthening the leg to achieve stability is problematic because it may result in nerve injury, a postoperative limp, lumbar pain, patient dissatisfaction, and possible litigation. Shortening the leg risks creating hip instability and may require overresection of the femoral neck and advancement of the greater trochanter, both of which add to the complexity of the procedure.

The surgical approach may determine the best method of assessing leg length during surgery. Any intraoperative change in leg length can be detected by measuring the distance between fixed points on the pelvis and the proximal femur before and after insertion of the trial components. The measurement can start from a fixed anatomic point or a screw or pin placed in a specific position. Many devices are available to ensure that the proper leg length is maintained during surgery, and computer navigation can be extremely helpful in estimating leg length. The intraoperative determination of leg length also can be affected by the method of anesthesia because stability is estimated based on soft-tissue tension. The extent of muscle relaxation varies depending on whether general or regional anesthesia is used. Greater relaxation is obtained with regional anesthesia unless specific motor paralytic agents are administered in addition to general anesthesia.

Most surgeons recommend that a preoperative physical examination, preoperative templating of hip radiographs, and intraoperative observation should be used in combination to obtain proper leg length. With a routine muscle-sparing posterolateral approach, the femoral head should sit approximately at the lip of the lateral rim of the acetabulum when the hip is dislocated, the trial components are in place, the hip is internally rotated to 90°, and no retractors are in position (Figure 5). A femoral head that sits significantly proximal to the lip often indicates that the leg is too long or the soft-tissue tension is too great. If the femoral head lies below the lip, the soft-tissue tension usually is inadequate. When the hip is reduced, the leg is carried through a range of motion, and soft-tissue tension is estimated by longitudinal traction on the located and extended femur. This qualitative determination provides a rough estimate of the abductor muscle tension. As a general rule, achieving good hip stability with a slight increase in soft-tissue laxity is preferable to excessive lengthening the leg. Any difference between the preoperative template and intraoperative anatomy should be recognized, and intraoperative radiographs should be obtained if the difference is substantial.

Acetabular Component Implantation

Determination of proper leg length, prevention of dislocation, and accurate acetabular component positioning are interrelated aspects that are critical for a successful THA. The correct anatomic position of the acetabular component is related to the patient's anatomy, the surgical approach, and the relative anteversion of the femoral component. To determine the position of the acetabular component, the surgeon must visualize the acetabulum in all planes and with specific reference to both its adduction or verticality and its forward flexion to the midcoronal plane. The sum of the acetabular forward flexion (anteversion) and the femoral anteversion should be approximately 45° in men and 40° in women when a standard posterolateral approach is used. This sum can be slightly lower when an anterolateral approach is used because of the low risk of posterior dislocation.

Proper positioning of the acetabular component can be ensured in several ways. If the patient is thin, it is relatively easy to orient the pelvis to the operating table and operating room and to build the abduction and forward flexion from this position. Many systems are available for securing the pelvis during the procedure. The patient is placed onto the nonsurgical side, and the pelvis is secured anteriorly by the pubic symphysis and posteriorly at the sacrum. To accommodate a male patient's typically greater shoulder width, a slight Trendelenburg position may be required to place the spine and pelvis parallel to the floor. Some female patients require placement in a slight reverse Trendelenburg position to obtain this alignment. If the patient is obese, it may be difficult to gain purchase on the bony pelvis, and anatomic landmarks or intraoperative radiographs must be relied on to assist in proper component positioning.

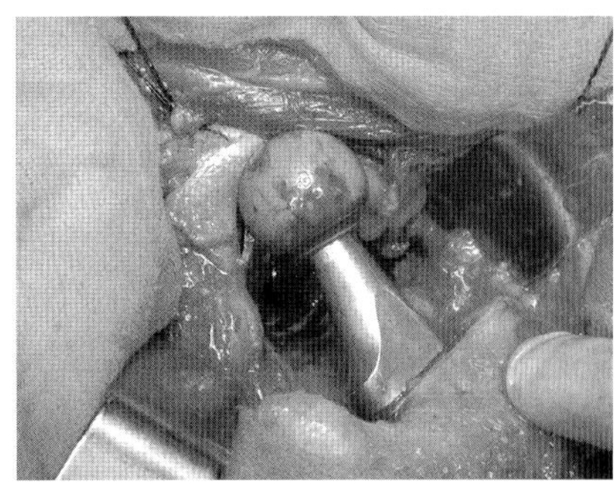

Figure 5 Intraoperative photograph of the posterolateral exposure showing the proper position of the trial femoral head component in relationship to the lateral lip of the acetabulum just before trial reduction.

After the acetabulum is exposed, it is important to remove the labrum and any portion of the capsule that may obscure the anterior or posterior walls, the lateral rim, or the transverse acetabular ligament. The typical arthritic hip has osteophytes that may obscure these anatomic landmarks; these must be removed to avoid malalignment or impingement. The osteoarthritic acetabulum tends to wear anteriorly and superiorly, and the anatomic position must be restored with the initial reaming so that firm purchase against the posterior wall can be obtained before the anterior wall becomes too thin to support the implant. Archbold and associates[33] found that the transverse acetabular ligament is a reproducible landmark that can guide proper orientation of the acetabular component; however, this landmark sometimes is obscured. If the patient has developmental dysplasia of the hip, there may be a significant anatomic variance that should be corrected rather than reproduced during surgery.

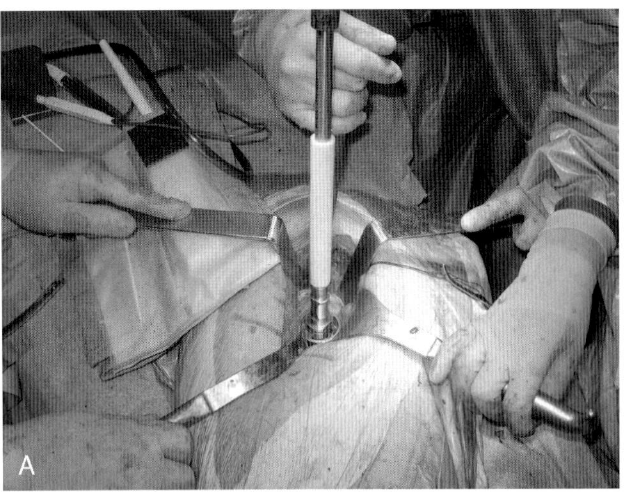

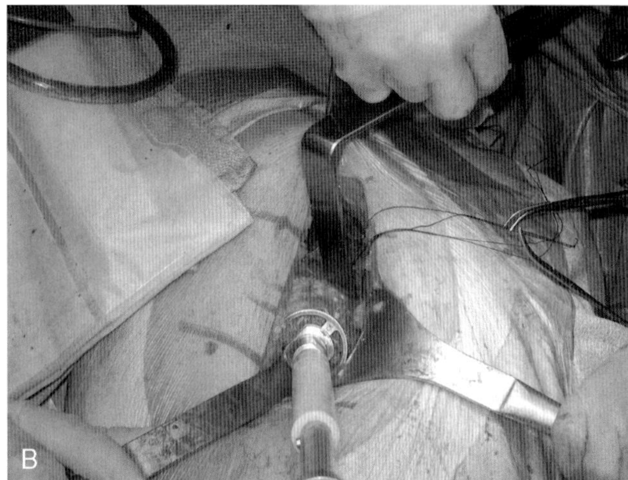

Figure 6 Intraoperative photographs showing acetabular reaming. **A,** The initial reaming is medial and just above the transverse acetabular ligament. **B,** Reaming is continued in the anatomic position until stability is obtained circumferentially, with most of the stability conferred by the posterior wall.

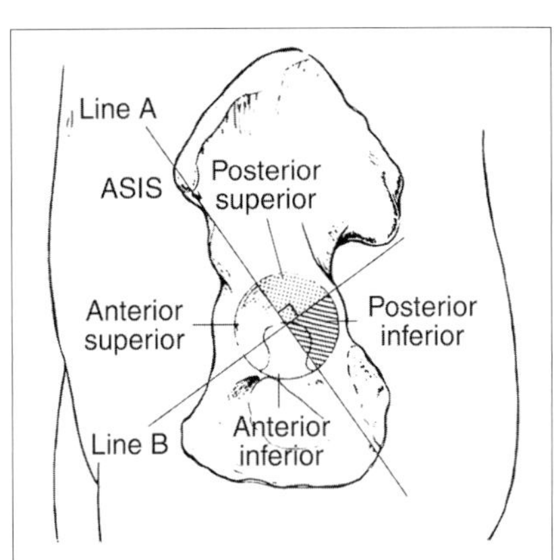

Figure 7 The acetabular quadrant system. The quadrants are formed by the intersection of lines A and B. Line A extends from the anterosuperior iliac spine (ASIS) through the center of the acetabulum to the posterior aspect of the fovea, dividing the acetabulum in half. Line B is drawn perpendicular to line A at the midpoint of the acetabulum, dividing it into four quadrants: the anterosuperior quadrant, the anteroinferior quadrant, the posterosuperior quadrant, and the posteroinferior quadrant. (Adapted with permission from Wasielewski RC, Cooperstein LA, Kruger MP, Rubash HE: Acetabular anatomy and the transacetabular fixation of screws in total hip arthroplasty. *J Bone Joint Surg Am* 1990; 72:501-508.)

The initial acetabular reaming should be directed medially and centered over the acetabular notch to prevent superoanterior reaming (Figure 6). It is important to remove the pulvinar before reaming so that the bottom of the notch (the medial wall of the pelvis) can be seen. At this point, the pelvis is reamed sequentially until anterior and posterior wall contact is achieved, as well as adequate osseous coverage. Most hip implant systems have attachments to the acetabular component inserter that are used to estimate the correct component position. The position is confirmed by palpation of anatomic landmarks, including the transverse acetabular ligament, and overall implant stability is tested with a trial reduction. If the position of the acetabular component is in question after implantation, it is wise to obtain an intraoperative radiograph. The use of computer navigation has facilitated accurate acetabular positioning. Fluoroscopy has been used with minimally invasive approaches to determine the correct positioning.[34]

The configuration and material properties of some types of implants require underreaming or line-to-line reaming. In a primary THA, the surgeon may choose not to use ancillary screw fixation or screw fixation directed into safe quadrants, avoiding anterior column screw placement[35] (Figure 7). The use of modular acetabular components allows the surgeon to choose among component liners that vary in material (polyethylene, metal, or ceramic) and geometry (neutral, lateralized, or extended lip). The selection of a modular liner is based on the intraoperative assessment of stability as well as the patient's age and activity level.

Femoral Component Implantation

All of the available types of femoral components (such as cemented, fully or proximally porous coated, or modular) have had satisfactory results.[36-39] Cementless implants are used for most femoral reconstructions in North America because they are easy to insert and have reliable results in patients of all ages. However, a cemented implant may be a better choice for a patient with extremely osteoporotic bone, if implant stability is of concern. Markedly distorted proximal anatomy requiring corrective osteotomy, as is found in a patient with developmental dysplasia, may be better treated with a modular implant or a fully porous-coated stem. A substantial number of primary THAs are done using a cementless tapered implant. The indications, preoperative templating, surgical technique, complications, and results of using a cementless tapered implant are discussed here.

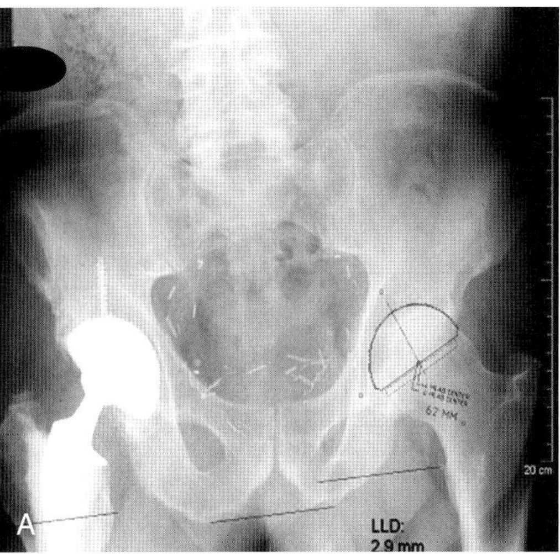

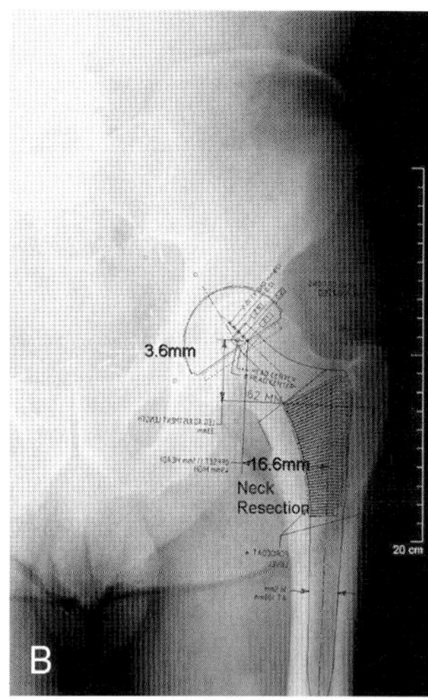

Figure 8 **A,** AP radiograph of the pelvis, with templating of an arthritic left hip. The planned hip center is marked, and the limb-length discrepancy (LLD) is documented. **B,** AP radiograph of the left hip, with the appropriate-size femoral component template placed in proper alignment and the level of neck resection determined.

Indications

The cementless tapered stem can be used for most patients who require THA. Durable fixation is likely in all bone types if the stem has a good ingrowth-ongrowth surface and the surgeon achieves implant stability.[40,41] A titanium stem with double or single tapering can provide excellent immediate axial and rotational stability. Circumferential, proximal porous coating, with or without hydroxyapatite, allows rapid bone ingrowth and protects the distal femur from osteolysis. There are pros and cons of using collared stems, but stems with or without a collar can be used successfully. Most available implants allow variable offset and neck length to accommodate the patient's anatomy.

Preoperative Templating

Preoperative templating is useful for estimating the size of the femoral component and facilitating surgical leg length restoration, proper offset, and component alignment. Good quality AP radiographs of the pelvis and femur are used to plan acetabular and femoral reconstruction (Figure 8). Leg length is measured at the hip, based on the relationship of the lesser trochanter to the transischial line, and this measurement is correlated with the clinically determined leg length. An appropriate-size femoral component template is placed on the radiograph to determine approximate fit and fill in neutral alignment and at a level to reproduce the leg length. The planned femoral neck resection is measured in millimeters above the lesser trochanter. The distance between the medial aspect of the implant and the calcar should be noted to obtain neutral alignment. The neck-shaft angle and offset of the prosthesis must be appropriate for restoring leg length and reproducing normal offset; the contralateral hip, if normal, is used for comparison.

It is important to remember that radiographic magnification and rotational factors can slightly distort the desired position of the femoral implant during templating. A marked discrepancy between the implant size selected based on the template and the size actually selected during surgery may indicate varus malpositioning of the femoral implant, undersizing of the femoral component, or an intraoperative fracture. The preoperative template can be correlated with an intraoperative radiograph to ensure that the leg length, offset, alignment, and hip center have been restored.

Surgical Technique

After surgical exposure and dislocation, the femoral head is resected above the lesser trochanter based on the preoperative template. The acetabulum is prepared, and either a trial component or the final component with a trial liner is placed. A retractor is placed under the proximal femur to elevate the femur out of the wound.

The canal is entered using a rongeur. The entry hole is typically placed in the posterolateral quadrant of the resected neck. Tapered reamers are then used to open the canal; the trajectory is directed toward the center of the knee in both the coronal and

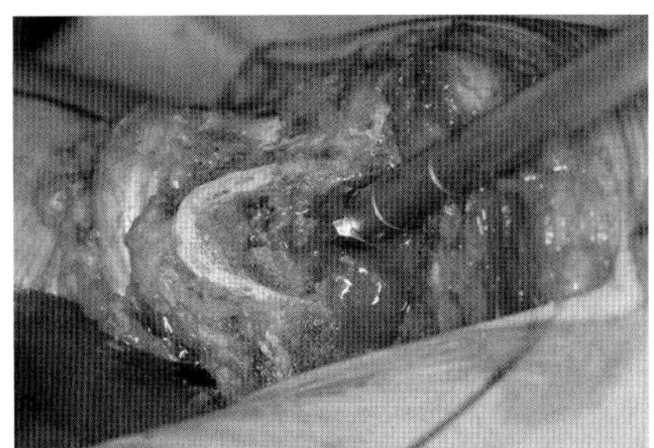

Figure 9 Intraoperative photograph showing a tapered reamer being passed down the medullary canal of the femur.

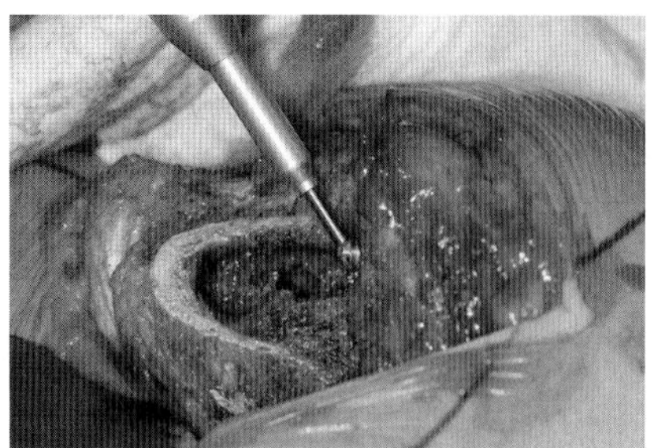

Figure 10 Intraoperative photograph showing a burr removing bone from the posterolateral aspect of the greater trochanter to ensure proper positioning of the femoral component.

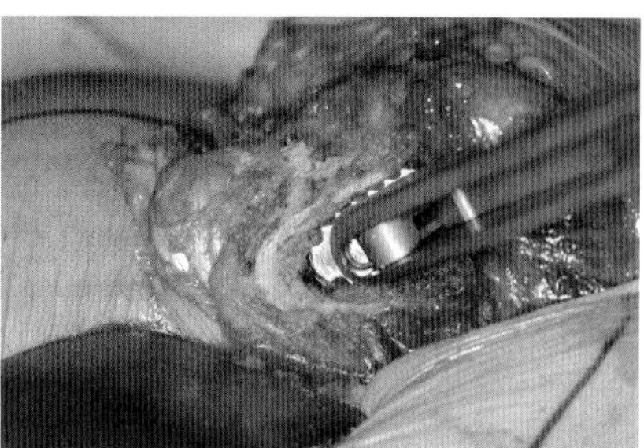

Figure 11 Intraoperative photograph showing placement of a broach to obtain a stable implant axially and rotationally.

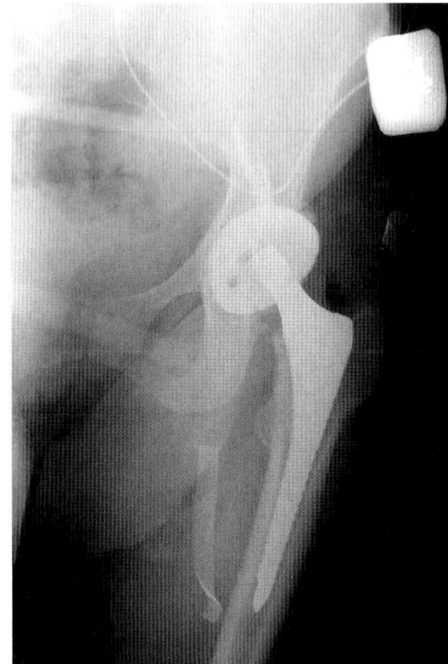

Figure 12 Intraoperative AP radiograph showing placement of the trial femoral component broach, neck, acetabular polyethylene, and femoral head.

sagittal planes. It is best to err laterally to avoid varus stem malposition. Power or hand reamers can be used; some surgeons prefer to prepare the canal by hand for better tactile feedback (Figure 9).

Broaches are used to contour the cancellous bone in the mediolateral and anteroposterior dimensions, in neutral axial alignment and 10° to 15° of femoral anteversion. A valgus thrust on the broach ensures good alignment. Occasionally a burr is used to remove the lateral bone to allow proper alignment of the broach (Figure 10). Anteversion should be kept constant, especially when contouring is almost complete. Broaches of increasing size are used until excellent axial and rotational stability is achieved (Figure 11).

A trial reduction is performed to assess leg length, stability, range of motion, and impingement of the hip joint. An intraoperative radiograph obtained with the broach in place can allow the surgeon to correct axial alignment, femoral sizing, and limb-length discrepancy with reference to the preoperative template, offset, and acetabular component position (Figure 12). The femoral head implant is selected based on intraoperative assessment of stability as well as the patient's age and activity level; implants are available in different materials (cobalt-chromium or ceramic) as well as different diameters. After successful trial reduction and final implant selection, the canal is cleaned of any debris, and the implant is inserted using multiple blows. A sudden change in the pitch or alignment of the implant may indicate an intraoperative fracture. If an intraoperative fracture is noticed, it is prudent to remove the implant, appropriately fix the fracture, reinsert the implant, and obtain an additional intraoperative radiograph. The trunnion is cleaned, and the final femoral head is impacted into place.

Postoperative Care

If the implant has good rotational and axial stability, most patients can bear weight on the extremity as tolerated. The use of bilateral crutches or a walker during the first 3 to 6 weeks after surgery is wise to protect against falling until the patient achieves adequate balance and a steady gait.

Complications and Results

The complications common to all types of THA can occur after a tapered femoral stem is used; they include infection, dislocation, deep venous thrombosis, and neurovascular conditions. Proximal femoral fracture may occur slightly more frequently during broaching or final stem insertion with a cementless tapered stem than with a cemented stem because tapered stems are placed with a relatively tight proximal fit.[42-45] A proximal longitudinal fracture is fixed with cerclage wire, and implant stability is ensured. Conversion to a procedure using a fully porous-coated stem may be necessary if the fracture is extensive.

Multiple centers have reported outstanding clinical and radiographic results in large series of patients, 10 to 15 years after THA using a cementless tapered stem.[46-54] Bone ingrowth is reliably obtained and appears to be quite durable.

Summary

The long-term success of primary THA requires a clear understanding of the technical aspects of the various surgical approaches available for the procedure. Accurate reproduction of leg length requires a preoperative physical examination and radiographic templating as well as intraoperative assessment. Precise surgical implantation of the acetabular and femoral components is necessary to ensure rigid fixation and avoid complications such as fracture, hip instability, and leg-length inequality.

References

1. Mallory TH, Lombardi AV Jr, Fada RA, Herrington SM, Eberle RW: Dislocation after total hip arthroplasty using the anterolateral abductor split approach. *Clin Orthop Relat Res* 1999;358:166-172.
2. Masonis JL, Bourne RB: Surgical approach, abductor function, and total hip arthroplasty dislocation. *Clin Orthop Relat Res* 2002;405:46-53.
3. Ritter MA, Harty LD, Keating ME, Faris PM, Meding JB: A clinical comparison of the anterolateral and posterolateral approaches to the hip. *Clin Orthop Relat Res* 2001;385:95-99.
4. Vicar AJ, Coleman CR: A comparison of the anterolateral, transtrochanteric, and posterior surgical approaches in primary total hip arthroplasty. *Clin Orthop Relat Res* 1984;188:152-159.
5. Bischoff R, Dunlap J, Carpenter L, DeMouy E, Barrack R: Heterotopic ossification following uncemented total hip arthroplasty: Effect of the operative approach. *J Arthroplasty* 1994;9:641-644.
6. Morrey BF, Adams RA, Cabanela ME: Comparison of heterotopic bone after anterolateral, transtrochanteric, and posterior approaches for total hip arthroplasty. *Clin Orthop Relat Res* 1984;188:160-167.
7. Hardinge K: The direct lateral approach to the hip. *J Bone Joint Surg Br* 1982;64:17-19.
8. Barber TC, Roger DJ, Goodman SB, Schurman DJ: Early outcome of total hip arthroplasty using the direct lateral versus the posterior surgical approach. *Orthopedics* 1996;19:873-875.
9. Moskal JT, Mann JW III: A modified direct lateral approach for primary and revision total hip arthroplasty: A prospective analysis of 453 cases. *J Arthroplasty* 1996;11:255-266.
10. Patiala H, Lehto K, Rokkanen P, Paavolainen P: Posterior approach for total hip arthroplasty: A study of postoperative course, early results and early complications in 131 cases. *Arch Orthop Trauma Surg* 1984;102:225-229.
11. Kwon MS, Kuskowski M, Mulhall KJ, Macaulay W, Brown TE, Saleh KJ: Does surgical approach affect total hip arthroplasty dislocation rates? *Clin Orthop Relat Res* 2006;447:34-38.
12. Pellicci PM, Bostrom M, Poss R: Posterior approach to total hip replacement using enhanced posterior soft tissue repair. *Clin Orthop Relat Res* 1998;355:224-228.
13. Weeden SH, Paprosky WG, Bowling JW: The early dislocation rate in primary total hip arthroplasty following the posterior approach with posterior soft tissue repair. *J Arthroplasty* 2003;18:709-713.
14. White RE Jr, Forness TJ, Allman JK, Junick DW: Effect of posterior capsular repair on early dislocation in primary total hip replacement. *Clin Orthop Relat Res* 2001;393:163-167.
15. Beaule PE, Griffin DB, Matta JM: The Levine anterior approach for total hip replacement as the treatment for an acute acetabular fracture. *J Orthop Trauma* 2004;18:623-629.
16. Judet J, Judet R: The use of an artificial femoral head for arthroplasty of the hip joint. *J Bone Joint Surg Br* 1950;32:166-173.
17. Judet R, Judet J: Technique and results with the acrylic femoral head prosthesis. *J Bone Joint Surg Br* 1952;34:173-180.
18. Light TR, Keggi KJ: Anterior approach to hip arthroplasty. *Clin Orthop Relat Res* 1980;152:255-260.
19. Matta JM, Shahrdar C, Ferguson T: Single-incision anterior approach for total hip arthroplasty on an orthopaedic table. *Clin Orthop Relat Res* 2005;441:115-124.
20. Siguier T, Siguier M, Bertrand B: Mini-incision anterior approach does not increase dislocation rate: A study of 1037 total hip replacements. *Clin Orthop Relat Res* 2004;426:164-173.
21. Siguier T, Siguier M, Judet T, Charnley G, Brumpt B: Partial resurfacing arthroplasty of the femoral head in avascular necrosis: Methods, indications, and results. *Clin Orthop Relat Res* 2001;386:85-92.
22. Bottner F, Delgado S, Sculco TP: Minimally invasive total hip replacement: The posterolateral approach. *Am J Orthop* 2006;35:218-224.
23. Toms A, Duncan CP: The limited incision, anterolateral, intermuscular technique for total hip arthroplasty. *Instr Course Lect* 2006;55:199-203.
24. Berger RA: The technique of minimally invasive total hip arthroplasty using the two-incision approach. *Instr Course Lect* 2004;53:149-155.
25. Berger RA: Total hip arthroplasty using the minimally invasive two-incision approach. *Clin Orthop Relat Res* 2003;417:232-241.
26. Berger RA, Duwelius PJ: The two-incision minimally invasive total hip arthroplasty: Technique and results. *Orthop Clin North Am* 2004;35:163-172.

27. Archibeck MJ, White RE Jr: Learning curve for the two-incision total hip replacement. *Clin Orthop Relat Res* 2004;429:232-238.

28. Bal BS, Haltom D, Aleto T, Barrett M: Early complications of primary total hip replacement performed with a two-incision minimally invasive technique. *J Bone Joint Surg Am* 2005;87:2432-2438.

29. Berry DJ, Berger RA, Callaghan JJ, et al: Minimally invasive total hip arthroplasty: Development, early results, and a critical analysis. *J Bone Joint Surg Am* 2003;85:2235-2246.

30. Pagnano MW, Leone J, Lewallen DG, Hanssen AD: Two-incision THA had modest outcomes and some substantial complications. *Clin Orthop Relat Res* 2005;441:86-90.

31. Mardones R, Pagnano MW, Nemanich TP, Trousdale RT: Muscle damage after total hip arthroplasty done with the two-incision and mini-posterior techniques. *Clin Orthop Relat Res* 2005;441:63-67.

32. Pagnano MW, Trousdale RT, Meneghini RM, Hanssen AD: Patients preferred a mini-posterior THA to a contralateral two-incision THA. *Clin Orthop Relat Res* 2006;453:156-159.

33. Archbold HA, Mockford B, Molloy D, McConway J, Ogonda L, Beverland D: The transverse acetabular ligament: An aid to orientation of the acetabular component during primary total hip replacement. A preliminary study of 1000 cases investigating postoperative stability. *J Bone Joint Surg Br* 2006;88:883-886.

34. Dorr LD, Malik A, Wan Z, Long WT, Harris M: Precision and bias of imageless computer navigation and surgeon estimates for acetabular component position. *Clin Orthop Relat Res* 2007;465:92-99.

35. Wasielewski RC, Cooperstein LA, Kruger MP, Rubash HE: Acetabular anatomy and the transacetabular fixation of screws in total hip arthroplasty. *J Bone Joint Surg Am* 1990;72:501-508.

36. Bobyn JD, Tanzer M, Krygier JJ, Dujovne AR, Brooks CE: Concerns with modularity in total hip arthroplasty. *Clin Orthop Relat Res* 1994;298:27-36.

37. Bourne RB, Rorabeck CH: Porous coated femoral fixation: The long and short of it! *Orthopedics* 2003;26:911-912.

38. Mulroy WF, Estok DM, Harris WH: Total hip arthroplasty with use of so-called second-generation cementing techniques: A fifteen-year-average follow-up study. *J Bone Joint Surg Am* 1995;77:1845-1852.

39. Smith SW, Estok DM II, Harris WH: Total hip arthroplasty with use of second-generation cementing techniques: An eighteen year average follow-up study. *J Bone Joint Surg Am* 1998;80:1632-1640.

40. Sharkey PF, Albert TJ, Hume EL, Rothman RH: Initial stability of a collarless wedge-shaped prosthesis in the femoral canal. *Semin Arthroplasty* 1990;1:87-90.

41. Keisu KS, Orozco F, Sharkey PF, Hozack WJ, Rothman RH, McGuigan FX: Primary cementless total hip arthroplasty in octogenarians: Two to eleven-year follow-up. *J Bone Joint Surg Am* 2001;83:359-363.

42. Fitzgerald RH Jr, Brindley GW, Kavanagh BF: The uncemented total hip arthroplasty: Intraoperative femoral fractures. *Clin Orthop Relat Res* 1988;235:61-66.

43. Parvizi J, Rapuri VR, Purtill JJ, Sharkey PF, Rothman RH, Hozack WJ: Treatment protocol for proximal femoral periprosthetic fractures. *J Bone Joint Surg Am* 2004;86(suppl 2):8-16.

44. Schwartz JT Jr, Mayer JG, Engh CA: Femoral fracture during non-cemented total hip arthroplasty. *J Bone Joint Surg Am* 1989;71:1135-1142.

45. Sharkey PF, Hozack WJ, Booth RE Jr, Rothman RH: Intraoperative femoral fractures in cementless total hip arthroplasty. *Orthop Rev* 1992;21:337-342.

46. Bourne RB, Rorabeck CH, Patterson JJ, Guerin J: Tapered titanium cementless total hip replacements: A 10 to 13-year follow-up study. *Clin Orthop Relat Res* 2001;393:112-120.

47. Burkart BC, Bourne RB, Rorabeck CH, Kirk PG: Thigh pain in cementless total hip arthroplasty: A comparison of two systems at 2 years' follow-up. *Orthop Clin North Am* 1993;24:645-653.

48. Garcia-Cimbrelo E, Cruz-Pardos A, Madero R, Ortega-Andreu M: Total hip arthroplasty with use of the cementless Zweymuller Alloclassic system: A 10 to 13 year follow-up study. *J Bone Joint Surg Am* 2003;85:296-303.

49. Hellman EJ, Capello WN, Feinberg JR: Omnifit cementless total hip arthroplasty: A 10-year average followup. *Clin Orthop Relat Res* 1999;364:164-174.

50. Martell JM, Pierson RH III, Jacobs JJ, Rosenberg AG, Maley M, Galante JO: Primary total hip reconstruction with a titanium fiber-coated prosthesis inserted without cement. *J Bone Joint Surg Am* 1993;75:554-571.

51. McLaughlin JR, Lee KR: Total hip arthroplasty with an uncemented femoral component: Excellent results at ten year follow-up. *J Bone Joint Surg Br* 1997;79:900-907.

52. Parvizi J, Keisu KS, Hozack WJ, Sharkey PF, Rothman RH: Primary total hip arthroplasty with an uncemented femoral component: A long-term study of the Taperloc stem. *J Arthroplasty* 2004;19:151-156.

53. Reitman RD, Emerson R, Higgins L, Head W: Thirteen year results of total hip arthroplasty using a tapered titanium femoral component inserted without cement in patients with type C bone. *J Arthroplasty* 2003;18:116-121.

54. Teloken MA, Bissett G, Hozack WJ, Sharkey PF, Rothman RH: Ten to fifteen year follow-up after total hip arthroplasty with a tapered cobalt-chromium femoral component (tri-lock) inserted without cement. *J Bone Joint Surg Am* 2002;84:2140-2144.

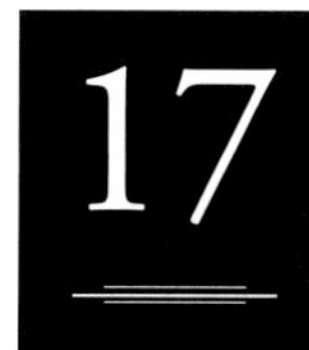

Achieving Stability and Lower Limb Length in Total Hip Arthroplasty

Keith R. Berend, MD
Scott M. Sporer, MD
Rafael J. Sierra, MD
Andrew H. Glassman, MD
Michael J. Morris, MD

Abstract

Total hip arthroplasty is an exceptionally cost-effective and successful surgical procedure. Dislocation, infection, osteolysis, and limb-length inequality are among the most common complications affecting the long-term success of total hip arthroplasty. Instability is a challenging complication to treat. The surgeon frequently must try to achieve a stable hip at the cost of increasing the length of the operated extremity. It is important to understand the factors associated with stability and limb length; the surgical options available; the effect and role of the various surgical approaches; and methods to manage instability, with and without limb-length inequality.

Total hip arthroplasty is an exceptionally cost-effective and successful surgical intervention.[1,2] Dislocation, infection, osteolysis, and limb-length inequality are among the most common complications affecting the long-term success of total hip arthroplasty.[2-8] Instability with dislocation is a complication that is costly to the patient, surgeon, and hospital.[9] The surgeon is frequently faced with the challenge of obtaining a stable hip at the cost of increasing the length of the lower extremity.[10] This chapter addresses the common issues that surround the achievement of both stability and limb-length equality with total hip arthroplasty. The preoperative patient education and factors associated with stability and limb length, the effect and role of various surgical approaches, the surgical techniques, and the management of instability with and without limb-length inequality are reviewed.

Instability

Dislocation rates are reported to be 0.3% to 10% after primary total hip arthroplasty and up to 28% after revision total hip arthroplasty. The incidence appears to be highest within the first year and rises at a rate of about 1% per 5 years to 7% at 25 years postoperatively.[11-21] A recent national database study reported that instability/dislocation was the most common diagnosis resulting in revision total hip arthroplasty in the United States.[3] There are patient-specific risk factors associated with in-

Dr. Berend or an immediate family member serves as a board member, owner, officer, or committee member of Mount Carmel New Albany Surgical Hospital and the American Association of Hip and Knee Surgeons Education Committee; has received royalties from Biomet; serves as a paid consultant to or is an employee of Biomet, Salient Surgical, and Synvasive; has received research or institutional support from Biomet; and owns stock or stock options in Angiotech. Dr. Sporer or an immediate family member is a member of a speakers' bureau or has made paid presentations on behalf of Zimmer; serves as a paid consultant to or is an employee of Zimmer; and has received research or institutional support from Zimmer. Dr. Sierra or an immediate family member is a member of a speakers' bureau or has made paid presentations on behalf of Biomet; serves as a paid consultant to or is an employee of Biomet; and has received research or institutional support from DePuy, Zimmer, and Stryker. Dr. Glassman or an immediate family member serves as a board member, owner, officer, or committee member of the Hip Society; has received royalties from Zimmer and Innomed; and owns stock or stock options in Stryker. Dr. Morris or an immediate family member has received research or institutional support from Biomet.

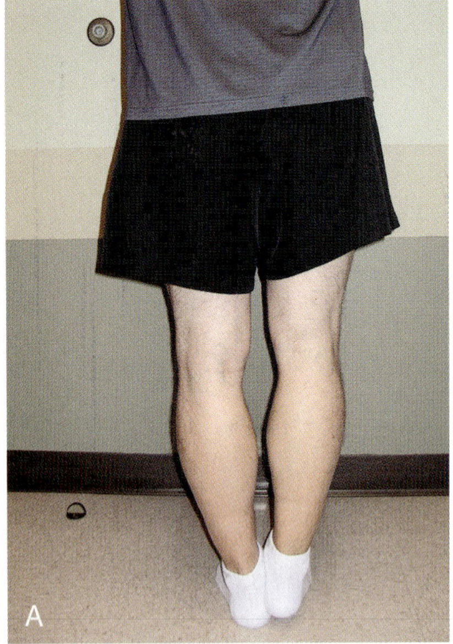

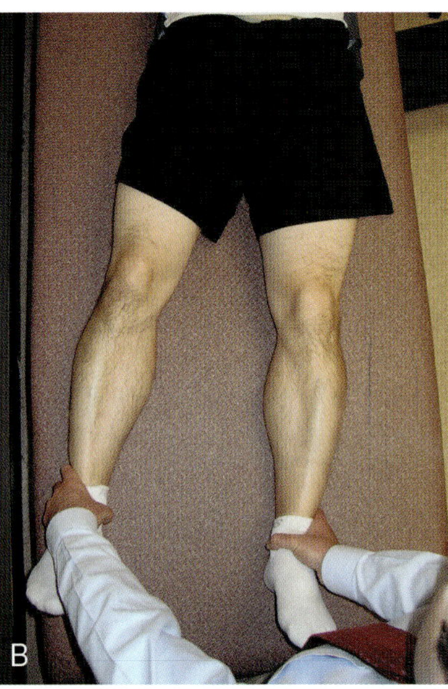

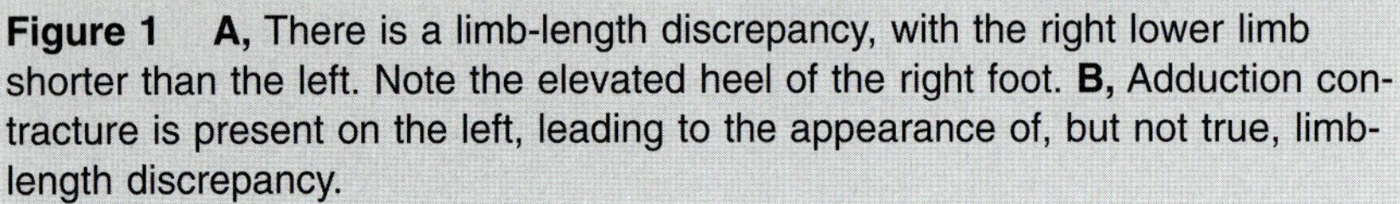

Figure 1 **A,** There is a limb-length discrepancy, with the right lower limb shorter than the left. Note the elevated heel of the right foot. **B,** Adduction contracture is present on the left, leading to the appearance of, but not true, limb-length discrepancy.

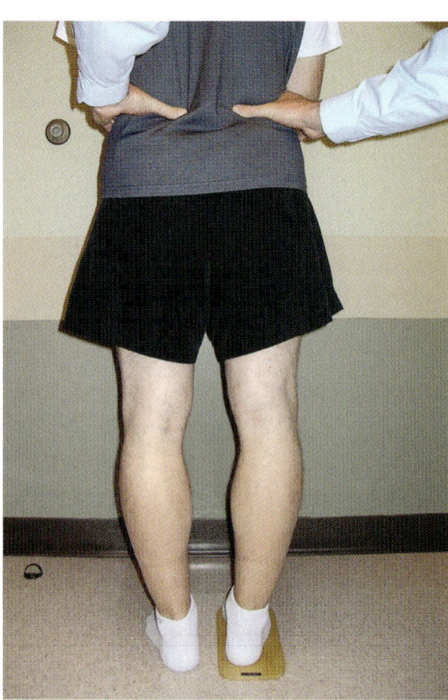

Figure 2 Standing evaluation of clinical limb length is performed by measuring the pelvic obliquity and limb-length difference. The examiner's hands palpate the superior iliac crests, and blocks are added under the short lower limb until the pelvis is level. The block height needed to level the pelvis is the limb-length difference.

stability, including female sex, increasing age, a diagnosis of osteonecrosis or femoral neck fracture, obesity, a high preoperative range of motion, and comorbidities.[5,13,15,22-33] There are variables under the surgeon's direct control, including the surgical approach, component position and orientation, femoral head size, restoration of offset, preservation of soft-tissue integrity, limb lengths, and prosthetic impingement. Surgeon experience is a variable, and the risk of instability is inversely related to the case volume of the operating surgeon.[5,13,15,30-32,34,35]

Preoperative Evaluation

Postoperative limb-length inequality and hip instability are common causes of litigation.[36-38] A thorough preoperative discussion establishes realistic patient expectations. A hierarchy of reconstruction goals should be outlined: first, well-fixed acetabular and femoral components; second, a dynamically stable construct; and third, equalization of limb lengths. The patient must understand and accept that lengthening of the lower limb may be required to achieve the first two goals.

A complete medical and surgical history should be obtained. Previous surgery on either extremity can create limb-length inequality that is not appreciated on a pelvic radiograph alone. Previous fracture, infection, physeal arrest, and various dysplasias may result in limb shortening. Abnormalities of the axial skeleton, such as prior spinal fusion, scoliosis, or neuromuscular disorders, or soft-tissue contractures associated with the hip or knee result in apparent limb-length discrepancy. The combination of "true" and "apparent" limb lengths contribute to the patient's subjective perception of limb-length inequality[39] (**Figure 1**).

Physical Examination

Observation of the patient's gait identifies pelvic obliquity, weak abductors, and dependence on assistive devices. The major muscles around the hip (abductors, adductors, and flexors) as well as the iliotibial band are assessed for contractures. The levels of the iliac crests are compared with the patient standing (**Figure 2**), and the thoracic and lumbar spine is assessed for coronal or sagittal deformity.

True limb length is determined by measuring the actual length of the extremity clinically or radiographically. The apparent limb length is determined by adding the effects of pelvic obliquity and soft-tissue contractures. Clinically, true limb length is measured from the anterior-superior iliac spine to the medial malleolus (**Figure 3**). Accurate identification of the osseous and anatomic landmarks can be difficult, especially in obese patients. A compensatory, flexible scoliosis may develop in the presence of a true limb-length inequality. The flexible deformities are corrected when a block is placed under the shorter extremity or when the patient sits. A

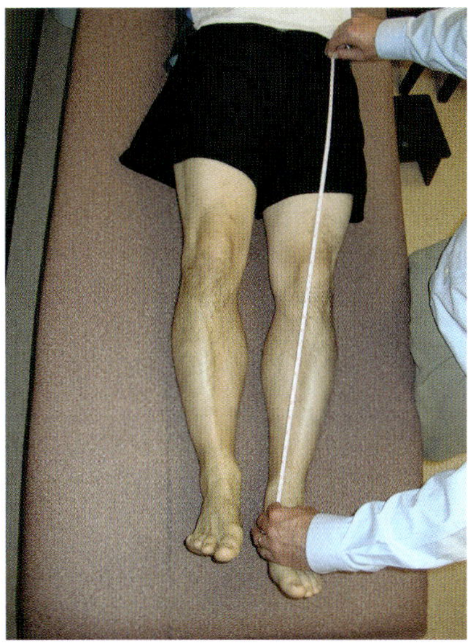

Figure 3 Supine evaluation of limb-length inequality is performed by measuring the distance between the anterior superior iliac spine and the medial malleolus with a tape measure.

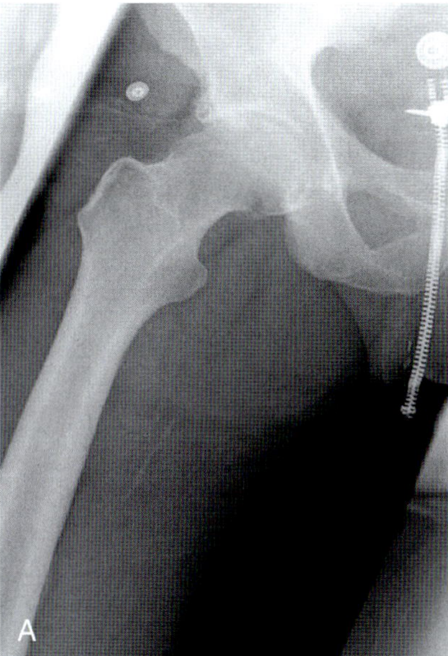

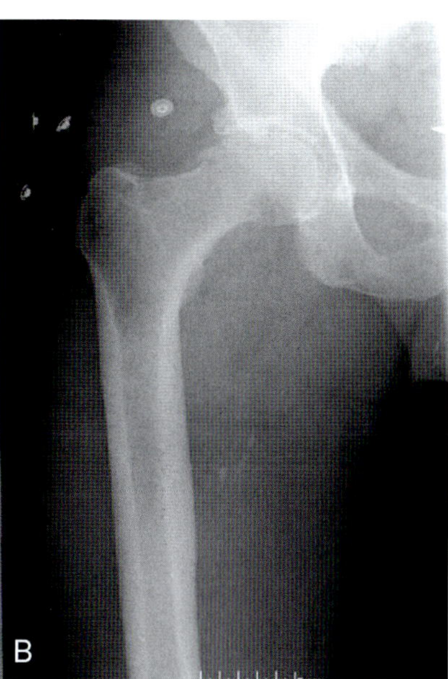

Figure 4 **A,** AP radiograph of a right femur in an externally rotated position. A false femoral offset is seen. **B,** AP radiograph of the same right femur with the hip in 20° of internal rotation. Note the marked femoral offset.

rigid coronal spinal deformity remains unchanged with these maneuvers.

Radiographic Assessment

Standing AP pelvic, AP femoral, and lateral femoral radiographs should be obtained. Because an arthritic hip frequently has an external rotation deformity, the AP pelvic and femoral radiographs should be made with the femur in 20° of internal rotation to avoid underestimation of femoral offset (**Figure 4**).

Preoperative radiographs provide an estimation of true limb-length inequality. A line drawn between the inferior aspects of the obturator foramina, ischia, or radiographic "teardrops" on a supine AP view of the pelvis is used as the pelvic reference. The distance between this line and a fixed point on the femur (the lesser or greater trochanter) can be compared with that of the contralateral hip. The difference between these two distances is the true limb-length inequality (**Figure 5**). This method is valid only if the limb lengths are equal below the chosen reference point and the two lower limbs are held in the same anatomic position.

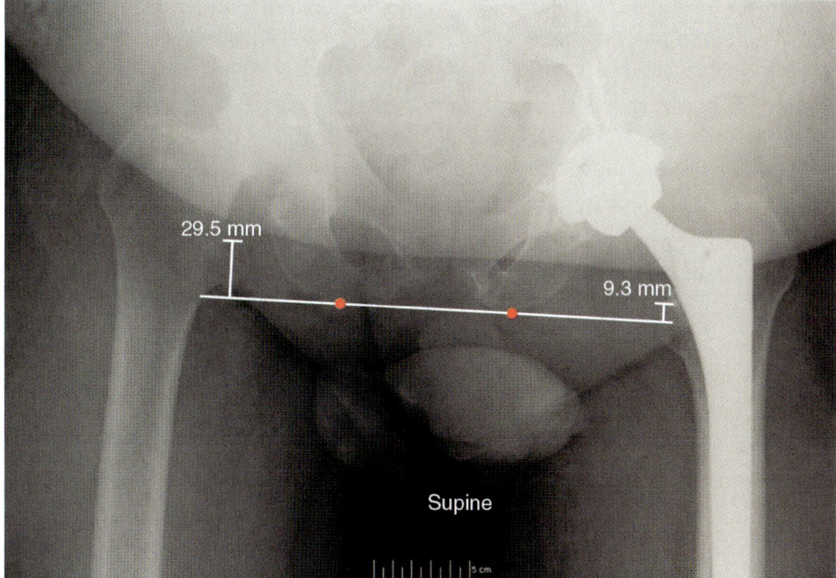

Figure 5 Preoperative AP pelvic radiograph made with the patient supine shows severe erosive arthritis of the right hip. A line is drawn at the most inferior portions of the ischia, providing the pelvic reference line. A perpendicular line is drawn bilaterally from the transischial line to the superior aspect of the lesser trochanter to determine the limb-length difference. The patient has a preoperative limb-length discrepancy of 2.0 cm.

Preoperative templating is essential to minimize limb-length inequality, restore offset, and therefore minimize

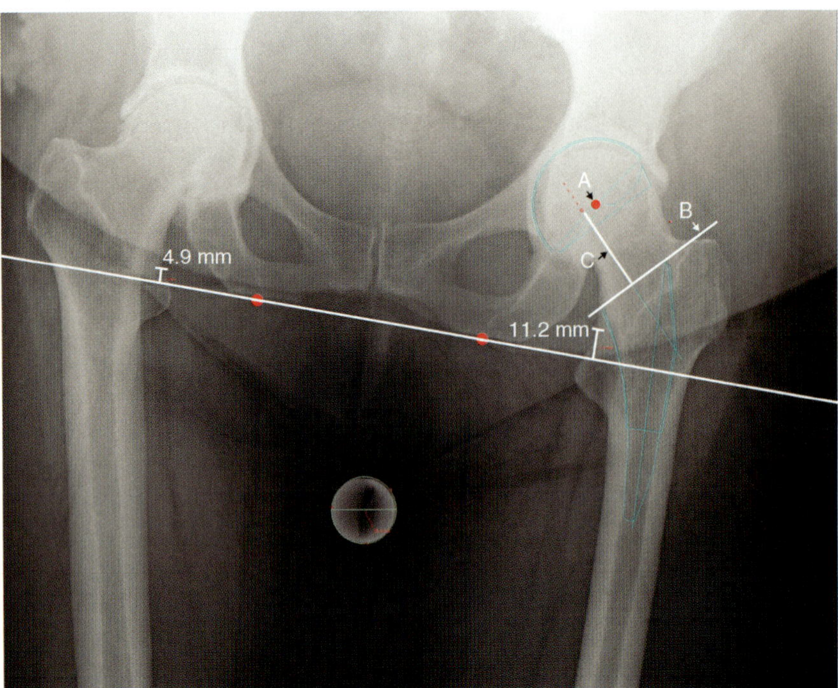

Figure 6 Preoperative templating can be performed with computerized radiology software. The new, anatomic center of rotation is templated (A), and the acetabular implant size is determined using the hip that is not being operated on. The appropriate femoral stem size and position are templated. The corresponding neck cut (B), prosthetic neck length (C), and limb-length difference are noted.

the possibility of instability (**Figure 6**). First, the new center of rotation for the hip is determined by selecting the optimal position of the acetabular component. In general, the inferomedial aspect of the acetabular component is placed in close approximation to the radiographic teardrop such that the inferiormost aspect of the acetabular implant template is aligned with the radiographic teardrop in the vertical plane.

With femoral templating, the examiner should determine (1) the prosthetic size (the fit and fill of the femur needed to achieve axial and rotational stability), (2) the component offset (extended-offset implants or a lateralized acetabular liner may be required to restore offset), and (3) limb length. Limb lengthening (or, rarely, shortening) is planned on the basis of the preoperative radiographic evaluation as well as the clinical assessment of apparent limb-length inequality.

Not all patients with a true limb-length inequality require lengthening. Patients with a fixed adduction contracture or a pelvic obliquity may believe that the limb is excessively long if the true limb length is restored. A common reason for dislocation is the failure to adequately restore offset, which is the distance between the center of hip rotation and the center of the femoral canal.[40] Technically, templating can be performed on the contralateral, normal hip, and changes in limb length or offset can be extrapolated to the hip that is to be operated on. Subsequently, femoral head-neck length and implant offset can be anticipated. Alternatively, templating of the hip that is to be operated on can allow immediate recognition of how much length or offset will be changed by anatomic placement of components, compared with the nonsurgical side.

Patient Expectations

Preoperative discussions about limb-length inequality and the possibility of hip dislocation are critical and should set realistic goals and reiterate the hierarchy of surgical priorities.[36] Patients must be aware that in some situations the lower limb must be lengthened to achieve component stability. Additionally, patients should be told that their lower limb will feel long immediately after the surgery and that this is a normal physiologic response following hip replacement. Patients who have a sense that the lower limb is longer preoperatively but actually have normal limb lengths, or those with a shortened extremity but the perception of equal limb lengths, are particularly at risk for perceiving that they have a discrepancy after surgery and should be appropriately warned preoperatively.[41]

Advantages and Disadvantages of Surgical Approaches in Terms of Limb Length and Stability

Anterior Approaches

The true anterior approaches expose the hip through the interval between the sartorius and tensor fascia femoris muscles, with several variations. The classic approach is the Smith-Petersen approach with either preservation or detachment of the direct head of the rectus femoris tendon. A variation of this approach—the Hueter approach (a fascial incision over the tensor fascia femoris)—has gained interest because of its theoretic ability to provide protection to the lateral femoral cutaneous nerve, which is at risk with the classic Smith-Petersen approach.[42-44]

Limb Length

A major advantage of the direct anterior approach is the ability to directly measure limb lengths because the patient is in the supine position and the true limb length can be measured at the ankle or heel. An intraoperative supine radiograph or fluoroscopy is helpful for measuring limb lengths and component position. Studies have shown an average mean limb-length discrepancy of 3.9 mm with this approach.[43,44] This small amount of lengthening is well tolerated and accepted by the patient, making this approach one of the most accurate in terms of limb-length reconstruction.

Stability

The direct anterior exposure is a true internervous plane between the sartorius (femoral nerve) and tensor fascia femoris (superior gluteal nerve). This approach minimizes soft-tissue damage about the hip and preserves the major abductor attachment. Only the anterior aspect of the capsule is excised. Advocates point out that no muscle detachment is necessary to deliver the femur anteriorly. The dislocation rate after a single-incision anterior approach ranges from 0.6% to 1.3%.[42-44]

Disadvantages

The approach is technically demanding and may or may not require the use of a specialized fracture table. There is a steep learning curve associated with the procedure.[42,45] The lateral femoral cutaneous nerve is always retracted, and the risk of injury to this nerve should be discussed with the patient preoperatively.

Two-Incision Technique

The two-incision technique was described by Light and Keggi[46] and was popularized by Berger.[47,48] It is basically an anterior Smith-Petersen approach with an additional posterior smaller incision for placement of the femoral component.

Limb Length

The advantages of this approach are similar to those of the direct anterior approach.

Stability

Excessive femoral anteversion is a risk because it is difficult to maintain anatomic version while inserting the femoral component through the small posterior incision. The reported dislocation rate after this procedure is relatively low (1.0%).[47-50]

Disadvantages

The two-incision approach is not popular because it is technically difficult, has a steep learning curve, and has a high intraoperative complication rate. In addition, there may be injury to the abductor muscles.[49,51-53]

Anterolateral, Direct Lateral, or Hardinge Approach

Direct lateral approaches include the Hardinge approach, in which the gluteus medius tendon is displaced with the vastus lateralis anteriorly and the hip is dislocated anteriorly.[54] Mallory et al[55] described a modified direct lateral approach in which the anterior portion of the gluteus medius is dissected and displaced anteriorly with the vastus lateralis.

Limb Length

Some surgeons perform this approach with the patient in the supine position, and this position may be advantageous in terms of obtaining equal limb lengths. The approaches that dislocate the hip anteriorly offer some additional protection against dislocation compared with posterolateral approaches.[56] Therefore, slight laxity in the hip to keep the lower limbs of equal length is acceptable.

Stability

The cumulative 10-year rate of dislocation has been reported to be 3.1% after anterolateral approaches but 6.9% after posterolateral approaches.[48,57,58]

Disadvantages

This approach violates the abductor mechanism and is sometimes associated with a postoperative limp. Damage to the superior gluteal nerve can occur and leads to denervation of the muscles that it enervates.[59] Heterotopic ossification is more common than it is with other approaches; this heterotopic bone has required removal in 1% of patients,[58] a rate that is higher than that associated with other approaches.

Posterolateral Approach

The posterolateral approach is the most extensile of all approaches, allowing complete exposure of the femur and acetabulum. It is the most commonly used approach in North America, primarily because it avoids damage to the abductor muscles.[50,60,61] Small-incision techniques have gained favor in recent years.[61] The debate over the clinical benefit and the effect on limb length and stability of this approach is beyond the scope of this chapter.[61,62]

Limb Length

When the posterolateral approach is used, the limb lengths are difficult to accurately measure with physical examination or radiographs, so some other means of determining limb length is necessary. Because of concerns about postoperative dislocation, it is not uncommon for the extremity to be overlengthened during the hip arthroplasty with this approach.[63]

Stability

The risk of dislocation associated with the posterior approach is higher than that found with transtrochanteric, anterolateral, and anterior-based approaches.[13,16,21,64] In a study of

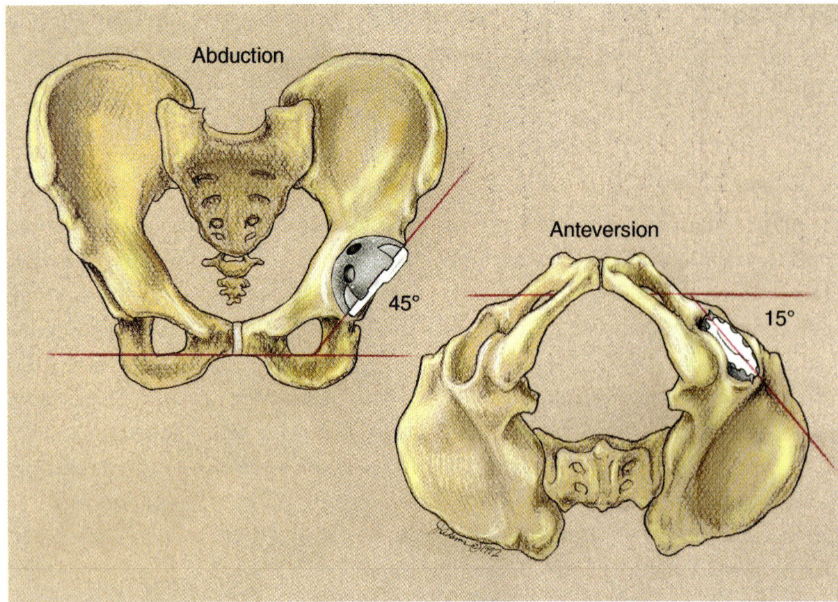

Figure 7 The so-called safe zone for orientation of the acetabular component. (Reproduced with permission of Joint Implant Surgeons, Inc, New Albany, Ohio.)

more than 21,000 primary total hip arthroplasties, Berry et al[13] reported dislocation rates at the time of a 10-year follow-up of 3.1%, 3.4%, and 6.9% for the anterolateral, transtrochanteric, and posterolateral approaches, respectively. A meta-analysis by Masonis and Bourne[64] suggested that the dislocation rate associated with the posterior approach is sixfold higher than that observed with a direct lateral approach. Proper repair of the capsule and short external rotators after a posterior approach reduces the incidence of dislocation.[60,64-69] Furthermore, Kim et al[70] advocated preserving the external rotators during the posterior approach, a technique that resulted in no dislocations.

Disadvantages

The risk of injury to the sciatic nerve with the posterior approach is reported to be 0.6%.[71,72] However, as a result of the proximity of the nerve with this approach, the risk of sciatic nerve injury is higher than that associated with all other surgical approaches.[59,70,73]

Surgical Technique

Implant Positioning: Acetabular Component

Implant malposition is a major contributor to instability and dislocation. Correct implant position decreases wear and reduces the risk of dislocation, but other factors play a role in hip stability.[74,75] Multiple investigators have attempted to define a safe zone of acetabular component anteversion and inclination, or abduction. It is widely believed that the acetabular component should be placed in approximately 45° (40° to 60°) of abduction and should be anteverted 15° to 20°[18] (**Figure 7**). The safe zone is 15° ± 10° of anteversion and 40° ± 10° of abduction.[18] Total hip arthroplasty components that dislocate anteriorly have mean anteversion and abduction angles that are greater than the safe zone, whereas those that dislocate posteriorly have mean anteversion and abduction angles that are less than the safe zone.[76] The position of the acetabular cup is not the only factor affecting instability and dislocation. Hassan et al[77] reported that 42% of total hip prostheses in which the acetabular cup was positioned outside the safe zone did not dislocate. Rittmeister and Callitsis[78] noted that although nearly 20% of acetabular cups were positioned outside the safe zone in their study, there was no increase in dislocations in that group.

Implant Positioning: Reference Landmarks

Landmarks are useful in assisting with positioning of the acetabular component. McCollum and Gray[79] investigated multiple external reference points for acetabular component positioning and found that significant changes in pelvic position and orientation occur when the patient is in the lateral decubitus position. Care must be taken to evaluate the effects of body position when using external cues for orientation of the acetabular component during surgery.

Fixed anatomic landmarks, in contrast to external aiming devices, are independent of patient positioning. Useful landmarks include the transverse acetabular ligament, the acetabular sulcus on the ischium, the most lateral prominence of the superior pubic rami (pubis), and the most superior aspect of the acetabulum.[80,81] These landmarks define a plane of orientation for acetabular component positioning that provides stability within a safe arc of motion.[81] An average cup position of 44° of abduction and 13° of anteversion can be achieved with use of these landmarks.[81]

Computer navigation, or computer-assisted orthopaedic surgery, has been proposed as a method for accurately determining correct acetabular component positioning. Computer-assisted orthopaedic surgery reduces outliers but is not totally reliable.[82-84] The cost and technical aspects of computer-assisted orthopaedic surgery currently prohibit its widespread use.

Implant Positioning: Femoral Component

The positioning of the femoral component affects limb length, offset, abductor tension, and stability. All other factors being equal, a distally placed femoral stem will result in a limb that is shorter than that resulting from a more proximally placed stem. The level of the femoral component has an equally important, albeit less obvious, effect on femoral offset. Femoral offset is defined as the distance from the center of rotation of the femoral head to a line bisecting the long axis of the femur. Reconstruction of the femoral offset is important for restoring the biomechanics of the hip and specifically the abductor lever arm. Proper restoration of offset enhances hip motion and reduces the risk of dislocation.[85] A high femoral neck resection can be combined with a short neck length to yield the same limb length as provided by a low femoral neck resection combined with a long modular head. However, the first combination yields less femoral offset and may be appropriate in the presence of coxa valga. The second combination yields greater offset and is better for hips with coxa vara. Varus or valgus malpositioning of the stem will increase or decrease offset and should be avoided. Rotational alignment of the stem to the appropriate femoral anteversion influences the amount of hip motion that is possible before impingement occurs as well as abductor tension. Herrlin et al[86] reported that femoral anteversion was significantly reduced in hips that dislocated after total hip arthroplasty. The ideal femoral anteversion is 15° to 20° in an osteoarthritic hip with otherwise normal anatomy. Acetabular deformity or deficiency may dictate less than ideal orientation of the acetabular component. To compensate for this, the femoral component may need to be placed in greater or less anteversion. In recognition of this possibility, the concept of combined acetabular and femoral component anteversion has been introduced. Using a mathematical model, Widmer and Zurfluh[87] determined that the acetabular component should be in 40° to 45° of inclination (abduction) and 20° to 28° of anteversion (forward flexion). This is combined with femoral anteversion such that the femoral anteversion multiplied by 0.7, plus the cup anteversion, should equal 37° to provide the greatest range of motion without impingement. Modular femoral components of various designs that allow adjustments in offset and anteversion without limb lengthening are now available from various manufacturers.[4,88]

There are some general rules of thumb for placing a femoral stem in the correct position. The proximal-distal position of the femoral stem is assessed in relation to the greater and lesser trochanters. Alternatively, the center of the femoral head in relation to the tip of the greater trochanter is noted. Additionally, the piriformis fossa can serve as a landmark for femoral neck resection. When the posterior approach is used, the templated neck resection can be easily reproduced by measuring the level of resection from the top of the lesser trochanter. This landmark is easily visualized on preoperative radiographs and intraoperatively, even through limited exposures. Woolson et al[89] described using the templated femoral neck and head segment as a guide for placing the femoral stem. By placing the femoral stem at that osteotomy level, they achieved an appropriate limb length in 97% of cases.

Soft-Tissue Balancing

By restoring femoral offset and limb length, proper balancing of the soft tissues around the hip minimizes postoperative instability, pain, and limp.[90,91] Inadequate restoration of femoral offset increases the risk of dislocation by decreasing soft-tissue tension.[91] Excessive limb lengthening can result when intraoperative instability caused by inadequate offset is inappropriately treated by increasing the neck length in an attempt to restore soft-tissue tension.[38] As mentioned previously, the combination of these factors is critical for understanding prosthetic hip stability.[19]

Better wear performance of the implants has been observed after femoral head medialization and femoral shaft lateralization. In addition, restoration of offset is associated with better functional and clinical results.[85,92,93] Bourne and Rorabeck[90] reviewed the available methods to restore offset. The most common approach is the use of a lateralized (high-offset) femoral stem (**Figure 8**). Another option is to use a lateralized acetabular liner. However, such liners decrease the abductor moment arm, increase the joint reactive force, and result in accelerated polyethylene wear.[90] A lower-level neck resection and more distal femoral stem placement combined with a longer neck segment can lateralize the femoral shaft without lengthening the limb. However, longer heads with skirts should be avoided because they decrease motion as a result of impingement.

Concerns have been raised that excessive femoral lateralization may increase the incidence of thigh pain and trochanteric bursitis or place undue strains on the bone-cement or biologic interfaces, leading to loosening. This latter concern has been refuted, and data show that, when indicated, a lateralized stem improves the accuracy of

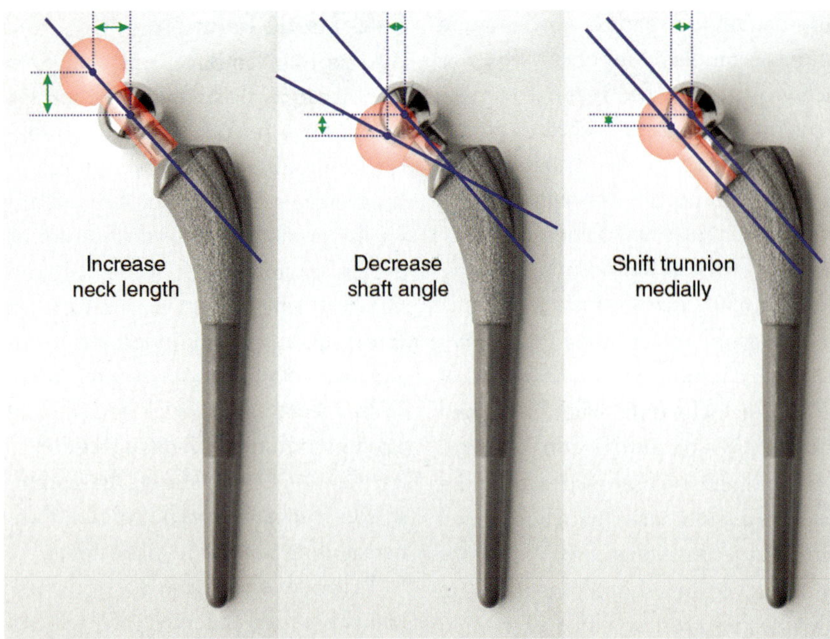

Figure 8 Various methods of restoring offset with use of the femoral stem. (Reproduced with permission of Joint Implant Surgeons, Inc, New Albany, Ohio.)

hip soft-tissue reconstruction and does not increase thigh pain, trochanteric pain, or loosening.[56] In fact, proper soft-tissue balancing, obtained with a lateralized stem, is associated with less thigh and trochanteric pain.[94] However, overlateralization should be avoided. Incavo et al[95] showed that excessive lateralization led to a 15% incidence of trochanteric pain. The value of intraoperative tests of soft-tissue balance, such as the shuck test or drop-kick test, is highly dependent on the surgical approach, the anesthetic technique, and surgeon experience.[90] These tests, however, can provide the surgeon with an assessment of the overall tightness of the reconstructed hip. The shuck test is performed by attempting to distract the total hip prosthesis in an inferior direction to assess soft-tissue tension. The drop-kick test is performed by placing the hip in extension, flexing the knee to 90°, and releasing the lower limb to assess the amount of recoil as the knee springs back toward extension. In addition, intraoperative motion of the hip is important to evaluate for potential bone or prosthetic impingement and prosthetic stability. These intraoperative assessments coupled with proper preoperative templating should allow the surgeon to restore proper hip offset and limb length.

Measuring Limb Length

Substantial limb-length discrepancy occurs after up to 3% of total hip arthroplasties, but the clinical relevance is not known.[69] The definition of clinically relevant limb-length discrepancy is not universally agreed on, with a range between 6 and 35 mm having been reported.[96-99] Most authors have agreed that discrepancies of less than 1 cm are well tolerated.[97] Edwards et al[71] reported average lengthening of 2.7 cm and 4.4 cm in 23 total hip arthroplasties complicated by peroneal and sciatic nerve palsy, respectively. White and Dougall[99] reported that lengthening of up to 35 mm does not affect clinical results. Edeen et al[37] reported that 32% of patients who had a total hip arthroplasty were aware of a limb-length inequality. Relevant limb-length discrepancy results in a limp, low back pain, and functional impairment and is a major cause of litigation.[38,100] There are several methods for the intraoperative assessment of limb length, with varied degrees of accuracy, technical difficulty, and expense. Many of the methods involve an intraoperative measuring device, which may also enable the measurement of offset.[41,63,101-103] These instruments measure from a fixed point on the pelvis to a fixed point on the femur and are used before femoral head dislocation and after total hip arthroplasty reconstruction. They are accurate if the position of the limb before the dislocation is correctly reproduced for the postarthroplasty measurement.[104] There is a learning curve with these devices as well as the need for additional expense and time for surgery. An average limb lengthening of 3.4 mm was observed with the use of one specific device; limb lengthening of more than 12 mm was observed in 5% of cases, and 7% had symptomatic lengthening requiring a heel lift.[103]

Alternatively, preoperative templating and intraoperative "well-leg" referencing for limb length is as accurate as other methods, with few radiographic outliers.[56] Preoperative templating is performed. The center of the acetabulum on the normal, contralateral side is identified with acetabular templates (**Figure 6**). The femoral component size and osteotomy level are determined, and the neck length is selected. The level of the femoral neck osteotomy is referenced intraoperatively with regard to the greater trochanter, the lesser trochanter, the piriformis fossa, or the distance from the center of the resected head. Direct measurement of limb length with the patient supine is performed before positioning for the total hip arthroplasty and preparation of the extremity. This measurement is correlated with the preoperative templating. The patient is positioned in the lateral decubitus position, and the uninvolved lower limb is used as a reference, with the relative difference felt at the patellar tendon (**Figure 9**). The relative difference is reassessed after trial components have been placed. In one series of 410 patients treated with a primary total hip arthroplasty, an average lengthening of 3.9 mm was seen and only 2 patients perceived a limb-length discrepancy.[56]

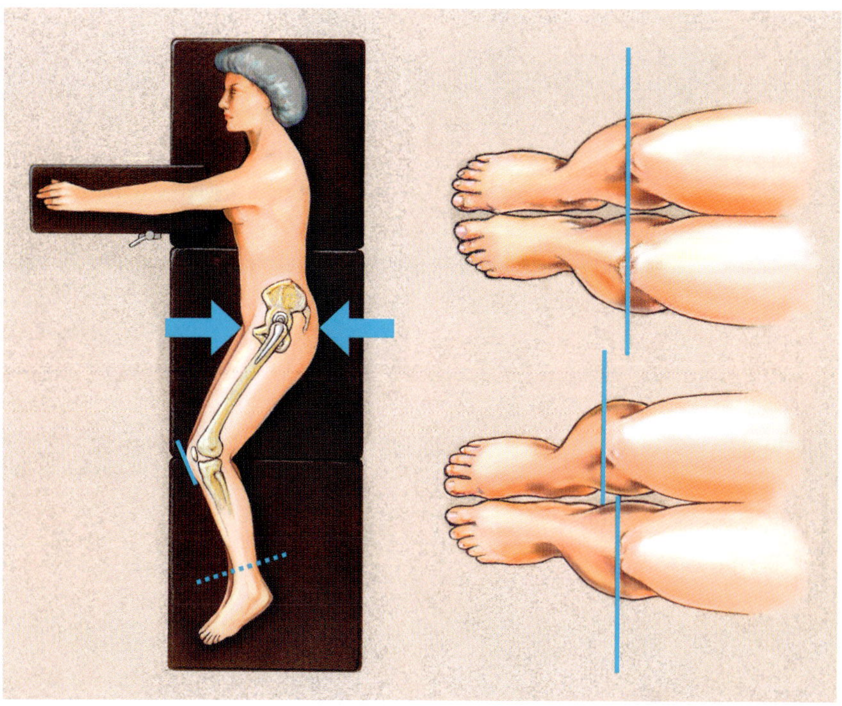

Figure 9 With the patient in a lateral position, the uninvolved lower limb is used to reference limb lengths intraoperatively. The pelvis needs to be perpendicular to the floor. With the feet symmetrically positioned, the patellar tendons are palpated, and the limb-length difference is assessed. The goal is to have symmetric positioning of the patellar tendons with the pelvis and feet. (Reproduced with permission of Joint Implant Surgeons, Inc., New Albany, Ohio.)

Implant-Related Factors

Femoral head size affects hip stability after a total hip arthroplasty.[13,105-107] Dislocation rates for all approaches decrease as femoral head size increases from 22 mm to 32 mm.[13] Smith et al[108] reported no dislocations when a 38-mm head had been used. Cuckler et al[109] also reported no dislocations with 38-mm heads, but 2.5% of the total hip prostheses with a 28-mm head dislocated. Peters et al[110] found no dislocations with 38-mm heads, a 0.4% rate with 38 to 56-mm heads, and a 2.5% rate with 28-mm heads. Smit[111] studied anatomically sized femoral heads (femoral heads with a size that was 6 mm less than the acetabular size) in primary total hip arthroplasties and reported no dislocations at 1-year follow-up. Others believe that a good capsular repair as well as a larger femoral head protects against a dislocation. Lachiewicz and Soileau[112] found that when a formal posterior capsular repair had been used, there was no change in the dislocation risk associated with 36- and 40-mm metal femoral heads compared with that for historic controls with standard-sized heads. Despite the overall impressive reduction in the dislocation rate associated with large femoral heads in these studies, Amstutz et al[113] reported a dislocation rate of 3.5% with large femoral heads in primary total hip arthroplasty. However, Amstutz et al[113] reported an advantage of using larger heads in revision total hip arthroplasties. In addition, the use of large heads increases volumetric wear, and a thinner polyethylene acetabular liner is needed to accommodate the larger head. To avoid the adverse mechanical and fatigue properties associated with thin liners, implant companies commonly offer offset liners to increase polyethylene thickness.[114] Offset liners may increase femoral offset, which affects the joint mechanics as previously discussed.

Management of Instability

An accurate and complete patient history is critical for defining the cause of hip instability. Surgical records are reviewed to determine the surgical approach, type of soft-tissue repair, and specific implant used, including the manufacturer's implant stickers if possible. The mechanism of the dislocation may be evaluated according to the direction of dislocation and the position of instability. Limb length, associated skeletal conditions such as scoliosis and contractures, neurologic function of both the affected limb and the abductors, and the overall neurologic function of the patient should be assessed. A thorough evaluation for infection is necessary.[115]

Radiographic studies are essential. AP and true lateral views of the hip and an AP view of the pelvis are the minimal imaging studies needed for these patients. Limb-length differences, femoral offset, the status of the greater trochanter, and the component orientation are noted. A preoperative CT scan to evaluate the position of the acetabular cup can provide important information regarding acetabular version.[116-119] Following evaluation and definition of the etiology of the dislocation, a treatment algorithm is established.[120,121]

The treatment options include closed reduction of the dislocated hip with or without bracing, total hip arthroplasty component revision, exchange of modular parts, cementing a liner into a well-fixed acetabular shell, bipolar or tripolar arthroplasty, use of a large femoral head, use of a constrained liner, advancement of the greater trochanter, and soft-tissue augmentation.[122-129] An understanding of the risk factors, the causes of dislocation, and management options enables the surgeon to effectively minimize the incidence of dislocation after total hip arthroplasty as well as to establish a strategy for treating a patient with an unstable total hip prosthesis.

Treatment Indications

Selection of the appropriate treatment option is guided by the cause and timing of the dislocation. Early dislocations occur within the first 3 to 6 months after the operation, and in most patients a single episode of dislocation can be adequately treated with closed reduction.[130] The role of cast-bracing or casting is controversial, and there are data supporting and refuting the use of this treatment after reduction of the hip.[123,126,129] Late dislocations are those that occur 5 years or more after the index procedure. Patients with a first-time late dislocation are at high risk for recurrent instability.[131] Late dislocations have multiple possible causes, including polyethylene wear, trauma, decline in neurologic function, increased soft-tissue laxity, or malposition of a total hip arthroplasty component.[132] Dislocations termed "intermediate" occur between 6 months and 5 years after the total hip arthroplasty. Patients in whom this is the first dislocation can usually be managed with closed reduction. Surgical management should be considered for patients with recurrent instability following the initial closed reduction.[73,132] Successful surgical management is critically dependent on accurate identification of the cause(s) of instability.[133]

Techniques and Results of Revision Total Hip Arthroplasty for Instability

Component revision is indicated when implants are seen to be malpositioned on radiographs, CT scans, or intraoperative evaluation.[118,119] Malpositioning of acetabular and femoral implants, limb-length inequality, and improper femoral offset can be corrected and restored in a reasonably predictable fashion with component revision.[11,58,120,134] Perhaps the easiest and most attractive option for managing recurrent instability in the presence of implants that appear to be in an appropriate position and alignment is modular component exchange, or so-called dry revision.[135] This option is indicated, however, only if the components are reasonably well positioned.[135] Increasing the head size and/or neck length and changing the acetabular liner are among the simplest solutions. Varying degrees of success with this approach have been reported in multiple small series. Toomey et al[135] successfully prevented recurrent dislocation with modular component exchange in 12 of 13 hips, although 3 hips dislocated once during the follow-up period. Importantly, these modular revisions also included excision of soft tissue and bone causing impingement in 10 hips. Nine of the hips were converted to either a lipped-bearing implant or an implant with a higher degree of lipped bearing. In another study, liner exchange was successful in 82% of cases of late instability associated with polyethylene wear.[136] In contrast, Barrack et al[88] reported multiple complications with modular component exchange, including liner dissociation and impingement, instability, and femoral head dislodgement from the stem trunnion. In cases of polyethylene wear-related instability, cementing a new liner into a well-fixed shell may provide an alternative to complete revision if the components are oriented correctly.[137,138]

High-walled liners can be valuable for treating or preventing dislocation of well-positioned components, as reported by Cobb et al[139] Similarly, in revision total hip arthroplasty, an augmentation device can act as an elevated-rim liner. McConway et al[140] reported a 1.6% dislocation rate in 307 patients treated with revision total hip arthroplasty with a posterior lip-augmentation device. Adding an augmentation device to the existing liner or socket has also been described and is effective in certain cases.[141-143] Currently, high-wall or lipped liners are used more sparingly because of concerns regarding impingement, wear, and limited hip motion.

Large femoral heads increase the head-neck ratio, thereby increasing the range of motion before impingement occurs, and increase the jump distance required for the head to dislocate.[107] In a series in which large femoral heads (36 mm and larger) were used, Beaulé et al[144] reported that more than 90% of the hips had no more instability after an average duration of follow-up of 6.5 years and only one had recurrent instability. Amstutz et al[113] reported that the dislocation rate after revisions for recurrent instability was higher than that after revisions for other etiologies. More troubling results were reported by Skeels et al,[145] who observed a 17% rate of recurrent dislocation in patients who had undergone revision surgery with a femoral head that was 36 mm or larger.

Another, less commonly used strategy to manage instability involves soft-tissue augmentation, or reinforcement of the hip abductor muscles and/or the posterior aspect of the hip capsule.[19] Reconstructions with an Achilles tendon allograft and a bone block, fascia lata, or a synthetic ligament have all been reported.[146-148] Indications for these procedures are unclear but may include deficiency of the hip abductor muscles or posterior aspect of the hip capsule in the setting of well-positioned, well-fixed total hip arthroplasty components.

Trochanteric advancement has been advocated for patients with well-positioned, well-fixed total hip arthroplasty implants.[124,149,150] Nonunion of the greater trochanter is a major concern, and trochanter-related hip pain is common. Ekelund[124] and Kaplan et al[150] independently reported 80% success rates with this approach in 21 patients each with recurrent dislocation and properly oriented components. Similarly, trochanteric osteotomy and advancement can be used for complex primary total hip arthroplasty to enhance stability.[151]

Bipolar arthroplasty is based on the principle of increasing the overall range of motion with articulation at two different bearing surfaces.[133,152,153] This provides a greater safe arc of motion before dislocation occurs and optimizes head-neck ratios while providing a larger jump distance. Parvizi and Morrey[133] reported the elimination of recurrent dislocation in 22 of 27 hips (81%). Attarian[152] and Ries and Wiedel[154] achieved 100% success using this technique. Medial and/or superior migration of the prosthesis, with resultant groin pain, is a concern if this technique is used.

Unconstrained tripolar hip arthroplasty uses a bipolar head to articulate with an acetabular shell and liner; this combination increases the head-neck ratio and the jump distance.[154-156] Grigoris et al[155] and Beaulé et al[154] used an unconstrained tripolar implant to successfully treat instability without compromising acetabular fixation in 95% of their patients. Levine et al[156] reported a 93% success rate in a series of 31 patients in whom an unstable total hip prosthesis had been treated with an unconstrained tripolar construct.

The final salvage option involves the use of a constrained acetabular liner.[19,157-169] Indications for this technique include hip abductor deficiency, neurologic impairment, low-demand patients with well-fixed components, instability for which the cause cannot be determined, and persistent intraoperative instability.[19,122,127,157,166,167] Constrained acetabular liners reduce the hip motion before impingement and therefore increase the risk of impingement and the acetabular shear stresses, which could lead to accelerated wear, loosening, or failure of fixation. These implants can be cemented into a well-fixed acetabular shell to reduce the morbidity of revision total hip arthroplasty.[137] Callaghan et al[162] reported no dislocations and two liner failures (a 94% success rate) with this technique in patients with a well-fixed, well-positioned, cementless acetabular shell. This procedure is considered a low-morbidity treatment option in the setting of a well-fixed, properly oriented acetabular component, especially in older, low-demand patients.[162]

Favorable results with the use of constrained devices have been reported in several studies, but these components should be considered only if no other treatment options are available.[170] At an average of 10.2 years after the use of 56 constrained tripolar devices, Goetz et al[163,164] reported a 7% failure rate secondary to recurrent dislocation, osteolysis, or aseptic loosening. Bremner et al[160] reported similar results, with a 6% failure rate secondary to recurrent dislocation or liner failure at 10.2 years. There is concern about the stability of fixation of constrained devices. Shrader et al[168] noted that, while no dislocations were seen, there were acetabular cup radiolucencies in 14% of their cases. Su and Pellicci[169] reported a 98% rate of success in terms of preventing instability in 85 hips with a constrained tripolar implant. There are modes of failure specific to tripolar constrained devices.[171-173] Guyen et al[172] reported 43 failures of tripolar constrained devices, with four types of failure: the bone-implant interface, the mechanism holding the constrained acetabular liner to the metal shell, the locking mechanism of the bipolar component, and dislocation of the head at the inner bearing. Methods for closed reduction of a constrained component have been described, but long-term outcomes have not yet been reported.[174]

Berend et al[158] reported on 755 alternatively designed constrained total hip arthroplasty components with a capture mechanism and locking ring design. The dislocation rate for the 667 hips followed for 10 years was 17.5%, and aseptic loosening of the cup and stem were also major long-term causes of failure that required a reoperation.[158] Newer designs allowing greater hip motion before impingement have been introduced. In another study, Berend et al[159] reported a 99% rate of success in terms of preventing recurrent dislocation in a group of 81 total hip arthroplasty revisions performed with a novel constrained device.

Summary

The intraoperative challenge of achieving stability and limb-length equality after total hip arthroplasty starts with preoperative planning, including physical examination, radiographic evaluation, templating, and aligning patient and surgeon expectations. Each surgical approach has advantages and disadvantages in terms of stability and limb length. It is the responsibility of the surgeon to be familiar with the benefits and drawbacks of each approach and use a method that most easily accomplishes the goals of a stable prosthetic construct, hip stability, and restoration of limb-length equality. Familiarity and experience with a total hip arthroplasty technique reduce the risk of dislocation and limb-length inequality. Intraoperatively, the prosthetic design, including the femoral head size and femoral offset, component orientation, and reconstruction of the hip soft tissues, are the critical variables for achieving success. Preoperative radiographic templating is paramount, and intraoperative maneuvers to determine limb length are important for obtaining the best result. Dislocation continues to be a major mode of failure of total hip arthroplasty. Obtaining a stable hip at the time of the initial total hip arthroplasty reduces the risk of this complication.

References

1. Bourne RB, Maloney WJ, Wright JG: An AOA critical issue: The outcome of the outcomes movement. *J Bone Joint Surg Am* 2004;86-A(3):633-640.
2. Chang RW, Pellisier JM, Hazen GB: A cost-effectiveness analysis of total hip arthroplasty for osteoarthritis of the hip. *JAMA* 1996;275(11):858-865.
3. Bozic KJ, Kurtz SM, Lau E, Ong K, Vail TP, Berry DJ: The epidemiology of revision total hip arthroplasty in the United States. *J Bone Joint Surg Am* 2009;91(1):128-133.
4. Goldstein WM, Gordon A, Branson JJ: Leg length inequality in total hip arthroplasty. *Orthopedics* 2005;28(9, Suppl):S1037-S1040.
5. Khatod M, Barber T, Paxton E, Namba R, Fithian D: An analysis of the risk of hip dislocation with a contemporary total joint registry. *Clin Orthop Relat Res* 2006; 447:19-23.
6. Kurtz S, Ong K, Lau E, Mowat F, Halpern M: Projections of primary and revision hip and knee arthroplasty in the United States from 2005 to 2030. *J Bone Joint Surg Am* 2007;89(4):780-785.
7. Levy RN, Levy CM, Snyder J, Digiovanni J: Outcome and long-term results following total hip replacement in elderly patients. *Clin Orthop Relat Res* 1995;316: 25-30.
8. Phillips CB, Barrett JA, Losina E, et al: Incidence rates of dislocation, pulmonary embolism, and deep infection during the first six months after elective total hip replacement. *J Bone Joint Surg Am* 2003;85-A(1):20-26.
9. Sanchez-Sotelo J, Haidukewych GJ, Boberg CJ: Hospital cost of dislocation after primary total hip arthroplasty. *J Bone Joint Surg Am* 2006;88(2):290-294.
10. Abraham WD, Dimon JH III: Leg length discrepancy in total hip arthroplasty. *Orthop Clin North Am* 1992;23(2):201-209.
11. Alberton GM, High WA, Morrey BF: Dislocation after revision total hip arthroplasty: An analysis of risk factors and treatment options. *J Bone Joint Surg Am* 2002; 84-A(10):1788-1792.
12. Berry DJ, von Knoch M, Schleck CD, Harmsen WS: The cumulative long-term risk of dislocation after primary Charnley total hip arthroplasty. *J Bone Joint Surg Am* 2004;86-A(1):9-14.
13. Berry DJ, von Knoch M, Schleck CD, Harmsen WS: Effect of femoral head diameter and operative approach on risk of dislocation after primary total hip arthroplasty. *J Bone Joint Surg Am* 2005;87(11):2456-2463.
14. Callaghan JJ, Templeton JE, Liu SS, et al: Results of Charnley total hip arthroplasty at a minimum of thirty years: A concise follow-up of a previous report. *J Bone Joint Surg Am* 2004;86-A(4):690-695.
15. Conroy JL, Whitehouse SL, Graves SE, Pratt NL, Ryan P, Crawford RW: Risk factors for revision for early dislocation in total hip arthroplasty. *J Arthroplasty* 2008;23(6):867-872.
16. Eftekhar NS: Dislocation and instability complicating low friction arthroplasty of the hip joint. *Clin Orthop Relat Res* 1976;121: 120-125.
17. Heithoff BE, Callaghan JJ, Goetz DD, Sullivan PM, Pedersen DR, Johnston RC: Dislocation after total hip arthroplasty: A single surgeon's experience. *Orthop Clin North Am* 2001;32(4):587-591, viii.
18. Lewinnek GE, Lewis JL, Tarr R, Compere CL, Zimmerman JR: Dislocations after total hip-replacement arthroplasties. *J Bone Joint Surg Am* 1978;60(2): 217-220.
19. Parvizi J, Picinic E, Sharkey PF: Revision total hip arthroplasty for instability: Surgical techniques and principles. *J Bone Joint Surg Am* 2008;90(5):1134-1142.
20. Ritter MA: Dislocation and subluxation of the total hip replacement. *Clin Orthop Relat Res* 1976; 121:92-94.
21. Woo RY, Morrey BF: Dislocations after total hip arthroplasty. *J Bone Joint Surg Am* 1982;64(9):1295-1306.
22. Sadr Azodi O, Adami J, Lindström D, Eriksson KO, Wladis A,

Bellocco R: High body mass index is associated with increased risk of implant dislocation following primary total hip replacement: 2,106 patients followed for up to 8 years. *Acta Orthop* 2008;79(1): 141-147.

23. Ekelund A, Rydell N, Nilsson OS: Total hip arthroplasty in patients 80 years of age and older. *Clin Orthop Relat Res* 1992;281:101-106.
24. Jibodh SR, Gurkan I, Wenz JF: In-hospital outcome and resource use in hip arthroplasty: Influence of body mass. *Orthopedics* 2004; 27(6):594-601.
25. Jolles BM, Zangger P, Leyvraz PF: Factors predisposing to dislocation after primary total hip arthroplasty: A multivariate analysis. *J Arthroplasty* 2002;17(3): 282-288.
26. Kim Y, Morshed S, Joseph T, Bozic K, Ries MD: Clinical impact of obesity on stability following revision total hip arthroplasty. *Clin Orthop Relat Res* 2006;453: 142-146.
27. Krenzel BA, Berend ME, Malinzak RA, et al: High preoperative range of motion is a significant risk factor for dislocation in primary total hip arthroplasty. *J Arthroplasty* 2010;25(6, Suppl): 31-35.
28. Lachiewicz PF, Soileau ES: Stability of total hip arthroplasty in patients 75 years or older. *Clin Orthop Relat Res* 2002;405:65-69.
29. Lee BP, Berry DJ, Harmsen WS, Sim FH: Total hip arthroplasty for the treatment of an acute fracture of the femoral neck: Long-term results. *J Bone Joint Surg Am* 1998;80(1):70-75.
30. Meek RM, Allan DB, McPhillips G, Kerr L, Howie CR: Epidemiology of dislocation after total hip arthroplasty. *Clin Orthop Relat Res* 2006;447:9-18.
31. Morrey BF: Instability after total hip arthroplasty. *Orthop Clin North Am* 1992;23(2):237-248.
32. Morrey BF: Difficult complications after hip joint replacement: Dislocation. *Clin Orthop Relat Res* 1997;344:179-187.
33. Zwartelé RE, Brand R, Doets HC: Increased risk of dislocation after primary total hip arthroplasty in inflammatory arthritis: A prospective observational study of 410 hips. *Acta Orthop Scand* 2004;75(6):684-690.
34. Battaglia TC, Mulhall KJ, Brown TE, Saleh KJ: Increased surgical volume is associated with lower THA dislocation rates. *Clin Orthop Relat Res* 2006;447:28-33.
35. Katz JN, Losina E, Barrett J, et al: Association between hospital and surgeon procedure volume and outcomes of total hip replacement in the United States medicare population. *J Bone Joint Surg Am* 2001;83-A(11):1622-1629.
36. Austin MS, Hozack WJ, Sharkey PF, Rothman RH: Stability and leg length equality in total hip arthroplasty. *J Arthroplasty* 2003; 18(3, Suppl 1):88-90.
37. Edeen J, Sharkey PF, Alexander AH: Clinical significance of leg-length inequality after total hip arthroplasty. *Am J Orthop (Belle Mead NJ)* 1995;24(4): 347-351.
38. Parvizi J, Sharkey PF, Bissett GA, Rothman RH, Hozack WJ: Surgical treatment of limb-length discrepancy following total hip arthroplasty. *J Bone Joint Surg Am* 2003;85-A(12):2310-2317.
39. Ranawat CS, Rodriguez JA: Functional leg-length inequality following total hip arthroplasty. *J Arthroplasty* 1997;12(4):359-364.
40. Charles MN, Bourne RB, Davey JR, Greenwald AS, Morrey BF, Rorabeck CH: Soft-tissue balancing of the hip: The role of femoral offset restoration. *Instr Course Lect* 2005;54:131-141.
41. Itokazu M, Masuda K, Ohno T, Itoh Y, Takatsu T, Wenyi Y: A simple method of intraoperative limb length measurement in total hip arthroplasty. *Bull Hosp Jt Dis* 1997;56(4):204-205.
42. Berend KR, Lombardi AV Jr, Seng BE, Adams JB: Enhanced early outcomes with the anterior supine intermuscular approach in primary total hip arthroplasty. *J Bone Joint Surg Am* 2009; 91(Suppl 6):107-120.
43. Kennon RE, Keggi JM, Wetmore RS, Zatorski LE, Huo MH, Keggi KJ: Total hip arthroplasty through a minimally invasive anterior surgical approach. *J Bone Joint Surg Am* 2003;85-A(Suppl 4):39-48.
44. Matta JM, Shahrdar C, Ferguson T: Single-incision anterior approach for total hip arthroplasty on an orthopaedic table. *Clin Orthop Relat Res* 2005;441:115-124.
45. Seng BE, Berend KR, Ajluni AF, Lombardi AV Jr: Anterior-supine minimally invasive total hip arthroplasty: Defining the learning curve. *Orthop Clin North Am* 2009;40(3):343-350.
46. Light TR, Keggi KJ: Anterior approach to hip arthroplasty. *Clin Orthop Relat Res* 1980;152: 255-260.
47. Berger RA: Total hip arthroplasty using the minimally invasive two-incision approach. *Clin Orthop Relat Res* 2003;417:232-241.
48. Berger RA: Mini-incision total hip replacement using an anterolateral approach: Technique and results. *Orthop Clin North Am* 2004; 35(2):143-151.
49. Archibeck MJ, White RE Jr: Learning curve for the two-incision total hip replacement. *Clin Orthop Relat Res* 2004;429: 232-238.
50. Berry DJ, Berger RA, Callaghan JJ, et al: Minimally invasive total hip arthroplasty: Development, early results, and a critical analysis. Presented at the Annual Meeting of the American Orthopaedic Association, Charleston,

South Carolina, USA, June 14, 2003. *J Bone Joint Surg Am* 2003; 85-A(11):2235-2246.

51. Bal BS, Haltom D, Aleto T, Barrett M: Early complications of primary total hip replacement performed with a two-incision minimally invasive technique. *J Bone Joint Surg Am* 2005; 87(11):2432-2438.
52. Mardones R, Pagnano MW, Nemanich JP, Trousdale RT: The Frank Stinchfield Award: Muscle damage after total hip arthroplasty done with the two-incision and mini-posterior techniques. *Clin Orthop Relat Res* 2005;441:63-67.
53. Pagnano MW, Leone J, Lewallen DG, Hanssen AD: Two-incision THA had modest outcomes and some substantial complications. *Clin Orthop Relat Res* 2005;441:86-90.
54. Hardinge K: The direct lateral approach to the hip. *J Bone Joint Surg Br* 1982;64(1):17-19.
55. Mallory TH, Lombardi AV Jr, Fada RA, Herrington SM, Eberle RW: Dislocation after total hip arthroplasty using the anterolateral abductor split approach. *Clin Orthop Relat Res* 1999;358:166-172.
56. Iagulli ND, Mallory TH, Berend KR, et al: A simple and accurate method for determining leg length in primary total hip arthroplasty. *Am J Orthop (Belle Mead NJ)* 2006;35(10):455-457.
57. Demos HA, Rorabeck CH, Bourne RB, MacDonald SJ, McCalden RW: Instability in primary total hip arthroplasty with the direct lateral approach. *Clin Orthop Relat Res* 2001;393:168-180.
58. Ritter MA, Harty LD, Keating ME, Faris PM, Meding JB: A clinical comparison of the anterolateral and posterolateral approaches to the hip. *Clin Orthop Relat Res* 2001;385:95-99.
59. Kenny P, O'Brien CP, Synnott K, Walsh MG: Damage to the superior gluteal nerve after two different approaches to the hip. *J Bone Joint Surg Br* 1999;81(6): 979-981.
60. Goldstein WM, Gleason TF, Kopplin M, Branson JJ: Prevalence of dislocation after total hip arthroplasty through a posterolateral approach with partial capsulotomy and capsulorrhaphy. *J Bone Joint Surg Am* 2001;83-A(Pt 1, Suppl 2):2-7.
61. Woolson ST, Mow CS, Syquia JF, Lannin JV, Schurman DJ: Comparison of primary total hip replacements performed with a standard incision or a mini-incision. *J Bone Joint Surg Am* 2004;86-A(7):1353-1358.
62. Ogonda L, Wilson R, Archbold P, et al: A minimal-incision technique in total hip arthroplasty does not improve early postoperative outcomes: A prospective, randomized, controlled trial. *J Bone Joint Surg Am* 2005;87(4): 701-710.
63. Huddleston HD: An accurate method for measuring leg length and hip offset in hip arthroplasty. *Orthopedics* 1997;20(4):331-332.
64. Masonis JL, Bourne RB: Surgical approach, abductor function, and total hip arthroplasty dislocation. *Clin Orthop Relat Res* 2002;405: 46-53.
65. Chiu FY, Chen CM, Chung TY, Lo WH, Chen TH: The effect of posterior capsulorrhaphy in primary total hip arthroplasty: A prospective randomized study. *J Arthroplasty* 2000;15(2): 194-199.
66. Pellicci PM, Bostrom M, Poss R: Posterior approach to total hip replacement using enhanced posterior soft tissue repair. *Clin Orthop Relat Res* 1998;355:224-228.
67. Sierra RJ, Raposo JM, Trousdale RT, Cabanela ME: Dislocation of primary THA done through a posterolateral approach in the elderly. *Clin Orthop Relat Res* 2005;441:262-267.
68. Suh KT, Park BG, Choi YJ: A posterior approach to primary total hip arthroplasty with soft tissue repair. *Clin Orthop Relat Res* 2004;418:162-167.
69. Weeden SH, Paprosky WG, Bowling JW: The early dislocation rate in primary total hip arthroplasty following the posterior approach with posterior soft-tissue repair. *J Arthroplasty* 2003;18(6): 709-713.
70. Kim YS, Kwon SY, Sun DH, Han SK, Maloney WJ: Modified posterior approach to total hip arthroplasty to enhance joint stability. *Clin Orthop Relat Res* 2008; 466(2):294-299.
71. Edwards BN, Tullos HS, Noble PC: Contributory factors and etiology of sciatic nerve palsy in total hip arthroplasty. *Clin Orthop Relat Res* 1987;218:136-141.
72. Navarro RA, Schmalzried TP, Amstutz HC, Dorey FJ: Surgical approach and nerve palsy in total hip arthroplasty. *J Arthroplasty* 1995;10(1):1-5.
73. Lachiewicz PF: Dislocation, in Hozack WJ, Parvizi J, Bender B, eds: *Surgical Treatment of Hip Arthritis: Reconstruction, Replacement, and Revision*. Philadelphia, PA, Saunders Elsevier, 2010, pp 429-436.
74. Kadakia NR, Noble PC, Sugano N, Paravic V: Posterior dislocation of the artificial hip joint: Effect of cup anteversion. *Orthop Trans* 1998-1999;22: 905-906.
75. Paterno SA, Lachiewicz PF, Kelley SS: The influence of patient-related factors and the position of the acetabular component on the rate of dislocation after total hip replacement. *J Bone Joint Surg Am* 1997;79(8):1202-1210.
76. Biedermann R, Tonin A, Krismer M, Rachbauer F, Eibl G, Stöckl B: Reducing the risk of dislocation after total hip arthroplasty: The effect of orientation of

the acetabular component. *J Bone Joint Surg Br* 2005;87(6):762-769.

77. Hassan DM, Johnston GH, Dust WN, Watson G, Dolovich AT: Accuracy of intraoperative assessment of acetabular prosthesis placement. *J Arthroplasty* 1998; 13(1):80-84.
78. Rittmeister M, Callitsis C: Factors influencing cup orientation in 500 consecutive total hip replacements. *Clin Orthop Relat Res* 2006;445:192-196.
79. McCollum DE, Gray WJ: Dislocation after total hip arthroplasty: Causes and prevention. *Clin Orthop Relat Res* 1990;261:159-170.
80. Archbold HA, Mockford B, Molloy D, McConway J, Ogonda L, Beverland D: The transverse acetabular ligament: An aid to orientation of the acetabular component during primary total hip replacement. A preliminary study of 1000 cases investigating postoperative stability. *J Bone Joint Surg Br* 2006;88(7):883-886.
81. Sotereanos NG, Miller MC, Smith B, Hube R, Sewecke JJ, Wohlrab D: Using intraoperative pelvic landmarks for acetabular component placement in total hip arthroplasty. *J Arthroplasty* 2006; 21(6):832-840.
82. Honl M, Schwieger K, Salineros M, Jacobs J, Morlock M, Wimmer M: Orientation of the acetabular component: A comparison of five navigation systems with conventional surgical technique. *J Bone Joint Surg Br* 2006; 88(10):1401-1405.
83. Jaramaz B, DiGioia AM III, Blackwell M, Nikou C: Computer assisted measurement of cup placement in total hip replacement. *Clin Orthop Relat Res* 1998; 354:70-81.
84. Spencer JM, Day RE, Sloan KE, Beaver RJ: Computer navigation of the acetabular component: A cadaver reliability study. *J Bone Joint Surg Br* 2006;88(7): 972-975.
85. McGrory BJ, Morrey BF, Cahalan TD, An KN, Cabanela ME: Effect of femoral offset on range of motion and abductor muscle strength after total hip arthroplasty. *J Bone Joint Surg Br* 1995; 77(6):865-869.
86. Herrlin K, Selvik G, Pettersson H, Kesek P, Onnerfält R, Ohlin A: Position, orientation and component interaction in dislocation of the total hip prosthesis. *Acta Radiol* 1988;29(4):441-444.
87. Widmer KH, Zurfluh B: Compliant positioning of total hip components for optimal range of motion. *J Orthop Res* 2004;22(4): 815-821.
88. Barrack RL, Burke DW, Cook SD, Skinner HB, Harris WH: Complications related to modularity of total hip components. *J Bone Joint Surg Br* 1993; 75(5):688-692.
89. Woolson ST, Hartford JM, Sawyer A: Results of a method of leg-length equalization for patients undergoing primary total hip replacement. *J Arthroplasty* 1999; 14(2):159-164.
90. Bourne RB, Rorabeck CH: Soft tissue balancing: the hip. *J Arthroplasty* 2002;17(4, Suppl 1):17-22.
91. Longjohn D, Dorr LD: Soft tissue balance of the hip. *J Arthroplasty* 1998;13(1):97-100.
92. Asayama I, Naito M, Fujisawa M, Kambe T: Relationship between radiographic measurements of reconstructed hip joint position and the Trendelenburg sign. *J Arthroplasty* 2002;17(6):747-751.
93. Sakalkale DP, Sharkey PF, Eng K, Hozack WJ, Rothman RH: Effect of femoral component offset on polyethylene wear in total hip arthroplasty. *Clin Orthop Relat Res* 2001;388:125-134.
94. Mineo R, Berend KR, Mallory TH, Lombardi AV Jr: A lateralized tapered titanium cementless femoral component does not increase thigh or trochanteric pain. *Surg Technol Int* 2007;16: 210-214.
95. Incavo SJ, Havener T, Benson E, McGrory BJ, Coughlin KM, Beynnon BD: Efforts to improve cementless femoral stems in THR: 2- to 5-year follow-up of a high-offset femoral stem with distal stem modification (Secur-Fit Plus). *J Arthroplasty* 2004;19(1): 61-67.
96. Bhave A, Paley D, Herzenberg JE: Improvement in gait parameters after lengthening for the treatment of limb-length discrepancy. *J Bone Joint Surg Am* 1999;81(4): 529-534.
97. Gurney B, Mermier C, Robergs R, Gibson A, Rivero D: Effects of limb-length discrepancy on gait economy and lower-extremity muscle activity in older adults. *J Bone Joint Surg Am* 2001; 83-A(6):907-915.
98. Maloney WJ, Keeney JA: Leg length discrepancy after total hip arthroplasty. *J Arthroplasty* 2004; 19(4, Suppl 1):108-110.
99. White TO, Dougall TW: Arthroplasty of the hip: Leg length is not important. *J Bone Joint Surg Br* 2002;84(3):335-338.
100. Ranawat CS, Rao RR, Rodriguez JA, Bhende HS: Correction of limb-length inequality during total hip arthroplasty. *J Arthroplasty* 2001;16(6):715-720.
101. Jasty M, Webster W, Harris W: Management of limb length inequality during total hip replacement. *Clin Orthop Relat Res* 1996; 333:165-171.
102. Matsuda K, Nakamura S, Matsushita T: A simple method to minimize limb-length discrepancy after hip arthroplasty. *Acta Orthop* 2006;77(3):375-379.
103. Shiramizu K, Naito M, Shitama T, Nakamura Y, Shitama H: L-shaped caliper for limb length measurement during total hip

arthroplasty. *J Bone Joint Surg Br* 2004;86(7):966-969.

104. Sarin VK, Pratt WR, Bradley GW: Accurate femur repositioning is critical during intraoperative total hip arthroplasty length and offset assessment. *J Arthroplasty* 2005;20(7):887-891.

105. Bartz RL, Nobel PC, Kadakia NR, Tullos HS: The effect of femoral component head size on posterior dislocation of the artificial hip joint. *J Bone Joint Surg Am* 2000;82(9):1300-1307.

106. Kung PL, Ries MD: Effect of femoral head size and abductors on dislocation after revision THA. *Clin Orthop Relat Res* 2007;465: 170-174.

107. Sariali E, Lazennec JY, Khiami F, Catonné Y: Mathematical evaluation of jumping distance in total hip arthroplasty: Influence of abduction angle, femoral head offset, and head diameter. *Acta Orthop* 2009;80(3):277-282.

108. Smith TM, Berend KR, Lombardi AV Jr, Emerson RH Jr, Mallory TH: Metal-on-metal total hip arthroplasty with large heads may prevent early dislocation. *Clin Orthop Relat Res* 2005;441: 137-142.

109. Cuckler JM, Moore KD, Lombardi AV Jr, McPherson E, Emerson R: Large versus small femoral heads in metal-on-metal total hip arthroplasty. *J Arthroplasty* 2004; 19(8, Suppl 3):41-44.

110. Peters CL, McPherson E, Jackson JD, Erickson JA: Reduction in early dislocation rate with large-diameter femoral heads in primary total hip arthroplasty. *J Arthroplasty* 2007;22(6, Suppl 2): 140-144.

111. Smit MJ: Hip stability in primary total hip arthroplasty using an anatomically sized femoral head. *Orthopedics* 2009;32(7):489.

112. Lachiewicz PF, Soileau ES: Dislocation of primary total hip arthroplasty with 36 and 40-mm femoral heads. *Clin Orthop Relat Res* 2006;453:153-155.

113. Amstutz HC, Le Duff MJ, Beaulé PE: Prevention and treatment of dislocation after total hip replacement using large diameter balls. *Clin Orthop Relat Res* 2004; 429:108-116.

114. Halley D, Glassman A, Crowninshield RD: Recurrent dislocation after revision total hip replacement with a large prosthetic femoral head: A case report. *J Bone Joint Surg Am* 2004;86-A(4): 827-830.

115. Spangehl MJ, Masri BA, O'Connell JX, Duncan CP: Prospective analysis of preoperative and intraoperative investigations for the diagnosis of infection at the sites of two hundred and two revision total hip arthroplasties. *J Bone Joint Surg Am* 1999;81(5):672-683.

116. Barmeir E, Dubowitz B, Roffman M: Computed tomography in the assessment and planning of complicated total hip replacement. *Acta Orthop Scand* 1982;53(4): 597-604.

117. Lasda NA, Levinsohn EM, Yuan HA, Bunnell WP: Computerized tomography in disorders of the hip. *J Bone Joint Surg Am* 1978;60(8):1099-1102.

118. Mian SW, Truchly G, Pflum FA: Computed tomography measurement of acetabular cup anteversion and retroversion in total hip arthroplasty. *Clin Orthop Relat Res* 1992;276:206-209.

119. Pierchon F, Pasquier G, Cotten A, Fontaine C, Clarisse J, Duquennoy A: Causes of dislocation of total hip arthroplasty: CT study of component alignment. *J Bone Joint Surg Br* 1994;76(1):45-48.

120. Dorr LD, Wan Z: Causes of and treatment protocol for instability of total hip replacement. *Clin Orthop Relat Res* 1998;355: 144-151.

121. Ritter MA: A treatment plan for the dislocated total hip arthroplasty. *Clin Orthop Relat Res* 1980; 153:153-155.

122. Cameron HU: Use of a constrained acetabular component in revision hip surgery. *Contemp Orthop* 1991;23:481-484.

123. Clayton ML, Thirupathi RG: Dislocation following total hip arthroplasty: Management by special brace in selected patients. *Clin Orthop Relat Res* 1983;177: 154-159.

124. Ekelund A: Trochanteric osteotomy for recurrent dislocation of total hip arthroplasty. *J Arthroplasty* 1993;8(6):629-632.

125. LaPorte DM, Mont MA, Pierre-Jacques H, Peyton RS, Hungerford DS: Technique for acetabular liner revision in a nonmodular metal-backed component. *J Arthroplasty* 1998;13(3):348-350.

126. Mallory TH, Vaughn BK, Lombardi AV Jr, Kraus TJ: Prophylactic use of a hip cast-brace following primary and revision total hip arthroplasty. *Orthop Rev* 1988; 17(2):178-183.

127. Russin LA, Sonni A: Indications for the use of a constrained THR prosthesis. *Orthop Rev* 1981;10: 81-84.

128. Sioen W, Simon JP, Labey L, Van Audekercke R: Posterior transosseous capsulotendinous repair in total hip arthroplasty: A cadaver study. *J Bone Joint Surg Am* 2002; 84-A(10):1793-1798.

129. Williams JF, Gottesman MJ, Mallory TH: Dislocation after total hip arthroplasty: Treatment with an above-knee hip spica cast. *Clin Orthop Relat Res* 1982;171:53-58.

130. Woolson ST, Rahimtoola ZO: Risk factors for dislocation during the first 3 months after primary total hip replacement. *J Arthroplasty* 1999;14(6):662-668.

131. von Knoch M, Berry DJ, Harmsen WS, Morrey BF: Late dislocation after total hip arthroplasty. *J Bone Joint Surg Am* 2002; 84-A(11):1949-1953.

132. Joshi A, Lee CM, Markovic L, Vlatis G, Murphy JC: Prognosis of dislocation after total hip arthroplasty. *J Arthroplasty* 1998; 13(1):17-21.

133. Parvizi J, Morrey BF: Bipolar hip arthroplasty as a salvage treatment for instability of the hip. *J Bone Joint Surg Am* 2000;82-A(8): 1132-1139.

134. Olerud S, Karlström G: Recurrent dislocation after total hip replacement: Treatment by fixing an additional sector to the acetabular component. *J Bone Joint Surg Br* 1985;67(3):402-405.

135. Toomey SD, Hopper RH Jr, McAuley JP, Engh CA: Modular component exchange for treatment of recurrent dislocation of a total hip replacement in selected patients. *J Bone Joint Surg Am* 2001;83-A(10):1529-1533.

136. Parvizi J, Wade FA, Rapuri V, Springer BD, Berry DJ, Hozack WJ: Revision hip arthroplasty for late instability secondary to polyethylene wear. *Clin Orthop Relat Res* 2006;447:66-69.

137. Beaulé PE, Ebramzadeh E, LeDuff M, Prasad R, Amstutz HC: Cementing a liner into a stable cementless acetabular shell: The double-socket technique. *J Bone Joint Surg Am* 2004; 86-A(5):929-934.

138. Heck DA, Murray DG: In vivo construction of a metal-backed, high-molecular-weight polyethylene cup during McKee-Farrar revision total joint arthroplasty: A case report. *J Arthroplasty* 1986; 1(3):203-206.

139. Cobb TK, Morrey BF, Ilstrup DM: The elevated-rim acetabular liner in total hip arthroplasty: Relationship to postoperative dislocation. *J Bone Joint Surg Am* 1996;78(1):80-86.

140. McConway J, O'Brien S, Doran E, Archbold P, Beverland D: The use of a posterior lip augmentation device for a revision of recurrent dislocation after primary cemented Charnley/Charnley Elite total hip replacement: Results at a mean follow-up of six years and nine months. *J Bone Joint Surg Br* 2007;89(12): 1581-1585.

141. Mogensen B, Arnason H, Jónsson GT: Socket wall addition for dislocating total hip: Report of two cases. *Acta Orthop Scand* 1986;57(4):373-374.

142. Rogers M, Blom AW, Barnett A, Karantana A, Bannister GC: Revision for recurrent dislocation of total hip replacement. *Hip Int* 2009;19(2):109-113.

143. Williamson JB, Galasko CS, Rowley DI: Failure of acetabular augmentation for recurrent dislocation after hip arthroplasty: Report of 3 cases. *Acta Orthop Scand* 1989;60(6):676-677.

144. Beaulé PE, Schmalzried TP, Udomkiat P, Amstutz HC: Jumbo femoral head for the treatment of recurrent dislocation following total hip replacement. *J Bone Joint Surg Am* 2002;84-A(2):256-263.

145. Skeels MD, Berend KR, Lombardi AV Jr: The dislocator, early and late: The role of large heads. *Orthopedics* 2009;32(9).

146. Barbosa JK, Khan AM, Andrew JG: Treatment of recurrent dislocation of total hip arthroplasty using a ligament prosthesis. *J Arthroplasty* 2004;19(3): 318-321.

147. Lavigne MJ, Sanchez AA, Coutts RD: Recurrent dislocation after total hip arthroplasty: Treatment with an Achilles tendon allograft. *J Arthroplasty* 2001;16(8, Suppl 1):13-18.

148. Strømsøe K, Eikvar K: Fascia lata plasty in recurrent posterior dislocation after total hip arthroplasty. *Arch Orthop Trauma Surg* 1995; 114(5):292-294.

149. Dennis DA, Lynch CB: Trochanteric osteotomy and advancement: A technique for abductor related hip instability. *Orthopedics* 2004; 27(9):959-961.

150. Kaplan SJ, Thomas WH, Poss R: Trochanteric advancement for recurrent dislocation after total hip arthroplasty. *J Arthroplasty* 1987;2(2):119-124.

151. Della Valle CJ, Berger RA, Rosenberg AG, Jacobs JJ, Sheinkop MB, Paprosky WG: Extended trochanteric osteotomy in complex primary total hip arthroplasty: A brief note. *J Bone Joint Surg Am* 2003;85-A(12):2385-2390.

152. Attarian DE: Bipolar arthroplasty for recurrent total hip instability. *J South Orthop Assoc* 1999;8(4): 249-253.

153. Ries MD, Wiedel JD: Bipolar hip arthroplasty for recurrent dislocation after total hip arthroplasty: A report of three cases. *Clin Orthop Relat Res* 1992;278:121-127.

154. Beaulé PE, Roussignol X, Schmalzried TP, Udomkiat P, Amstutz HC, Dujardin FH: Tripolar arthroplasty for recurrent total hip prosthesis dislocation. *Rev Chir Orthop Reparatrice Appar Mot* 2003;89(3):242-249.

155. Grigoris P, Grecula MJ, Amstutz HC: Tripolar hip replacement for recurrent prosthetic dislocation. *Clin Orthop Relat Res* 1994;304:148-155.

156. Levine BR, Della Valle CJ, Deirmengian CA, et al: The use of a tripolar articulation in revision total hip arthroplasty: A minimum of 24 months' follow-up. *J Arthroplasty* 2008;23(8):1182-1188.

157. Anderson MJ, Murray WR, Skinner HB: Constrained acetabular components. *J Arthroplasty* 1994; 9(1):17-23.

158. Berend KR, Lombardi AV Jr, Mallory TH, Adams JB, Russell JH, Groseth KL: The long-term outcome of 755 consecutive constrained acetabular components in total hip arthroplasty examining the successes and fail-

ures. *J Arthroplasty* 2005;20(7, Suppl 3):93-102.

159. Berend KR, Lombardi AV Jr, Welch M, Adams JB: A constrained device with increased range of motion prevents early dislocation. *Clin Orthop Relat Res* 2006;447:70-75.

160. Bremner BR, Goetz DD, Callaghan JJ, Capello WN, Johnston RC: Use of constrained acetabular components for hip instability: An average 10-year follow-up study. *J Arthroplasty* 2003;18(7, Suppl 1):131-137.

161. Callaghan JJ, O'Rourke MR, Goetz DD, Lewallen DG, Johnston RC, Capello WN: Use of a constrained tripolar acetabular liner to treat intraoperative instability and postoperative dislocation after total hip arthroplasty: A review of our experience. *Clin Orthop Relat Res* 2004;429: 117-123.

162. Callaghan JJ, Parvizi J, Novak CC, et al: A constrained liner cemented into a secure cementless acetabular shell. *J Bone Joint Surg Am* 2004;86-A(10): 2206-2211.

163. Goetz DD, Bremner BR, Callaghan JJ, Capello WN, Johnston RC: Salvage of a recurrently dislocating total hip prosthesis with use of a constrained acetabular component: A concise follow-up of a previous report. *J Bone Joint Surg Am* 2004;86-A(11):2419-2423.

164. Goetz DD, Capello WN, Callaghan JJ, Brown TD, Johnston RC: Salvage of a recurrently dislocating total hip prosthesis with use of a constrained acetabular component: A retrospective analysis of fifty-six cases. *J Bone Joint Surg Am* 1998;80(4): 502-509.

165. Goetz DD, Capello WN, Callaghan JJ, Brown TD, Johnston RC: Salvage of total hip instability with a constrained acetabular component. *Clin Orthop Relat Res* 1998;355:171-181.

166. Lombardi AV Jr, Mallory TH, Kraus TJ, Vaughn BK: Preliminary report on the S-ROM constraining acetabular insert: A retrospective clinical experience. *Orthopedics* 1991;14(3):297-303.

167. Padgett DE, Warashina H: The unstable total hip replacement. *Clin Orthop Relat Res* 2004;420: 72-79.

168. Shrader MW, Parvizi J, Lewallen DG: The use of a constrained acetabular component to treat instability after total hip arthroplasty. *J Bone Joint Surg Am* 2003; 85-A(11):2179-2183.

169. Su EP, Pellicci PM: The role of constrained liners in total hip arthroplasty. *Clin Orthop Relat Res* 2004;420:122-129.

170. Kaper BP, Bernini PM: Failure of a constrained acetabular prosthesis of a total hip arthroplasty: A report of four cases. *J Bone Joint Surg Am* 1998;80(4):561-565.

171. Fisher DA, Kiley K: Constrained acetabular cup disassembly. *J Arthroplasty* 1994;9(3):325-329.

172. Guyen O, Lewallen DG, Cabanela ME: Modes of failure of Osteonics constrained tripolar implants: A retrospective analysis of forty-three failed implants. *J Bone Joint Surg Am* 2008;90(7): 1553-1560.

173. Robertson WJ, Mattern CJ, Hur J, Su EP, Pellicci PM: Failure mechanisms and closed reduction of a constrained tripolar acetabular liner. *J Arthroplasty* 2009; 24(2):322, e5-e11.

174. McPherson EJ, Costigan WM, Gerhardt MB, Norris LR: Closed reduction of dislocated total hip with S-ROM constrained acetabular component. *J Arthroplasty* 1999;14(7):882-885.

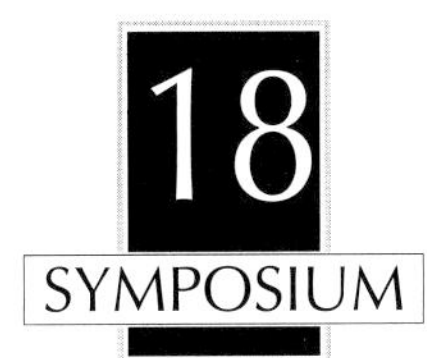

Hot Topics and Controversies in Arthroplasty: Cementless Femoral Fixation in Elderly Patients

Andrew Dutton, FRCS
*Harry E. Rubash, MD

Abstract

Cementless femoral fixation has been established as the gold standard for hip arthroplasty in young patients because of its exceptional longevity. Because older Americans are living longer and staying active, cementless femoral fixation for hip arthroplasty should be considered in all patients who have good bone quality. Numerous studies have shown excellent results using cementless fixation for hip arthroplasty in elderly patients. Histologic analysis, radiographic review, and dual-energy x-ray absorptiometry have shown solid osseointegration for biologic fixation and minimal bone loss. Cementless fixation provides superb functional outcomes with results comparable to those achieved using cemented fixation for hip arthroplasty. Additional advantages of cementless femoral fixation include shorter surgical times and substantial savings in health care costs.

Total hip arthroplasty (THA) can provide patients with an exceptional quality of life.[1-3] The femoral component may be cemented or cementless. Cementless femoral stems are proximally or fully coated to provide biologic fixation. Despite similar long-term results compared with cemented fixation, cementless femoral fixation provides additional benefits, including decreased morbidity and improved cost-effectiveness. Cementless femoral implants for THAs are an excellent choice for the elderly patient population.

The Aging Population: Implant Considerations

Elderly individuals are becoming an increasingly large proportion of the US population.[4] In 2000, 12.4% of the US population was older than 65 years. It is estimated that this percentage will increase to 16.3% by 2020. According to data from 2003 from the US Department of Health and Human Services, the life expectancy at birth was 75.3 years for males and 80.1 years for females.[4] At 75 years of age, the mean life expectancy was 10.5 years for males and 12.6 years for females (Table 1). Trends show an increase in life expectancy projections[4] (Table 2).

A study by Ritter and associates[5] compared the life expectancy of patients treated with THA to that of the general population. The 10-year life expectancy rate for women who were treated with THA at age 71 to 80 years was 75%, and 58% for those older than 80 years at the time of THA. In contrast, women in the general population age 71 to 80 years had a 10-year life expectancy rate of 60%, and those older than 80 years had a 10-year life expectancy rate of 27%. This improved life expectancy rate may be due in part to the medical screening of patients prior to THA and to the health status of those who are eligible for the procedure. Because patients undergoing THA have the potential for a long life, it is important that implants used in THA will properly function throughout the patient's lifetime.

Advantages of Cementless Implants

Implant Survival

The biologic fixation provided by cementless stems has led to excellent

Harry Rubash, MD or the department with which he is affiliated has received research or institutional support and royalties from Zimmer.

long-term implant survival (Table 3). Pieringer and associates[6] retrospectively reviewed the clinical and radiologic results of 80 patients (87 hips) who were older than 80 years at the time of cementless THA. A grit-blasted, titanium alloy femoral stem (Alloclassic SL; Centerpulse, Winterthur, Switzerland) was used in all patients; mean follow-up was 69.3 months. No femoral stems were removed for aseptic loosening during this period. One intraoperative femoral fracture occurred. Deep infection occurred in two patients, with one patient requiring repeat surgery with a liner and femoral head exchange. Two early postoperative dislocations occurred and were treated successfully with closed reduction. Keisu and associates[7] performed 123 cementless THAs using a plasma-sprayed, titanium alloy femoral stem (Taperloc; Biomet, Warsaw, IN) in patients 80 to 89 years of age. Ninety-two hips (86 patients) had a mean follow-up of 5 years. There were no femoral revisions. One patient who had recurrent dislocations was again treated with closed reduction. Two late periprosthetic fractures occurred; one was treated with open reduction and internal fixation and the other was treated with traction. No perioperative deaths occurred, but the rate of medical complications was 24%. Complications included pulmonary emboli in 6.5% of patients and cardiac abnormalities in 2.4%. McAuley and associates[8] reviewed 159 cementless THAs that used the fully porous-coated Anatomic Medullary Locking femoral stem (DePuy, Johnson and Johnson, Warsaw, IN) in patients with a mean age of 71 years and a mean follow-up of 8.5 years. One intraoperative, periprosthetic fracture occurred and was treated with cerclage wiring. There was one femoral revision for aseptic loosening at 2.3 years, which was revised successfully to a larger stem. Nine hips dislocated postoperatively, with only one requiring a revision. Two other revisions were needed, one for sepsis and another for an avulsion fracture of the greater trochanter secondary to osteolysis. In another study, Bourne and associates[9] reviewed 307 cementless THAs using a proximally plasma-sprayed, titanium alloy femoral stem (Mallory Head; Biomet Inc, Warsaw, IN) in patients with a mean age of 64 years. With a follow-up period of 10 to 13 years, two femoral revisions were needed; one revision was for a periprosthetic fracture and the other for sepsis. Berend and associates[10] reviewed the outcome of 49 cementless THAs using the Mallory Head femoral component in patients with a mean age of 79 years. With a mean follow-up of 5 years,

Table 1
Life Expectancy in the United States in 2003[4]

	Male (years)	Female (years)
Birth	75.3	80.1
Age 65	16.8	19.8
Age 75	10.5	12.6
Age 85	5.7	6.9

Table 2
Life Expectancy at Birth (Based on Year of Birth)[4]

Year of Birth	Male	Female
1900	46.3	48.3
1950	65.6	71.1
1990	71.8	78.8
2000	74.3	79.7

Table 3
Results of Cementless THAs in Elderly Patients

Study	Patient Age (Years)	Number of Hips	Femoral Stem Type	Follow-up (Years)	Stem Survival	Resurgery (Number and Reason)
Pieringer et al[6]	> 80	87	Grit-blasted titanium alloy (Alloclassic SL)	Mean 5.8	100%	2 PPFXs 1 Sepsis
Keisu et al[7]	80 to 89	92	Plasma-sprayed titanium tapered (Taperloc)	Mean 5	100%	1 PPFX
McAuley et al[8]	Mean 71	159	Fully coated anatomic (Anatomic Medullary Locking)	Mean 8.5	98%	1 Loose 1 Dislocation 1 Sepsis 1 PPFX
Bourne et al[9]	Mean 64	307	Plasma-sprayed titanium tapered (Mallory Head)	10 to 13	100%	1 Sepsis 1 PPFX
Berend et al[10]	Mean 79	49	Plasma-sprayed titanium tapered (Mallory Head)	Mean 5	100%	1 Pain

PPFX = periprosthetic fracture

no femoral revisions for aseptic loosening occurred. One intraoperative femoral fracture was treated with cerclage wiring, and one femoral stem was revised unsuccessfully for unexplained leg (not thigh) pain; intraoperatively, the stem was noted to be well fixed. These studies show excellent results for the survival of cementless femoral components in elderly patients; these results are comparable to the results achieved using cemented femoral implants.

Preservation of Femoral Bone Stock

The preservation of femoral bone stock is desirable in elderly patients with osteoporosis. The variety of stem geometries and surface coatings available with cementless femoral stems allow biologic fixation in a variety of femoral canal geometries. Grit-blasted, titanium femoral components have shown excellent histologic osseointegration.[11] Marshall and associates[12] radiographically reviewed 200 cementless THAs using plasma-sprayed, titanium alloy femoral stems (Integral, Biomet). Spot welds were seen in 99.3% of the stems, and endosteal bone formation around the tip was noted in 51%. Cortical hypertrophy in zones 2, 3, 5, and 6 was noted in 26%. Akhavan and associates[13] reviewed the results of THA using a cementless stem consisting of a cobalt-chromium core surrounded by polyaryletherketone and titanium mesh (Epoch; Zimmer, Warsaw, IN). Twenty-eight patients were followed for an average of 6.2 years. There was no radiographic evidence of femoral loosening. Although there was a small, initial decrease in bone mass at the proximal zones of 1, 2, 6, and 7 on dual-energy x-ray absorptiometry, bone mass did not decrease significantly over time. Minimal bone loss was noted in the distal zones. There was one femoral revision for a periprosthetic fracture. Cementless femoral components allow excellent biologic fixation and minimize bone loss.

Modularity and Geometry of Femoral Stems

Cementless femoral stems also provide the necessary modularity and geometry for fixation in most types of femoral canals. With aging, there is significant remodeling of the femur, which is most pronounced in women.[14] Radiographic analysis of cadaveric femurs revealed an average of 3° of varus remodeling of the femoral neck with aging. At the isthmus, canal expansion averaged 0.092 mm per year. The femoral canal changes from a so-called champagne flute shape to that resembling a stovepipe. Because of these morphologic changes, using a cemented generic femoral component in an elderly woman may compromise the proximal medial cement mantle. To avoid this complication, the stem may be downsized; however, this leads to an excessively thick cement mantle. The option of multiple cementless femoral stem geometries can accommodate the variations in femoral morphology associated with aging.

Cost Implications

THAs performed in the increasingly larger elderly population have substantial economic implications. From 1990 to 2002, the number of THAs performed has increased by 46%.[15] Health cost assessment and minimization is essential in orthopaedic procedures.[1] Barrack and associates[16] analyzed 50 cases to compare the cost of implanting cemented versus cementless femoral stems. The cases were divided into two groups: uncomplicated, primary, cementless THAs or hybrid THAs. Femoral cementation involved extra equipment including a canal water pik and brush, canal plug, stem centralizer, and cement. Cemented THAs required longer surgical times (average increase, 20 minutes) that were related to cement insertion and setting. Overall, cementless femoral fixation was approximately 8% less costly than cemented fixation.

Functional Outcomes

Functional outcomes for cementless THAs in elderly patients have been excellent. Zimmerman and associates[17] compared functional outcomes of cementless versus hybrid THAs in 272 patients older than 65 years. Assessment at 2, 6, and 12 months postoperatively found no differences in pain level, walking speed, and lower extremity function in performing activities of daily living between the two groups. In a study analyzing the clinical results of cementless THAs in patients with an average age of 79 years and an average follow-up of 5 years, 71% of patients were able to walk more than two blocks, 44% did not require an assistive device, 35% required a cane, and 19% used a walker.[10] Jones and associates[18] reviewed the functional outcomes of 454 patients treated with THA. Using the Western Ontario and McMaster Universities Osteoarthritis Index and the Medical Outcomes Society 36-Item Short Form survey, they determined that age was not related to functional outcome. Cementless femoral THA has superb and comparable functional results to cemented THA.

Complications: Considerations of Cementless Versus Cemented THAs

Cemented femoral fixation has distinct disadvantages compared with cementless fixation. Data from the Norwegian Arthroplasty Register show that patients with cemented THAs have a significantly increased risk (1.8 times higher) of infection compared with patients with cementless THAs.[19] This finding may be related to bone necrosis secondary to either direct cement toxicity or from heat generated from cement polymerization. Elderly patients are often susceptible to infection because of medical comorbidities.

Elderly patients are more susceptible to cardiopulmonary compromise resulting from the pulmonary emboli related to cemented femoral fixation. Clark and associates[20] evaluated 20 patients age 59 to 83 years who were treated with cemented hemiarthroplasty and monitored with a transesophageal Doppler probe. During cementation, patients had a 33% reduction in cardiac output and a 44% reduction in stroke volume. Hagio and associates[21] evaluated 88 patients treated with a hybrid THA who were monitored with a transesophageal echocardiograph. Severe embolic events (cascade of fine emboli or embolic masses) occurred in 61.5% of patients in the hybrid THA group compared with 5.9% of patients in the group treated with cementless THA. These events were associated with significant decreases in arterial oxygen saturation and systolic blood pressure. Parvizi and associates[22] reviewed the records of 23 patients who died during surgery from cardiorespiratory compromise during THA. These deaths represented 0.06% of THAs performed at the authors' institution. The mean patient age was 80.9 years, and all patients had undergone cemented femoral component fixation. Autopsies were performed in 13 patients. Bone marrow microemboli were found in the lungs of 11 patients, and methylmethacrylate particles were found in 3 patients.

Hemodynamic changes caused by cementation may be associated with a higher rate of postoperative confusion in elderly patients. Pagnano and associates[23] reviewed the clinical outcome of THAs in 47 patients older than 90 years. Twenty-two patients had 35 medical complications; 9 were caused by transient postoperative confusion. These serious adverse effects of femoral cementation can be particularly problematic in elderly patients with underlying cardiac and pulmonary pathology.

Cemented femoral fixation in THA is associated with prolonged surgical times. The mean surgical time for cementless THA was 120 minutes compared with 140 minutes for cemented THA.[16] The Norwegian Arthroplasty Register noted that surgical times for cementless THAs were on average 15 minutes shorter than for cemented THAs.[19] Smabrekke and associates[24] further analyzed the Register's data and noted that cemented implants with surgical times of less than 51 minutes and more than 90 minutes were associated with an increased risk of revision because of aseptic loosening. Prolonged surgical times (> 150 minutes) were associated with an increased risk of revision because of infection. Because cemented femoral fixation in THA is associated with longer surgical times, operating room and anesthesia costs are increased, as well as the risk of infection.

Another disadvantage of cement fixation is the difficulty encountered in revision surgery. Removing the cement mantle of a femoral stem is challenging and time consuming.[25] Cement removal may necessitate bone damage secondary to procedures such as an extended trochanteric osteotomy or the creation of a cortical window.[26,27] Thirteen percent of intraoperative fractures occur during cement removal.[28] The use of specialized instruments to remove cement also carry inherent risks, including the risk of femoral perforation, thermal tissue damage with the use of an ultrasonic device, and increased infection risk secondary to contaminated aerosols from a burr device.[29,30] The preservation of bone stock by avoiding stress shielding can be valuable in the revision setting.

Summary

The use of cementless femoral prostheses should be considered for THA in all patients with good bone quality. These implants allow biologic fixation with physiologic loading of the bone to minimize stress shielding and have excellent survivorship in elderly patients with all types of bone morphology. With an increasingly large elderly population, cementless femoral prostheses have demonstrated superior cost-effectiveness compared with cemented prostheses. Cementless THA is not associated with the disadvantages of cemented femoral fixation that include cement-related emboli, longer surgical times, increased infection risk, and the difficulties inherent in cement extraction. Cementless femoral implants for THA are an excellent choice for elderly patients.

References

1. Bozic KJ, Saleh KJ, Rosenberg AG, Rubash HE: Economic evaluation in total hip arthroplasty: Analysis and review of the literature. *J Arthroplasty* 2004;19:180-189.

2. Chang RW, Pelliser JM, Hazen GB: Cost-effectiveness analysis of total hip arthroplasty for osteoarthritis of the hip. *JAMA* 1996;275:858-865.

3. Brander VA, Malhotra S, Jet J, Heinemann AW, Stulberg DS: Outcome of hip and knee arthroplasty in persons aged 80 years and older. *Clin Orthop Relat Res* 1997;345:67-78.

4. Centers for Disease Control Website. National Center for Health Statistics. Available at: www.cdc.gov/nchs/fastats/lifexpec.html. Accessed March, 2007.

5. Ritter MA, Albohm MJ, Keating M, Faris P, Meding JB: Life expectancy after total hip arthroplasty. *J Arthroplasty* 1998;13:874-875.

6. Pieringer H, Labek G, Auersperg V, Bohler N: Cementless total hip arthroplasty in patients older than 80 years of age. *J Bone Joint Surg Br* 2003;85:641-645.

7. Keisu KS, Orozco F, Sharkey PF, Hozack WJ, Rothman RH: Primary cementless total hip arthroplasty in octogenarians: Two to eleven year follow-up. *J Bone Joint Surg Am* 2001; 83-A:359-363.

8. McAuley JP, Moore KD, Culpepper WJ II, Engh CA: Total hip arthroplasty with porous coated prostheses fixed without cement in patients who are sixty-five years of age and older. *J Bone Joint Surg Am* 1998;80:1648-1655.

9. Bourne RB, Rorabeck CH, Patterson JJ, Guerin J: Tapered titanium cementless total hip replacements: A 10 to 13 year follow-up. *Clin Orthop Relat Res* 2001;393:112-120.

10. Berend KR, Lombardi AV, Mallory TH, Dodds KL, Adams JB: Cementless double-tapered total hip arthroplasty in patients 75 years of age and older. *J Arthroplasty* 2004;19: 288-295.

11. Feighan JE, Goldberg VM, Davy D, Parr JA, Stevenson S: The influence of surface-blasting on the incorporation of titanium-alloy implants in a rabbit intramedullary model. *J Bone Joint Surg Am* 1995;77:1380-1395.

12. Marshall AD, Mokris JG, Reitman RD, Dandar A, Mauerhan DR: Cementless titanium tapered-wedge femoral stem: 10-15 year follow-up. *J Arthroplasty* 2004;19:546-552.

13. Akhavan S, Matthiesen MM, Schulte L, et al: Clinical and histologic results related to a low-modulus composite total hip replacement. *J Bone Joint Surg Am* 2006;88:1308-1314.

14. Noble PC, Box GG, Kamaric E, Fink MJ, Alexander JW, Tullos HS: The effect of aging on the shape of the proximal femur. *Clin Orthop Relat Res* 1995;316:31-44.

15. Kurtz S, Mowat F, Ong K, Chan N, Lau E, Halpern M: Prevalence of primary and revision total hip and knee arthroplasty in the United States from 1990 through 2002. *J Bone Joint Surg Am* 2005;87:1487-1497.

16. Barrack RL, Castro F, Guinn S: Cost of implanting a cemented versus cementless femoral stem. *J Arthroplasty* 1996;11:373-376.

17. Zimmerman S, Hawkes WG, Hudson JI, et al: Outcomes of surgical management of total hip replacement in patients aged 65 years and older: Cemented versus cementless femoral component and lateral or anterolateral versus posterior anatomical approach. *J Orthop Res* 2002;20:182-191.

18. Jones CA, Voaklander DC, Johnston DW, Suarez-Almazor ME: The effect of age on pain, function, and quality of life after total hip and knee arthroplasty. *Arch Intern Med* 2001;161: 454-460.

19. Engesaeter LB, Espehaug B, Lie SA, Furnes O, Havelin LI: Does cement increase the risk of infection in primary total hip arthroplasty? Revision rates in 56,275 cemented and uncemented primary THAs followed for 0-16 years in the Norwegian Arthroplasty Register. *Acta Orthop* 2006;77: 351-358.

20. Clark DI, Ahmed AB, Baxendale BR, Moran CG: Cardiac output during hemiarthroplasty of the hip: A prospective, controlled trial of cemented and uncemented prostheses. *J Bone Joint Surg Br* 2001;83:414-418.

21. Hagio K, Sugano N, Takashina M, Nishii T, Yoshikawa H, Ochi T: Embolic events during total hip arthroplasty: An echocardiographic study. *J Arthroplasty* 2003;18:186-192.

22. Parvizi J, Holiday A, Ereth M, Lewallen DG: Sudden death during primary hip arthroplasty. *Clin Orthop Relat Res* 1999;369:39-48.

23. Pagnano MW, McLamb LA, Trousdale RT: Primary and revision total hip arthroplasty for patients 90 years of age and older. *Mayo Clin Proc* 2003; 78:285-288.

24. Smabrekke A, Epehaug B, Havelin LI, Furnes O: Operating time and survival of primary total hip replacements: An analysis of 31,745 primary cemented and uncemented total hip replacements from local hospitals reported to the Norwegian Arthroplasty Register 1987-2001. *Acta Orthop Scand* 2004;75:524-532.

25. Schurman DJ, Maloney WJ: Segmental cement extraction at revision total hip arthroplasty. *Clin Orthop Relat Res* 1992;285:158-163.

26. Taylor JW, Rorabeck CH: Hip revision arthroplasty: Approach to the femoral side. *Clin Orthop Relat Res* 1999;369:208-222.

27. Paprosky WG, Weeden SH, Bowling JW: Component removal in revision total hip arthroplasty. *Clin Orthop Relat Res* 2001;393:181-193.

28. Meek RM, Garbuz DS, Masri BA, Greidanus NV, Duncan CP: Intraoperative fracture of the femur in revision total hip arthroplasty with a diaphyseal fitting stem. *J Bone Joint Surg Am* 2004;86-A:480-485.

29. Nogler M, Lass-Florl C, Wimmer C, Mayr E, Bach C, Ogon M: Contamination during removal of cement in revision hip arthroplasty: A cadaver study using ultrasonic and high speed cutters. *J Bone Joint Surg Br* 2003;85: 436-439.

30. Brooks AT, Nelson CL, Stewart CL, Skinner RA, Siems ML: Effect of an ultrasonic device on temperatures generated in bone and on bone-cement structure. *J Arthroplasty* 1993; 8:413-418.

Postoperative Pain Management Techniques in Hip and Knee Arthroplasty

Javad Parvizi, MD, FRCS
Manny Porat, MD
Kishor Gandhi, MD, MPH
*Eugene R. Viscusi, MD
*Richard H. Rothman, MD, PhD

Abstract

Adequate control of postoperative pain following hip and knee arthroplasty can be a challenging task fraught with potential complications. Postoperative pain is perceived by the patient via a complex network and a multitude of molecular messengers in both the peripheral and central nervous systems. This allows the physician to modulate pain via an array of medications that act on different sites within the body. Using both contemporary and traditional pain modulators, the delivery and timing of these medications can affect postoperative pain and, ultimately, rehabilitation of the arthroplasty patient. Current techniques for controlling pain use both multimodal and preemptive analgesia to improve the outcome of the surgery while minimizing the potential adverse effects of the medications given.

Adequate control of postoperative pain following hip and knee arthroplasty can be a challenging task.[1,2] Previous studies have shown that more than 50% of patients undergoing surgery report postoperative pain as a major concern.[3] Consequences of uncontrolled pain can lead to myocardial ischemia and infarctions, pulmonary infections, paralytic ileus, urinary retention, thromboembolisms, and impaired immune function, as well as anxiety. In addition, inadequate control of pain may result in patient dissatisfaction, impaired patient rehabilitation, and prolonged hospitalization.[3] The negative influence of postoperative pain on rehabilitation is a cause of concern for patients undergoing joint arthroplasty. Functional recovery and return of muscle strength are dependent on the ability of these patients to comply with rehabilitation. The drawbacks of inadequate rehabilitation are especially cumbersome in hip and knee surgeries because faster mobilization leads to quicker discharge from the hospital. Furthermore, studies have shown that in comparison with recovery from hip replacement, recovery from knee arthroplasty is prolonged up to 50 days postoperatively.[4] Pain control is especially important for knee arthroplasty patients to allow recovery of range of motion and muscle strength for ambulation.[5] Because the adverse outcomes from uncontrolled pain can be potentially devastating after arthroplasty, adequate pain management is critical. Two current and critical elements of contemporary pain management include preemptive analgesia and preventive multimodal techniques. A better understanding of pain pathways and newer drugs will help to bring about pain-free joint arthroplasty and faster postoperative rehabilitation.

Eugene R. Viscusi, MD or the department with which he is affiliated has received research or institutional support from Pfizer and Merck. Richard H. Rothman, MD, PhD or the department with which he is affiliated has received research or institutional support and royalties from Stryker and is a consultant for or an employee of Stryker.

Preemptive Analgesia

The concept of preemptive analgesia was introduced in the late 1980s. The strategy incorporated the delivery of medication before the offending insult, an action that ultimately would reduce the requirement for analgesics given after the insult-related inflammation developed. The opiate receptors at the dorsal horn, if premedicated before the injury, would reduce the transmission of the stimulus. Standard practice currently has shown the benefits of administering shorter-acting opiates at the time of induction instead of during the postinflammatory state.[6] Several studies have demonstrated the benefits of regional anesthesia before surgery, with a significant decrease in postoperative pain in patients undergoing total joint arthroplasty.[7]

In addition to opiates, other drugs have been useful in preemptive treatment. To engage both the peripheral sensory as well as the central neurons, nonsteroidal anti-inflammatory drugs (NSAIDs) have been effective. Although the timing of the medications is still under investigation, α2-agonists such as clonidine and α2δ-subunit ligands such as gabapentin and pregabalin have been shown to be effective in reducing pain and pain medication requirements when administered before the surgical procedure. When combined with opioids preoperatively, they can dramatically improve the postoperative rehabilitation and, ultimately, the outcome of the patient.

Multimodal Analgesia

The value of multimodal analgesia is understated in the literature.[8] Most reports on the control of postoperative pain consist of unimodal therapies. However, the combination of multiple analgesic drugs with different mechanisms and pathways of action is the best way to achieve maximal control of pain after hip and knee arthroplasty.[9] Kehlet and Dahl first described the concept of combining multiple analgesic techniques in 1993 as a method of improving outcome following colon surgery.[8] Multimodal analgesia was used to improve analgesia intraoperatively and postoperatively and ultimately reduced the need for opioids along with the risks of their adverse effects. Adverse events from the use of opioids include nausea, vomiting, respiratory depression, sedation, and pruritus. By using different types of medications, the synergistic effects reduce the necessity for larger opioid doses, lowering the incidence of common adverse effects. In addition to decreasing adverse effects and improving postoperative pain, multimodal analgesia may shorten hospitalization time and improve recovery, which decreases health care costs following total joint arthroplasty.[10] Common adjuvant medications include NSAIDs, ketamine, local anesthetics, α2-agonists, and α2δ-ligands. Recent studies have demonstrated the benefits of using cyclooxygenase-2 (COX-2) inhibitors with regional anesthesia in the treatment of the total knee arthroplasty patient. In one study, there was a reduction in epidural analgesic use, in-hospital opioid consumption, and pain scores in patients who received COX-2 inhibitors.[11] Patients also had improved range of motion of the knee at the time of discharge and 1-month follow-up. Similar beneficial effects have been seen in patients undergoing spinal fusion and anterior cruciate ligament reconstruction.

Pain Pathway

Multimodal analgesia requires an understanding of the molecular mechanisms of pain pathways. Postoperative pain is a consequence of tissue injury, nerve irritation, and the resulting cascade of neurohumeral events that follow. After a painful stimulus, chemical mediators such as prostaglandins and bradykinin are released at the site of tissue injury. These chemical mediators stimulate nociceptors, peripheral pain receptors that respond to trauma and high temperatures. These nociceptors form pain fibers that enter the spinal cord via the dorsal root ganglion. Pain receptors that are principally responsible for noxious stimulation in the dorsal horn of the spinal cord are N-methyl D-aspartate (NMDA) receptors. Painful stimulus is propagated by central NMDA receptors in the spinal cord by way of the spinothalamic tract to the brain. Through this complex pathway, the brain experiences pain after trauma inflicted to the site of tissue injury caused by surgery. The concept of multimodal analgesia relies on understanding these complex neurohumeral interactions. Analgesia after surgery can be achieved by using a combination of drugs that inhibit this complex pathway at multiple sites (Figure 1).

Preoperative Period

The preemptive strategy behind multimodal analgesia must begin in advance of the surgical incision. Pain control for patients undergoing knee and hip arthroplasty can be achieved with a combination of drugs used prior to surgery (NSAIDs, COX-2 inhibitors, anticonvulsants, and ketamine).

NSAIDs and COX-2 Inhibitors

The use of nonopioid drugs during the preoperative period can reduce excess intraoperative opioid usage and the possible subsequent effect of opioid-induced hyperalgesia seen after surgery.[12] Opioid-induced hyperalgesia is a complex phenomenon that can follow rapid escalation in opioids during or following a surgical procedure; this condition can paradoxically lower the pain threshold and result in greater opioid requirements. Research has shown that activation of NMDA receptors in the central nervous system results in hyperalgesia associated with opioids. This phenomenon may be minimized by limiting opioids and maximizing nonopioid drugs. The use of NSAIDs is recommended as a multimodal approach to pain management as part of most acute pain management guidelines.[13]

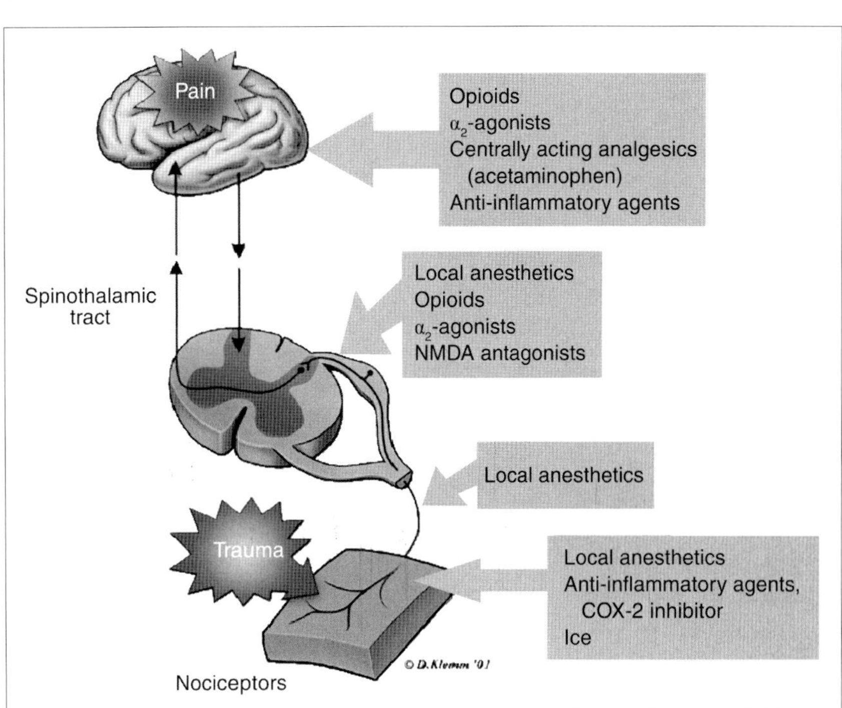

Figure 1 Pain pathways and multimodal analgesic therapy. (Adapted with permission from Gottschalk A, Smith DS: New concepts in acute pain therapy: Preemptive analgesia. *Am Fam Physician* 2001;63:1979-1984.)

The use of preoperative NSAIDs and COX-2 inhibitors also has a significant effect on opioid requirements following surgery. This has been referred to as an "opioid-sparing effect." The clinical significance of this may be the reduction of opioid-related side effects, improved analgesia, and better patient satisfaction. The primary site of action of NSAIDs and COX-2 inhibitors are in the periphery where they inhibit prostaglandin synthesis and the stimulation of nociceptors (Figure 1). Through this inhibition, they target peripheral pain pathways (peripheral sensitization). Recent findings show elevation of prostaglandins in the central nervous system, which also may play a role in central sensitization syndrome.[14] Furthermore, the hypersensitivity of injured tissue also may produce a secondary hyperalgesic effect on uninjured tissue.[15] Prostaglandins have been demonstrated to lower pain thresholds in both the central and peripheral nervous system. NSAIDs or COX-2 inhibitors can be used preoperatively to effectively reduce the occurrence of central and peripheral sensitization syndrome after surgery.

Preemptive treatments with NSAIDs such as ketorolac and ibuprofen are shown to have the advantage of decreasing postoperative pain scores, opioid requirements, and nausea after surgery.[16] Some surgeons are concerned about the use of NSAIDs before surgery because of a decrease in platelet aggregation and a potential increase in bleeding time.[17] Consequently, NSAIDs are commonly discontinued 7 to 10 days before surgery to reduce perioperative bleeding, particularly with hip arthroplasty.[18] Other concerns associated with NSAIDs include gastritis and peptic ulcer disease, renal impairment, and poor wound and bone healing. Because of these concerns, COX-2 selective inhibitors may have advantages over NSAIDs in the acute postoperative setting.

COX-2 selective inhibitors provide selective inhibition of prostaglandins, thereby reducing bleeding and gastric adverse effects seen with NSAIDs. COX-2 selective inhibitors allow for dosage on an empty stomach before surgery, with low risk of bleeding during surgery. Recently, COX-2 inhibitors have fallen out of favor because of concerns for the potential increased risk of cardiovascular adverse effects with long-term usage. Rofecoxib has been withdrawn from the market because of its cardiovascular adverse effects. However, the COX-2 selective inhibitors have not been implicated for cardiovascular side effects with short-term use such as in postoperative analgesia. Many studies have demonstrated benefits of using these agents in the perioperative setting.

One study using preoperative dosing of COX-2 inhibitors 1 hour before arthroscopic knee surgery

Table 1
Dosage Recommendations for Individual Nonopioid Agents That May Be Administered as Part of Multimodal Analgesia

Drug	Dose	Route of Administration	Time Before Surgery	Time After Surgery
NSAIDs				
Ketorolac	15-30 mg	PO/IV	1-2 h	15-30 mg every 6 h
Ibuprofen	800 mg	PO	1-2 h	800 mg every 6 h
COX-2 Inhibitors				
Celecoxib	400 mg	PO	1 h	200 mg × 1 (2 h after surgery)
Valdecoxib	40 mg	PO	1 h	Twice daily
Antineuropathics				
Gabapentin	1,200 mg	PO	1-2 h	1,200 mg × 1 (24 h after surgery)
Pregabalin	150 mg	PO	1 h	150 mg × 1 (12 h after surgery)
Analgesics				
Propacetamol	2 g	PO/IV PO/IV	15 min	2 g every 4 h
Acetaminophen	1 g	PO/IV PO/IV	15 min	1 g every 4 h

NSAIDs = nonsteroidal anti-inflammatory drugs; COX = cyclooxygenase; IV = intravenous; PO = orally.

showed significant reduction in pain scores compared with placebo at 1 hour, 2 hours, and 24 hours after surgery.[19] These patients had a significantly longer duration postoperatively before requiring analgesics, and the 24-hour consumption of opioids was significantly lower than patients who were offered the same drug postoperatively. Another study using rofecoxib 24 hours and 1 hour before surgery with continued postoperative drug administration for 14 days had better outcomes in total knee arthroplasty.[20] These patients showed reduced opioid requirements, faster time to physical rehabilitation, reduced nausea and vomiting, better sleep patterns, and greater patient satisfaction after surgery. In addition, an opioid-sparing effect has been demonstrated with the preoperative use of celecoxib and rofecoxib after spinal fusion surgery.[21] In this study, rofecoxib (50 mg) showed an extended benefit for 24 hours after surgery. Both NSAIDs and COX-2 inhibitors may be continued after the patient is discharged from the hospital for optimal pain management. Dosage recommendations for preoperative treatments are given in Table 1.

Gabapentin and Pregabalin

Gabapentin and pregabalin are alkylated aminobutyric acid analogs initially used as antiepileptic medications. Gabapentin, introduced in 1993, has been used to treat painful neuropathies and postherpetic neuralgia. The mechanism of action of these drugs is to bind to the presynaptic voltage-gated calcium channels in the dorsal root ganglia and the spinal cord. They work by inhibiting the release of excitatory neurotransmitters such as substance P, glutamate, and noradrenaline. Gabapentin is not metabolized by the body and is excreted in the urine. Gabapentin reaches peak plasma level approximately 3 hours after loading dose, unlike pregabalin, which has dose-independent absorption. Gabapentinoids have been used recently to reduce acute postoperative pain. Because of their ability to reduce central sensitization, these drugs have shown promising results when administered preoperatively. In several studies, doses from 800 mg to 1,200 mg have been administered 1 to 2 hours after common orthopaedic surgeries. As a result, preoperative anxiety was reduced, and postoperative range of motion was improved in patients who underwent anterior cruciate ligament reconstruction.[22]

Studies have shown that preoperative administration of gabapentin leads to a reduction in postoperative pain and morphine consumption.[23-25] Synergistic benefits are seen up to 72 hours when COX-2 inhibitors and gabapentin are used together before surgery for lower abdominal and spinal fusion surgeries.[23,26] Pregabalin also had a synergistic effect with COX-2 inhibitors in clinical studies involving patients undergoing spinal fusion.[27] The combination of the two drugs reduced postoperative pain, morphine consumption at 24 hours, and opioid-induced adverse effects. Improvements in outcome were greater when these drugs were used in combination than either of the drugs used alone. Studies continue to determine optimal timing of these drugs for the surgical patient. Common adverse effects include dizziness, somnolence, and peripheral edema.

Ketamine

Ketamine is a noncompetitive antagonist of the NMDA receptors. Ketamine's proposed mechanism of action is to prevent the progressive nociceptive response by blocking NMDA receptor–related pain transmission from incisional and inflammatory injury. It has been studied in various formats, given both preoperatively and postoperatively in patients undergoing major orthopaedic surgeries. According to one study, administration of ketamine improved passive knee mobilization 24 hours after arthroscopic anterior ligament reconstruction and improved postoperative functional outcomes with knee arthroscopy.[28] In a study by Adam and associates,[29] perioperative ketamine administration to patients undergoing total knee arthroplasty decreased morphine consumption by 35% and improved early rehabilitation with similar incidences of adverse effects. However, they did not find any long-term improvements in functional recovery. In another study, a small dose of ketamine, in addition to local anesthetic, was administered via an epidural catheter preoperatively to patients scheduled for total knee arthroplasty.[30] Based on their results, the authors suggest that this may decrease injury-induced pain sensitization and may provide better postoperative analgesia alone than with local anesthetics.[30] Other studies investigating the use of ketamine with opioids in the perioperative period have not found any substantial benefit compared with opioids alone.[31] Common adverse effects from ketamine use include nausea/vomiting, nystagmus, hypersalivation, and hallucinations.

Table 2
Dose Recommendations for Agents That May Be Used as Adjuncts Perioperatively

Agent	Dose	Onset
Spinal Block		
Epinephrine	0.1-0.6 mg	Rapid
Meperidine	1.2-1.5 mg/kg	Rapid
Morphine	100-300 mg	20-30 min
Fentanyl	5-25 mg	45-75 min
Clonidine	75 mg	5-10 min
Intravenous		
Ketamine	5-6 mg/kg/min	Rapid

Primary Intraoperative Period

Spinal and Epidural Analgesia

Regional anesthesia usually is preferred over general anesthesia in the United States. Regional anesthesia provides optimal surgical conditions and analgesia extending into the postoperative period. The motor block achieved by spinal anesthesia is unsurpassed by any other technique. The modest reduction in arterial blood pressure contributes to reduced surgical blood loss. Regional analgesia also may result in reduced postoperative nausea and vomiting, less respiratory and cardiac depression, and decreased risks of thromboembolism.[32-34] Regional anesthesia has the advantage of blunting stress response in surgery and decreasing morbidity and mortality in high-risk surgical patients.[35,36] Regional analgesia uses local anesthetics (such as bupivicaine, ropivacaine, or tetracaine) as the primary agent for the blockade of central sensory and motor receptors. The onset of analgesia is dependent on characteristics of the local anesthetic (lipid solubility, pK_a, and dosage and volume of anesthetic used), patient anatomy (age, weight, height, and gender), and technique used (site of injection, type of needle used, and direction of the needle) (Table 2). Local anesthetics in regional anesthesia block nociceptive transmission in the peripheral nervous system (via peripheral nerve block) and the central nervous system (via spinal/epidural blocks) (Figure 1). Some agents may be coadministered with local anesthetics in an attempt to enhance the quality of the neural blockade. Agents commonly used include vasoconstrictors (epinephrine), opioids (morphine or fentanyl), α2-receptor agonists (clonidine), NSAIDs (ketorolac), or COX-2 inhibitors.[37] Although many studies have demonstrated a benefit to this practice, the use of some agents is equivocal. Also, the addition of some agents introduces other adverse effects. Hence, the risk-benefit ratio always must be individualized to the specific patient.

Regional analgesia during the perioperative period involves the use of spinal analgesia, combined spinal-epidural analgesia, or peripheral nerve blockade for pain control during and after surgery. Spinal anesthesia commonly used for total joint arthroplasty uses a spinal needle to place drugs (local anesthetics) into the intrathecal (subarachnoid) space. The onset of spinal anesthesia is rapid because the cerebrospinal fluid quickly carries the drug to various sites in the spinal cord. The intensity and height of the spinal blockade depends on the baricity (compared with spinal fluid) and the volume of the local anesthetic used. Opioids such as morphine and fentanyl may be added to the intrathecal mixture to prolong postoperative pain control. Fentanyl, because of its lipophilic properties, produces rapid onset (10 to 15 minutes) but short duration (2 to 4 hours) of analgesia, whereas morphine, with its hydrophilic properties, has a longer duration (18 to 24 hours) of action into the postoperative period.[37] Relatively small does of intrathecal morphine (0.2 mg) are effective for providing prolonged analgesia after hip arthroplasty. For optimal postoperative pain relief as part of multimodal analgesia, morphine has a higher degree of patient satisfaction because of its prolonged analgesic effect. Randomized controlled studies with patients undergoing total hip replacement show significant reduction in postoperative intravenous morphine requirements for patients who received 0.1 to 0.3 mg of intrathecal morphine.[38] The same dose of morphine with total knee replacement did not significantly reduce the need for supplemental intravenous morphine in the postoperative period. The most common side effects of intrathecal morphine reported after the surgery were pruritus, nausea, vomiting, and oxygen desaturation. Older patients undergoing hip arthroplasty may benefit from a more conservative dose of 100 μg of morphine added to the spinal anesthetic because serious adverse effects such as oversedation and delayed respiratory depression are minimized.[39] Nonetheless, intrathecal morphine has a long record of safety when moderate doses are tailored to the specific patient.

The administration of clonidine with spinal local analgesics can decrease the need for postoperative morphine consumption. Clonidine is a α2-adrenergic agonist that potentiates the sensory and motor blocks of local anesthetics in the spinal cord. The combination of clonidine and morphine in an intrathecal regimen results in significant improvements in postoperative pain and decreased morphine requirements for 12 hours after total knee arthroplasty;[40] however, hypotension was reported in some of these patients.

Epidural anesthesia is preferred by some clinicians. Epidural anesthesia and analgesia requires placing a specially designed needle into the epidural space. Drugs may be injected directly through the needle, or an epidural catheter may be inserted. Subsequent postoperative analgesia may use continuous drug infusion or injection of a single drug. A variety of other agents have been added to epidural infusions. Epinephrine can induce a synergistic analgesic on the spinal cord as well as elicit vasoconstriction on the blood vessels for decreased absorption of a local anesthetic.[41] Other multimodal approaches have used small doses of ketamine, an NMDA antagonist in the spinal cord, for sensory blockade and the prevention of central sensitization of nociceptors.[42]

The benefits of epidural analgesia and surgical outcomes have been well documented in the literature.[43] Compared with parenteral opioid use after surgery, the use of continuous infusion with epidural analgesia provides superior relief in postoperative pain with few adverse outcomes. The limitations of epidural analgesia often involve failed or dislodged catheters, unilateral blocks, and incompatibility in patients who are anticoagulated. There is a risk of spinal hematomas with patients who are receiving anticoagulants with an indwelling epidural catheter. Other limitations related to local anesthetics include hypotension and motor impairment in these patients.

Some of these issues related to epidural catheters or the local anesthetics themselves may be addressed by using an extended-release epidural morphine (EREM) formulation.[43] DepoDur (Endo Pharmaceuticals, Chadds Ford, PA), recently approved by the US Food and Drug Administration, uses microscopic multivesicular liposomal spherical particles with internal aqueous chambers containing morphine. Patients given a single epidural injection of EREM have experienced a 48-hour period of analgesia.[44] Patients given EREM in clinical trials after hip replacement had a significantly lower supplemental opioid requirement after surgery than placebo.[44] Furthermore, the need for rescue medications was minimal, with fewer instances of hypotension. Other potential advantages of EREM include no epidural catheter or pump-related issues, which can create gaps in analgesia postoperatively. The absence of epidural and patient-controlled analgesia (PCA) pump technology theoretically reduces opportunities for medication errors and pump programming errors. The adverse effects of EREM are similar to those of other opioids, including nausea, vomiting, constipation, and respiratory depressions. Ideally, the use of EREM in a multimodal analgesic approach and with appropriate patient selection may result in analgesia without the need for any tethering pump technology.

Peripheral Nerve Blocks

Peripheral nerve blocks (PNBs) represent an increasingly popular technique for anesthesia and pain management for total joint arthroplasty. Some clinicians prefer PNBs in patients who will receive anticoagulation therapy because of concerns for epidural hematomas. PNBs also may reduce the incidence of arterial hypotension or urinary retention compared with spinal or epidural techniques. The psoas compartment block of the lumbar plexus is an effective analgesic block for total hip arthroplasty. Anesthesia for total knee arthroplasty requires block of both the lumbar plexus (femoral or psoas compartment) and the lumbosacral plexus (sciatic nerve). However, adequate postoperative analgesia is usually achieved with a lumbar plexus block alone. Peripheral nerve blocks can be achieved with a single injection of a local anesthetic or with a catheter that uses continuous infusion of a local anesthetic.

Some studies show that a continuous femoral nerve block (FNB) has efficacy equal to epidural analgesia in patients undergoing total hip arthroplasty.[45] Although there were no significant differences between the two techniques, some of the adverse effects seen with epidural blocks, such as hypotension and spinal hematomas may be avoided with FNBs. The authors concluded that PNBs may be superior to epidural blocks because of the decreased systemic adverse effects seen with these blocks.

In studies involving total knee arthroplasty, both epidural analgesia and continuous FNB had better pain relief and faster knee rehabilitation compared with intravenous PCA usage after surgery.[46] The efficacy of FNBs alone is questioned by some because the sciatic nerve innervates the posterior and lateral aspect of the knee. Although it is necessary to combine both femoral and sciatic nerve blocks for total knee arthroplasty anesthesia, adequate postoperative analgesia is usually achieved with an FNB. A combination of continuous sciatic nerve block and FNB has been used in patients undergoing total knee arthroplasty.[47] In one study, adding a sciatic nerve block significantly decreased morphine requirements up to 36 hours.[47] However, one randomized study found minimal benefits of adding a sciatic nerve block to FNB.[48] There were no differences in morphine consumption with FNBs and the combined sciatic-femoral block. The authors concluded that sciatic innervation of the posterior knee may be a minor contributor of postoperative pain following total knee arthroplasty. Furthermore, blocking the obturator nerve in a psoas block also may give limited benefit.[49] There was limited benefit in analgesic requirements in a psoas block and no difference in functional outcome when compared to femoral and sciatic blocks. No block is without risk; hence clinicians must carefully evaluate the individual risk-benefit ratio of adding the sciatic block solely for postoperative analgesia.

All nerve blocks previously discussed may be performed with a single injection of local anesthetic or with a continuous infusion through an indwelling catheter. The benefits offered by a continuous infusion may include better analgesia through the second postoperative day; however, one study did not demonstrate a difference in length of hospital stay and functional recovery.[50] The limitations of a continuous catheter include additional time, cost, and skills required to manage the catheter, along with potential risks of infection and nerve injury. External infusion pump technology also introduces the potential for technical failures and requires additional surveillance. For these reasons, some clinicians avoid this approach.

Postoperative Period

Intravenous PCA

Intravenous PCA is the most widely used form of postoperative analgesia offered to patients after surgery.[51] PCA uses infusion pumps to deliver patient-activated fixed and small doses of opioids based on demand and a lockout period with an hourly maximal dose. Opioids commonly used in PCA include morphine, hydromorphone, and fentanyl. For PCA to be successful, patients have to be willing to actively participate in their care. Patients must comprehend the operation of the device and be able to give themselves a bolus when needed. Effective PCA treatment involves initial clinician titration by bolus to establish analgesia. PCA is intended to maintain analgesia, not to achieve analgesia. Opioid-related adverse effects are common. Elderly patients are particularly vulnerable to confusion and delirium after PCA use. Multimodal analgesia in combination with PCA may reduce opioid requirements, resulting in better pain control and fewer adverse effects. The complexity of standard PCA pumps may consume valuable health care resources, including nursing and pharmacy time and materials. PCA pumps have been implicated in medication errors and programming errors that may lead to patient harm. Hence, strict protocols need to be in place to prevent these errors.

Transdermal PCA

Transdermal PCA is a novel approach to the postoperative delivery of opioids without venous access, external infusion pumps, or the potential for programming errors. Transdermal PCA uses iontophoresis technology to deliver drugs through the skin by use of an external electrical field.[52] The fentanyl iontophoretic transdermal system (ITS) has recently been approved for the treatment of postoperative pain.[53,54] This system consists of a preprogrammed, needle-free credit card–sized system that is applied to the patient's upper outer arm or chest for 24 hours. The system uses an on-demand delivery dose of 40 μg of fentanyl for 10 minutes, up to 6 doses per hour with a maximum of 80 doses. The system shuts down after 80 doses or 24 hours (whichever comes first). Randomized placebo-controlled trials demonstrated that the fentanyl ITS was superior to placebo for pain control in the first 24 hours following surgery. Patients who received the fentanyl ITS had lower pain scores and fewer drug discontinuations compared to placebo. The side effect profiles were also similar between control patients and those who received fentanyl ITS. Another randomized study conducted on patients undergoing abdominal and orthopaedic surgeries in Europe showed fentanyl ITS to be just as effective as morphine PCA.[55] However, the iontophoretic system had greater ease of use and was less time-consuming than traditional PCA. The fentanyl ITS may be particularly attractive for total joint arthroplasty patients as it eliminates the need for a bulky infusion pump and tethering intravenous tubing that may impede patient activity and participation in physical therapy. Further studies will be needed to identify the benefits of less invasive technologies.

Acetaminophen (Paracetamol)

Acetaminophen is a popular adjuvant to opioids as part of multimodal analgesia in acute postoperative pain management. It also has an opioid-sparing effect, especially when used in combination with NSAIDs. Acetaminophen has no associated postoperative bleeding and is a cost-effective, centrally acting analgesic (Figure 1). An intravenous formulation of acetaminophen is available in many parts of the world and is currently under development in the United States. The intravenous acetaminophen formulation has had great efficacy in total joint arthroplasty patients.[56] The use of the drug also resulted in reduced morphine requirements and was better tolerated in elderly and high-risk patients.

Capsaicin

Capsaicin, an ingredient that can be isolated from chili peppers, is known to be highly pungent to the palate, often in dilute amounts. It is an agonist of the transient receptor potential vanilloid family receptor type 1 (TRPV1). The receptor is a nonselective cation channel that is responsible for the large release of calcium into the cell. The receptor can be activated by several ligands, including capsaicin, as well as various temperature changes.[57] The TRPV receptor is found in various tissues often associated with inflammatory states, including inflammatory bowel disease, irritable bowel syndrome, gastroesophageal reflux disease, and injured brachial plexus fibers and skin nerve fibers in women with chronic breast tenderness.[57] Activation of the TRPV1 receptor by agonists has been associated with transient local irritation followed by analgesic properties inducing a desensitization of the nerve. In addition, TRPV1 antagonists have been studied for their potential analgesic properties and potential clinical use in patients with chronic pain. Capsaicin has been used to treat neuropathic pain, burn wounds, stump pain from amputations, joint arthritic pain, and postoperative pain. Deal and associates,[58] in a double-blinded controlled study, demonstrated that capsaicin topical cream was effective in treating patients with knee osteoarthritis. The results of the study demonstrated a mean reduction in pain by 33% after 4 weeks of treatment. However, 40% of patients reported local burning, stinging, or erythema from the treatments. Other studies have demonstrated positive results in patients when injected with various forms and concentrations of capsaicin.[57] In a study by Davis and associates,[59] the protocol had patients intraoperatively injected with Adlea (Anesiva Inc, South San Francisco, CA), a capsaicin derivative, while undergoing unilateral knee arthroplasty. In the study, the patients reported decreased pain on first ambulation. Because of the dearth of clinical studies, further information is needed to determine the efficacy of capsaicin as a potent and viable analgesic in the arthroplasty patient.

An Institutional Approach to Multimodal Analgesia

Protocols and pathways can be used to apply multimodal techniques for total joint arthroplasty. Our protocols use multiple modalities administered at different times before and after surgery (Figure 2). These protocols are reduced to order sets with preselected options available for physician computer order entry. Although the options are adjusted to the needs of a particular patient, the availability of standard pathways facilitates application to a large number of patients in a high-volume orthopaedic practice. Patient outcomes are tracked, and these protocols are adjusted over time based on these findings and other emerging evidenced-based techniques.

Summary

Multimodal analgesia offers many benefits to patients undergoing total joint arthroplasty. Opioids remain an integral part of most analgesic plans, but techniques that reduce opioid requirements typically improve pain control both at rest and with motion, reduce opioid-related adverse effects, provide better patient satisfaction, and, according to a recent study, may reduce the incidence of long-term pain following surgery.[10] Well-designed pathways incorporating multimodal analgesia may affect the length of a hospital stay and functional outcome of these patients with prosthetic joints. Effective multimodal regimens require an understanding of the multiple pathways of pain. Optimal application of these techniques often is best served by developing institutional pathways for specific procedures.

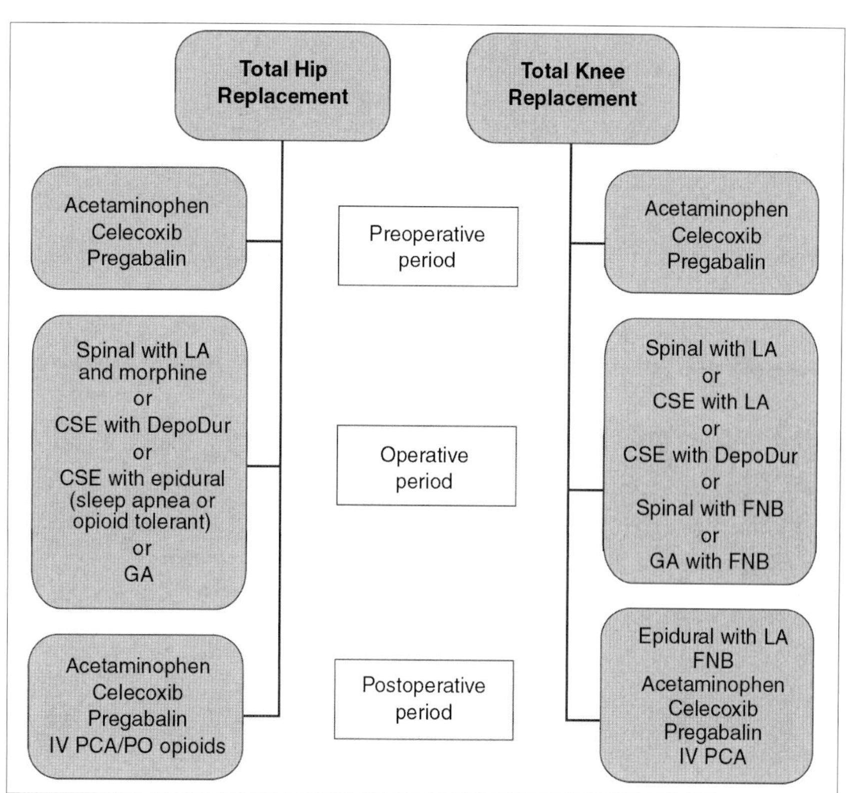

Figure 2 Multimodal analgesia algorithm for hip and knee arthroplasty at Thomas Jefferson University Hospital and Rothman Institute for Orthopaedics. GA = general anesthesia; IV = intravenous; LA = local anesthetic; CSE = combined spinal and epidural; PO = orally.

References

1. Apfelbaum JL, Chen C, Mehta SS, Gan TJ: Postoperative pain experience: Results from a national survey suggest postoperative pain continues to be undermanaged. *Anesth Analg* 2003;97:534-540.
2. Warfield CA, Kahn CH: Acute pain management: Programs in U.S. hospitals and experiences and attitudes among U.S. adults. *Anesthesiology* 1995;83:1090-1094.
3. Joshi GP, Ogunnaike BO: Consequences of inadequate postoperative pain relief and chronic persistent postoperative pain. *Anesthesiol Clin North America* 2005;23:21-36.
4. Salmon P, Hall GH, Peerbhoy D, Shenkin A, Parker C: Recovery from hip and knee arthroplasty: Patients' perspective on pain, function, quality of life, and well-being up to 6 months postoperatively. *Arch Phys Med Rehabil* 2001;82:360-366.
5. Shoji H, Solomonow M, Yoshino S, et al: Factors affecting postoperative flexion in total knee arthroplasty. *Orthopedics* 1990;13:643-649.
6. Bromley L: Pre-emptive analgesia and protective premedication: What is the difference? *Biomed Pharmacother* 2006;60:336-340.
7. Klasen J, Haas M, Graf S, et al: Impact on postoperative pain of long-lasting pre-emptive epidural analgesia before total hip replacement: A prospective randomized double-blind study. *Anaesthesia* 2005;60:118-123.
8. Kehlet H, Dahl JB: The value of "multimodal" or "balanced analgesia" in postoperative pain treatment. *Anesth Analg* 1993;77:1048-1056.
9. White PF: The changing role of non-opioid analgesic techniques in the management of postoperative pain. *Anesth Analg* 2005;101:S5-S22.
10. Reuben SS, Buvanendran A: Preventing the development of chronic pain after orthopaedic surgery with preventive multimodal analgesic techniques. *J Bone Joint Surg Am* 2007;89:1343-1358.
11. Buvanendran A, Kroin JS, Tuman KJ, et al: Effects of perioperative administration of a selective cyclooxygenase 2 inhibitor on pain management and recovery of function after knee replacement: A randomized controlled trial. *JAMA* 2003;290:2411-2418.
12. Mercadante S, Ferrera P, Villari P, Arcuri E: Hyperalgesia: An emerging iatrogenic syndrome. *J Pain Symptom Manage* 2003;26:769-775.
13. Practice guidelines for acute pain management in the perioperative setting: A report by the American Society of Anesthesiologists Task Force on Pain Management, Acute Pain Section. *Anesthesiology* 1995;82:1071-1081.

14. Samad TA, Moore KA, Sapirstein A, et al: Interleukin-1 β-mediated induction of Cox-2 in the CNS contributes to inflammatory pain hypersensitivity. *Nature* 2001;410:471-475.

15. Woolf CJ, Chong MS: Preemptive analgesia: Treating postoperative pain by preventing the establishment of central sensitization. *Anesth Analg* 1993;77:362-379.

16. Comfort VK, Code WF, Rooney ME, Yip RW: Naproxen premedication reduces postoperative tubal ligation pain. *Can J Anesthesiol* 1992;4:349-352.

17. Souter AJ, Fredman B, White PF: Controversies in the perioperative use of nonsteroidal antiinflammatory drugs. *Anesth Analg* 1994;79:1178-1180.

18. Robinson CM, Christie J, Malcon-Smith N: Nonsteroidal anti-inflammatory drugs, perioperative blood loss, and transfusion requirements in elective hip arthroplasty. *J Arthroplasty* 1993;8:607-610.

19. Reuben SS, Bhopatkar S, Maciolek H, Joshi W, Sklar J: The preemptive analgesic effect of rofecoxib after ambulatory arthroscopic knee surgery. *Anesth Analg* 2002;94:55-59.

20. Buvanendran A, Kroin JS, Tuman KJ, et al: Effects of perioperative administration of a selective cyclooxygenase 2 inhibitor on pain management and recovery of function after knee replacement: A randomized controlled trial. *JAMA* 2003;290:2411-2418.

21. Reuben SS, Connelly NR: Postoperative analgesic effects of celecoxib or rofecoxib after spinal fusion surgery. *Anesth Analg* 2000;91:1221-1225.

22. Tiippana EM, Hamunen K, Kontinen VK, Kalso E: Do surgical patients benefit from perioperative gabapentin/pregabalin? A systematic review of efficacy and safety. *Anesth Analg* 2007;104:1545-1556.

23. Turan A, Karamanlioglu B, Memis D, et al: Analgesic effect of gabapentin after spinal surgery. *Anesthesiology* 2004;100:935-938.

24. Turan A, Karamanlioglu B, Memis D, et al: The analgesic effects of gabapentin after total abdominal hysterectomy. *Anesth Analg* 2004;98:1370-1373.

25. Dierking G, Duedahl TH, Rasmussen ML, et al: Effects of gabapentin on postoperative morphine consumption and pain after abdominal hysterectomy: A randomized, double-blind trial. *Acta Anaesthesiol Scand* 2004;48:322-327.

26. Turan A, White PF, Karamanlioglu B, et al: Gabapentin: An alternative to the cyclooxygenase-2 inhibitors for perioperative pain management. *Anesth Analg* 2006;102:175-181.

27. Reuben SS, Buvanendran A, Kroin JS, Raghunathan K: The analgesic efficacy of celecoxib, pregabalin, and their combination for spinal fusion surgery. *Anesth Analg* 2006;103:1271-1277.

28. Menigaux C, Guignard B, Fletcher D, et al: Intraoperative small dose ketamine enhances analgesia after outpatient knee arthroscopy. *Anesth Analg* 2001;93:606-612.

29. Adam F, Chauvin M, Manoir B, Langlois M, Sessler DI, Fletcher D: Small dose ketamine infusion improves postoperative analgesia and rehabilitation after total knee arthroplasty. *Anesth Analg* 2005;100:475-480.

30. Himmelseher S, Pithamitsis D, Argiriadou H, Martin J, Esselborn S, Kochs E: Small dose S(+)-ketamine reduces postoperative pain when applied with ropivacaine in epidural anesthesia for total knee arthroplasty. *Anesth Analg* 2001;92:1290-1295.

31. Sveticic G, Farzanegan F, Zmoos P, Zmoos S, Eichenberger U, Curatolo M: Is the combination of morphine with ketamine better than morphine alone for postoperative intravenous patient-controlled analgesia? *Anesth Analg* 2008;106:287-293.

32. Modig J, Boreg T, Karlstrom G, Maripuu E, Sahlstedt B: Thromboembolism after total hip replacement: Role of epidural and general anesthesia. *Anesth Analg* 1983;62: 174-180.

33. Thorburn J, Louden JR, Vallance R: Spinal and general anesthesia in total hip replacement: Frequency of deep vein thrombosis. *Br J Anaesth* 1980;52:1117.

34. Christopherson R, Beattie C, Frank SM, et al: Perioperative morbidity in patients randomized to epidural or general anesthesia for lower extremity vascular surgery. *Anesthesiology* 1993;79:422-434.

35. Kehlet H: The stress response to surgery: Release mechanisms and the modifying effect of pain relief. *Acta Chir Scand Suppl* 1989;550:22-28.

36. Yeager MP, Glass DD, Neff RK, Brinck-Johnsen T: Epidural anesthesia and analgesia in high-risk surgical patients. *Anesthesiology* 1987;66:729-736.

37. Rathmell JP, Lair TR, Nauman B: The role of intrathecal drugs in the treatment of acute pain. *Anesth Analg* 2005;101:S30-S43.

38. Rathmell JP, Pin CA, Taylor R, Patrin T, Viani BA: Intrathecal morphine for postoperative analgesia: A randomized, controlled, dose-range study after hip and knee arthroplasty. *Anesth Analg* 2003;97:1452-1457.

39. Murphy PM, Stack D, Kinirons B, Laffey JG: Optimizing the dose of intrathecal morphine in older patients undergoing hip arthroplasty. *Anesth Analg* 2003;97:1709-1715.

40. Sites BD, Beach M, Biggs R, et al: Intrathecal clonidine added to a bupivacaine-morphine spinal anesthetic improves postoperative analgesia for total knee arthroplasty. *Anesth Analg* 2003;96:1083-1088.

41. Huang KS, Tseng CH, Cheung KS, Hui YL, Tan PP: Influence of epinephrine as an adjuvant to epidural morphine for postoperative analgesia. *Ma Zui Xue Za Zhi* 1993;31:245-248.

42. Chia YY, Liu K, Liu YC, Chang HC, Wong CS: Adding ketamine in a multimodal patient-controlled epidural regimen reduces postoperative pain and analgesic consumption. *Anesth Analg* 1998;86:1245-1249.

43. Viscusi ER: Emerging techniques in the management of acute pain: Epi-

dural analgesia. *Anesth Analg* 2005; 101:S23-S29.

44. Viscusi ER, Martin G, Hartrick CT, et al: 48 hours of postoperative pain relief following total hip arthroplasty with a novel, extended-release epidural morphine formulation. *Anesthesiology* 2005;102:1014-1022.

45. Singelyn FJ, Ferrant T, Malisse MF, Joris D: Effects of intravenous patient-controlled analgesia with morphine, continuous epidural analgesia, and continuous femoral nerve sheath block on rehabilitation after unilateral total-hip arthroplasty. *Reg Anesth Pain Med* 2005;30:452-457.

46. Singelyn FJ, Deyaert M, Jorist D, Pendeville E, Gouverneur JM: Effects of intravenous patient-controlled analgesia with morphine, continuous epidural analgesia, and continuous three-in-one block on postoperative pain and knee rehabilitation after unilateral total knee arthroplasty. *Anesth Analg* 1998;87:88-92.

47. Pham Dang C, Gautheron E, Guilley J, et al: The value of adding sciatic block to continuous femoral block for analgesia after total knee replacement. *Reg Anesth Pain Med* 2005;30:128-133.

48. Allen HW, Liu SS, Ware PD, Nairn CS, Owens BD: Peripheral nerve blocks improve analgesia after total knee replacement surgery. *Anesth Analg* 1998;87:93-97.

49. Morin AM, Kratz CD, Eberhart LH, et al: Postoperative analgesia and functional recovery after total-knee replacement: Comparison of a continuous posterior lumbar plexus (psoas compartment) block, a continuous femoral nerve block, and the combination of a continuous femoral and sciatic nerve block. *Reg Anesth Pain Med* 2005;30:434-445.

50. Salinas FV, Liu SS, Mulroy MF: The effect of single-injection femoral nerve block versus continuous femoral nerve block after total knee arthroplasty on hospital length of stay and long-term functional recovery within an established clinical pathway. *Anesth Analg* 2006;102:1234-1239.

51. Grass JA: Patient-controlled analgesia. *Anesth Analg* 2005;101:S44-S61.

52. Ashburn MA, Strisand J, Zhang J, et al: The iontophoresis of fentanyl citrate in humans. *Anesthesiology* 1995; 82:1146-1153.

53. Viscusi ER, Reynolds L, Taint S, Melson T, Atkinson LE: An iontophoretic fentanyl patient-activated analgesic delivery system for postoperative pain: A double-blind, placebo-controlled trial. *Anesth Analg* 2006; 102:188-194.

54. Viscusi ER, Reynolds L, Chung F, Atkinson LE, Khanna S: Patient-controlled transdermal fentanyl hydrochloride vs intravenous morphine pump for postoperative pain: A randomized controlled trial. *JAMA* 2004;291:1333-1341.

55. Grond S, Hall J, Spacek A, Hoppenbrouwers M, Richarz U, Bonnet F: Iontophoretic transdermal system using fentanyl compared with patient-controlled intravenous analgesia using morphine for postoperative pain management. *Br J Anaesth* 2007;98: 806-815.

56. Sinatra RS, Jahr JS, Reynolds LW, Viscusi ER, Groudine SB, Payen-Champenois C: Efficacy and safety of single and repeated administration of 1 gram intravenous acetaminophen injection (paracetamol) for pain management after major orthopedic surgery. *Anesthesiology* 2005;102:822-831.

57. Knotkova H, Pappagallo M, Szallasi A: Capsaicin (TRPV1 agonist) therapy for pain relief: Farewell or revival? *Clin J Pain* 2008;24:142-154.

58. Deal CL, Schnitzer TJ, Lipstein E, et al: Treatment of arthritis with topical capsaicin: A double-blind trial. *Clin Ther* 1991;13:383-395.

59. Davis J, Williams H, Bramlett K, et al: Enduring and well tolerated analgesia for total knee arthroplasty postsurgical pain produced by a single, rapidly-eliminated, intraoperative instillation of 4975. *J Pain* 2007;8:546.

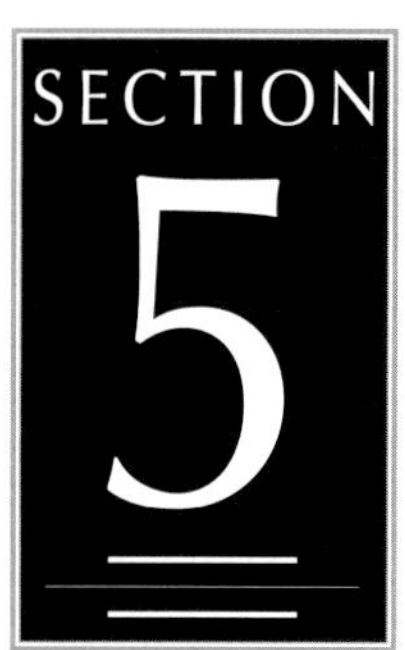

Managing Complications

Managing Complications

It is well recognized that total hip and knee replacements are among the most cost-effective surgical procedures for adding quality years of life, yet there remains some risk to patients treated with total hip or total knee arthroplasty. The chapters in this section describe some of the risks for complications faced by patients and managed by their treating surgeons.

Three chapters focus on hematologic issues in joint replacement. The chapter by Clark discusses blood management for patients treated with hip and knee replacement, whereas the chapters by Haas and associates and Friedman discuss the challenging topic of venous thromboembolic (VTE) disease and its prevention. The other chapters in this section, by Della Valle and associates and Richards and associates, present a thorough review of the management of periprosthetic fractures about the hip and the knee.

Clark presents a comprehensive summary of perioperative blood management strategies for patients treated with hip and knee replacement. The key message is to avoid routine postoperative transfusion triggers by adopting a more comprehensive approach to blood management. This approach includes identifying the preoperative factors (most importantly, preoperative hemoglobin levels) and the intraoperative factors (anticipated difficulty of the case) that may increase the need for a blood transfusion. Good discussions of perioperative blood salvage and methods for preoperatively identifying patients who may be at increased risk for transfusion are presented.

Blood management strategies have evolved since the publication of this chapter. The most notable change, only briefly mentioned in the chapter, is the increasing use of antifibrinolytic agents. Tranexamic acid is the most commonly used antifibrinolytic agent in joint replacement surgery. Recent studies have shown decreased transfusion rates in patients who receive tranexamic acid, although controversy remains on the optimal dose and timing of administration.[1-3] The theoretic concern about increased thromboembolic events in patients who receive tranexamic acid has not been proven. In some studies, tranexamic acid has been given to all patients without increasing the complication rate, whereas other investigators have adopted a more cautious approach and do not administer tranexamic acid in patients with a history of prior thromboembolic diseases or those with cardiac stents.

Since the publication of the Clark chapter, there has been an increasing awareness of the negative consequences of blood transfusions. It is well recognized that allogenic blood is an immunosuppressant. There is growing evidence in the literature of increased infection rates in orthopaedic patients who receive allogeneic blood.[4] There is also good evidence that restrictive transfusion practices (allowing hemoglobin levels to drop below 8 mg/dL in patients who do not have active ischemic cardiac disease) are not associated with increased perioperative medical complications and poorer postoperative function.[5-7]

The chapters by Haas and associates and Friedman discuss the complex topic of VTE disease and its prevention. Managing this problem is a balancing act for surgeons who wish to prevent a thromboembolism while avoiding the potential bleeding complications that may be associated with too aggressive pharmacologic prophylaxis. The ideal method of VTE prevention, which should be safe, effective, easy to use, and cost effective, remains elusive. As patients continue to recover more quickly from joint replacement procedures, with shorter hospital stays and faster return to day-to-day activities, the occurrence of thromboembolic events may decrease (although this theory remains unproven). The shorter duration of hospitalization after hip and knee arthroplasty has, for the most part, shifted the prevention of VTE disease from the hospital to the outpatient setting.

Haas and associates provide a comprehensive review of VTE disease after total hip and knee arthroplasty. The authors outline various mechanical and pharmacologic methods of prophylaxis, including multimodal prevention methods. The American College of Chest Physicians (ACCP) guidelines for prophylaxis against deep venous thrombosis and the American Academy of Orthopaedic Surgeons (AAOS) guideline for preventing pulmonary embolism are discussed. This section of the chapter is less relevant because the ACCP guidelines have been updated,[8] and the AAOS published a new guideline in 2011 for preventing VTE disease in patients undergoing elective hip and knee arthroplasty.[9] The first part of this chapter remains relevant, with an excellent discussion on the mechanisms of action of current pharmacologic and mechanical methods of VTE prophylaxis.

For the readers interested in a more detailed description of new oral anticoagulants for VTE prophylaxis after orthopaedic surgery, the chapter by Friedman provides a detailed review of newer marketed agents with more widespread clinical use. The chapter provides a worthwhile review of the coagulation cascade and the points at which various agents inhibit this pathway.

The last two chapters in this section, by Della Valle and associates and Richards and associates, address the increasingly prevalent and challenging task of managing periprosthetic fractures about the hip and knee. Because of the increasing prevalence of joint replacements, periprosthetic fractures are increasing in number and now represent the third most common reason for revision hip surgery (after surgery for osteolysis and instability). The need for successful management is critical. Both chapters describe a practical, stepwise approach to managing periprosthetic fracture complications. Without such an approach, patients may require repeat surgeries, which can result in poor function and increase the risks for further complications.

The chapter by Della Valle and associates provides a comprehensive review of periprosthetic fracture about the hip and knee. The chapter outlines important trends for treating periprosthetic femoral hip fractures, including the use of uncemented, long, fluted, tapered stems for managing fractures with loose implants (Vancouver type B2 and some type B3 fractures) and the use of locking plates for type B1 fractures with stable implants. With improved plating technology (the ability to use locking screws together with standard compression screws and cables) the need for allograft struts has decreased. The addition of allograft struts is not typically required when stable plate fixation is obtained; their use may lead to further devascularization of the fracture and knee stiffness secondary to quadriceps scarring.

The high complication rate in periprosthetic patellar fractures is an important consideration. Many patellar fractures identified on routine radiographic follow-up examinations are asymptomatic or minimally symptomatic and have an intact extensor mechanism. Surgery is not required for asymptomatic patients; symptomatic patients can typically be managed with a short course of immobilization and protected weight bearing. Surgery is indicated for patients with extensor mechanism disruption with lag and weakness or those with symptoms caused by a loose patellar implant. Repeated attempts at extensor mechanism repair are discouraged, and failed attempts at open reduction and internal fixation are best managed with extensor mechanism reconstruction.

The final chapter in this section, by Richards and associates, discusses the more focused topic of Vancouver type B3 periprosthetic femoral hip fractures (a loose implant with severe bone loss). Management of these fractures is divided into three broad groups: reconstruction of the femur using an impaction allografting technique or strut grafting of the deficient femur in conjunction with distal fixation of an uncemented stem; replacement of the proximal femur with either a proximal femoral prosthesis or allograft prosthetic composite; or the use of a long, uncemented implant (typically with a long, fluted stem) with distal fixation around which the remaining proximal femur is secured. In this type of reconstruction, it is intended that the proximal bone will remodel and reconstitute to some degree. Provided that sufficient bone is present for distal fixation, the use of a long, fluted, tapered implant with cerclage cable fixation of the remaining proximal femur is preferred because of its improved rate of success, versatility, and shorter surgical time compared with the other techniques. It should be noted that patients with Vancouver type B3 fractures may have a deficient abductor mechanism and are at increased risk for instability. Large femoral heads, an unconstrained tripolar bearing, or a constrained liner into a well-fixed cup should be used for these patients.

Mark J. Spangehl, MD
Assistant Professor
Department of Orthopaedic Surgery
Mayo Clinic
Phoenix, Arizona

References

1. Alshryda S, Sarda P, Sukeik M, Nargol A, Blenkinsopp J, Mason JM: Tranexamic acid in total knee replacement: A systematic review and meta-analysis. *J Bone Joint Surg Br* 2011;93(12):1577-1585.
2. Sukeik M, Alshryda S, Haddad FS, Mason JM: Systematic review and meta-analysis of the use of tranexamic acid in total hip replacement. *J Bone Joint Surg Br* 2011;93(1):39-46.
3. Charoencholvanich K, Siriwattanasakul P: Tranexamic acid reduces blood loss and blood transfusion after TKA: A prospective randomized controlled trial. *Clin Orthop Relat Res* 2011;469(10):2874-2880.
4. Innerhofer P, Klingler A, Klimmer C, Fries D, Nussbaumer W: Risk for postoperative infection after transfusion of white blood cell-filtered allogeneic or autologous blood components in orthopedic patients undergoing primary arthroplasty. *Transfusion* 2005;45(1): 103-110.
5. Hébert PC, Wells G, Blajchman MA, et al: A multicenter, randomized, controlled clinical trial of transfusion requirements in critical care: Transfusion Requirements in Critical Care Investigators, Canadian Critical Care Trials Group. *N Engl J Med* 1999;340(6):409-417.
6. Vuille-Lessard E, Boudreault D, Girard F, Ruel M, Chagnon M, Hardy JF: Postoperative anemia does not impede functional outcome and quality of life early after hip and knee arthroplasties. *Transfusion* 2012;52(2):261-270.
7. So-Osman C, Nelissen R, Brand R, Brand A, Stiggelbout AM: Postoperative anemia after joint replacement surgery is not related to quality of life during the first two weeks postoperatively. *Transfusion* 2011;51(1):71-81.
8. Falck-Ytter Y, Francis CW, Johanson NA, et al; American College of Chest Physicians: Prevention of VTE in orthopedic surgery patients: Antithrombotic therapy and prevention of thrombosis, 9th ed. American College of Chest Physicians Clinical Practice Guideline. *Chest* 2012;141(2, suppl):e278S-e325S.
9. American Academy of Orthopaedic Surgeons. *Clinical Practice Guideline on Preventing Venous Thromboembolic Disease in Patients Undergoing Elective Hip and Knee Arthroplasty*. Rosemont, IL, American Academy of Orthopaedic Surgeons, September 2011.http://www.aaos.org/research/guidelines/VTE/VTE_guideline.asp.

Dr. Spangehl or an immediate family member has received research or institutional support from Stryker, and serves as a board member, owner, officer, or committee member of the American Academy of Orthopaedic Surgeons.

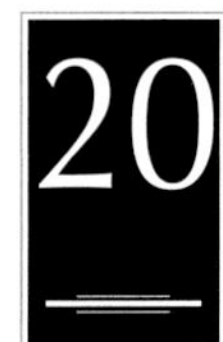

Perioperative Blood Management in Total Hip Arthroplasty

*Charles R. Clark, MD

Abstract

Blood management during total hip arthroplasty is a critical component of successful patient care, and an overall strategy is necessary. Multiple options for blood management are available, including the use of predeposited autologous blood, perioperative blood salvage, hemodilution techniques, erythropoietic agents, hemostatic agents, and allogeneic blood. Rather than relying on automatic so-called transfusion triggers, the surgeon should identify patient-specific risk factors such as the anticipated difficulty of the procedure, preoperative hemoglobin level, comorbidities, and a plan for blood management.

Blood management is an important consideration in total hip arthroplasty (THA) that is critical to the successful management of patients undergoing total joint arthroplasty. Important considerations include the safety of blood or blood products, the efficacy of oxygen delivery to the tissues, cost, and convenience. Patient-specific factors are integral to the decision process. The ultimate objective is to minimize the use of allogeneic blood transfusion and its associated risks.

Bierbaum and associates[1] described current blood usage in their review of 9,482 patients, 5,741 (61%) of whom had predonated autologous blood before total joint arthroplasty. Interestingly enough, 4,464 of 9,920 units (45%) were not used. Patients undergoing primary total hip or knee arthroplasty and revision total knee arthroplasty had the greatest number of so-called wasted units. In addition, 9% of patients (503 of 5,741) who had predonated blood needed to have an allogeneic blood transfusion. The frequency of allogeneic transfusion was highest in patients undergoing revision THA, bilateral total knee arthroplasty, and patients with a baseline hemoglobin level of 13 g/dL or less.

With respect to clinical factors, Pola and associates[2] analyzed the factors associated with the risk of requiring an allogeneic blood transfusion and evaluated clinical variables such as age, gender, the presence of hypertension, and body mass index. The authors performed a simultaneous analysis of parameters and stratified patients with different risks. The goal was to increase the efficacy of, as well as reduce the cost associated with, blood management. The authors found that these various parameters may be synergistic. There was a significantly increased risk of blood transfusion when two or more of these clinical parameters were present ($P = 0.02$).

Salido and associates[3] also evaluated clinical factors associated with the need for allogeneic blood transfusion after hip and knee arthroplasty and found that the preoperative hemoglobin and weight of the patient significantly predicted the need for transfusion. As shown in Figure 1, all patients with a preoperative hemoglobin level less than 11 g/dL required a blood transfusion, whereas the percentage of patients receiving transfusions with a hemoglobin level greater than 15 g/dL was 13%. Furthermore, these authors found that with a hemoglobin level less than 13 g/dL, there was a four times greater risk of requiring a

**Charles R. Clark, MD or the department with which he is affiliated has received research or institutional support from Zimmer and is a consultant for or an employee of Zimmer.*

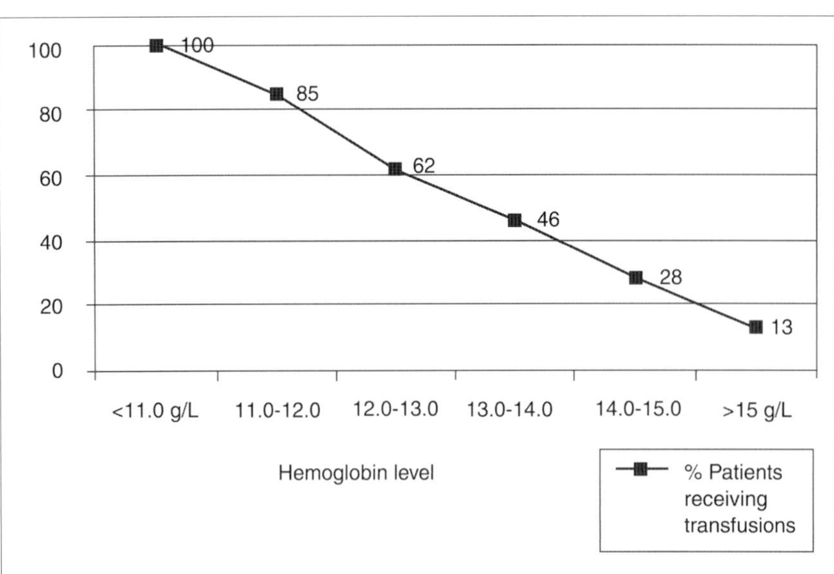

Figure 1 Relationship between the preoperative hemoglobin levels and the percentage of patients who received a blood transfusion. (Reproduced with permission from Salido JA, Marin LA, Gomez LA, Zorrilla P, Martinez C: Perioperative hemoglobin levels and the need for transfusion after prosthetic hip and knee surgery. *J Bone Joint Surg Am* 2002;84:216-220.)

blood transfusion compared with a hemoglobin level from 13 to 15 g/dL; when the hemoglobin level was less than 13 g/dL, there was a 15.3-fold greater risk of requiring a blood transfusion than in patients with a hemoglobin level greater than 15 g/dL.

The risks associated with blood transfusion are a major consideration. Many patients fear receiving an allogeneic blood transfusion because of the risk of virally transmitted diseases, such as hepatitis C and human immunodeficiency virus (HIV). The risk of acquiring hepatitis C, however, is approximately 1 in 100,000 blood transfusions, and the risk of acquiring HIV is approximately 1 in 500,000 transfusions. Fatal hemolytic reactions caused by ABO blood-type incompatibility occur in approximately 1 in 600,000 patients. One way of putting this information in perspective is to consider that a patient has a 1 in 200 chance of dying related to smoking if the patient smokes one pack of cigarettes per day.

The use of allogeneic blood transfusion has declined; however, the safety of the blood supply has improved. Other important factors to consider relate to the cost and inventory of blood supply on hand; consequently, so-called transfusion triggers can be reconsidered in view of patient-specific factors.

Blood Management Strategies

Preoperative Autologous Donation

Preoperative autologous blood was rarely used before the recognition of HIV. The patient donates blood, typically two units within 42 days of surgery. Such donation decreases a patient's hemoglobin level by approximately 1.2 to 1.5 g/dL per donated unit. Hatzidakis and associates[4] analyzed the risk factors for allogeneic transfusions in patients who had donated autologous blood before total joint arthroplasty. The authors reviewed 489 consecutive patients, 271 of whom underwent THA and 247 underwent total knee arthroplasty. The authors found that preoperative autologous donation significantly reduced the need for banked blood. They recommend identifying patients who are at low risk for transfusion and found that patients with a preoperative hemoglobin level greater than 15 g/dL and patients with a hemoglobin level from 13 to 15 g/dL who were younger than 65 years were at low risk for requiring a banked blood transfusion. Billote and associates[5] performed a prospective randomized study of preoperative autologous donation in patients undergoing THA and found that autologous donation was of no benefit for nonanemic patients (Hg > 12 g/dL in this study) undergoing primary THA.

Furthermore, cost is a consideration. At the University of Iowa Hospitals and Clinics, the patient charge for a unit of autologous blood in 1999 was approximately $500; in 2008, the charge for a unit of banked blood was $730 and a unit of autologous blood cost $760.

Perioperative Blood Salvage

The options for perioperative blood salvage include the use of an intraoperative cell saver, postoperative blood salvage, and a technique that includes combined intraoperative and postoperative cell salvage. The principle is to collect lost blood and return it to the patient. Perioperative salvage has the advantage of returning the patient's own blood. Zarin and associates[6] analyzed the efficacy of intraoperative blood collection and reinfusion in patients undergoing THA. The authors reviewed

126 patients who underwent revision THA. They found that intraoperative collection and reinfusion significantly reduced the net perioperative blood loss in two groups of patients—patients who had revision of both the acetabular and femoral components and patients who had revision of the acetabular component alone.

Grosvenor and associates[7] analyzed the efficacy of postoperative blood salvage following primary THA in patients with or without predeposited autologous units. They found that postoperative salvage significantly reduced the risk of allogeneic transfusion among patients undergoing primary THA, whether or not the patients had predeposited autologous blood ($P = 0.001$). As shown in Figure 2, patients without postoperative salvage were approximately 10 times more likely to require allogeneic transfusion than were patients who had the reinfusion drain.

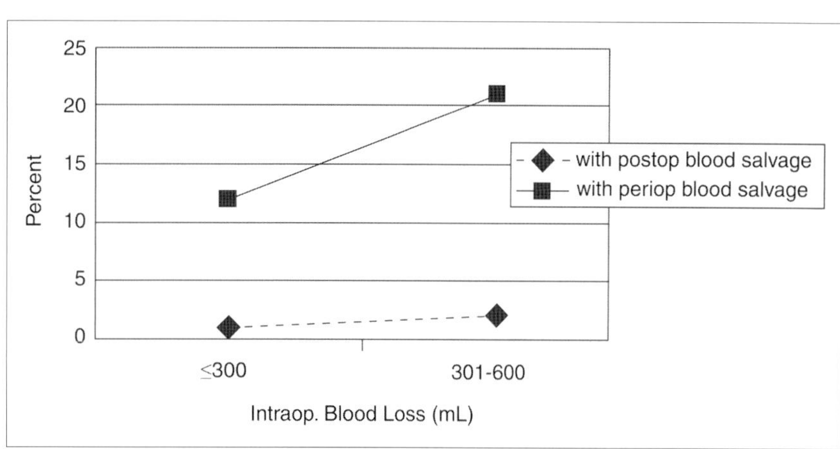

Figure 2 Graph illustrating the likelihood of allogeneic transfusion in a 60-year-old man with one unit of deposited autologous blood, a preoperative hematocrit of 0.35, and a cementless prosthesis. Postop = postoperative; periop = perioperative; intraop = intraoperative. (Reproduced with permission from Grosvenor D, Goyal V, Goodman S: Efficacy of postoperative blood salvage following total hip arthroplasty in patients with and without deposited autologous units. *J Bone Joint Surg Am* 2000;82: 951-954.)

Colwell and associates[8] analyzed erythrocyte viability in blood salvage during intraoperative (from a cell saver) cemented total joint arthroplasty. They used a double isotope-labeling technique and found that the mean erythrocyte viability was 88%, which is well above the American Association of Blood Banks standards for banked and preoperative autologous-donated blood of 70%. The values for three subjects are shown in Figure 3.

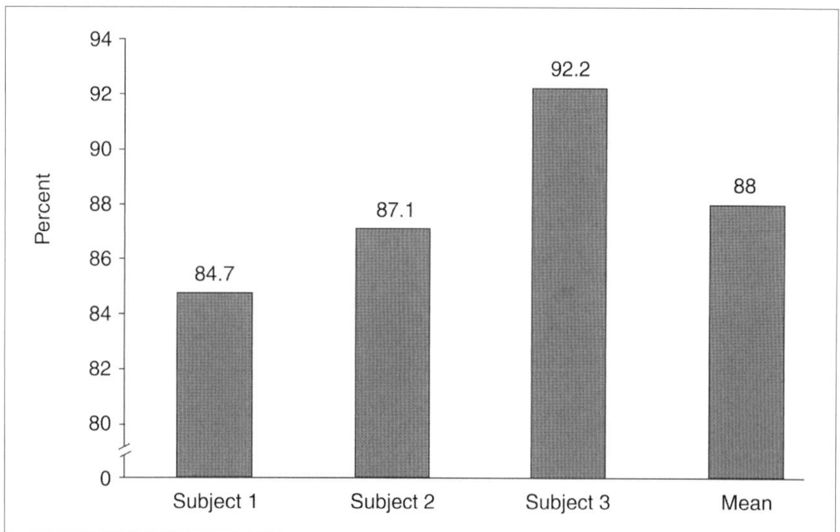

Figure 3 Erythrocyte viability for three patients at 24 hours after surgery. (Reproduced with permission from Colwell CW Jr, Beutler E, West C, Hardwick ME, Morris BA: Erythrocyte viability and blood salvage during total joint arthroplasty with cement. *J Bone Joint Surg Am* 2002;84:23-25.)

A combined technique of intra- and postoperative salvage can be performed with a device known as OrthoPAT (Haemonitics, Braintree, MA). Clark and associates[9] reviewed their experience with this perioperative autotransfusion device in 398 patients undergoing total hip and total knee arthroplasty. They used a decision-tree analysis; included in the study group were patients who underwent primary and revision total knee and total hip arthroplasties as well as bilateral simultaneous total knee arthroplasties. Some patients underwent preoperative autologous donations and others used the OrthoPAT device. Overall, the authors found that all patients undergoing total hip and total knee arthroplasty with the reinfusion device had a significant relative risk reduction with regard to the use of banked blood. There is a cost involved with this device, however, and it is helpful to have a dedicated

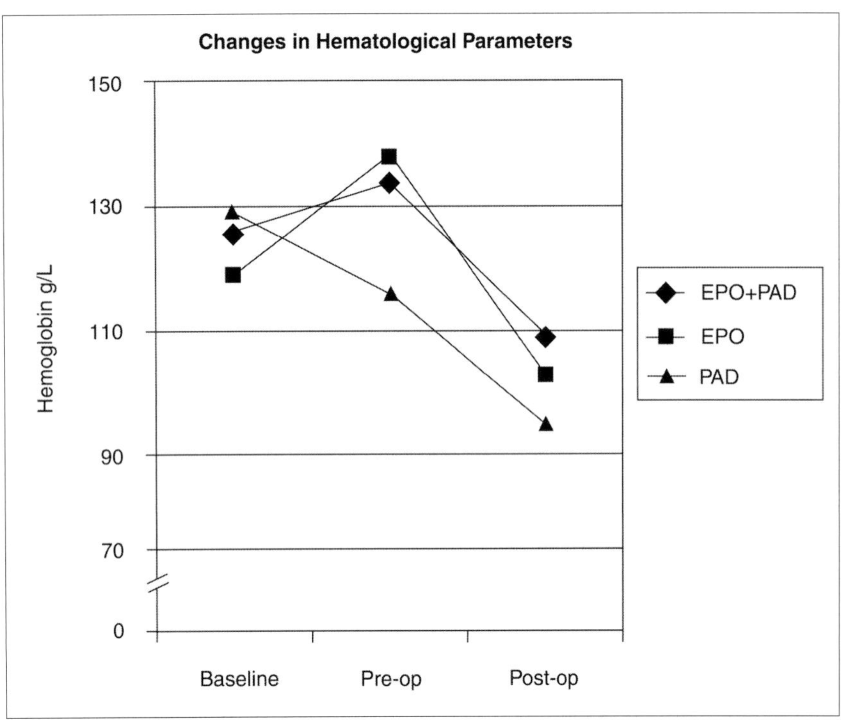

Figure 4 Graphic representation of the changes in hematologic parameters (from baseline to immediately preoperative to the lowest postoperative level) in each group. EPO = erythropoietin, PAD = preoperative autologous donation. (Reproduced with permission from Bezwada HP, Nazarian DG, Henry DH, Booth RE Jr: Preoperative use of recombinant human erythropoietin before total joint arthroplasty. *J Bone Joint Surg Am* 2003;85:1795-1800.)

team of nurses and/or technicians to troubleshoot technical problems with the device that may arise.

Hemodilution

A technique for diluting the patient's blood is known as acute normovolemic hemodilution. Blood is collected immediately preoperatively for immediate postoperative reinfusion. The volume removed is replaced with crystallite and colloid, with the rationale that intraoperative blood loss will have a lower hematocrit level and transfused cells will be healthier. Carless and associates[10] performed a meta-analysis of nine randomized controlled trials and found no reduction in the requirement for allogeneic blood transfusion with the use of acute normovolemic hemodilution. They did, however, recommend its use in conjunction with other blood conservation techniques.

Hematopoiesis

There are two basic techniques for hematopoiesis: the use of iron and erythropoietin α. Although in use for many years, iron is slow acting and is less effective than erythropoietin α. Oral iron preparations are relatively inexpensive; however, some patients do not tolerate their use over the long term. Recombinant human erythropoietin is more effective than iron for stimulating the differentiation of progenitor cells to become a dedicated red blood cell line, but it is much more expensive than oral iron. Sparling and associates[11] reviewed the use of erythropoietin in five Jehovah's Witness patients who underwent revision THA. Each received 100 IU/week of erythropoietin preoperatively over an average of 26 days. Hematocrit level was monitored and was held at greater than 45%. The authors found no complications due to blood loss, and no patient underwent a blood transfusion. Bezwada and associates[12] analyzed the preoperative use of recombinant human erythropoietin before total joint arthroplasty. They concluded that the preoperative use of erythropoietin in conjunction with preoperative autologous donation reduced the need for allogeneic blood transfusion associated with total joint arthroplasty and was more effective than either erythropoietin or preoperative autologous donation alone (Figure 4).

Indications for the use of erythropoietin include a hemoglobin level less than 13 g/dL and greater than 10 g/dL. Further, it may be considered for patients unable or unwilling to predeposit autologous blood and for patients undergoing simultaneous bilateral total hip or total knee arthroplasty. The strategy may also be useful in revision cases and patients with religious concerns regarding the receipt of blood.

Hemostasis Agents

Hemostasis agents are pharmacologic agents and include topically active agents (such as thrombin, collagen, and fibrin glue) as well as antifibrinolytics. Levy and associates[13] analyzed their use of fibrin tissue adhesive following total knee arthroplasty and found that it was associated with a significant reduction in blood loss following total knee arthroplasty. Antifibrinolytic agents are controversial, however, because of their high cost and associated thromboembolic complications.

Allogeneic Blood Transfusion

It is important to note the increased safety of the allogeneic blood supply now that blood banks are able to screen for various viruses. Further, the surgeon should not have so-called automatic triggers, based on a specific hemoglobin or hematocrit level, for blood transfusion. Rather, patient-specific factors need to be considered, including the patient's comorbidities and age as well as procedure-specific factors such as an anticipated difficult revision arthroplasty or bilateral simultaneous arthroplasties.

Along with an increased risk of infection, allogeneic blood is associated with immunomodulation, and the T cells and macrophages are suppressed by its presence. Patients may inquire about having a designated donor with regard to allogeneic blood. However, there has been an increased risk of hepatitis B and C as well as HIV in comparison with the transfusion of standard banked blood. Furthermore, waste of the blood product remains an issue because it is expensive; designator donor blood is wasted if not given to the designated patient.

Pierson and associates[14] used a blood conservation algorithm in patients undergoing total hip and total knee arthroplasty. These authors found a reduced need for allogeneic blood transfusion in patients in whom the algorithm was used. They studied a consecutive series of 500 patients undergoing total hip and total knee arthroplasty, 433 of whom followed the algorithm and 67 did not. When the algorithm was followed (Figure 5), there was a 2.1% rate of banked blood transfusion. When the algorithm was not followed, the banked blood transfusion rate rose to 16.4% ($P = 0.001$).

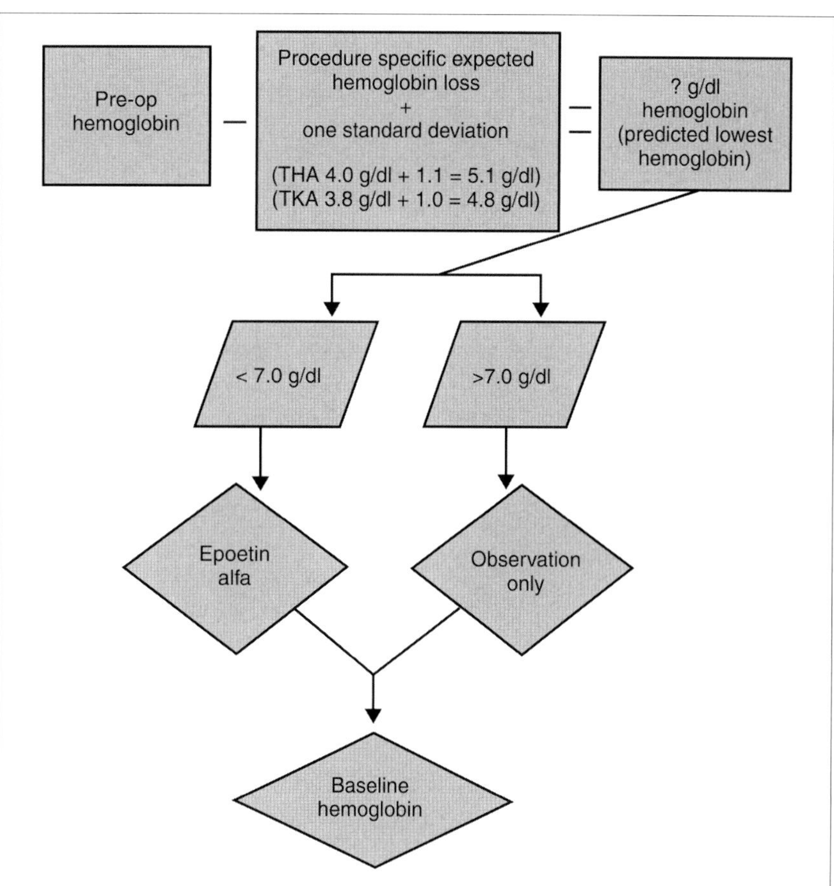

Figure 5 Flowchart illustrating patient-specific recommendations. TKA = total knee arthroplasty. (Reproduced with permission from Pierson JL, Hannon TJ, Earles DR: A blood-conservation algorithm to reduce blood transfusion after total hip and knee arthroplasty. *J Bone Joint Surg Am* 2004;86:1512-1518.)

Author's Preferred Hemogenous Management

Factors assessed preoperatively include medical comorbidities and baseline hemoglobin and hematocrit values, as well as the anticipated difficulty of the procedure.

Typically, in a healthy patient with minor comorbidities who has a normal baseline hemoglobin level and is undergoing a primary THA, preoperative blood salvage is the primary blood management technique; autologous blood is administered if needed.

Higher blood loss is anticipated with bilateral procedures and revision procedures, as well as difficult primary procedures. Additional blood management strategies may be necessary.

In patients who are Jehovah's Witnesses, perioperative blood salvage typically is the primary blood management technique if they agree to comply with its use. Erythropoietin is another option.

Summary

It is important to have an overall strategy for blood management. Although allogeneic blood is safer than it has been in the past, multiple other options are available, including the use of predeposited autologous blood, perioperative blood salvage, hemodilution techniques, erythropoietic agents, hemostatic agents, and allogeneic blood.

The surgeon should not have an automatic transfusion trigger. Rather, patient-specific risk factors should be identified, such as an anticipated difficult revision or simultaneous bilateral procedures and the patient's preoperative hemoglobin level, and a patient-specific plan developed.

References

1. Bierbaum BE, Callaghan JJ, Galante JO, Rubash HE, Tooms RE, Welch RB: An analysis of blood management in patients having a total hip or knee arthroplasty. *J Bone Joint Surg Am* 1999;81:2-10.
2. Pola E, Papaleo P, Santoliquido A, Gasparini G, Aulisa L, De Santis E: Clinical factors associated with an increased risk of perioperative blood transfusion in nonanemic patients undergoing total hip arthroplasty. *J Bone Joint Surg Am* 2004;86:57-61.
3. Salido JA, Marin LA, Gomez LA, Zorrilla P, Martinez C: Perioperative hemoglobin levels and the need for transfusion after prosthetic hip and knee surgery. *J Bone Joint Surg Am* 2002;84:216-220.
4. Hatzidakis AM, Mendlick RM, McKillip T, Reddy RL, Garvin KL: Preoperative autologous donation for total joint arthroplasty: An analysis of risk factors for allogenic transfusion. *J Bone Joint Surg Am* 2000;82:89-100.
5. Billote DB, Glisson SN, Green D, Wixson RL: A prospective randomized study of preoperative autologous donation for hip replacement surgery. *J Bone Joint Surg Am* 2002;84:1299-1304.
6. Zarin J, Grosvenor D, Schurman D, Goodman S: Efficacy of intraoperative blood collection and reinfusion in revision total hip arthroplasty. *J Bone Joint Surg Am* 2003;85:2147-2151.
7. Grosvenor D, Goyal V, Goodman S: Efficacy of postoperative blood salvage following total hip arthroplasty in patients with and without deposited autologous units. *J Bone Joint Surg Am* 2000;82:951-954.
8. Colwell CW Jr, Beutler E, West C, Hardwick ME, Morris BA: Erythrocyte viability and blood salvage during total joint arthroplasty with cement. *J Bone Joint Surg Am* 2002;84:23-25.
9. Clark CR, Spratt KF, Blondin M, Craig S, Fink L: Perioperative autotransfusion in total hip and knee arthroplasty. *J Arthroplasty* 2006;21:23-35.
10. Carless P, Moxey A, O'Connell D, Henry D: Autologous tranfusion techniques: A systematic review of their efficacy. *Transfus Med* 2004;14:123-144.
11. Sparling EA, Nelson CL, Lavender R, Smith J: The use of erythropoietin in the management of Jehovah's Witnesses who have revision total hip arthroplasty. *J Bone Joint Surg Am* 1996;78:1548-1552.
12. Bezwada HP, Nazarian DG, Henry DH, Booth RE Jr: Preoperative use of recombinant human erythropoietin before total joint arthroplasty. *J Bone Joint Surg Am* 2003;85:1795-1800.
13. Levy O, Martinowitz U, Oran A, Tauber C, Horoszowski H: The use of fibrin tissue adhesive to reduce blood loss and need for blood transfusion after total knee arthroplasty: A prospective, randomized, multicenter study. *J Bone Joint Surg Am* 1999;81:1580-1588.
14. Pierson JL, Hannon TJ, Earles DR: A blood-conservation algorithm to reduce blood transfusion after total hip and knee arthroplasty. *J Bone Joint Surg Am* 2004;86:1512-1518.

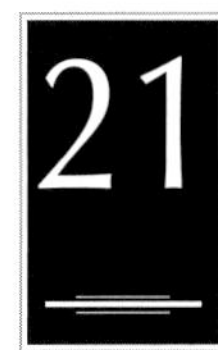

Venous Thromboembolic Disease After Total Hip and Knee Arthroplasty

Steven B. Haas, MD, MPH
Robert L. Barrack, MD
Geoffrey Westrich, MD

Abstract

A variety of pharmacologic and mechanical means can be used to prevent thromboembolic disease following total hip or knee arthroplasty. The existing pharmacologic options are parenteral heparin, fondaparinux, oral warfarin, and oral acetylsalicylic acid. An oral form of heparin as well as direct thrombin inhibitors of factors IIa, IXa, and Xa are being developed in the hope of discovering an agent that effectively prevents thrombi formation but carries a low risk of bleeding complications. Mechanical prophylaxis devices include foot pumps, calf pumps, and calf and thigh pumps for standard pneumatic compression, sequential compression, or rapid inflation compression. Although an ideal prophylaxis does not exist, a multimodal approach incorporating pharmacologic and mechanical prophylaxis has been proved safe and effective.

The published recommendations of the American College of Chest Physicians (ACCP) for deep venous thrombosis prophylaxis of total joint patients are widely used throughout the world. These ACCP guidelines have a rigorous foundation in evidence-based medicine and meet the requirements of many oversight groups; some recommendations also meet the standards of certain state and federal programs. In the view of many orthopaedic surgeons, however, these ACCP guidelines have some notable disadvantages. The routine use of relatively aggressive pharmacologic prophylaxis has led to complication rates higher than those reported in the studies used by the ACCP. Equivalent results have been achieved in reducing symptomatic deep venous thrombosis, pulmonary embolisms, and deaths with less aggressive, less expensive prophylaxis protocols that still meet the requirements of recently enacted federal programs that monitor deep venous thrombosis.

This chapter and chapter 74, "Prevention of Symptomatic Pulmonary Embolism in Patients Undergoing Total Hip and Knee Arthroplasty: Clinical Guideline of the American Academy of Orthopaedic Surgeons," were published as a combined text with the title "Venous Thromboembolic Disease After Total Hip and Knee Arthroplasty" in the Journal of Bone and Joint Surgery Am, *December 2008.*

Thromboembolic disease continues to pose a major threat to patients undergoing total hip and knee arthroplasty. Despite a great deal of research, there is still controversy concerning the best prophylactic regimen. This chapter outlines the various methods of mechanical and pharmacologic prophylaxis and describes the pros and cons of the American College of Chest Physicians (ACCP) guidelines for the prevention of deep venous thrombosis.

Prophylactic Modalities: Mechanical and Pharmacologic

The ideal prophylaxis modality for the high-risk population of patients undergoing total hip or knee arthroplasty would be clinically effective without side effects, be practical and easy to use, require no monitoring, and be cost-effective. Unfortunately, this ideal method of prophylaxis does not exist. The use of anticoagulants requires constant balancing of the risk of clots against the risk of bleeding. Some of these issues can be overcome with a multimodal approach, which is the closest to an "ideal" method that is currently available.

Pharmacologic Prophylaxis

Parenteral heparin, fondaparinux, oral warfarin, and oral acetylsalicylic acid are the major existing pharmacologic prophylaxis agents. Desirudin, a hirudin derivative, has also been approved by the US Food and Drug Administration (FDA) for the prevention of venous thromboembolism. There are many more medications in various stages of development, including oral heparin and direct thrombin inhibitors of factors IIa, IXa, and Xa such as indraparinux, dabigatran, apixaban, and rivaroxaban.

Parenteral Heparin

Three different types of parenteral or low-molecular-weight heparin have been approved by the FDA. Enoxaparin (Lovenox; Sanof-Aventis, Bridgewater, NJ) is the most commonly used and has been approved for patients undergoing total hip or knee arthroplasty. In addition, ardeparin (Normiflo; Wyeth-Ayerst Laboratories, Philadelphia, PA) has been approved for patients undergoing total knee arthroplasty, and dalteparin (Fragmin; Pfizer, New York, NY) has been approved for patients undergoing total hip arthroplasty.

Low-molecular-weight heparin has many advantages, including rapid antithrombotic action. There is limited variability in its effects among different individuals, and prothrombin time and activated partial thromboplastin time have little influence. The drug has linear pharmacokinetics and a half-life of 4.5 hours. No monitoring is required, which allows more practical outpatient use, and the drug can be effective when given every 12 or 24 hours.

The major disadvantages are the cost and risks of complications and bleeding. At our institution, low-molecular-weight heparin therapy costs $31 per day, compared with $9 per day for subcutaneous unfractionated heparin or less than $1 per day for warfarin. The presence of an epidural catheter is a contraindication to the use of low-molecular-weight heparin because such catheters increase the possibility of epidural hematomas and neurologic deficits associated with regional anesthesia. The evidence regarding the greater risk of bleeding complications is inconclusive, although it is still a cause for concern. One trial demonstrated a higher prevalence of bleeding complications, and another showed increased blood loss associated with low-molecular-weight heparin therapy.[1,2] A large randomized prospective study showed that the overall prevalences of symptomatic deep venous thrombosis and pulmonary embolism in patients with unilateral primary hip arthroplasty were similar in a group that received low-molecular-weight heparin and a group treated with warfarin, with most patients having received the study medication for 1 to 7 days.[3] Just over 1% of 1,516 patients (18) who received enoxaparin and 0.5% (8) of 1,495 patients (8) who received warfarin had major bleeding events. The prevalence of minor bleeding events was significantly higher (P = 0.021) in the patients treated with enoxaparin (140 of 1,516; 9.2%) than it was in those treated with warfarin (106 of 1,495; 7.1%). Francis and associates[4] reported that the prevalence of bleeding complications at the surgical site and the rate of postoperative transfusions in patients treated with low-molecular-weight heparin were significantly higher (P = 0.03 and P = 0.001, respectively) than the prevalences in patients treated with warfarin, but they did not find any significant differences between the groups with respect to the decrease in the hematocrit, intraoperative or postoperative blood loss, or the prevalence of major bleeding complications.

Oral Warfarin

The pharmacologic agent most commonly used for anticoagulation is warfarin (Coumadin; Bristol-Myers Squibb, New York, NY). The widely accepted and extensively proven efficacy of this compound and the low risk of bleeding complications are major benefits. It is also effective for secondary prophylaxis, even in patients in whom clots developed while warfarin was being used as the primary prophylaxis.[5] The oral administration allows easy continued use in the outpatient setting.

Limitations of warfarin include the still-present risk of bleeding complications and possible inferiority of its effectiveness for primary prevention of thrombosis compared with that of low-molecular-weight heparin.[1] It also requires monitoring to ensure therapeutic but safe international normalized ratios. Previous findings indicate that an international normalized ratio of between 2.0 and 2.5 is associated with the lowest rates of bleeding complications, with retention of efficacy.[6-8] The prevalence of deep venous thrombosis after total knee arthroplasty in patients treated with warfarin alone remains as high as 35% to 55%, indicating that warfarin on its own is not sufficient for clot prevention.[9] Several studies have shown that warfarin is more effective for prophylaxis against proximal deep venous thrombosis than it is for the prevention of distal deep venous thrombosis in patients treated with total hip replacement.[10-12]

Acetylsalicylic Acid

Acetylsalicylic acid, commonly known as aspirin, is a simple, inexpensive oral anticoagulant that does not require monitoring. It is extremely safe and has the added benefit of reducing heterotopic ossification. Most studies have shown it to be less effective than both low-molecular-weight heparin and warfarin, but it may provide sufficient prophylaxis against thromboembolic disease when it is used in combination with mechanical prophylaxis.[9,13] Westrich and associates[14] conducted a randomized prospective study comparing treatment with low-molecular-weight heparin and a calf mechanical compression device with treatment with acetylsalicylic acid and the same device in patients undergoing total knee arthroplasty. The rates of deep venous thrombosis, as assessed with ultrasonography, were not significantly different between the two groups, showing that aspirin in combination with mechanical compression may be as effective as, and safer than, more aggressive anticoagulant therapy.

Oral Heparin

One promising new pharmacologic agent that is being developed for anticoagulation is oral heparin. The goal of this new formulation is to attain the highly effective clot-prevention ability of parenteral heparin with an easily administered oral form of the drug. This could be achieved by combining unfractionated heparin and a carrier molecule, sodium N-(8 [2-hydroxybenzoyl] amino) caprylate, allowing greater gastrointestinal absorption. A recent multicenter, randomized, double-blind phase III study showed that oral heparin decreased the prevalence of postoperative thrombi with a low frequency of bleeding complications in a large population of patients treated with total hip arthroplasty.[15]

Other Agents

The other major focus of new research is the development of compounds that are able to directly or indirectly inhibit factors IIa (thrombin), IXa, or Xa in the coagulation pathway.

Ximelagatran (Exanta and Exarta; AstraZeneca PLC, Wilmington, DE), an oral direct factor IIa inhibitor, initially showed promise, but marketing and foreign-distribution efforts in the United States were halted in 2006 because of unacceptable levels of hepatotoxicity. Prior to this, conflicting efficacy results had been shown. Cohen and associates[16] found no overall advantage of ximelagatran over low-molecular-weight heparin in patients treated with hip or knee surgery, but Colwell and associates[17] found the efficacy of ximelagatran to be superior to that of warfarin. Although ximelagatran had unacceptable serious side effects, there may be other direct thrombin inhibitors that can be effective with fewer side effects.

Recombinant hirudin and its derivative desirudin (Iprivask; Canyon Pharmaceutical, Hunt Valley, MD) are direct factor IIa inhibitors in an injectable form. Hirudin naturally occurs as a peptide in the salivary glands of medicinal leeches. Early research showed that the prevalence of deep venous thrombosis associated with desirudin was lower than that associated with enoxaparin or unfractionated heparin and that the bleeding risks were similar.[18,19] Desirudin is currently approved for use for the prevention of thromboembolic disease.

Dabigatran etexilate (Rendix and Pradaxa; Boehringer Ingelheim, Ingelheim, Germany), an oral direct factor IIa inhibitor, is currently being assessed in phase III trials. Completed phase II research studies comparing dabigatran etexilate, started 1 to 4 hours postoperatively, with enoxaparin, started 12 hours preoperatively, showed that the rates of pulmonary embolism and deep venous thrombosis associated with the highest doses of dabigatran were significantly lower than those associated with enoxaparin ($P = 0.0007$).[20] The risk of serious bleeding complications increased in a dose-dependent manner. The overall efficacy with regard to the prevention of venous thromboembolism and the risk of bleeding events were similar to those associated with enoxaparin.

Fondaparinux (Arixtra; GlaxoSmithKline, London, England) is the first synthetic inhibitor of factor Xa. It is a single chemical entity created through a total chemical synthesis process, which enables batch-to-batch consistency. It has a single molecular target within the coagulation cascade, and there is no risk of pathogen contamination. It is administered subcutaneously in daily doses. Bauer and associates[21] performed a multicenter, randomized, double-blind trial comparing fondaparinux (2.5 mg once daily) with enoxaparin (30 mg twice daily). The primary outcome was the development of venous thromboembolism, which was assessed up to 11 days postoperatively in 724 patients. The patients who received fondaparinux had a significantly lower prevalence of thromboembolic complications ($P < 0.001$), although their risk of major bleeding was significantly higher ($P = 0.006$). Fondaparinux is FDA approved and currently available.

Idraparinux is a hypermethylated fondaparinux derivative. As an indirect inhibitor of factor Xa, it requires antithrombin as a cofactor. Idraparinux is administered subcutaneously once a week. A phase II study demonstrated a treatment effect similar to that of warfarin, with less bleeding than warfarin at a dose of 2.5 mg but an unacceptable risk of major bleeding at a dose of 10 mg.[22] Further phase III research is in progress.

Oral factor Xa inhibitors are also being developed. One of these, apixaban, is currently being evaluated in phase III trials to compare it with acetylsalicylic acid and warfarin for the prevention of stroke and systemic embolism.[23] A previous study on apixaban therapy in patients treated with total knee replacement showed a promising risk-benefit profile when the drug was given at dosages of 2.5 mg twice a day and 5 mg once a day.[24]

Rivaroxaban (Xarelto; Bayer HealthCare, Leverkusen, Germany) is another oral factor Xa inhibitor. It has a rapid onset, high oral bioavailability, and predictable pharmacokinetics.[25] Phase II studies showed it to be well tolerated and effective in the prevention of thromboembolic disease following orthopaedic surgery.[25-27] A phase III study of patients treated with total knee replacement showed it to be significantly superior to enoxaparin in terms of efficacy ($P = 0.01$), with a similar risk of bleeding.[25] Currently, four separate trials are being performed to assess rivaroxaban: two involving patients treated with total hip replacement and two involving patients treated with total knee replacement.

Mechanical Prophylaxis

Mechanical devices help to prevent venous thromboembolic disease by increasing fibrinolysis and decreasing stasis with accelerated venous emptying. Their efficacy has been proven in the fields of general surgery and neurosurgery as well as orthopaedic surgery. Foot pumps, calf pumps, and calf/thigh pumps are the three major types of mechanical prophylaxis devices. The type of pneumatic compression also varies. It may be standard pneumatic compression, sequential, or rapid inflation. Although these compression devices are associated with extremely low complication rates, compliance issues may decrease their effectiveness. Research on these devices has been less extensive than that on pharmacologic agents, but several studies have been conducted to compare the prophylaxis efficacy and compliance rates associated with different device types and compression types.

In a randomized prospective study by Westrich and Sculco,[28] the combination of pneumatic plantar compression and acetylsalicylic acid was compared with acetylsalicylic acid alone for prophylaxis for patients treated with total knee replacement. The trial included 164 knees in 121 patients (78 treated with a unilateral total knee arthroplasty and 43 with a bilateral total knee arthroplasty). The rate of deep venous thrombosis in the group treated with compression and acetylsalicylic acid (27%, 22 of 81) was significantly lower ($P < 0.001$) than that in the group treated with acetylsalicylic acid alone (59%, 49 of 83). There was also a direct relationship between compliance with use of the mechanical compression device and the efficacy of the device with regard to the prevention of deep venous thrombosis, as assessed with venography (or, if a venogram was unattainable or contraindicated, venous Doppler ultrasound). In another recent randomized prospective study, Ryan and associates[29] compared the efficacy of an impulse mechanical compression device with that of prophylactic stockings for the prevention of pelvic and proximal deep venous thrombosis, as assessed with magnetic resonance venography, in 100 patients treated with total hip replacement. The mechanical compression led to a significantly lower rate of deep venous thrombosis (8%, 4 of 55) compared with that associated with the use of prophylactic stockings (22%, 11 of 50; $P < 0.05$).

In 2004, Lachiewicz and associates[30] conducted a randomized prospective study of 423 patients who had a total of 472 knee replacements. The patients were randomized to treatment with either a rapid-inflation asymmetric compression device or a sequential circumferential compression device. The prevalence of thrombi in the patients treated with the rapid-inflation asymmetric compression device (6.9%, 16 of 206) was significantly lower ($P = 0.007$) than that in the patients treated with the sequential circumferential compression device (15.0%, 36 of 217).

The hemodynamics in patients treated with total hip or total knee arthroplasty were examined in two other studies.[31,32] One study, in patients who underwent total knee replacement, tested three calf-and-thigh pump designs, two foot pump designs, one foot-and-calf pump design, and one calf pump design.[31] The greatest increase in venous volume and velocity (below the saphenous vein) was found in the patients treated with a device that incorporated rapid calf compression.

In the other study, involving patients who underwent total hip replacement, three calf-and-thigh pump designs, two foot pump designs, one foot-and-calf pump design, and one calf pump design were tested.[32] The greatest increase in peak venous velocity occurred with pulsatile calf and calf-and-foot pneumatic compression with a rapid inflation time. The final key finding was that, because of compliance issues, simple and easy-to-apply efficacious devices have the greatest chance of success.

A prospective study of 100 patients showed that the rate of compliance with the use of a foot-pump pneumatic compression device (PlexiPulse; Hygia Health Services, Birmingham, AL) after total knee arthroplasty was 90.1%.[33] Patients found the device to be relatively comfortable and easy to apply and remove, and nurses rated this device highly in comparison with other pneumatic compression devices. Because a device is effective only when it is used as directed, it is important to consider ease of use and likelihood of staff and patient compliance, not just "ideal" use, when evaluating different types of mechanical compression devices.

Inferior Vena Cava Filters

Inferior vena cava filters do not prevent deep venous thrombosis, but they can prevent pulmonary embolization. They are often inserted in patients with a history of venous thromboembolic disease and those with substantial traumatic injuries before other prophylaxis methods can be initiated. Inferior vena cava filters are recommended if pharmacologic anticoagulant therapy is clearly contraindicated or if the patient has had thromboembolic complications despite adequate anticoagulation in the past.[34] The cost of these filters is substantial, and the application is an invasive procedure that requires the use of contrast agents, exposing the patient to a risk of complications.[35] A promising development has been the introduction of retrievable inferior vena cava filters, which may decrease the risks of complications associated with permanent filter placement. Early data have shown that retrievable filters are effective in preventing pulmonary embolism, with a low rate of insertion-related complications.[36,37] These filters can be left in place permanently or removed when they are no longer needed; however, because of clots lodged in the filter or difficulty with capturing the filter, planned removal may not always be possible.[38]

Multifactorial Approach

A review of 50 studies involving a total of 10,929 patients who had undergone total hip replacement revealed deep venous thrombosis rates of 48% in patients treated with a placebo, 31% in those treated with acetylsalicylic acid, 23% in those treated with warfarin, 21% in those treated with pneumatic compression, and 18% in those treated with low-molecular-weight heparin.[39] The lowest rate of distal deep venous thrombosis was in the pneumatic compression group, and this rate was significantly lower than that in the aspirin group and the warfarin group ($P = 0.0007$ and $P = 0.0001$, respectively). Proximal deep venous thrombosis was significantly less common in the warfarin group and the low-molecular-weight heparin group ($P = 0.0004$ and $P = 0.0059$, respectively) than it was in the pneumatic compression group. The overall prevalence of symptomatic pulmonary embolism was less than 1% in the low-molecular-weight heparin, warfarin, and pneumatic compression groups, but the aspirin group had a significantly higher rate of symptomatic pulmonary embolism than the warfarin and low-molecular-weight heparin groups ($P < 0.0083$).

In another extensive review article, the authors examined 23 trials that included 6,001 patients treated with total knee replacement.[40] They found a deep venous thrombosis rate of 53% in association with aspirin therapy, 45% in association with warfarin, 29% in association with low-molecular-weight heparin, and 17% in association with pneumatic compression. This study did not include a placebo group, and the rates of proximal and distal deep venous thrombosis were not examined separately. Patients who received low-molecular-weight heparin or pneumatic compression were significantly less likely to have a deep venous thrombosis than were patients who received aspirin ($P < 0.0001$) or warfarin ($P < 0.0001$). The patients treated with aspirin had a significantly higher rate of pulmonary embolism than the patients who received any other means of prophylaxis ($P < 0.05$). In both of the meta-analyses, the rates of deep venous thrombosis with the use of each singular modality were substantially higher than rates that have been associated with a combination of chemical and mechanical means. Trials of the use of compression devices in conjunction with postoperative aspirin therapy have shown this combination to be as effective as low-molecular-weight heparin for the prevention of proximal and distal deep venous thrombosis, with a decreased risk of major bleeding complications.[9,39,40]

Our institution uses and advocates a multifactorial approach to prevent venous thromboembolism that has been validated by extensive research.[14,35,40-42] The protocol includes a combination of preoperative, intraoperative, and postoperative prophylaxis techniques. Preoperative assessment involves a full medical evaluation with special attention paid to coagulation risk factors such as a current malignant tumor, a history of pulmonary embolism or deep venous thrombosis, estrogen therapy, oral contraceptive use, and tobacco use. Patients must discontinue the use of any procoagulant medication before admission. Autologous blood donation is also encouraged because it has been proven to significantly reduce the prevalence of deep venous thrombosis after total hip and total knee arthroplasty ($P = 0.003$ and $P < 0.01$, respectively).[43,44]

There are intraoperative techniques that may reduce the risk of thromboembolic complications. Using regional anesthesia decreases blood loss and the rate of deep venous thrombosis, and intraoperative pneumatic compression decreases venous stasis and the risk of clotting.[45-47] A surgical duration of less than 70 minutes also decreased the rate of deep venous thrombosis in patients treated with total knee arthroplasty.[48] A single intraoperative dose of unfractionated heparin may decrease the rate of deep venous thrombosis after total hip arthroplasty, but the data with regard to total knee arthroplasty are less conclusive.[9,49]

The standard inpatient postoperative prophylaxis includes intermittent pneumatic compression and pharmacologic prophylaxis (usually warfarin, or aspirin if warfarin is contraindicated). Furthermore, it is important for prophylaxis to continue following discharge from the hospital and for the patient to be aware of the symptoms of venous thromboembolism postdischarge. Pellegrini and associates[5] found that secondary prophylaxis with extended warfarin therapy reduced the rates of readmission for the treatment of pulmonary embolism, deep venous thrombosis, or bleeding after total knee replacement, and they recommended that patients continue to take warfarin following discharge. Another recent study showed that even if screening tests reveal negative findings, discharging patients without continuing prophylaxis after a total hip or knee arthroplasty is not cost-effective.[13]

In a large study from our institution, González Della Valle and associates[41] found that a multimodal approach of preoperative and intraoperative measures combined with pneumatic compression, knee-high elastic stockings, early mobilization, and chemoprophylaxis with acetylsalicylic acid (83% of patients) or warfarin (17%) for 4 to 6 weeks following total hip arthroplasty was safe and efficacious. The study included 1,947 consecutive patients (2,032 total hip arthroplasties) who were observed prospectively for 3 months. The first 171 patients had a 6.4% prevalence of asymptomatic deep venous thrombosis as assessed with ultrasound, and the other 1,776 patients had a 2.5% prevalence of clinical deep venous thrombosis. Nonfatal symptomatic pulmonary embolism occurred in 0.6% (12) of the 1,947 patients. The low rates of thromboembolic complications in this high-risk population are evidence that routine anticoagulation with chemoprophylactic agents that may increase the risk of bleeding, such as low-molecular-weight heparin, is unnecessary. The authors of a review of prophylaxis following total knee arthroplasty concurred,[35] finding that "no one method of prophylaxis has been shown to be ideal and there is little doubt that more than one modality focusing on both mechanical and chemical means of prevention need to be employed."

Pros and Cons of the ACCP Guidelines for Prophylaxis Against Deep Venous Thrombosis After Total Joint Arthroplasty

In 2004, the recommendations of the Seventh ACCP Conference on Antithrombotic and Thrombolytic Therapy for prophylaxis against deep venous thrombosis were published.[50] These recommendations were based on a systematic review of the literature by experts in the field, with use of strict, well-defined criteria for inclusion of studies. Because the recommendations of the ACCP are frequently used as a standard, it is important to understand the methodology as well as the advantages and disadvantages of these guidelines.[51] The criteria for inclusion of studies that form the basis of the recommendations included a defined patient population that was identified as belonging to the group at risk, a sample size of at least 10 patients in each group, and an identifiable end point normally consisting of the prevalence of deep venous thrombosis as demonstrated by contrast venography. Only randomized clinical trials were assessed for the determination of prophylaxis efficacy. Final recommendations were based on comments from 5 to 10 external reviewers. The rationale for prophylaxis for hospitalized patients was based on the high prevalence of venous thromboembolism, the adverse consequence of sequelae of deep venous thrombosis, and the efficacy and effectiveness of thromboprophylaxis. Patients undergoing total joint arthroplasty were considered to be either at high risk or at the highest risk depending on their age, the presence of additional risk factors, and the high-risk nature of arthroplasty surgery.

Additional rationales for routine thromboprophylaxis for patients undergoing total joint arthroplasty were that most postoperative deep venous thrombi and pulmonary emboli are clinically silent; it is difficult to predict whether symptomatic deep venous thrombosis or pulmonary embolism will develop in a particular patient; and identifying at-risk patients with either physical examination or screening modalities has proven to be generally ineffective. Also, the cost of diagnosing and treating the sequelae of venous thromboembolic disease is substantial. In addition to the risk and cost of treating a disease that could have been prevented, there is an increased future risk of recurrent disease and its sequelae, such as chronic postthrombotic syndrome. The underlying assumptions regarding the effectiveness of thromboprophylaxis include evidence that prophylaxis is very effective in lowering the prevalence of deep venous thrombosis, that prophylaxis can prevent both symptomatic pulmonary embolism and fatal pulmonary embolism, and that prophylaxis against deep venous thrombosis is cost-effective. Also underlying these recommendations are the facts that many cases of symptomatic venous thromboembolic disease occur after discharge, failure to prevent venous thromboembolic disease results in therapeutic anticoagulation with additional substantial risks, and venous thrombi can result in several sequelae that are frequently overlooked. These sequelae include postthrombotic syndrome, which can cause leg swelling, dermatitis, and ulcers; venous insufficiency; and persistent venous occlusion. The clinical diagnosis of venous thromboembolic disease is unreliable, and routine screening of asymptomatic patients has not been cost-effective. There is a strong case, therefore, for primary prophylaxis on a routine basis. Of all practices reviewed by the Agency for Healthcare Research and Quality, in terms of their ability to reduce adverse events while decreasing overall costs, prophylaxis against deep venous thrombosis has received the highest safety rating.

The end point selected for the clinical trials on thromboprophylaxis by the ACCP was venographically proven deep venous thrombosis. Although it is recognized that most asymptomatic deep venous thrombi are not clinically relevant, there is allegedly a strong concordance between the surrogate outcome of asymptomatic deep venous thrombosis and clinically important deep venous thrombosis, with a ratio estimated to range from 5:1 to 10:1. The use of a decrease in mortality or the rate of symptomatic pulmonary embolism alone as an end point has been termed problematic.[50]

On the basis of these underlying assumptions and the rigorous methodology, evidence-based guidelines, rated as either grade 1 (defined as strong and indicative of benefits that outweigh risk, burden, and cost) or grade 2 (defined as being less certain with regard to the magnitude of benefits, risks, and costs), were released. Grade 1 recommendations were subdivided into grade 1A recommendations, which are based on randomized clinical trials with consistent results that provide unbiased recommendations; grade 1B recommendations, which are based on randomized clinical trials with inconsistent results or with major methodologic weaknesses; and grade 1C recommendations, which are based on observational studies or on generalization from one group of patients included in randomized clinical trials to a different, but somewhat similar, group of patients who did not participate in those trials.[52] The grade 1A recommendations for prophylaxis for hip replacement included administration of warfarin with a target international normalized ratio of 2.5 (range, 2 to 3), low-molecular-weight heparin, or fondaparinux, for a minimum of 10 days. The recommendations were the same for knee replacement but included pneumatic compression devices as a grade 1B recommendation. There was a grade 1A recommendation against the use of aspirin alone following elective hip or knee arthroplasty. A prolonged course of treatment, for 4 to 5 weeks, was recommended for patients at highest risk.

In addition to the rigorous, well-described methodology underlying the ACCP guidelines, an advantage of these recommendations is that they meet the criteria of virtually every oversight group, including hospitals, health maintenance organizations, and insurance companies, and therefore following them minimizes medicolegal exposure. The ACCP grade 1A recommendations also meet requirements of state and federal programs, including the Surgical Care Improvement Project and the Center for Medicare and Medicaid Services Pay-for-Performance program initiative. The Surgical Care Improvement Project has a goal of reducing surgical complications by 25% by 2010.[53,54] Four areas have been targeted, one of which is minimizing venous thromboembolism. The Pay-for-Performance program was implemented by the Tax Relief and Health Care Act of 2006.[55] In 2007, the Physician Quality Reporting Initiative identified numerous health-quality measures, including venous thromboembolism prophylaxis for all patients for whom it is indicated. Reporting that three performance measures were met for 80% of eligible patients qualified physicians for a 1.5% bonus, whereas failure to report or comply in the future will in all likelihood result in a decreased reimbursement.[56] Although the ACCP recommendations for prophylaxis against deep venous thrombosis after hip and knee arthroplasty meet the requirements of the federal programs, following these recommendations is not necessary to satisfactorily meet the requirements of those programs. According to the manual for National Hospital Quality Measures, the use of low-molecular-weight heparin, factor Xa inhibitor, or warfarin meets the requirement for both total hip replacement and total knee replacement.[57] In addition, pneumatic compression devices meet the requirement for elective total knee arthroplasty. Of note is the fact that neither the dose nor the duration of pharmacologic prophylaxis is specified; this is especially relevant for warfarin, for which lower-dose protocols are often embraced by orthopaedic surgeons and shorter durations of prophylaxis have occasionally been used successfully as well. Aspirin alone is not recommended for prophylaxis against deep venous thrombosis.

Potential problems with following grade 1A protocols have been noted in recent studies. Reviews of the available literature, particularly studies related to hip and knee arthroplasty, have resulted in differing conclusions. One major issue is whether the prevalence of deep venous thrombosis should be used as a surrogate marker for effectiveness because deep venous thrombosis does not correlate with symptomatic pulmonary embolism or death rates following hip and knee arthroplasty. Deep venous thrombosis is two to three times more common after knee replacement than it is after hip replacement, but the prevalence of pulmonary embolism following total knee arthroplasty is equivalent or reduced compared with that after total hip arthroplasty.[58] Also of crucial importance is the observation, supported by several clinical studies, that the more effective reduction of deep venous thrombosis achieved with the aggressive use of chemoprophylactic agents leads to a higher risk of bleeding and subsequent morbidity. One recent study showed that converting to an ACCP grade 1A protocol actually substantially increased complications and decreased efficacy compared with the outcomes associated with a previously used protocol that did not meet any of the criteria set forth by the ACCP.[59] Prior to 2004, 705 patients were treated with a short course (7 days) of low-dose Coumadin (warfarin), with a target international normalized ratio of 2 to 2.5, and routine predischarge ultrasound screening. This course was shorter than the 10-day minimum recommended by the ACCP, the target international normalized ratio was lower than that recommended by the ACCP, and the use of routine screening was in disagreement with a grade 1A ACCP negative recommendation. Despite this, the efficacy of the pre-2004 protocol was high, with no deaths and only one symptomatic pulmonary embolism (0.1%). Patient acceptance of the protocol was high, with most patients receiving most or all of their prophylactic treatment while they were in the hospital, so the cost of the protocol to the patient was usually zero. On the basis of the ACCP recommendations, the protocol at the institution was changed in conjunction with an institutional review board–approved prospective study in which a 10-day course of low-molecular-weight heparin was used for all eligible patients.[50] Data on wound drainage, symptomatic deep venous thrombosis and pulmonary embolism, hospital readmission, injection site complications, heparin-induced thrombocytopenia, and patient satisfaction and compliance were collected prospectively. Complete data were collected on 290 consecutive patients treated with total joint arthroplasty. The original study design called for more than 2,000 patients, but the study was terminated prematurely because of a concern about patient safety. The results were compared with those from a previous study.[59] Major complications occurred in 9%; symptomatic deep venous thrombosis in 7%; pulmonary embolism in 1.6%; hematoma and a revision in 2.3%; local wound problems in 6.2%; and heparin-induced thrombocytopenia in 0.8%. The rate of major complications was significantly higher and the efficacy was significantly lower than those with the non-ACCP protocol used immediately before the institution of this study[50,59] (Table 1). In addition, the rate of minor complications, including prolonged hospitalization, was 7%.

Complications associated with the use of more aggressive protocols for prophylaxis against deep venous thrombosis have recently been re-

Table 1
Comparison of Efficacy and Complications With an ACCP Grade 1A Protocol With Previous Results With a Non-ACCP Protocol in Patients Treated With Total Hip Arthroplasty

	ACCP Grade 1A Protocol With Lovenox (Enoxaparin)	Non-ACCP Protocol With Coumadin (Warfarin)	*P* Value
Major complications	11/129 (9%)	15/705 (2.1%)	< 0.001
Symptomatic deep venous thrombosis	9/129 (7%)	11/705 (1.6%)	< 0.001
Pulmonary embolism	2/129 (1.6%)	1/705 (0.1%)	< 0.01
Hematoma/revision	3/129 (2.3%)	2/705 (0.3%)	< 0.01
Local wound problems	8/129 (6.2%)	4/705 (0.6%)	< 0.001
Heparin-induced thrombocytopenia	1/129 (0.8%)		

Table 2
Results of Lower-Dose Warfarin Protocols for Patients Treated With Joint Arthroplasty

Study	No. of Cases	Target	Pulmonary Embolism	Death
Vresilovic et al[63]	852	Prothrombin time, 1.2-1.4 × control	6 (0.7%)	0
Paiement et al[64]	268	Prothrombin time, 1.25-1.5 × control	2 (0.7%)	0
Lieberman et al[65]	1,099	Prothrombin time, 14-17 seconds	12 (1.1%)	1 (0.09%)
Pellegrini et al[66]	1,972	International normalized ratio, 2.0	14 (0.7%)	3 (0.15%)
Pellegrini et al[5]	1,321	International normalized ratio, 2.0	9 (0.7%)	2 (0.15%)
Keeney et al[67]	705	International normalized ratio, 2-2.5	5 (0.7%)	0
Total	6,217		48 (0.77%)	6 (0.1%)

ported at other centers. Patel and associates[60] reported prolonged wound drainage and subsequent associated complications following primary hip and knee replacement. The proportion of patients who still had wound drainage on the fifth postoperative day was significantly higher in the group that received low-molecular-weight heparin than it was in the groups treated with the other studied modalities ($P = 0.003$); each day of prolonged wound drainage increased the risk of wound infection by 42% following a total hip arthroplasty and by 29% following a total knee arthroplasty. Parvizi and associates[61] studied the effect of excessive anticoagulation on the subsequent prevalence of periprosthetic infection. For the patients in whom infection developed following hip or knee replacement, the factors that were strongly associated with that complication were wound hematoma, wound drainage, or an international normalized ratio of more than 1.5 at the time of discharge. Novicoff and associates[62] noted that implementation of a protocol based on ACCP grade 1A recommendations led to a substantial increase in the prevalence of complications as compared with the rate associated with a previously used low-dose warfarin protocol.

Several orthopaedic studies of less aggressive pharmacologic prophylaxis for patients treated with hip or knee replacement have demonstrated excellent results when the end points were death and symptomatic pulmonary embolism. The largest body of data relates to the use of lower-dose warfarin protocols with a target international normalized ratio of 2.0 or less. Extremely low prevalences of symptomatic pulmonary embolism and death have been noted in several studies from leading total joint arthroplasty centers over the past 15 years[5,63-67] (Table 2). Bern and associates[68] reported on more than 1,000 patients treated with total hip arthroplasty and an ultra-low-dose warfarin protocol consisting of 1 mg/day for 7 days before surgery, a variable dose with a target international normalized ratio of 1.5 to 2 while the patient was in the hospital, and 1 mg/day for 4 to 6 weeks following discharge. There were only two cases of symptomatic deep venous thrombosis and one nonfatal pulmonary embolism, with a follow-up rate of more than 99%.

The other deep venous thrombosis prophylaxis regimen that has received some support in the orthopaedic literature is the use of aspirin. Although there is an ACCP grade 1A recommendation against the use of aspirin alone, Lotke and Lonner[69] reported a prevalence of pulmonary embolism of only 0.06% after more than 3,000 total knee arthroplasties with aspirin prophylaxis. More recently, Callaghan and associates[70] reported no deaths after 427 total knee arthroplasties, 73% of which were low-risk procedures, in patients treated with aspirin, foot pumps, and screening ultrasound. In a study of a large total joint arthroplasty database of patients treated with various prophylactic modalities, including aspirin (4,719), warfarin (51,923), and low-molecular-weight heparin or fondaparinux (37,198), Bozic and associates[71] reported no difference in mortality rates but substantially less bleeding in the aspirin group.

Many arthroplasty surgeons disagree with some of the major conclusions and recommendations of the ACCP guidelines. The two major issues are the use of venographically proven deep venous thrombosis as the end point of prophylaxis against venous thromboembolic disease and the measure of efficacy of prophylactic regimens. These criteria generally favor aggressive pharmacologic prophylaxis and correlate poorly with the prevalences of death and symptomatic pulmonary embolism following hip and knee arthroplasties. Largely because of this issue, the American Academy of Orthopaedic Surgeons formed a task force to recommend clinical guidelines specifically for prophylaxis against deep venous thrombosis in patients treated with lower extremity total joint arthroplasty. This task force chose prevention of symptomatic pulmonary embolism, rather than reduction in the prevalence of deep venous thrombosis, as the end point.[72] Use of this different end point led to different recommendations regarding appropriate regimens for prophylaxis against deep venous thrombosis. Probably the greatest difference of opinion, however, is over the prevalence of complications related to the use of aggressive pharmacologic prophylaxis. Many orthopaedic surgeons have observed a higher prevalence of prolonged wound drainage with the use of the more aggressive anticoagulation protocols. Pharmacologic prophylactic protocols resulting in a high risk of wound drainage also have been associated with hematoma formation, prolonged hospitalization, and other complications that can compromise the clinical result. The number of total joint procedures is expected to increase dramatically in the immediate future, with the increase in knee arthroplasties predicted to be much greater than that in hip arthroplasties and the highest rate of increase expected among younger patients, who tend to be healthier and at lower risk for deep venous thrombosis.[73] The use of aggressive pharmacologic protocols on a routine basis, therefore, may put an increasingly higher number of patients with a low risk for deep venous thrombosis at risk for complications from the prophylaxis; therefore, it is less likely to be cost-effective. The clinical success of less aggressive protocols and the increasing number of young, healthy patients who are undergoing hip and knee replacements seem to indicate that selective use of these aggressive pharmacologic protocols, with an emphasis on identifying patients who are at risk and more judicious use of aggressive prophylaxis against deep venous thrombosis, is prudent.

References

1. RD heparin compared with warfarin for prevention of venous thromboembolic disease following total hip or knee arthroplasty: RD Heparin Arthroplasty Group. *J Bone Joint Surg Am* 1994;76:1174-1185.
2. Hull R, Raskob G, Pineo G, et al: A comparison of subcutaneous low-molecular-weight heparin with warfarin sodium for prophylaxis against deep-vein thrombosis after hip or knee implantation. *N Engl J Med* 1993;329:1370-1376.
3. Colwell CW Jr, Collis DK, Paulson R, et al: Comparison of enoxaparin and warfarin for the prevention of venous thromboembolic disease after total hip arthroplasty: Evaluation during hospitalization and three months after discharge. *J Bone Joint Surg Am* 1999;81:932-940.
4. Francis CW, Pellegrini VD Jr, Totterman S, et al: Prevention of deep-vein thrombosis after total hip arthroplasty: Comparison of warfarin and dalteparin. *J Bone Joint Surg Am* 1997; 79:1365-1372.
5. Pellegrini VD Jr, Donaldson CT, Farber DC, Lehman EB, Evarts CM: The Mark Coventry Award: Prevention of readmission for venous thromboembolism after total knee arthroplasty. *Clin Orthop Relat Res* 2006; 452:21-27.
6. Hirsch J: Therapeutic range for the control of oral anticoagulant therapy. *Arch Intern Med* 1985;145:1187-1188.
7. Hirsh J: Oral anticoagulant drugs. *N Engl J Med* 1991;324:1865-1875.
8. Hirsh J, Levine MN: The optimal intensity of oral anticoagulant therapy. *JAMA* 1987;258:2723-2726.
9. Sculco TP, Colwell CW Jr, Pellegrini VD Jr, Westrich GH, Böttner F: Prophylaxis against venous thromboembolic disease in patients having a total hip or knee arthroplasty. *J Bone Joint Surg Am* 2002;84:466-477.
10. Paiement G, Wessinger SJ, Waltman AC, Harris WH: Low-dose warfarin versus external pneumatic com-

pression for prophylaxis against venous thromboembolism following total hip replacement. *J Arthroplasty* 1987;2:23-26.

11. Paiement GD, Beisaw NE, Harris WH, Wessinger SJ, Wyman EM: Advances in prevention of venous thromboembolic disease after elective surgery. *Instr Course Lect* 1990; 39:413-421.
12. Francis CW, Pellegrini VD Jr, Marder VJ, et al: Comparison of warfarin and external pneumatic compression in prevention of venous thrombosis after total hip replacement. *JAMA* 1992; 267:2911-2915.
13. Lieberman JR, Hsu WK: Prevention of venous thromboembolic disease after total hip and knee arthroplasty. *J Bone Joint Surg Am* 2005;87:2097-2112.
14. Westrich GH, Bottner F, Windsor RE, et al: VenaFlow plus Lovenox vs VenaFlow plus aspirin for thromboembolic disease prophylaxis in total knee arthroplasty. *J Arthroplasty* 2006; 21(6, suppl 2)139-143.
15. Arbit E, Goldberg M, Gomez-Orellana I, Majuru S: Oral heparin: Status review. *Thromb J* 2006;4:6.
16. Cohen AT, Hirst C, Sherrill B, Holmes P, Fidan D: Meta-analysis of trials comparing ximelagatran with low molecular weight heparin for prevention of venous thromboembolism after major orthopaedic surgery. *Br J Surg* 2005;92:1335-1344.
17. Colwell CW Jr, Berkowitz SD, Lieberman JR, et al: Oral direct thrombin inhibitor ximelagatran compared with warfarin for the prevention of venous thromboembolism after total knee arthroplasty. *J Bone Joint Surg Am* 2005;87:2169-2177.
18. Eriksson BI, Wille-Jørgenson P, Kälebo P, et al: A comparison of recombinant hirudin with a low-molecular-weight heparin to prevent thromboembolic complications after total hip replacement. *N Engl J Med* 1997;337:1329-1335.
19. Eriksson BI, Ekman S, Lindbratt S, et al: Prevention of thromboembolism with use of recombinant hirudin: Results of a double-blind, multicenter trial comparing the efficacy of desirudin (Revasc) with that of unfractionated heparin in patients having a total hip replacement. *J Bone Joint Surg Am* 1997;79:326-333.
20. Eriksson BI, Dahl OE, Büller HR, et al: A new oral direct thrombin inhibitor, dabigatran etexilate, compared with enoxaparin for prevention of thromboembolic events following total hip or knee replacement: The BISTRO II randomized trial. *J Thromb Haemost* 2005;3:103-111.
21. Bauer KA, Eriksson BI, Lassen MR, Turpie AG; Steering Committee of the Pentasaccharide in Major Knee Surgery Study: Fondaparinux compared with enoxaparin for the prevention of venous thromboembolism after elective major knee surgery. *N Engl J Med* 2001;345:1305-1310.
22. Motsch J, Walther A, Bock M, Böttiger BW: Update in the prevention and treatment of deep vein thrombosis and pulmonary embolism. *Curr Opin Anaesthesiol* 2006;19:52-58.
23. Hirsh J, O'Donnell M, Eikelboom JW: Beyond unfractionated heparin and warfarin: Current and future advances. *Circulation* 2007;116: 552-560.
24. Lassen MR, Davidson BL, Gallus A, et al: The efficacy and safety of apixaban, an oral, direct factor Xa inhibitor, as thromboprophylaxis in patients following total knee replacement. *J Thromb Haemost* 2007;5:2368-2375.
25. Perzborn E, Kubicza D, Misselwitz F: Rivaroxaban: A novel, oral, direct factor Xa inhibitor in clinical development for the prevention and treatment of thromboembolic disorders. *Hamostaseologie* 2007;27:282-289.
26. Laux V, Perzborn E, Kubitza D, Misselwitz F: Preclinical and clinical characteristics of rivaroxaban: A novel, oral, direct factor Xa inhibitor. *Semin Thromb Hemost* 2007;33: 515-523.
27. Fisher WD, Eriksson BI, Bauer KA, et al: Rivaroxaban for thromboprophylaxis after orthopaedic surgery: Pooled analysis of two studies. *Thromb Haemost* 2007;97:931-937.
28. Westrich GH, Sculco TP: Prophylaxis against deep venous thrombosis after total knee arthroplasty: Pneumatic plantar compression and aspirin compared with aspirin alone. *J Bone Joint Surg Am* 1996;78:826-834.
29. Ryan MG, Westrich GH, Potter HG, et al: Effect of mechanical compression on the prevalence of proximal deep venous thrombosis as assessed by magnetic resonance venography. *J Bone Joint Surg Am* 2002;84:1998-2004.
30. Lachiewicz PF, Kelley SS, Haden LR: Two mechanical devices for prophylaxis of thromboembolism after total knee arthroplasty: A prospective, randomised study. *J Bone Joint Surg Br* 2004;86:1137-1141.
31. Westrich GH, Specht LM, Sharrock NE, et al: Venous haemodynamics after total knee arthroplasty: Evaluation of active dorsal to plantar flexion and several mechanical compression devices. *J Bone Joint Surg Br* 1998,80.1057-1066.
32. Westrich GH, Specht LM, Sharrock NE, et al: Pneumatic compression hemodynamics in total hip arthroplasty. *Clin Orthop Relat Res* 2000; 372:180-191.
33. Westrich GH, Jhon PH, Sánchez PM: Compliance in using a pneumatic compression device after total knee arthroplasty. *Am J Orthop* 2003;32: 135-140.
34. Merli GJ: Prevention of thrombosis with warfarin, aspirin, and mechanical methods. *Clin Cornerstone* 2005;7: 49-56.
35. Boscainos PJ, McLardy-Smith P, Jinnah RH: Deep vein thrombosis prophylaxis after total-knee arthroplasty. *Curr Opin Orthop* 2006;17:60-67.
36. Dentali F, Ageno W, Imberti D: Retrievable vena cava filters: Clinical experience. *Curr Opin Pulm Med* 2006; 12:304-309.
37. Imberti D, Ageno W, Carpenedo M: Retrievable vena cava filters: A

review. *Curr Opin Hematol* 2006;13: 351-356.

38. Seshadri T, Tran H, Lau KK, Tan B, Gan TE: Ins and outs of inferior vena cava filters in patients with venous thromboembolism: The experience at Monash Medical Centre and review of the published reports. *Intern Med J* 2008;38:38-43.

39. Freedman KB, Brookenthal KR, Fitzgerald RH Jr, Williams S, Lonner JH: A meta-analysis of thromboembolic prophylaxis following elective total hip arthroplasty. *J Bone Joint Surg Am* 2000;82:929-938.

40. Westrich GH, Haas SB, Mosca P, Peterson M: Meta-analysis of thromboembolic prophylaxis after total knee arthroplasty. *J Bone Joint Surg Br* 2000; 82:795-800.

41. González Della Valle A, Serota A, Go G, et al: Venous thromboembolism is rare with a multimodal prophylaxis protocol after total hip arthroplasty. *Clin Orthop Relat Res* 2006; 444:146-153.

42. Westrich GH, Rana AJ, Terry MA, et al: Thromboembolic disease prophylaxis in patients with hip fracture: A multimodal approach. *J Orthop Trauma* 2005;19:234-240.

43. Bae H, Westrich GH, Sculco TP, Salvati EA, Reich LM: The effect of preoperative donation of autologous blood on deep-vein thrombosis after total hip arthroplasty. *J Bone Joint Surg Br* 2001;83:676-679.

44. Anders MJ, Lifeso RM, Landis M, et al: Effect of preoperative donation of autologous blood on deep-vein thrombosis following total joint arthroplasty of the hip or knee. *J Bone Joint Surg Am* 1996;78:574-580.

45. Lieberman JR, Huo MM, Hanway J, et al: The prevalence of deep venous thrombosis after total hip arthroplasty with hypotensive epidural anesthesia. *J Bone Joint Surg Am* 1994;76:341-348.

46. Miric A, Lombardi P, Sculco TP: Deep vein thrombosis prophylaxis: A comprehensive approach for total hip and total knee arthroplasty patient populations. *Am J Orthop* 2000;29: 269-274.

47. Westrich GH, Farrell C, Bono JV, et al: The incidence of venous thromboembolism after total hip arthroplasty: A specific hypotensive epidural anesthesia protocol. *J Arthroplasty* 1999;14:456-463.

48. Sharrock NE, Hargett MJ, Urquhart B, et al: Factors affecting deep vein thrombosis rate following total knee arthroplasty under epidural anesthesia. *J Arthroplasty* 1993;8:133-139.

49. DiGiovanni CW, Restrepo A, González Della Valle AG, et al: The safety and efficacy of intraoperative heparin in total hip arthroplasty. *Clin Orthop Relat Res* 2000;379:178-185.

50. Geerts WH, Pineo GF, Heit JA, et al: Prevention of venous thromboembolism: The Seventh ACCP Conference on Antithrombotic and Thrombolytic Therapy. *Chest* 2004;126 (suppl 3):338S-400S.

51. Schünemann HJ, Munger H, Brower S, et al: Methodology for guideline development for the Seventh American College of Chest Physicians Conference on Antithrombotic and Thrombolytic Therapy: The Seventh ACCP Conference on Antithrombotic and Thrombolytic Therapy. *Chest* 2004;126(suppl 3):174S-178S.

52. Guyatt G, Schünemann HJ, Cook D, Jaeschke R, Pauker S: Applying the grades of recommendation for antithrombotic and thrombolytic therapy: The Seventh ACCP Conference on Antithrombotic and Thrombolytic Therapy. *Chest* 2004;126 (suppl 3): 179S-187S.

53. Bratzler DW, Hunt DR: The surgical infection prevention and surgical care improvement projects: National initiatives to improve outcomes for patients having surgery. *Clin Infect Dis* 2006;43:322-330.

54. Medicare Quality Improvement Community Website: SCIP measures table. http://www.qualitynet.org/dcs/ContentServer?pagename=Medqic/Search/SearchResults&siteVersion=null&sort=_CONFIDENCE_&sortdir=ascending¤tsearch=aQIOOnly,0,MQAttributes,QIOOnly,FF1,No,SearchText,1,MQAttributes,SearchText,scip%20measures,0.01,0,¤tsearch2=aFile,1,MQAttributes,File,scip%20measures,0.01,0,¤tsearchPage=aQIOOnly,0,MQAttributes,QIOOnly,FF1,No,SearchText,1,MQAttributes,SearchText,scip%20measures,0.01,0,&cntntTpsToSrch=MQReports,MQStories,MQNews MQTests,MQWeblinks,MQTools,MQ Presentat. Accessed October 10, 2006.

55. Haralson RH III: Getting your share of the CMS P4P 2007 bonus payments. American Academy of Orthopaedic Surgeons Website. http://www.aaos.org/news/bulletin/janfeb0 7/reimbursement2.asp. Accessed January 25, 2008.

56. American Academy of Orthopaedic Surgeons Website: Background paper: Medicare. http://www3.aaos.org/Govern/Federal/Issues/Medicare/06medicarebg.cfm. Accessed October 20, 2008.

57. Specifications manual for National Hospital Quality Measures. http://www.medqic.org. Accessed April 15, 2007.

58. Callaghan JJ, Dorr LD, Engh GA, et al: Prophylaxis for thromboembolic disease: Recommendations from the American College of Chest Physicians. Are they appropriate for orthopaedic surgery? *J Arthroplasty* 2005;20:273-274.

59. Burnett RS, Clohisy JC, Wright RW, et al: Failure of the American College of Chest Physicians-1A protocol for lovenox in clinical outcomes for thromboembolic prophylaxis. *J Arthroplasty* 2007;22:317-324.

60. Patel VP, Walsh M, Sehgal B, et al: Factors associated with prolonged wound drainage after primary total hip and knee arthroplasty. *J Bone Joint Surg Am* 2007;89:33-38.

61. Parvizi J, Ghanem E, Joshi A, et al: Does "excessive" anticoagulation predispose to periprosthetic infection? *J Arthroplasty* 2007;22(6, suppl 2): 24-28.

62. Novicoff WM, Brown TE, Cui Q, Mihalko WM, Slone HS, Saleh KJ: Mandated venous thromboembolism prophylaxis: Possible adverse outcomes. *J Arthroplasty* 2008;23:(6, suppl 1)15-19.

63. Vresilovic EJ Jr, Hozack WJ, Booth RE, Rothman RH: Incidence of pulmonary embolism after total knee arthroplasty with low-dose Coumadin prophylaxis. *Clin Orthop Relat Res* 1993;286:27-31.

64. Paiement GD, Wessinger SJ, Hughes R, Harris WH: Routine use of adjusted low-dose warfarin to prevent venous thromboembolism after total hip replacement. *J Bone Joint Surg Am* 1993;75:893-898.

65. Lieberman JR, Wollaeger J, Dorey F, et al: The efficacy of prophylaxis with low-dose warfarin for prevention of pulmonary embolism following total hip arthroplasty. *J Bone Joint Surg Am* 1997;79:319-325.

66. Pellegrini VD Jr, Donaldson CT, Farber DC, Lehman EB, Evarts CM: The John Charnley Award: Prevention of readmission for venous thromboembolic disease after total hip arthroplasty. *Clin Orthop Relat Res* 2005;441:56-62.

67. Keeney JA, Clohisy JC, Curry MC, Maloney WJ: Efficacy of combined modality prophylaxis including short-duration warfarin to prevent venous thromboembolism after total hip arthroplasty. *J Arthroplasty* 2006;21:469-475.

68. Bern M, Deshmukh RV, Nelson R, et al: Low-dose warfarin coupled with lower leg compression is effective prophylaxis against thromboembolic disease after hip arthroplasty. *J Arthroplasty* 2007;22:644-650.

69. Lotke PA, Lonner JH: The benefit of aspirin chemoprophylaxis for thromboembolism after total knee arthroplasty. *Clin Orthop Relat Res* 2006;452:175-180.

70. Callaghan JJ, Warth LC, Hoballah J, Liu S, Wells C: Abstract: Low-morbidity low-cost deep vein thrombosis prophylaxis in low-risk patients undergoing total knee arthroplasty. *The Journal of Arthroplasty*. New York, NY, Elsevier, 2008, p 320.

71. Bozic KJ, Auerbach A, Maselli J, Smith A, Vail TP: Abstract: Is there a role for aspirin in venous thromboembolism prophylaxis after total knee arthroplasty? *The Journal of Arthroplasty*. New York, NY, Elsevier, 2008, p 317.

72. American Academy of Orthopaedic Surgeons Website: American Academy of Orthopaedic Surgeons clinical guideline on prevention of pulmonary embolism in patients undergoing total hip or knee arthroplasty. May, 2007. http://www.aaos.org/Research/guidelines/PE_guideline.pdf. Accessed October 20, 2008.

73. Kurtz S, Ong K, Lau E, Mowat F, Halpern M: Projections of primary and revision hip and knee arthroplasty in the United States from 2005 to 2030. *J Bone Joint Surg Am* 2007;89:780-785.

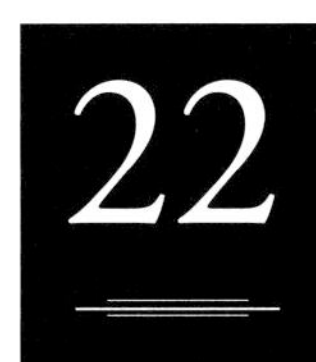

New Oral Anticoagulants for Venous Thromboembolism Prophylaxis in Orthopaedic Surgery

Richard J. Friedman, MD, FRCSC

Abstract

Anticoagulant drugs reduce the risk of venous thromboembolic events after total hip and knee arthroplasty. However, the use of current drugs, such as low-molecular-weight heparins, is hampered by their subcutaneous administration. The use of a vitamin K antagonist, such as warfarin, is hampered by the required routine coagulation monitoring and dose titration to provide effective anticoagulation without an increased risk of bleeding. Numerous possible food and drug interactions must also be considered. New classes of oral anticoagulant agents have been developed that have a fixed dose, do not require coagulation monitoring, do not have food and drug interactions, and demonstrate similar or better efficacy and safety profiles when compared with current agents.

In the United States, in 2007, the number of total hip arthroplasties (THAs) and total knee arthroplasties (TKAs) performed was approximately 300,000 and 500,000, respectively.[1] The number of THAs is expected to increase to 572,000 and the number of TKAs to 3.48 million by 2030. As has been well documented, patients treated with THA or TKA are at significant risk of developing venous thromboembolism (VTE), comprising deep venous thrombosis and (DVT) and pulmonary embolism (PE).[2] Without thromboprophylaxis, 42% to 57% of patients treated with THA have venographically confirmed total (proximal or distal) DVT. In patients treated with TKA without thromboprophylaxis, 41% to 85% have venographically confirmed total DVT.

The appropriate use of antithrombotic agents has been shown to reduce the risk of VTE after THA and TKA; guidelines by several organizations, such as the American College of Chest Physicians (ACCP) and the American Academy of Orthopaedic Surgeons (AAOS), recommend their routine use after this type of surgery. More information on the guideline recommendations is available in chapter 26. However, symptomatic clinical events still occur in approximately 2% to 4% of patients and occur at a mean of 9.7 days after TKA and 21.5 days after THA[3] (**Figure 1**). With the current trend toward shorter hospital stays, which average fewer than 3 days for THA and TKA, VTE prophylaxis has become essentially an outpatient issue.

Pharmacologic Prophylaxis

Options and Limitations

Recommended pharmacologic options for thromboprophylaxis after THA or TKA include vitamin K antagonists (such as warfarin), low-molecular-weight heparins (such as enoxaparin and dalteparin), and an indirect factor Xa inhibitor (fondaparinux). The limitations of warfarin include the requirement for regular coagulation monitoring, the potential for food and drug interactions, and a delayed onset of action.[3,4] Parenteral anticoagulants, such as enoxaparin and fondaparinux, may be less convenient than those administered orally. There is also a risk of heparin-induced thrombocytopenia with low-molecular-weight heparins.[5]

Although warfarin offers the convenience of oral administration, its use in

Dr. Friedman or an immediate family member serves as a board member, owner, officer, or committee member of the AAOS, the American Shoulder and Elbow Surgeons, and the BOS; has received royalties from DJ Orthopaedics and CRC Press; serves as a paid consultant to or is an employee of Johnson & Johnson, Astellas US, Boehringer Ingelheim, and DJO Surgical; and has received research or institutional support from Astellas US.

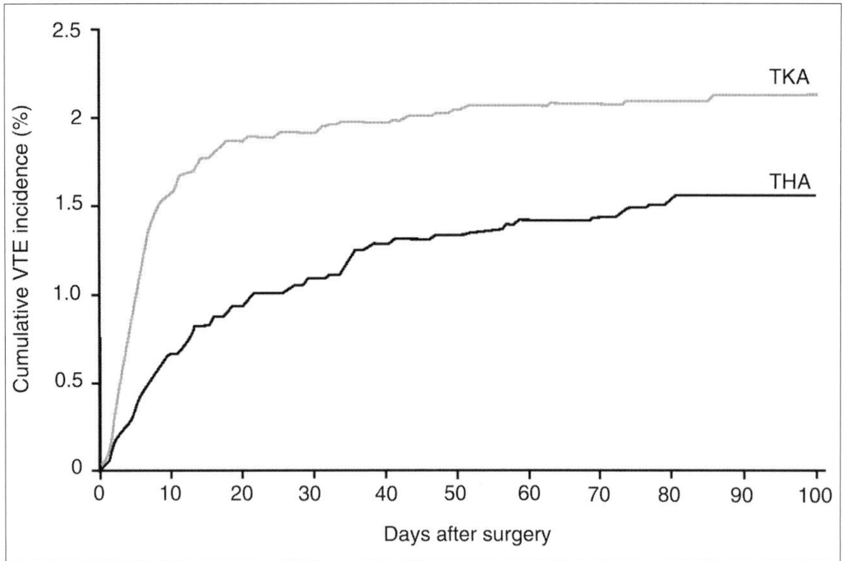

Figure 1 Graph showing the cumulative incidence of VTE, with the mean time to a symptomatic event after TKA being 9.7 days and 20.5 days after THA. (Reproduced with permission from Warwick D, Friedman W, Agnelli G, et al: Insufficient duration of venous thromboembolism prophylaxis after total hip or knee replacement when compared with the time course of thromboembolic events. *J Bone Joint Surg Br* 2007;89:799-807.)

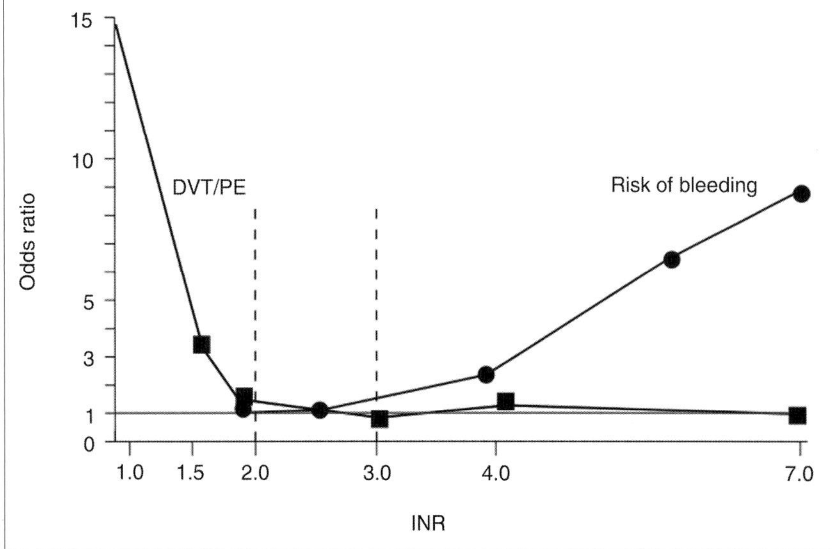

Figure 2 Graph showing the narrow therapeutic range of warfarin. (Adapted with permission from Friedman RJ: Prevention of thrombophlebitis in total knee arthroplasty, in Scott WN: *Surgery of the Knee*, ed 4. Philadelphia, PA, Churchill-Livingstone, 2006, vol 2, pp 1837-1847.)

clinical practice can be complicated. It has a narrow therapeutic window and shows considerable individual variability in its dose-response relationship[6] (**Figure 2**). With a narrow therapeutic window, an international normalized ratio (INR) of less than 2.0 is associated with a low risk of bleeding but reduced efficacy and therefore an increased risk for DVT and PE. If the INR rises above 3.0, the risk for thromboembolic complications is low, but the risk of surgical site and remote bleeding rises exponentially. Warfarin is subject to numerous dietary and drug interactions, and the need for regular dose adjustments to achieve and maintain a target INR can lead to additional problems, such as nonadherence to the medication regimen or communication difficulties between the physician and the patient.[6] These factors make it difficult for the patient to achieve and maintain adherence to the narrow therapeutic window of efficacy and safety.

New Oral Anticoagulant Agents

To overcome these limitations, new oral anticoagulants that do not require regular coagulation monitoring, are unlikely to interact with food and drugs, and have a fast onset and offset of action are being developed. Because patients often need to self-administer injectable thromboprophylaxis at home, an ideal anticoagulant would allow easier administration. Oral anticoagulants have a clear advantage over parenteral agents.

Several new oral anticoagulants in development have shown promising benefit-risk profiles in clinical trials with similar or better efficacy and safety profiles compared with current agents.[7-10] Clinical studies have focused on the use of oral, direct factor Xa inhibitors (such as apixaban and rivaroxaban) and a direct thrombin inhibitor (dabigatran etexilate) for thromboprophylaxis following THA and TKA. At the time of this writing, these agents are classified by the Food and Drug Administration as investigational and have not been cleared for clinical use in the United States.

Because currently available anticoagulant drugs are administered subcutaneously or require monitoring and dose adjustment to provide effective anticoagulation without increasing bleeding risk, their use presents a clinical challenge for orthopaedic surgeons. It is hoped that new drugs will meet the needs of orthopaedic surgeons in providing improved VTE prophylaxis for their patients.

An ideal anticoagulant should be efficacious without increasing bleeding risk, safe, convenient to use, and administered orally once daily with fixed dosing—factors that could potentially improve patient compliance. The most promising new oral anticoagulants are the direct thrombin inhibitors and the direct factor Xa inhibitors. These agents directly target a single coagulation factor in the coagulation cascade (**Figure 3**). Dabigatran is approved for use in Europe, Canada, and other countries. It is dosed at 110 mg within 1 to 4 hours of surgery and then 220 mg once daily for 28 to 35 days after THA and 10 days after TKA, for VTE prophylaxis after elective THA and TKA.[11] Rivaroxaban is also approved in Europe, Canada, and numerous other countries for the prevention of VTE in patients after elective THA or TKA at a dose of 10 mg 6 to 10 hours after surgery and then once daily for 35 days after THA and 14 days after TKA.[12] These two drugs represent the first new oral agents for VTE prophylaxis in THA and TKA in more than 50 years.

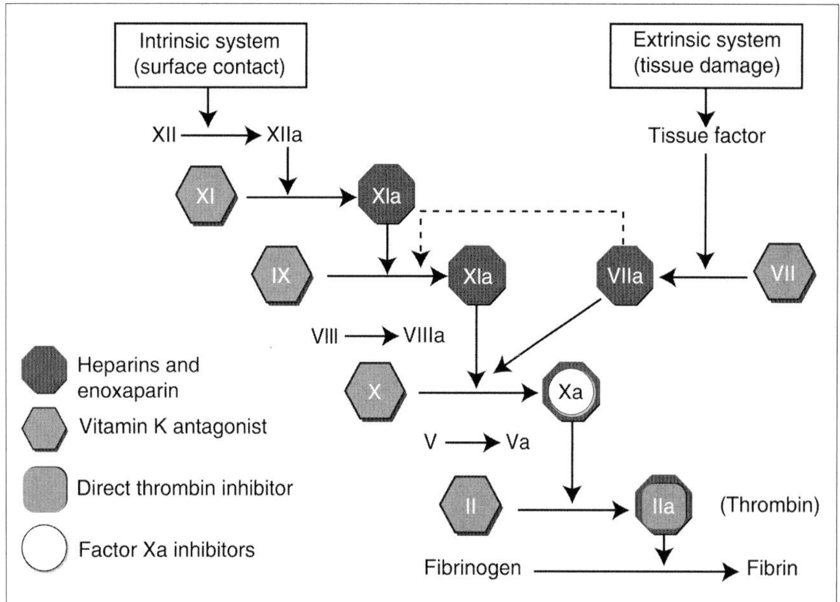

Figure 3 Schematic diagram of the simplified coagulation cascade showing sites of action of anticoagulant drugs used in thromboprophylaxis. (Adapted with permission from Friedman RJ: Prevention of thrombophlebitis in total knee arthroplasty, in Scott WN: *Surgery of the Knee*, ed 4. Philadelphia, PA, Churchill-Livingstone, 2006, vol 2, pp 1837-1847.)

Direct Thrombin Inhibitors

Mode of Action

Thrombin is an enzyme that catalyzes the conversion of fibrinogen to fibrin, which leads to thrombus formation. Direct thrombin inhibitors bind to thrombin and block the interaction of thrombin with its substrate, thereby preventing the conversion of fibrinogen to fibrin.[4] Direct thrombin inhibitors offer some potential advantages over indirect thrombin inhibitors. Because of low levels of plasma protein binding, direct inhibitors offer a more predictable anticoagulant effect than indirect inhibitors and also are effective against both circulating and clot-bound thrombin (whereas heparins are ineffective against clot-bound thrombin, which remains biologically active). An important advantage of direct thrombin inhibitors is their oral administration, which (as with the oral direct factor Xa inhibitors) provides added convenience and may encourage patient compliance.

Dabigatran Etexilate

Dabigatran etexilate is rapidly absorbed and converted to its active form, dabigatran.[13] The bioavailability of dabigatran after oral administration is low (6% to 7%). After oral administration of a 200-mg dose of dabigatran, the half-life is approximately 9 hours. The predominant elimination pathway is renal excretion, through which more than 80% of the systemically available dabigatran is eliminated. Because renal function declines with increasing age, dabigatran elimination would be expected to be prolonged in elderly patients with compromised renal function. In a pharmacokinetic study of healthy individuals age 65 years or older, dabigatran dosed at 150 mg twice daily for 6 days and once on day 7 resulted in a half-life of 12 to 14 hours.[14]

The sex of the patient has not been shown to have any clinically important effects on dabigatran pharmacokinetics, and there is limited clinical experience in patients with extreme body weight.[14] Food consumption delays the time to peak plasma concentration by 2 hours but does not affect the extent of absorption.[15] Comedications (such as diuretics, drugs that accelerate the gastrointestinal transit time, acetaminophen, and CYP3A4 inhibitors), demographics, and standard laboratory parameters had no relevant effect on standard coagulation tests in a population pharmacodynamic analysis in patients treated with THA.[16] The

CYP450 system does not appear to play an important role in the pharmacodynamics of dabigatran; therefore, drugs that are metabolized by this system are unlikely to interact with therapeutic doses of dabigatran.[3] Dabigatran does not require regular coagulation monitoring.[17]

Three phase III studies have been completed for dabigatran.[18-20] The RE-NOVATE study was conducted in patients treated with THA, and the RE-MODEL and RE-MOBILIZE studies in patients treated with TKA. All three studies were prospective, randomized, double-blind, double-dummy, controlled trials. The primary efficacy end point in the three studies was the composite of total VTE (venographic or symptomatic DVT or symptomatic PE) and death.

In the RE-NOVATE THA study of 3,494 patients, dabigatran (150 mg or 220 mg once daily) was compared with enoxaparin (40 mg once daily), with both drugs administered for 28 to 35 days.[18] The primary efficacy end point occurred in 8.6% of the 150-mg group (absolute risk difference versus enoxaparin, 1.9%), 6.0% of the 220-mg group (absolute risk difference versus enoxaparin, –0.7%), and 6.7% of the enoxaparin group. Both doses of dabigatran were noninferior to enoxaparin ($P < 0.0001$ for noninferiority for both doses). Symptomatic DVT occurred in 0.8% of the 150-mg group, 0.5% of the 220-mg group, and 0.1% of the enoxaparin group. Rates of major bleeding were 1.3% for the 150-mg group ($P = 0.60$), 2.0% for the 220-mg group ($P = 0.44$), and 1.6% for the enoxaparin group. Clinically relevant, nonmajor bleeding occurred in 4.7%, 4.2%, and 3.5% of the dabigatran 150 mg, dabigatran 220 mg, and enoxaparin groups, respectively. The rate of wound complications was 3% in each of the dabigatran groups and 4% in the enoxaparin group. Bleeding events leading to reoperation occurred in 0.3% of patients receiving dabigatran 150 mg, 0.2% of patients receiving dabigatran 220 mg, and 0.3% of patients receiving enoxaparin.

In the RE-MODEL TKA study of 2,101 patients, dabigatran (150 mg and 220 mg once daily) was compared with enoxaparin (40 mg once daily; n = 699).[19] The primary efficacy end point occurred in 40.5% of patients in the 150-mg group (absolute risk difference versus enoxaparin, 2.8%; $P = 0.017$ for noninferiority), 36.4% of the dabigatran 220 mg group (absolute risk difference versus enoxaparin, –1.3%; $P = 0.0003$ for noninferiority), and 37.7% of the enoxaparin group. Rates of major bleeding were 1.3% for the 150-mg group ($P = 1.0$), 1.5% for the 220-mg group ($P = 0.82$), and 1.3% for the enoxaparin group. Symptomatic DVT occurred in 0.4% of patients in the 150-mg group, 0.1% of patients the 220-mg group, and 1.2% of patients in the enoxaparin group. Clinically relevant, nonmajor bleeding occurred in 6.8% of the dabigatran 150-mg group, 5.9% of the dabigatran 220-mg group, and 5.3% of the enoxaparin group. Bleeding leading to reoperation occurred in 0.1% of patients receiving dabigatran 150 mg, 0.4% of patients receiving dabigatran 220 mg, and 0.1% of patients receiving enoxaparin.

In the RE-MOBILIZE TKA study of 2,615 patients, dabigatran (150 mg and 220 mg once daily) was compared with enoxaparin (30 mg twice daily).[20] Dabigatran did not meet the noninferiority criteria for either dose. The primary efficacy outcome occurred in 33.7% of the 150-mg group, 31.1% of the 220-mg group, and 25.3% of the enoxaparin group. For the 150-mg group, the risk difference was 8.4% ($P = 0.0009$), and for the 220-mg group, the risk difference was 5.8% ($P = 0.0234$) compared with enoxaparin. Major bleeding occurred in 0.6% of the 150-mg group, 0.6% of the 220-mg group, and 1.4% of the enoxaparin group. Clinically relevant, nonmajor bleeding occurred in 2.5%, 2.7%, and 2.4% of the dabigatran 150 mg, dabigatran 220 mg, and enoxaparin groups, respectively. No patients in the dabigatran arm experienced bleeding that led to reoperation, but one patient in the enoxaparin group required reoperation because of bleeding.

Dabigatran showed noninferiority to the enoxaparin 40-mg once-daily regimen after THA and TKA but failed to meet the noninferiority criteria compared with the North American enoxaparin 30-mg twice-daily regimen after TKA. In all three studies, the incidence of liver enzyme elevations (alanine aminotransferase > 3 times the upper limit of the normal range) and acute coronary events was similar between the three groups.

A meta-analysis of the three trials has been completed.[10] A meta-analysis of the dabigatran 220-mg dose showed no significant differences between dabigatran 220 mg and enoxaparin in any of the end points when all three trials were included in the analysis. Major bleeding rates did not differ significantly when the RE-MODEL and RE-NOVATE studies were analyzed ($P = 0.41$ for random effect and fixed effect analyses) or when RE-MOBILIZE was included in the analysis ($P = 0.85$ for random effects and $P = 0.95$ for fixed effects). Clinically relevant, nonmajor bleeding also did not differ significantly in the two-trial analysis ($P = 0.34$ for random effects and $P = 0.33$ for fixed effects) or when all three trials were analyzed together ($P = 0.31$ for both random effect and fixed effect analyses). These findings support the conclusions of RE-MODEL and RE-NOVATE that dabigatran 220 mg is noninferior to enoxaparin 40 mg once daily, with a similar safety profile.

Based on this information, 2,055 patients treated with THA were entered in the RE-NOVATE II study, a double-blind, noninferiority trial, in which patients were randomized to treatment for 28 to 35 days with oral dabigatran, 220 mg once daily, starting with a half dose 1 to 4 hours after surgery; or subcutaneous enoxaparin 40 mg once daily.[21] The primary efficacy outcome was a composite of total VTE (venographic or symptomatic) and death from all causes. The main secondary composite outcome was major VTE (proximal DVT or nonfatal PE) plus VTE-related death. The main safety outcome was major bleeding during treatment. The primary efficacy outcome occurred in 61 of 792 patients (7.7%) in the dabigatran group versus 69 of 785 patients (8.8%) in the enoxaparin group (absolute risk difference –1.1%, 95% confidence interval [CI], –3.8% to 1.6%; $P < 0.0001$) for the prespecified noninferiority margin. The main secondary efficacy outcome occurred in 18 of 805 patients (2.2%) in the dabigatran group versus 33 of 794 patients (4.2%) in the enoxaparin group (absolute risk difference –1.9%; 95% CI, –3.6% to –0.2%; $P = 0.03$). Major bleeding occurred in 1.4% of the dabigatran group and 0.9% of the enoxaparin group ($P = 0.40$). The incidence of adverse events, including liver and cardiac events, did not differ significantly between the groups. Extended prophylaxis with oral dabigatran 220 mg once daily was as effective as subcutaneous enoxaparin 40 mg once daily in reducing the risk of VTE after THA. The risk of bleeding and the safety profiles were similar.

Direct Factor Xa Inhibitors

Mode of Action

The enzyme factor X is an attractive target for inhibition because it occupies a critical junction between the intrinsic and extrinsic coagulation cascade pathways and is essential for the conversion of prothrombin to thrombin, which leads to thrombus formation[22,23] (**Figure 3**). In response to vascular injury, factor X is activated to factor Xa by either the contact (intrinsic pathway) or by the tissue factor/factor VIIa (extrinsic pathway). Factor Xa combines with its cofactor, factor Va, on phospholipid membranes to form the prothrombinase complex. This complex converts prothrombin to thrombin, which leads to the amplified generation of thrombin.

The indirect factor Xa inhibitors, such as subcutaneous fondaparinux, showed that factor Xa is an effective target for anticoagulation. Direct factor Xa inhibitors have some advantages over indirect factor Xa inhibitors. Unlike indirect factor Xa inhibitors, which catalyze factor Xa inhibition by antithrombin, direct factor Xa inhibitors bind directly to factor Xa, thus preventing the subsequent reactions leading to thrombin generation.[22,23] In addition, they inhibit both free and platelet-bound factor Xa and factor Xa bound to the prothrombinase complex. Some direct factor Xa inhibitors in development are administered parenterally (for example, DX-9065a), whereas others (for example, apixaban and rivaroxaban) are orally active.

Apixaban

Apixaban is an oral, direct factor Xa inhibitor that has no food and relatively few drug interactions. Peak concentrations occur 3 to 4 hours after oral administration, and the terminal half-life is 9 to 12 hours. Bioavailability is 50%, and there is a dual mode of excretion, with 25% excreted renally. A phase II study of apixaban was used to establish the dose to be used for the phase III clinical development program.[24] In this study, 1,238 patients were randomized to one of six double-blind apixaban doses (5, 10, or 20 mg once daily or 2.5, 5, or 10 mg twice daily), enoxaparin (30 mg twice daily subcutaneously), or open-label warfarin (titrated to an INR of 1.8 to 3.0) for 10 to 14 days. The primary efficacy outcome (the composite of VTE and all cause mortality) decreased with an increasing apixaban dose ($P = 0.09$ with once- or twice-daily regimens combined; $P = 0.19$ for once-daily and $P = 0.13$ for twice-daily dosing). There was a significant dose-related increase of total adjudicated bleeding events for the once-daily ($P = 0.01$) and twice-daily ($P = 0.02$) regimens. The authors concluded that apixaban administered at 2.5 mg twice daily and 5 mg once daily might have a promising risk–benefit profile compared with enoxaparin 30 mg twice daily and warfarin.

The ADVANCE-1 phase III study of 3,195 patients compared apixaban 2.5 mg twice daily with the enoxaparin regimen commonly used in North America of 30 mg twice daily for the prevention of VTE after TKA.[8] The primary efficacy outcome (composite of venographic DVT; symptomatic, objectively confirmed DVT; nonfatal PE; or death from any cause) occurred in 9.0% of patients receiving apixaban and 8.9% of patients receiving enoxaparin (relative risk, 1.02; 95% CI, 0.78 to 1.32; $P = 0.06$ for noninferiority; absolute risk difference, 0.1%; 95% CI, –2.2 to 2.44; $P < 0.001$ for noninferiority) during the treatment period. The rates of PE were 1.0% in the apixaban group and 0.4% in the enoxaparin group; two PEs were fatal in the apixaban group, and none were fatal in the enoxaparin group. Major or clinically relevant nonmajor bleeding occurred in 2.9% and 4.3% of patients receiving apixaban and enoxaparin, respectively ($P = 0.03$). Major bleeding occurred in 0.7% and 1.4% of patients receiving apixaban and enoxaparin, respectively ($P = 0.05$). One patient in the enoxaparin group died from bleeding; no patients in the apixaban group died from bleeding.

In the ADVANCE-2 study, which compared apixaban 2.5 mg twice daily with enoxaparin 40 mg once daily in 3,057 patients treated with TKA, it was hypothesized that apixaban would be noninferior to enoxaparin based on a prespecified margin for the primary efficacy outcome in which the upper limit of the two-sided 95% CI is less than 1.25 for relative risk and less than 0.056 for the absolute risk difference.[7] The primary efficacy end point (the same as in ADVANCE-1 study) occurred in 15.1% of the apixaban group and 24.4% of the enoxaparin group (relative risk 0.62; 95% CI, 0.51 to 0.74; $P < 0.001$; absolute risk difference, –9.3%; 95% CI, –12.7 to –5.8; $P < 0.001$). Major VTE, the composite of proximal DVT, PE, and VTE death, was also significantly less in the apixaban group (1.1%) versus the enoxaparin group (2.2%) (relative risk, 0.50; 95% CI, 0.26 to 0.97; $P = 0.019$). The rates of PE were 0.26% in the apixaban group and 0.0% in the enoxaparin group; one PE was fatal in the apixaban group, and none was fatal in the enoxaparin group. Major or clinically relevant, nonmajor bleeding occurred in 3.5% and 4.8% of patients receiving apixaban and enoxaparin, respectively ($P = 0.09$). Major bleeding occurred in 0.6% and 0.9% of patients receiving apixaban and enoxaparin, respectively ($P = 0.3$).

In the ADVANCE-3 THA study, 5,407 patients were randomized to receive either apixaban 2.5 mg twice daily or enoxaparin 40 mg for 35 days.[25] The same primary and secondary efficacy outcomes were used as in the previous two studies. Total VTE occurred in 1.4% of the apixaban patients compared with 3.9% of the enoxaparin patients (relative risk 0.36; 95% CI, 0.22 to 0.54; $P < 0.0001$; absolute risk difference, 2.5; 95% CI, 1.5 to 3.5; $P < 0.0001$). The secondary efficacy endpoint, major VTE, occurred in 0.5% of the apixaban patients and 1.1% in the enoxaparin patients (relative risk, 0.40; 95% CI, 0.15 to 0.80; $P < 0.0001$; absolute risk difference, 0.7; 95% CI, 0.2 to 1.3; $P < 0.0001$). Major or clinically relevant, nonmajor bleeding occurred in 4.8% and 5.0% of patients receiving apixaban and enoxaparin, respectively ($P = 0.72$). Major bleeding occurred in 0.8% and 0.7% of patients receiving apixaban and enoxaparin, respectively ($P = 0.54$). After THA, one major VTE is prevented for each of the 146 patients treated with apixaban compared with enoxaparin, without an increased risk of bleeding. Symptomatic rates were extremely low for both groups, 0.15% for apixaban versus 0.37% for enoxaparin.

In all three studies, there were no differences in the occurrence of liver function enzyme elevations, thrombocytopenia, or cardiac events (stroke or myocardial infarction). The findings of these studies suggest that apixaban 2.5 mg daily is superior to the 40-mg once-daily enoxaparin regimen at reducing the composite of DVT, PE, and death by any cause and similar to the 30-mg twice-daily dosing, with a trend toward decreased bleeding.

Rivaroxaban

Rivaroxaban is an oral, direct factor Xa inhibitor, which is rapidly absorbed and has a mean terminal half-life of 7 to 11 hours.[12] It exhibits a predictable pharmacokinetic and pharmacodynamic profile and does not require dose adjustment for age, sex, or weight.[26,27] Rivaroxaban and its metabolites have a dual route of elimination: one third of the administered drug is cleared as unchanged active drug by the kidneys, one third is metabolized to inactive metabolites and then excreted by the kidneys, and one third is metabolized to inactive metabolites and then excreted by the fecal route.[28]

Rivaroxaban has a low propensity for drug-drug interaction with frequently used concomitant medications such as naproxen, aspirin, or clopidogrel, and no interaction with the cardiac glycoside digoxin.[29-32] Dietary restrictions are not necessary, and rivaroxaban was given with or without food in the phase III VTE prevention studies (RECORD studies 1 to 4). Phase II studies showed that all investigated rivaroxaban dose regimens had similar efficacy to enoxaparin, and the incidence of major bleeding was not significantly different compared with enoxaparin across a fourfold dose range (5 to 20 mg total daily rivaroxaban dose).[33-36]

The RECORD program consisted of four phase III studies investigating the efficacy and safety of rivaroxaban in 12,500 patients treated with THA and TKA.[37-40] All patients received rivaroxaban 10 mg once daily 6 to 8 hours after surgery, and there was no upper age or weight limit for participation. The primary efficacy end point was the composite of DVT (as detected by mandatory bilateral venography) nonfatal PE, and all-cause mortality up to days 30 to 42 after surgery for RECORD1 and RECORD2, up to days 13 to 17 for RECORD3, and up to day 17 for RECORD4. The secondary efficacy end points were the incidence of major VTE (composite of proximal DVT, nonfatal PE, or death from VTE). Any DVT, symptomatic VTE during treatment and follow-up, and death during follow-up were also evaluated.

The main safety end point was the incidence of treatment-emergent (observed no later than 2 days after the last dose of the study drug) major bleeding events, which were defined as fatal events, bleeding into a critical organ (for example, retroperitoneal, intracranial, intraocular, and intraspinal bleeding) requiring reoperation, clinically overt extra surgical-site bleeding associated with a fall in hemoglobin of at least 2 g/dL, or needing transfusion of two or more units of whole blood or packed cells. Clinically relevant, nonmajor bleeding events (defined as multiple-source bleeding, excessive wound hematomas, nose bleeding for more than 5 minutes, gingival bleeding for more than 5 minutes, macroscopic hematuria, rectal bleeding, coughing of blood, hematemesis, vaginal bleeding, intra-articular bleeding with trauma, surgical-site bleeding, unexpected hematoma or blood in semen), hemorrhagic wound complications, and postoperative wound infection were among the other outcomes reported.[37-40]

RECORD1 showed that 5 weeks of extended-duration rivaroxaban (10 mg once daily for 31 to 39 days after surgery) was significantly more effective than enoxaparin (40 mg once daily for 31 to 39 days) for extended-duration prophylaxis in patients treated with THA (1.1% versus 3.7% for the primary efficacy end point, $P < 0.001$).[37] Major bleeding events did not differ significantly between the groups (0.3% for the rivaroxaban group versus 0.1% for the enoxaparin group, $P = 0.18$). Clinically relevant nonmajor bleeding occurred in 2.9% of the rivaroxaban group versus 2.4% of the enoxaparin group; hemorrhagic wound complications in 1.5% versus 1.7% of patients; and postoperative wound infections in 0.4% of patients in both groups. The incidence of symptomatic VTE during treatment was not significantly different between the groups (0.3% for the rivaroxaban group versus 0.5% for the enoxaparin group, $P = 0.22$).

RECORD2 showed that extended-duration rivaroxaban prophylaxis (10 mg once daily for 31 to 39 days after surgery) was significantly more effective than short-duration prophylaxis with enoxaparin (40 mg once daily for 10 to 14 days) followed by placebo in patients treated with THA (2.0% for the rivaroxaban group versus 9.3% for the enoxaparin group for the primary efficacy end point, $P < 0.0001$).[38] The incidence of bleeding was comparable between extended-regimen rivaroxaban and short-duration enoxaparin. Major bleeding events occurred in fewer than 0.1% of patients in both groups. Clinically relevant nonmajor bleeding was recorded in 3.3% of the rivaroxaban group versus 2.7% of the enoxaparin group; hemorrhagic wound complications in 1.6% versus 1.7% of patients; and postoperative wound infections in 0.7% versus 0.5% of patients, respectively. Significantly fewer patients in the rivaroxaban group had symptomatic VTE (0.2%) than in the enoxaparin group (1.2%, $P = 0.004$) during the active study period.

In RECORD3, rivaroxaban prophylaxis (10 mg once daily for 10 to 14 days) was significantly more effective than the European enoxaparin regimen for prophylaxis (40 mg once daily) in patients treated with TKA (9.6% versus 18.9% for the primary efficacy end point, $P < 0.001$), with a similar safety profile.[39] Rates of major bleeding were similar in the rivaroxaban and enoxaparin groups (0.6% versus 0.5%, $P = 0.77$). Clinically relevant, nonmajor bleeding occurred in 2.7% of rivaroxaban versus 2.3% of enoxaparin patients, hemorrhagic wound complications in 2.0% versus 1.9%, and postoperative wound infections in 0.6% versus 0.9%, respectively. There was a significant reduction in the number of symptomatic VTE events in the rivaroxaban group (0.7% versus 2.0%, $P = 0.005$).

In RECORD4, rivaroxaban showed significantly better efficacy than the enoxaparin regimen (30 mg every 12 hours) commonly used in North America for short-term prophylaxis after TKA (6.9% versus 10.1%, respectively for the primary efficacy end point, $P = 0.0118$).[40] The rates of major bleeding were 0.7% versus 0.3% ($P = 0.1096$) respectively, and major and clinically relevant nonmajor bleeding 3.0% versus 2.3% ($P = 0.179$), respectively. The observed incidences of symptomatic VTE in those receiving rivaroxaban or enoxaparin were 0.7% versus 1.2% ($P = 0.187$), respectively.

In the four studies comparing rivaroxaban with enoxaparin, rivaroxaban demonstrated superior efficacy compared with enoxaparin. In addition, extended thromboprophylaxis with rivaroxaban was significantly more effective than short-term enoxaparin plus placebo in the prevention of total, major, and symptomatic VTE after THA. The incidence of treatment-emergent major and clinically relevant nonmajor bleeding was low for rivaroxaban and enoxaparin ($P = 0.21$ for RECORD1, P value not reported for RECORD2, $P = 0.44$ for RECORD3, and $P = 0.18$ for RECORD4). There was no evidence of compromised liver function or rebound cardiovascular events associated with rivaroxaban.

In a pooled analysis of the RECORD1, 2, and 3 studies (which compared rivaroxaban with enoxaparin 40 mg once daily after THA and TKA), the prespecified primary efficacy outcome (the composite of symptomatic VTE [DVT or PE] and all-cause mortality at 2 weeks) was 0.4% and 0.8%, respectively ($P = 0.005$).[41] The rates were 0.5% and 1.3%, respectively, at the end of the planned medication period ($P < 0.001$). Rates of on-treatment major bleeding were 0.2% for both drugs at 2 weeks ($P = 0.662$), and 0.3% for rivaroxaban and 0.2% for enoxaparin at the end of the planned medication period ($P = 0.305$). Rates of clinically relevant, nonmajor bleeding were 2.6% for rivaroxaban and 2.3% for enoxaparin at 2 weeks, and 3.0% and 2.5%, respectively, at the end of the planned medication period.

In a pooled analysis of the four RECORD studies, the primary efficacy end point (the composite of symptomatic VTE [DVT or PE] and death) was significantly reduced for the rivaroxaban regimens compared with enoxaparin regimens at day 12 ± 2 (0.5% versus 1.0%, $P = 0.001$) and in the planned treatment period (0.6% versus 1.3%, $P < 0.001$).[9] Rates of treatment-emergent major bleeding were not significantly different between the groups at any of the time points analyzed. The composite of major and clinically relevant, nonmajor bleeding for the rivaroxaban and enoxaparin regimens were 2.9% versus 2.5% ($P = 0.186$) at day 12 ± 2 and 3.2% versus 2.6% ($P = 0.039$), respectively, in the planned treatment period. Rates of the composite of PE and death were lower for rivaroxaban compared with enoxaparin in the planned treatment period and at follow-up (0.5% versus 0.8%, $P = 0.039$).[42]

Summary

It is difficult to achieve a good balance between efficacy and safety when administering prophylaxis for orthopaedic surgical procedures. With insufficient anticoagulation prophylaxis, the patient is at increased risk of VTE, whereas too much anticoagulation prophylaxis places the patient at increased risk for a bleeding event. Although guidelines (such as the ACCP and AAOS) for thromboprophylaxis are available, a substantial proportion of orthopaedic patients still do not receive adequate prophylaxis.[43] The discovery of new oral anticoagulants with promising benefit-risk profiles for VTE prevention after THA and TKA could be an important advance for orthopaedic surgeons and patients. Research has focused on oral direct factor Xa inhibitors and direct thrombin inhibitors, which have several advantages over conventional agents. Phase III studies have shown that some of these new agents can improve the benefit-risk ratio. With the convenience of oral dosing and the potential for simplified postoperative management of patients, it is possible that these new agents will replace the more conventional anticoagulants currently in clinical practice.

References

1. Kurtz S, Ong K, Lau E, Mowat F, Halpern M: Projections of primary and revision hip and knee arthroplasty in the United States from 2005 to 2030. *J Bone Joint Surg Am* 2007;89(4):780-785.
2. Geerts WH, Bergqvist D, Pineo GF, et al: Prevention of venous thromboembolism: American College of Chest Physicians Evidence-Based Clinical Practice Guidelines (8th edition). *Chest* 2008;133(6, Suppl):381S-453S.
3. Warwick D, Friedman RJ, Agnelli G, et al: Insufficient duration of venous thromboembolism prophylaxis after total hip or knee replacement when compared with the time course of thromboembolic events: Findings from the Global Orthopaedic Registry. *J Bone Joint Surg Br* 2007;89 (6):799-807.
4. Weitz JI, Hirsh J, Samama MM; American College of Chest Physicians: New antithrombotic drugs: American College of Chest Physicians Evidence-Based Clinical Practice Guidelines (8th Edition). *Chest* 2008;133(6, Suppl):234S-256S.
5. Hirsh J, Bauer KA, Donati MB, et al: Parenteral anticoagulants: American College of Chest Physicians Evidence-Based Clinical Practice Guidelines (8th edition). *Chest* 2008;133(6, Suppl):141S-159S.
6. Ansell J, Hirsh J, Hylek E, et al: Pharmacology and management of the vitamin K antagonists: American College of Chest Physicians Evidence-Based Clinical Practice Guidelines (8th edition). *Chest* 2008;133(6, Suppl):S160-S198.
7. Lassen MR, Raskob GE, Gallus AS, et al: Apixaban versus enoxaparin for thromboprophylaxis after knee replacement (ADVANCE-2): A randomised double-blind trial. *Lancet* 2010; 375(9717):807-815.
8. Lassen MR, Raskob GE, Gallus A, Pineo G, Chen D, Portman RJ: Apixaban or enoxaparin for thromboprophylaxis after knee replacement. *N Engl J Med* 2009; 361(6):594-604.
9. Turpie AGG, Lassen MR, Kakkar AK et al: A pooled analysis of four pivotal studies of rivaroxaban for the prevention of venous thromboembolism after orthopaedic surgery: Effect on symptomatic venous thromboembolism and death, and bleeding. *Haematologica* 2009;94(Suppl 2):439.
10. Wolowacz SE, Roskell NS, Plumb JM, Caprini JA, Eriksson BI: Efficacy and safety of dabigatran etexilate for the prevention of venous thromboembolism following total hip or knee arthroplasty: A meta-analysis. *Thromb Haemost* 2009;101(1):77-85.
11. Summary of Product Characteristics. Pradaxa Website. http://www.pradaxa.com/Include/media/pdf/Pradaxa_SPC_EMEA.pdf. Accessed May 10, 2010.
12. Summary of Product Characteristics. Xarelto Website. http://www.xarelto.com/html/

downloads/Xarelto_Summary_of_Product_ Characteristics_May2009.pdf. Accessed May 10, 2010.

13. Blech S, Ebner T, Ludwig-Schwellinger E, Stangier J, Roth W: The metabolism and disposition of the oral direct thrombin inhibitor, dabigatran, in humans. *Drug Metab Dispos* 2008;36(2):386-399.
14. Stangier J, Stähle H, Rathgen K, Fuhr R: Pharmacokinetics and pharmacodynamics of the direct oral thrombin inhibitor dabigatran in healthy elderly subjects. *Clin Pharmacokinet* 2008;47(1):47-59.
15. Stangier J, Eriksson BI, Dahl OE, et al: Pharmacokinetic profile of the oral direct thrombin inhibitor dabigatran etexilate in healthy volunteers and patients undergoing total hip replacement. *J Clin Pharmacol* 2005;45(5):555-563.
16. Eriksson BI, Quinlan DJ, Weitz JI: Comparative pharmacodynamics and pharmacokinetics of oral direct thrombin and factor Xa inhibitors in development. *Clin Pharmacokinet* 2009;48(1):1-22.
17. Stangier J: Clinical pharmacokinetics and pharmacodynamics of the oral direct thrombin inhibitor dabigatran etexilate. *Clin Pharmacokinet* 2008;47(5):285-295.
18. Eriksson BI, Dahl OE, Rosencher N, et al: Dabigatran etexilate versus enoxaparin for prevention of venous thromboembolism after total hip replacement: A randomised, double-blind, non-inferiority trial. *Lancet* 2007;370(9591):949-956.
19. Eriksson BI, Dahl OE, Rosencher N, et al: Oral dabigatran etexilate vs. subcutaneous enoxaparin for the prevention of venous thromboembolism after total knee replacement: The RE-MODEL randomized trial. *J Thromb Haemost* 2007;5(11):2178-2185.
20. RE-MOBILIZE Writing Committee; Ginsberg JS, Davidson BL, et al: Oral thrombin inhibitor dabigatran etexilate vs the North American enoxaparin regimen for the prevention of venous thromboembolism after knee arthroplasty surgery. *J Arthroplasty* 2009;24(1):1-9.
21. Eriksson B, Dahl OE, Kurth AA, et al: Oral dabigatran versus enoxaparin for thromboprophylaxis after primary total hip arthroplasty: The RE-NOVATE II randomised trial (Abstract OC645). *Pathophysiol Haemost Thromb* 2010;37(Suppl 1):A20.
22. Leadley RJ Jr: Coagulation factor Xa inhibition: Biological background and rationale. *Curr Top Med Chem* 2001;1(2):151-159.
23. Mann KG, Butenas S, Brummel K: The dynamics of thrombin formation. *Arterioscler Thromb Vasc Biol* 2003;23(1):17-25.
24. Lassen MR, Davidson BL, Gallus A, Pineo G, Ansell J, Deitchman D: The efficacy and safety of apixaban, an oral, direct factor Xa inhibitor, as thromboprophylaxis in patients following total knee replacement. *J Thromb Haemost* 2007;5(12):2368-2375.
25. Lassen MR, Gallus A, Raskob GE, Pineo G, Chen D, Ramirez LM: ADVANCE-3 Investigators: Randomized double blind comparison of apixaban and enoxaparin for thromboprophylaxis after hip replacement. The ADVANCE-3 trial (Abstract #OC356). *Pathophysiol Haemost Thromb* 2010;37(Suppl 1):A20.
26. Kubitza D, Becka M, Mueck W, Zuehlsdorf M: The effect of extreme age, and gender, on the pharmacology and tolerability of rivaroxaban, an oral, direct factor Xa inhibitor. *Blood* 2006;108(11):905.
27. Kubitza D, Becka M, Zuehlsdorf M, Mueck W: Body weight has limited influence on the safety, tolerability, pharmacokinetics, or pharmacodynamics of rivaroxaban (BAY 59-7939) in healthy subjects. *J Clin Pharmacol* 2007;47(2):218-226.
28. Weinz C, Schwarz T, Kubitza D, Mueck W, Lang D: Metabolism and excretion of rivaroxaban, an oral, direct factor Xa inhibitor, in rats, dogs, and humans. *Drug Metab Dispos* 2009;37(5):1056-1064.
29. Kubitza D, Becka M, Mueck W, Zuehlsdorf M: Rivaroxaban (BAY 59-7939), an oral direct factor Xa inhibitor, has no clinically relevant interaction with naproxen. *Br J Clin Pharmacol* 2007;63(4):469-476.
30. Kubitza D, Becka M, Mueck W, Zuehlsdorf M: Safety, tolerability, pharmacodynamics, and pharmacokinetics of rivaroxaban, an oral direct factor Xa inhibitor, are not affected by aspirin. *J Clin Pharmacol* 2006;46(9):981-990.
31. Kubitza D, Becka M, Mueck W, Zuehlsdorf M: Co-administration of rivaroxaban, a novel, oral, direct factor Xa inhibitor, and clopidogrel in healthy subjects. *Eur Heart J* 2007;28:1272.
32. Kubitza D, Becka M, Zuehlsdorf M: No interaction between the novel, oral direct factor Xa inhibitor BAY 59-7939 and digoxin. *J Clin Pharmacol* 2006;46:702.
33. Eriksson BI, Borris LC, Dahl OE, et al: Dose-escalation study of rivaroxaban (BAY 59-7939), an oral, direct Factor Xa inhibitor, for the prevention of venous thromboembolism in patients undergoing total hip replacement. *Thromb Res* 2007;120(5):685-693.
34. Eriksson BI, Borris LC, Dahl OE, et al: Oral, direct factor Xa inhibition with BAY 59-7939 for the prevention of venous thromboembolism after total hip replacement. *J Thromb Haemost* 2006;4(1):121-128.

35. Eriksson BI, Borris LC, Dahl OE, et al: A once-daily, oral, direct factor Xa inhibitor, rivaroxaban (BAY 59-7939), for thromboprophylaxis after total hip replacement. *Circulation* 2006;114(22): 2374-2381.

36. Turpie AG, Fisher WD, Bauer KA, et al: BAY 59-7939: An oral, direct factor Xa inhibitor for the prevention of venous thromboembolism in patients after total knee replacement. A phase II dose-ranging study. *J Thromb Haemost* 2005;3(11): 2479-2486.

37. Eriksson BI, Borris LC, Friedman RJ, et al: Rivaroxaban versus enoxaparin for thromboprophylaxis after hip arthroplasty. *N Engl J Med* 2008;358(26):2765-2775.

38. Kakkar AK, Brenner B, Dahl OE, et al: Extended duration rivaroxaban versus short-term enoxaparin for the prevention of venous thromboembolism after total hip arthroplasty: A double-blind, randomised controlled trial. *Lancet* 2008;372(9632):31-39.

39. Lassen MR, Ageno W, Borris LC, et al: Rivaroxaban versus enoxaparin for thromboprophylaxis after total knee arthroplasty. *N Engl J Med* 2008;358(26): 2776-2786.

40. Turpie AG, Lassen MR, Davidson BL, et al: Rivaroxaban versus enoxaparin for thromboprophylaxis after total knee arthroplasty (RECORD4): A randomised trial. *Lancet* 2009;373(9676):1673-1680.

41. Eriksson BI, Kakkar AK, Turpie AG, et al: Oral rivaroxaban for the prevention of symptomatic venous thromboembolism after elective hip and knee replacement. *J Bone Joint Surg Br* 2009;91(5): 636-644.

42. Friedman RJ, Turpie AG, Lassen MR, et al: A pooled analysis of four pivotal studies of rivaroxaban for the prevention of venous thromboembolism after hip or knee arthroplasty. *122nd Annual Meeting of the American Orthopaedic Association Proceedings*. Rosemont, IL, American Orthopaedic Association, 2009, p 62.

43. Friedman RJ, Gallus AS, Cushner FD, Fitzgerald G, Anderson FA Jr; Global Orthopaedic Registry Investigators: Physician compliance with guidelines for deep-vein thrombosis prevention in total hip and knee arthroplasty. *Curr Med Res Opin* 2008;24(1): 87-97.

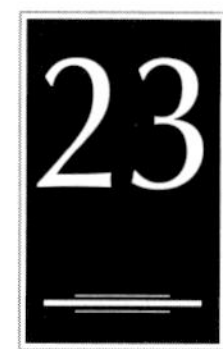

Periprosthetic Fractures of the Hip and Knee: A Problem on the Rise But Better Solutions

Craig J. Della Valle, MD
George J. Haidukewych, MD
John J. Callaghan, MD

Abstract

The absolute number of periprosthetic fractures seen by the orthopaedic surgeon is increasing. The basic principles of fracture management include preoperative patient optimization and determining the stability of the associated components. Loose components require revision, whereas fractures associated with well-fixed implants are generally treated with internal fixation. Although these fractures are challenging to manage, advances in surgical techniques, including the use of locking plates for internal fixation and improved revision systems and biomaterials (such as highly porous metals), offer the surgeon enhanced tools for treating these complex clinical disorders.

The number of periprosthetic fractures associated with total hip arthroplasties (THAs) and total knee arthroplasties (TKAs) are increasing in number secondary to the increase in the total number of these procedures being performed annually; the concomitant increase in the number of implants in service, which may be affected by prosthetic loosening or osteolysis; the increase in the number of revision surgeries; and an aging population, which is at a higher risk for osteoporosis. Data from the Swedish hip registry suggest that since the year 2000, periprosthetic fractures of the femur are the third most common reason (following only aseptic loosening and recurrent instability) for revision surgery after THA. Periprosthetic fractures account for 6% of revision surgeries.[1] These fractures are the second leading cause of implant failure requiring revision surgery in patients 4 years or more after THA. It is estimated that the cumulative risk of a periprosthetic fracture occurring following THA within the first 10 years is 0.64% and up to 2.3% for patients in certain high risk categories, such as elderly patients, those with inflammatory arthritis or osteoporosis, and patients previously treated with prosthetic replacement for a hip fracture.[2,3]

The treatment of periprosthetic fractures following both THA and TKA is challenging and associated with a high rate of orthopaedic and systemic complications. Lindahl and associates[4] reported that 10-year implant survivorship without the need for surgery of the ipsilateral hip was 69.9%. The early failure rate (nearly 50% of all resurgeries occurred within 1 year) was particularly high,

Dr. Della Valle or an immediate family member is a member of a speakers' bureau or has made paid presentations on behalf of Angiotech; serves as a paid consultant to or is an employee of Zimmer; serves as an unpaid consultant to Biomet and Kinamed; has received research or institutional support from Zimmer; and has received nonincome support (such as equipment or services), commercially derived honoraria, or other non–research-related funding (such as paid travel) from Smith & Nephew and Stryker. Dr. Haidukewych or an immediate family member serves as a board member, owner, officer, or committee member of the Florida Orthopaedic Institute; has received royalties from DePuy and Zimmer; is a member of a speakers' bureau or has made paid presentations on behalf of DePuy; serves as a paid consultant to or is an employee of DePuy; has received research or institutional support from DePuy; and has stock or stock options held in Surmodics. Dr. Callaghan or an immediate family member has received royalties from DePuy; serves as an unpaid consultant to DePuy; has received research or institutional support from Arthrex and Smith & Nephew; and has received nonincome support (such as equipment or services), commercially derived honoraria, or other non–research-related funding (such as paid travel) from Wolters Kluwer Health–Lippincott Williams & Wilkins.

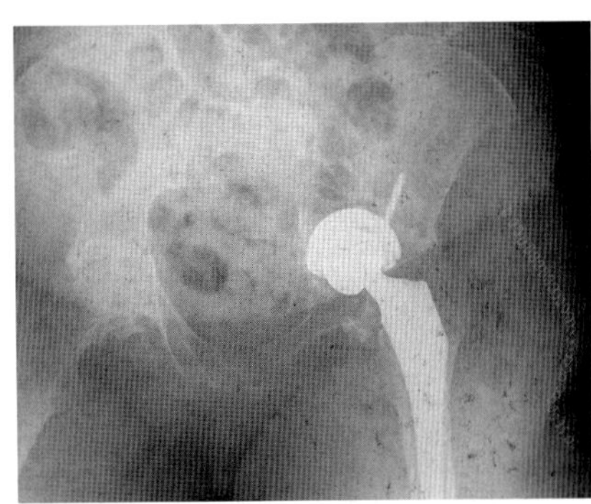

Figure 1 Radiograph showing an acute periprosthetic fracture of the pelvis following a primary THA with a fracture of the posterior column and a pelvic discontinuity treated with plating of the posterior column of the pelvis and staged revision of the acetabular component.

with most failures attributed to attempts at internal fixation as opposed to prosthetic revision in treating a loose femoral implant. Bhattacharyya and associates[5] reviewed the results of the treatment of 106 periprosthetic fractures of the femur associated with THA and found that 11% of the patients died within 1 year, which is similar to (albeit lower than) the mortality rate for patients with a fracture of the native proximal femur. Mortality increased among patients when surgery was delayed for more than 2 days. Patients treated with open reduction and internal fixation as opposed to femoral component revision also had a higher mortality rate (33% to 12%, respectively).

Risk Factors

The predominant risk factors for a periprosthetic fracture of the hip or knee are factors related to poor bone quality (female sex, older age, inflammatory arthritis) that increase the risks of fractures in general. Patients at high risk for falls, including those with poor vision and balance or neurologic disorders, have an increased risk for periprosthetic fractures. Most periprosthetic fractures are associated with low-energy trauma. Other factors that increase the risks include loose implants with associated bone loss and large osteolytic lesions. These risk factors highlight the need for radiographic surveillance of all patients treated with THA or TKA, even those who are asymptomatic.

Specific risk factors associated with a periprosthetic fracture of the femur following THA include a preoperative diagnosis of a proximal femoral fracture, certain implant types (those associated with high rates of osteolysis), and revision surgery compared with primary THA.[2] Intraoperative and early postoperative fractures are increasing in number secondary to the increased use of cementless rather than cemented implants in both primary and revision surgery.[6]

Periprosthetic Fractures of the Acetabulum

Acute Fractures in Primary THA

Periprosthetic fractures of the acetabulum are relatively rare and seem to be iatrogenic in nature, with a prevalence of less than 1%.[7] These fractures are a relatively recent phenomenon and are associated with the now common practice of underreaming the acetabulum and inserting a press-fit cementless acetabular component, particularly in an attempt to avoid the use of screws for adjunctive fixation. In a cadaver study, underreaming of the acetabulum by 2 mm was associated with a periprosthetic fracture in 26% of specimens, whereas underreaming by 4 mm was associated with a fracture in 93% of specimens.[8] The authors also reported that substantial impaction forces of 2,000 N were required to fully seat the components, and fractures were difficult to detect using plain radiographs only.

Clinical studies also have identified poor bone quality as an important risk factor in periprosthetic fractures of the acetabulum; this risk factor is common in older women and in patients with rheumatoid arthritis.[9] A more recent report identified more periprosthetic fractures of the acetabulum in elliptic compared with hemispheric acetabular components, with a particularly high rate in monoblock (as opposed to modular) elliptic shells.[7] If identified intraoperatively, the stability of the component should be carefully assessed. If the component is unstable, it should be removed and replaced with a component that can be fixed with multiple screws. Stable components have been associated with a high rate of osteointegration without the need for additional intervention, although bone graft from the acetabular reaming was placed in the fracture site in all patients in one study.[7] Rarely, an unstable intraoperative fracture may involve the acetabular columns and require plating of the posterior and, in some instances, the anterior column (Figure 1).

Stress Fractures of the Pelvis

Stress fractures of the pubic rami also occur following THA and can be an uncommon cause of groin pain after an otherwise successful THA.[10] These fractures typically occur in women with poor bone quality who were treated with THA using a cementless acetabular component. It is hypothesized that the patient's increased ambulatory capacity after successful THA is the cause of these fractures; they have been shown to heal reliably with nonsurgical treatment. Although early plain radiographs may be normal following the onset of pain, the fracture can be diagnosed with a bone scan or with serial radiographs over time. Stress fractures also may be associated with extensive retroacetabular osteolysis. If the component is stable, treatment should include exchange of the modular bearing surface and grafting of the osteolytic lesion.[11]

Pelvic Discontinuity

Pelvic discontinuity typically occurs in association with a loose acetabular component and can be considered a "chronic periprosthetic fracture of the acetabulum" in which the superior and inferior portions of the pelvis are separated by an area of bone loss.[12] Pelvic discontinuity is most commonly associated with female sex and a diagnosis of inflammatory arthritis.[13] Radiographic characteristics of a pelvic discontinuity include a transverse fracture line, medial translation of the inferior hemipelvis (with a break in the ilioischial line), and asymmetry of the obturator foramen. Vertical migration of the loose component of more than 3 cm is common[14] (Figure 2).

Traditional treatment includes extensive bone grafting, plating of the posterior column, and using a reconstruction cage that spans from the ilium to the ischium.[13] A recent report describes the successful use, at short-term follow-up, of trabecular metal acetabular components with augments.[15] The use of custom-made, porous-coated, triflanged components also has been described as a successful technique for reconstruction.[16]

Springer and associates[17] recently described a variant of a pelvic discontinuity associated with well-fixed components following revision THA, in which a trabecular metal acetabular component was used. All seven of the patients in the study were female and presented with groin pain. Five of the seven patients had a displaced fracture that was treated surgically; four required plating and bone grafting of the posterior column, and one was treated with a reconstruction cage to stabilize the pelvis.

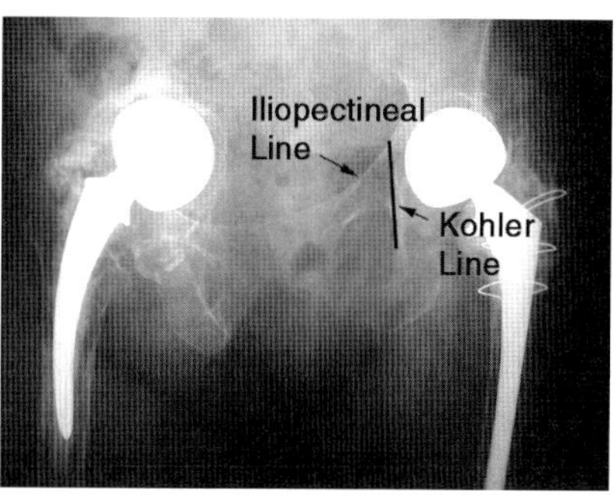

Figure 2 Pelvic discontinuity of the right hemipelvis. Note the break in the iliopectineal and ilioischial (Kohler) lines with significant superior and medial migration of the acetabulum, a transverse fracture line, and ischial lysis. Rotation of the inferior hemipelvis is seen as asymmetry of the obturator ring when compared with the contralateral side. Normal radiographic landmarks are shown on the left hemipelvis. (Reproduced from Della Valle CJ, Momberger NG, Paprosky WG: Periprosthetic fractures of the acetabulum associated with a total hip arthroplasty. *Instr Course Lect* 2003;52:281-290.)

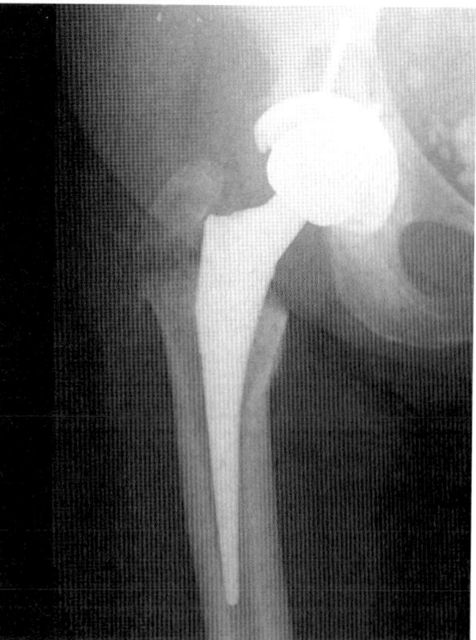

Figure 3 Radiograph showing a Vancouver type A periprosthetic fracture of the greater trochanter.

Periprosthetic Fractures of the Femur Associated With THA

Classification

The Vancouver classification system was developed for cemented prostheses and is clinically helpful in guiding treatment of periprosthetic femoral fractures. It is based on the location of the fracture, the fixation status of the femoral component, and the quality of the remaining bone stock. Vancouver type A fractures involve the greater or lesser trochanter and are almost always associated with osteolysis (Figure 3). Vancouver type B fractures occur around the stem and are the most common type of periprosthetic femoral fracture. Type B1 fractures occur around a well-fixed implant (Figure 4), type B2 fractures occur around a loose implant with good remaining bone stock (Figure 5), and type B3 fractures are associated with a loose implant and poor remaining proximal bone stock. Vancouver type C fractures occur well distal to the femoral component, and the component is almost always well fixed[18] (Figure 6).

Vancouver Type A Periprosthetic Fractures

The mainstay of managing Vancouver type A fractures is treating the associated osteolysis, typically with a modular polyethylene liner exchange. Osteolytic lesions can be grafted with cancellous allograft, and unstable greater trochanteric fractures should be stabilized; tension band techniques have been rec-

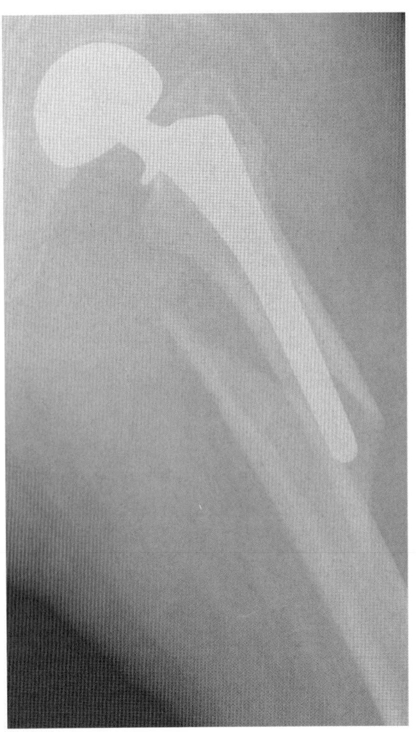

Figure 4 Radiograph showing a Vancouver type B1 fracture with a well-fixed femoral component.

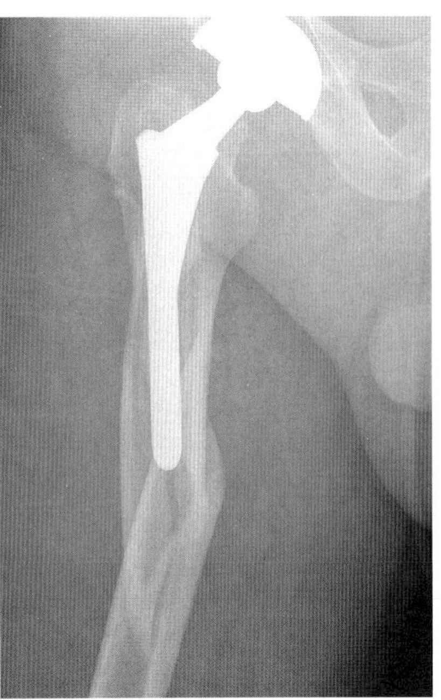

Figure 5 Radiograph showing a Vancouver type B2 periprosthetic fracture of the femur. A review of early postoperative radiographs showed clear subsidence of the femoral component, indicating loosening.

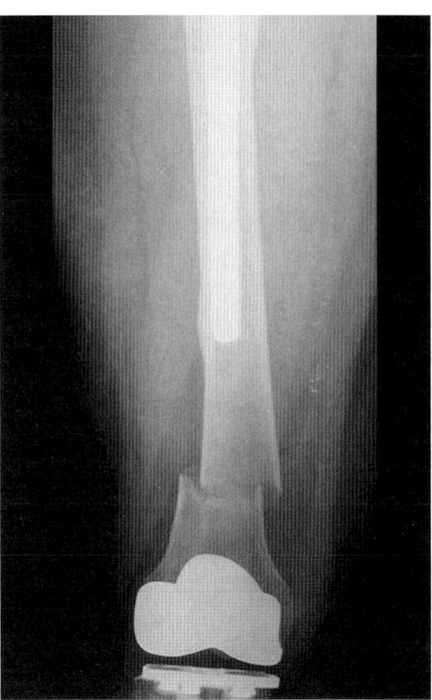

Figure 6 Radiograph showing a Vancouver type C periprosthetic fracture of the hip.

ommended using wire or heavy braided suture. It is important to understand that bone quality is typically poor because the trochanter has been "hollowed out" by the lytic process. If displaced and unstable, heavy suture fixation into the abductor tendon is recommended, which typically provides robust fixation. Internal fixation of the greater trochanter alone, without treating the wear problem with bearing exchange and bone grafting, will not resolve the underlying disorder and will likely lead to fixation failure. An abduction brace and protected weight bearing are recommended after trochanteric fixation.

Vancouver Type B1 Fractures

For type B1 fractures around a well-fixed implant, internal fixation with a plate with or without an allograft strut is recommended. It is critical to ensure that that stem is well fixed because treating a periprosthetic fracture of the femur with internal fixation when the femoral component is loose is a common cause of failure.

During internal fixation of type B1 fractures, obtaining stable proximal fixation is paramount. A lateral locked plate with a combination of unicortical locked screws and proximal cables generally provides adequate fixation. Proximal cable fixation alone is often inadequate because cables alone provide limited resistance to rotation. In general, three cables and three locked screws proximally and four bicortical screws distally (using a combination of locked and traditional screws) are used to achieve balanced internal fixation above and below the fracture (Figure 7). The authors of a cadaver study concluded that a combination of locked screws and cables is preferable.[19] The particular fracture geometry and length of the proximal segment will ultimately determine how many points of proximal fixation are possible. All proximal unicortical screws should be locked. It is important to preserve fracture biology and avoid medial dissection because most of the vascularity of the femur is medially based. The use of broad-based retractors and periosteal stripping is discouraged. It is important, however, to avoid fracture distraction when locked plating techniques are used. If possible, compression should be achieved to allow load sharing with the available bone; however, load sharing will vary with fracture geometry and the degree of comminution present. The use of hybrid plating techniques distally, using traditional nonlocked screws for compression and then locking the construct with bicortical locking screws, can facilitate obtaining a stable, compressed construct.

The use of supplementary allograft struts remains controversial. Struts were routinely used with good results before the advent of modern locked plating devices because some form of orthogonal bony support was necessary to minimize screw toggle and fixation failure. In the past, some authors have advocated "strut only" fixation constructs; however, in an era of modern locked plating devices, such constructs have generally fallen from favor. The need for strut augmentation is now typically based on bone quality. If a strut is used, it should be contoured with a high-speed burr to provide broad-based contact with the underlying host bone. Orthogonal placement of a locked plate (strut anterior on the femur) is generally preferred because medial dissection is avoided. Anterior placement can irritate the quadriceps and lead to knee stiffness, so careful attention is needed to prevent this potential postoperative complication, which can affect rehabilitation. The use of an allograft strut can be particularly problematic in thin patients of small stature in whom struts can add substantial bulk to the construct. Struts also add considerable expense and surgical time but carry a low risk of disease transmission. It is likely that as internal fixation implants and techniques evolve, the use of allograft struts for this indication will continue to decrease.

Vancouver Type B2 and B3 Fractures

Vancouver type B2 and B3 fractures are periprosthetic fractures of the femur associated with a loose implant. Treatment must include both revision of the femoral component and fracture fixation. A type B3 fracture is differentiated from type B2 by the presence of severe bone loss of the femur that further complicates treatment; however, a continuum of severity of femoral bone loss exists, and this differentiation is somewhat subjective.

For most type B2 fractures, the principal strategy for treatment includes the use of a cementless femoral component to achieve distal fixation beyond the fracture, effectively performing an intramedullary rodding of the femur. This treatment strategy is supported by the general success achieved with distally fixed, cementless femoral components, and reports suggest that the use of cemented femoral components for treating periprosthetic fractures is associated with a higher rate of failure.[20,21] Success with the use of impaction grafting has been reported.[22]

The first challenge in treating type B2 periprosthetic femoral fractures is removing the loose femoral component and the retained cement. Authors have described the successful use of an extended trochanteric osteotomy to facilitate cement removal, exposure, and implantation of the revision component.[23-25] The osteotomy is made distal to the tip of the fracture, the intact femoral diaphysis is prepared, the revision stem is implanted, and the proximal fragments are wrapped around the revision implant[23-25] (Figure 8). The amount of intact femoral diaphysis available for distal fixation and the diameter of the revision implant are important considerations in selecting an appropriate revision component. Cylindric, fully porous-coated stems have been shown to have higher rates of failure when less than 4 cm is available for distal fixation (in Paprosky type IIIB and type IV femoral defects). When the diameter of the implant is greater than 19 mm, a modular, titanium, fluted stem may be associated with a higher rate of success.[26,27]

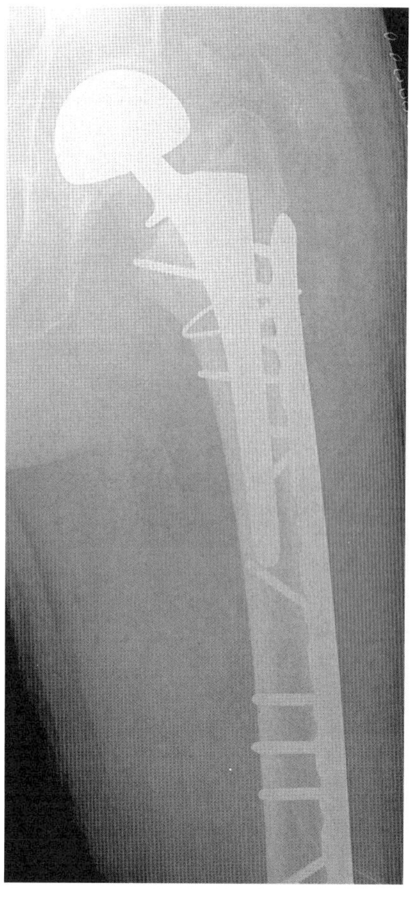

Figure 7 Postoperative radiograph of the fracture shown in Figure 4. Proximal fixation was achieved using a combination of unicortical and bicortical locking and unlocked screws as well as a cerclage cable.

Type B3 periprosthetic fractures of the femur have been successfully treated with the methods previously described for type B2 fractures, although other authors have advocated the use of proximal femoral replacement using an allograft-prosthetic composite or a tumor-type proximal femoral prosthesis.[28,29] If either of these treatment

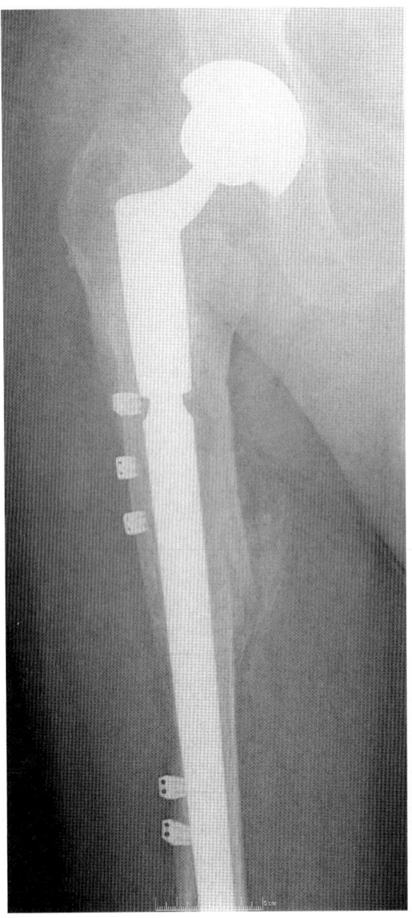

Figure 8 Postoperative radiograph of the fracture shown in Figure 5. An extended trochanteric osteotomy was used to remove the failed femoral component and facilitate implantation of the revision stem. The modular tapered revision femoral component was inserted first, achieving distal fixation, and the proximal fragments were wrapped around the revision femoral component.

options is considered, abductor deficiency can lead to instability, and a constrained acetabular liner should be considered.

Vancouver Type C Fractures

The principles of internal fixation of Vancouver type C injuries are similar to those of an osteopenic distal femoral fracture, with the added difficulty of proximally treating a potential stress riser from the existing

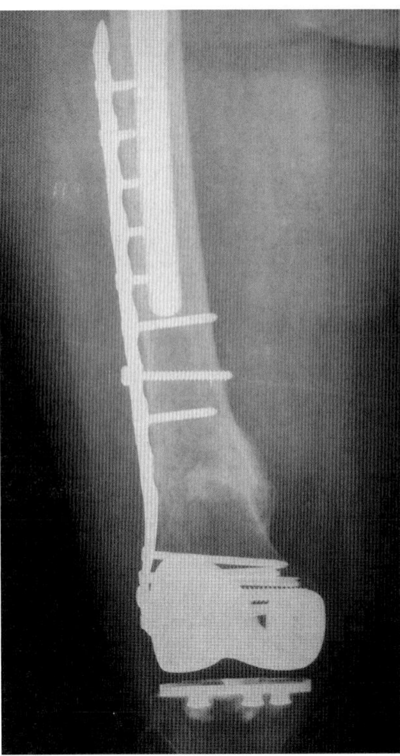

Figure 9 Postoperative radiograph of the fracture shown in Figure 6. A locked plate applied laterally was used to fix this Vancouver type C fracture.

femoral component. If a sufficient length of femoral diaphysis (at least 12 cm) is available between supracondylar fixation and the tip of the femoral stem, a short plate may be considered without bypassing the stem proximally. However, this situation is exceedingly rare and typically occurs only in tall patients with long femurs and very distal fractures. In most situations, it is preferable to bypass the femoral stem by two cortical diameters with the proximal part of the plate (Figure 9). Short retrograde nails are discouraged in this setting, and a long, locked plate that bypasses the tip of the ipsilateral femoral component is the treatment of choice.

The use of long, locked plates has been facilitated with modern jig-driven targeting of screws that avoids elevation of the vastus lateralis. This method theoretically preserves fracture vascularity and improves the rate of union. These concepts have generally been supported by the available trauma literature on distal femoral fractures.[30-33] With modern implants and biologically friendly implantation techniques, it is quite easy to insert a long plate that bypasses the femoral stem above without excessive soft-tissue dissection. An incision is made distally over the femoral condyles and another is made proximally below the greater trochanter. The plate is inserted submuscularly and extraperiosteally and is then stabilized with locked screw fixation proximally and distally, effectively bridging the fracture zone. Recent data have shown high union rates with such strategies without the need for the routine use of a femoral strut allograft.[34] After internal fixation, patients are mobilized postoperatively, and full weight bearing is typically delayed for at least 6 to 8 weeks until progressive radiographic healing is evident. Ambulatory aids are used for 12 weeks.

Periprosthetic Fractures of the Femur Associated With TKA

Important Considerations and Classification

The goals of treating periprosthetic femoral fractures after TKA include obtaining bony union; maintaining correct limb alignment, length, and rotation; and avoiding both local and systemic complications. Obstacles to achieving stable distal fixation include the often short, osteopenic distal bony fragments; fracture comminution; areas of osteolysis; and achieving fixation around the femoral component and associated stem, if present. Periprosthetic femoral fractures usually require an internal fixation device that provides coronal plane stability to avoid deformity (typically varus collapse) that can occur during the healing process. In general, nonsurgical treatment should be considered only for patients with nondisplaced or minimally displaced fractures that are associated with well-fixed implants, those at high risk of perioperative mortality, or patients who were nonambulatory before the fracture. The risks of both systemic (such as thromboembolic and other complications related to recumbency and immobilization) and local complications (such as a stiff knee joint and malunion of the fracture) must be carefully weighed against the risks of surgery. The Lewis and Rorabeck system is the most commonly used classification for periprosthetic fractures of the distal femur[35] (Table 1). As with other periprosthetic fractures, implants that are loose require revision for successful treatment.

Retrograde Nailing

Intramedullary nailing has been successfully used to manage complex periprosthetic distal femoral fractures. It limits soft-tissue disruption and provides excellent biomechanical stability.[36-41] Among the challenges to successful union with intramedullary techniques is that locking screws (even modern nail-locking screw clusters) provide marginal distal fixation of the typically comminuted, osteopenic distal bony fragments. Intramedullary nailing is not practical for use with implants that substitute for the posterior cruciate ligament because the femoral housing precludes access to the intramedullary canal. Intramedullary techniques are typically reserved for treating fractures located above cruciate-retaining femoral components with sufficient distal bone to allow purchase with a minimum of two distal locking screws. Recent biomechanical evidence suggests that in the presence of medial comminution, retrograde intramedullary nails may be mechanically more stable than laterally placed locking plates; however, this stability is based on achieving good distal fixation.[42] Occasionally, antegrade femoral nailing can be used for periprosthetic distal femur fractures if a sufficiently long distal fragment is present. The main challenges with antegrade techniques are obtaining appropriate alignment and stable distal fixation. With antegrade nailing techniques, an area of high stress concentration is created between the distal end of the nail and the femoral component. If a nailing strategy is chosen, a long retrograde nail may represent a more attractive option secondary to the benefits of distal locking bolts further from the fracture site.

Traditional Plate Fixation

In the past, devices such as the 95° blade plate and dynamic condylar screw have been used with mixed results.[36,38,39,43-47] Because of the extremely distal nature of these fractures, the blade of the blade plate or the lag screw of the dynamic condylar screw often must be inserted more proximally to avoid portions of the femoral component; thus, distal fixation is often suboptimal. Traditional condylar buttress plates offer more freedom of angulation of distal screws but no coronal plane stability. Unacceptable rates of varus collapse have been reported when this device is used for unstable fractures.[47,48] These implants have been largely abandoned in favor of static or polyaxial locked plates.

Table 1
Lewis and Rorabeck Classification of Periprosthetic Fractures of the Distal Femur

Type I	Prosthesis stable, fracture nondisplaced
Type II	Prosthesis stable, fracture displaced (most common)
Type III	Prosthesis loose

Locking Plate Fixation

Locking plate technology has been used for managing complex periarticular fractures about the knee for more than a decade.[30-33,49-55] Threads on the screw heads are threaded into corresponding threads in the plate holes, forming a fixed-angle construct and providing coronal plane stability.[56] These devices have been used with excellent results for managing complex periarticular injuries and provide reliable distal fixation. Such devices allow multiple locked screws to be placed around and between portions of the femoral component, improving distal fixation[51,57] (Figure 9). In a study of 38 periprosthetic fractures treated with the Less Invasive Stabilization System (LISS; Synthes, Paoli, PA), Kregor and associates[53] reported two failures (5%); one patient required revision knee arthroplasty and one required bone grafting to achieve a solid union. Ultimately, 37 of 38 fractures (97%) healed. Medical and orthopaedic complications were infrequent. To ensure predictable healing with this technique, the metaphyseal comminution should remain undisturbed to preserve the vascularity of the fragments.

In addition to providing excellent mechanical stability, several locked plating designs offer the theoretic biologic advantage of percutaneous insertion, which minimizes the need for additional large incisions

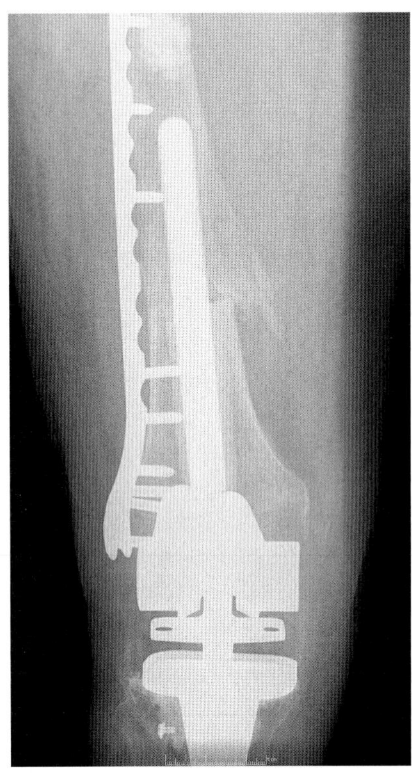

Figure 10 Radiograph showing nonunion of an allograft-prosthetic composite.

around the knee and potentially minimizes the soft-tissue complications and stiffness associated with traditional exposures used for open reduction and internal fixation.[30,51] When percutaneous techniques are used, vigilance is required to avoid malalignment, typically valgus positioning and hyperextension of the distal fragment.[51] Many commercially available locked plating designs offer the surgeon the option of either open or percutaneous insertion. When possible, percutaneous internal fixation takes advantage of the mechanical stability of a locking plate and the theoretic biologic advantages of percutaneous insertion.[58]

Prosthetic Revision

A periprosthetic fracture of the distal femur associated with a loose femoral component (type III) requires revision of the components and concomitant treatment of the fracture. Management of these injuries is particularly difficult because the remaining bone stock of the femur can be of particularly poor quality. Prosthetic revision can be performed with standard revision components that include a stem, the use of a distal femoral replacing hinged prosthesis, or an allograft-prosthetic composite.

If prosthetic revision with stemmed components is the selected treatment, the stem used should bypass the fracture by at least two cortical diameters.[35] Although a long, fully cemented stem can be considered, it may be difficult to prevent cement from entering the fracture site; this intrusion could lead to fracture nonunion. If a cementless stem is chosen, it must be of adequate length and diameter to provide both axial and rotational stability at the fracture site; augmentation with a plate or strut allograft can be considered if stability is not achieved intraoperatively.

Replacing the distal femur with a hinged, tumor-type prosthesis allows immediate weight bearing. Fracture healing is not required for successful treatment because the distal femur is removed. Although this strategy has been described as a successful treatment option, there is a substantial risk of complications, and it is probably best reserved for low-demand patients. This treatment option also has been described for patients with type II fractures (associated with a well-fixed prosthesis) when difficulties with distal fixation secondary to a small or osteopenic distal fragment are encountered.

The principles of using an allograft-prosthetic composite include cementing the allograft to the prosthesis and achieving union at the graft-host junction with a plate or strut allograft and typically a cementless stem that is placed into the retained more proximal aspect of the distal femur (Figure 10). Reattachment of the collateral ligaments to the allograft can be attempted; however, instability is a recognized complication of this approach, and the use of a constrained condylar insert or a resurfacing hinge-type implant should be strongly considered.

Periprosthetic Fractures of the Tibia

Periprosthetic fractures of the tibia are a relatively infrequent occurrence and are typically associated with loose components and/or extensive osteolysis. Because the components are either loose or the bone stock of the proximal tibia is compromised secondary to osteolysis, component revision is required. The primary goal of treatment is to bypass the fracture with a stemmed revision component if the component is loose. Because loss of proximal tibial bone stock is prevalent in this injury pattern, restoration of bone stock with impaction grafting has been described as a successful revision technique.[59] Although a fully cemented tibial stem can be used, interdigitation of cement at the fracture site may occur and inhibit bony healing. Consequently, a cementless, canal-filling stem is preferred, with cementation only in the metaphyseal region of the stem. Periprosthetic fractures of the tibia may be associated with well-fixed components in high-energy traumatic injuries or in elderly patients. In these scenarios, locked or standard plating techniques from the lateral side can be used (Figure 11).

Periprosthetic Fractures of the Patella

Periprosthetic fractures of the patella are relatively uncommon and occur in association with approximately 1% of TKAs.[60] Most of these fractures seem to occur without an identifiable traumatic event, and many are noted incidentally on routine follow-up radiographs without associated symptoms.[60] Surgical treatment of periprosthetic fractures of the patella have a high rate of complications (approximately 50% in most studies); therefore, surgical treatment is discouraged unless the extensor mechanism is disrupted or the patellar component is loose.[60-62] The most commonly reported complications include nonunion, recurrent extensor lag, painful hardware, and infection. The high rate of complications associated with surgical treatment is probably related to several factors, including damage to the blood supply of the patellar remnant secondary to a prior medially based arthrotomy (in some cases, a lateral retinacular release) and the potential difficulty of achieving rigid fixation in the thin patellar remnant. It also is difficult to balance the immobilization required for fracture healing against the stiffness that may result from extended periods of immobilization.

Risk Factors and Prevention

The primary patient-related factors associated with periprosthetic fractures of the patella include male sex, obesity, high activity levels, inflammatory arthritis, revision as opposed to primary procedures, and high range of motion. Several prosthetic design features, including the use of a metal-backed patella, cementless patellar components, and one large central peg as opposed to designs with three smaller pegs, have been associated with a higher prevalence of this complication.

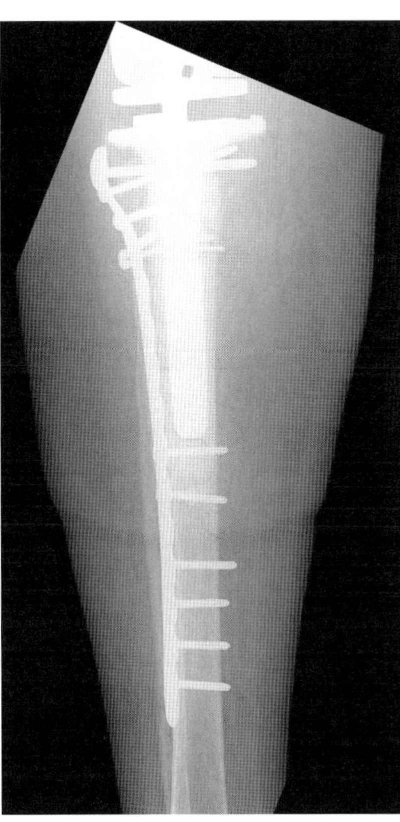

Figure 11 Radiograph showing a periprosthetic fracture of the tibia associated with a well-fixed component that was treated with a lateral locking plate.

Care in preparing both the patella itself and the tibiofemoral components are important in preventing periprosthetic fractures of the patella.[63] Appropriate external rotation and lateralization of the tibial and femoral components as well as medialization of the patellar component assist in patellar tracking and lower the risk of patellar complications. Patellae that are cut too thin (particularly less than 12 mm in thickness), remain too thick, or are cut asymmetrically seem to increase the risk of a periprosthetic fracture of the patella.[64] Lateral retinacular release, particularly with sacrifice of the superolateral geniculate artery, also has been associated with an increased risk of a periprosthetic fracture of the patella.[65]

Table 2
Classification of Periprosthetic Fractures of the Patella

Type I	Extensor mechanism intact, prosthesis stable (most common)
Type II	Extensor mechanism disrupted
Type III	Extensor mechanism intact, prosthesis loose
Type IIIA	"Reasonable" remaining bone stock (rare)
Type IIIB	Bone stock unsatisfactory for internal fixation and/or another resurfacing procedure

Classification

The most important considerations in treating a periprosthetic fracture of the patella include whether the extensor mechanism is intact or disrupted and if the patellar component itself is well fixed or loose. If the extensor mechanism is disrupted, surgery is required to restore active knee extension. The most commonly cited classification is that of Ortiguera and Berry[60] (Table 2).

Type I Fractures

In a type I periprosthetic fracture of the patella, the extensor mechanism is intact, and the patellar component is well fixed. These are often incidental radiographic findings that do not require specific treatment. If the patient is symptomatic, recommended treatment is a short course of immobilization followed by progressive, protected range of motion in a hinged knee brace. Surgical treatment is discouraged, regardless of the radiographic findings, because of the high rate of failure and complications. Nonsurgical treatment of type I fractures is associated with a high rate of success.[60]

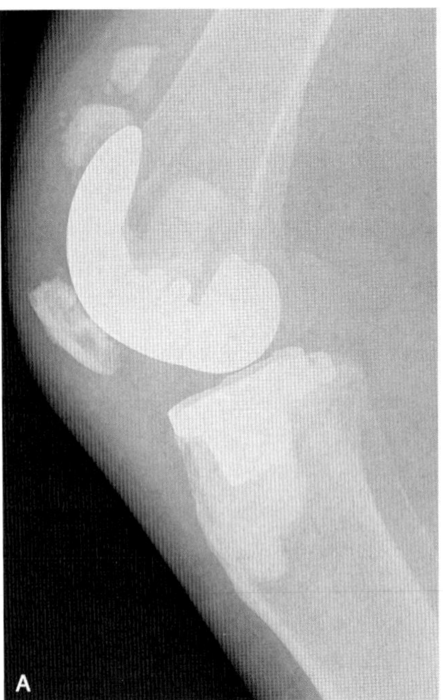
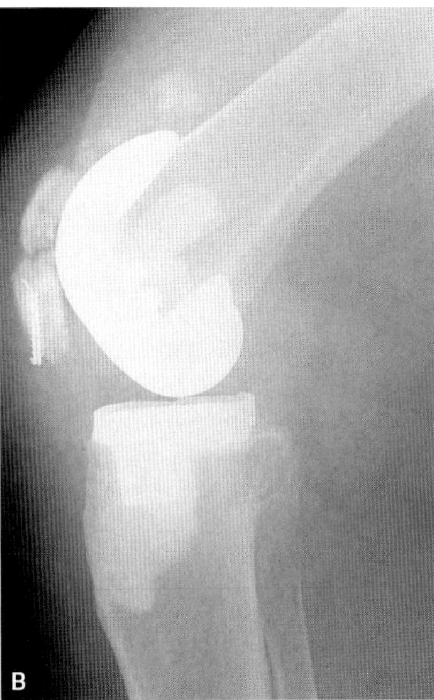

Figure 12 **A,** Radiograph of a type II periprosthetic fracture of the patella in a 57-year-old woman with rheumatoid arthritis. **B,** Despite fixation with cannulated lag screws, a tension band, and a cerclage wire, a nonunion developed.

Type II Fractures

If the extensor mechanism is not intact, surgical treatment is required to restore continuity and active knee extension. Patients who sustain this type of injury must be counseled preoperatively that the risk of complications is high but that surgical treatment is necessary to enable active knee extension and restore knee stability (Figure 12). Because there is a high risk of infection, it is critical to ensure that the skin overlying the knee is intact (and not abraded) before proceeding with surgery. Although the use of cannulated, partially threaded screws with a tension band running through them is the strongest construct biomechanically, it may be difficult to use this type of technique if the remaining patellar bone is thin; alternative methods, such as a standard tension band with a circumferential cerclage wire, may be required.[66] If the displaced fragment is small or otherwise unrepairable to the main body of the patella, excision of the fragment with primary soft-tissue repair of the extensor mechanism can be performed. Postoperative immobilization in a cast should be considered to allow bony union or soft-tissue healing. It must be recognized that concomitant tibiofemoral component revision may be required to correct rotational malalignment, which is a predisposing risk factor for the fracture; preoperative CT scans to objectively identify component rotation should be considered.[67]

Type III Fractures

In a type III fracture, the patellar component is loose, and the extensor mechanism is intact (fractures with a loose component and a disrupted extensor mechanism are classified as type II). Many of these fractures are associated with osteonecrosis of the patella. If the patellar component is loose and the patient can perform a straight leg raise, an initial course of nonsurgical treatment is recommended, particularly if the initial presentation was associated with a traumatic event. If the patient is persistently symptomatic, the component can be revised if there is adequate remaining bone stock. In most instances, however, the component is simply removed and the remaining bone contoured to optimize patellar tracking.

Management of Treatment Failures

If open reduction and internal fixation or attempts at primary extensor mechanism repair have failed, repeated attempts at repair are not recommended because of the high risk of infection and the low likelihood that repeated attempts at repair will result in restoration of extensor mechanism function. In these situations, a complete extensor mechanism allograft is recommended to restore active knee extension.[68]

Summary

Periprosthetic fractures are increasing common and are difficult clinical entities to treat. Challenges faced by the orthopaedic surgeon include gaining fracture fixation around a prosthesis that is implanted in bone that is often of poor quality or revising components in the setting of bone loss. These fractures also present biologic challenges because of prior damage to the endosteal blood supply. Postoperative treatment of some patients may be difficult because of medical comorbidities. A thorough understanding of the common pitfalls in treating and strategies for avoiding those pitfalls is paramount to achieving successful outcomes.

References

1. Lindahl H, Malchau H, Herberts P, Garellick G: Periprosthetic femoral fractures classification and demographics of 1049 periprosthetic femoral fractures from the Swedish National Hip Arthroplasty Register. *J Arthroplasty* 2005;20:857-865.
2. Lindahl H, Malchau H, Odén A, Garellick G: Risk factors for failure after treatment of a periprosthetic fracture of the femur. *J Bone Joint Surg Br* 2006;88:26-30.
3. Lowenhielm G, Hansson LI, Kärrholm J: Fracture of the lower extremity after total hip replacement. *Arch Orthop Trauma Surg* 1989;108:141-143.
4. Lindahl H, Oden A, Garellick G, Malchau H: The excess mortality due to periprosthetic femur fracture: A study from the Swedish national hip arthroplasty register. *Bone* 2007;40:1294-1298.
5. Bhattacharyya T, Chang D, Meigs JB, Estok DM II, Malchau H: Mortality after periprosthetic fracture of the femur. *J Bone Joint Surg Am* 2007;89:2658-2662.
6. Berry DJ: Epidemiology: Hip and knee. *Orthop Clin North Am* 1999;30:183-190.
7. Haidukewych GJ, Jacofsky DJ, Hanssen AD, Lewallen DG: Intraoperative fractures of the acetabulum during primary total hip arthroplasty. *J Bone Joint Surg Am* 2006;88:1952-1956.
8. Kim YS, Callaghan JJ, Ahn PB, Brown TD: Fracture of the acetabulum during insertion of an oversized hemispherical component. *J Bone Joint Surg Am* 1995;77:111-117.
9. Sharkey PF, Hozack WJ, Callaghan JJ, et al: Acetabular fracture associated with cementless acetabular component insertion: A report of 13 cases. *J Arthroplasty* 1999;14:426-431.
10. Christiansen CG, Kassim RA, Callaghan JJ, Marsh JL, Schmidt AH: Pubic ramus insufficiency fractures following total hip arthroplasty: A report of six cases. *J Bone Joint Surg Am* 2003;85:1819-1822.
11. Sánchez-Sotelo J, McGrory BJ, Berry DJ: Acute periprosthetic fracture of the acetabulum associated with osteolytic pelvic lesions: A report of 3 cases. *J Arthroplasty* 2000;15:126-130.
12. Della Valle CJ, Momberger NG, Paprosky WG: Periprosthetic fractures of the acetabulum associated with a total hip arthroplasty. *Instr Course Lect* 2003;52:281-290.
13. Berry DJ, Lewallen DG, Hanssen AD, Cabanela ME: Pelvic discontinuity in revision total hip arthroplasty. *J Bone Joint Surg Am* 1999;81:1692-1702.
14. Paprosky WG, Perona PG, Lawrence JM: Acetabular defect classification and surgical reconstruction in revision arthroplasty: A 6-year follow-up evaluation. *J Arthroplasty* 1994;9:33-44.
15. Sporer SM, Paprosky WG: Acetabular revision using a trabecular metal acetabular component for severe acetabular bone loss associated with a pelvic discontinuity. *J Arthroplasty* 2006;21:87-90.
16. DeBoer DK, Christie MJ, Brinson MF, Morrison JC: Revision total hip arthroplasty for pelvic discontinuity. *J Bone Joint Surg Am* 2007;89:835-840.
17. Springer BD, Berry DJ, Cabanela ME, Hanssen AD, Lewallen DG: Early postoperative transverse pelvic fracture: A new complication related to revision arthroplasty with an uncemented cup. *J Bone Joint Surg Am* 2005;87:2626-2631.
18. Brady OH, Garbuz DS, Masri BA, Duncan CP: Classification of the hip. *Orthop Clin North Am* 1999;30:215-220.
19. Dennis MG, Simon JA, Kummer FJ, Koval KJ, DiCesare PE: Fixation of periprosthetic femoral shaft fractures occurring at the tip of the stem: A biomechanical study of 5 techniques. *J Arthroplasty* 2000;15:523-528.
20. Maloney WJ, Herzwurm P, Paprosky W, Rubash HE, Engh CA: Treatment of pelvic osteolysis associated with a stable acetabular component inserted without cement as part of a total hip replacement. *J Bone Joint Surg Am* 1997;79:1628-1634.
21. Springer BD, Berry DJ, Lewallen DG: Treatment of periprosthetic femoral fractures following total hip arthroplasty with femoral component revision. *J Bone Joint Surg Am* 2003;85:2156-2162.
22. Tsiridis E, Narvani AA, Haddad FS, Timperley JA, Gie GA: Impaction femoral allografting and cemented revision for periprosthetic femoral fractures. *J Bone Joint Surg Br* 2004;86:1124-1132.
23. Levine BR, Della Valle CJ, Lewis P, Berger RA, Sporer SM, Paprosky W: Extended trochanteric osteotomy for the treatment of Vancouver B2/B3 periprosthetic fractures of the femur. *J Arthroplasty* 2008;23:527-533.
24. Stiehl JB: Extended osteotomy for periprosthetic femoral fractures in total hip arthroplasty. *Am J Orthop* 2006;35:20-23.
25. Ko PS, Lam JJ, Tio MK, Lee OB, Ip FK: Distal fixation with Wagner revision stem in treating Vancouver type B2 periprosthetic femur fractures in geriatric patients. *J Arthroplasty* 2003;18:446-452.
26. Della Valle CJ, Paprosky WG: Classification and an algorithmic approach to the reconstruction of femoral deficiency in revision total hip arthroplasty. *J Bone Joint Surg Am* 2003;85:1-6.
27. Sporer SM, Paprosky WG: Extensively coated cementless femoral components in revision total hip arthroplasty: An update. *Surg Technol Int* 2005;14:265-274.
28. Maury AC, Pressman A, Cayen B, Zalzal P, Backstein D, Gross A: Proximal femoral allograft treatment of Vancouver type-B3 periprosthetic femoral fractures after total hip arthroplasty. *J Bone Joint Surg Am* 2006;88:953-958.

29. Klein GR, Parvizi J, Rapuri V, et al: Proximal femoral replacement for the treatment of periprosthetic fractures. *J Bone Joint Surg Am* 2005;87:1777-1781.

30. Kregor PJ: Distal femur fractures with complex articular involvement: Management by articular exposure and submuscular fixation. *Orthop Clin North Am* 2002;33:153-175.

31. Kregor PJ, Stannard J, Zlowodzki M, Cole PA, Alonso J: Distal femoral fracture fixation utilizing the Less Invasive Stabilization System (L.I.S.S.): The technique and early results. *Injury* 2001;32:SC32-SC47.

32. Schandelmaier P, Partenheimer A, Koenemann B, Grün OA, Krettek C: Distal femoral fractures and LISS stabilization. *Injury* 2001;32:SC55-SC63.

33. Schütz M, Müller M, Krettek C, et al: Minimally invasive fracture stabilization of distal femoral fractures with the LISS: A prospective multicenter study. Results of a clinical study with special emphasis on difficult cases. *Injury* 2001;32:SC48-SC54.

34. Ricci WM, Bolhofner BR, Loftus T, Cox C, Mitchell S, Borrelli J Jr: Indirect reduction and plate fixation, without grafting, for periprosthetic femoral shaft fractures about a stable intramedullary implant. *J Bone Joint Surg Am* 2005;87:2240-2245.

35. Rorabeck CH, Taylor JW: Periprosthetic fractures of the femur complicating total knee arthroplasty. *Orthop Clin North Am* 1999;30:265-277.

36. Ayers DC: Supracondylar fractures adjacent to total knee implants. *Instr Course Lect* 1997;46:197-203.

37. Engh GA, Ammeen DJ: Periprosthetic fractures adjacent to total knee implants: Treatment and clinical results. *Instr Course Lect* 1998;47:437-448.

38. Healy WL, Siliski JM, Incavo SJ: Operative treatment of distal femoral fractures proximal to total knee replacements. *J Bone Joint Surg Am* 1993;75:27-34.

39. Chen F, Mont MA, Bachner RS: Management of ipsilateral supracondylar femur fractures following total knee arthroplasty. *J Arthroplasty* 1994;9:521-526.

40. Henry SL, Busconi B, Gold S: Management of supracondylar femur fractures proximal to total knee prostheses with the GSH supracondylar intramedullary nail. *Orthop Trans* 1995;19:153.

41. Henry SL: Management of supracondylar fractures proximal to total knee arthroplasty with the GSH supracondylar nail. *Contemp Orthop* 1995;31:231-238.

42. Bong MR, Egol KA, Koval KJ, et al: Comparison of the LISS and a retrograde-inserted supracondylar intramedullary nail for fixation of a periprosthetic distal femur fracture proximal to a total knee arthroplasty. *J Arthroplasty* 2002;17:876-881.

43. Mulvey TJ, Thornhill TS, Kelly MA, Healy WL: Complications associated with total knee arthroplasty, in Pellici PM, Tria AJ Jr, Garvin KL, eds: *Orthopaedic Knowledge Update 2: Hip and Knee Reconstruction*. Rosemont, IL, American Academy of Orthopaedic Surgeons, 2000, pp 323-337.

44. Ayers DC, Dennis DA, Johanson NA, Pellegrini VD Jr: Common complications of total knee arthroplasty. *J Bone Joint Surg Am* 1997;79:278-311.

45. Sanders R, Regazzoni P, Ruedi TP: Treatment of supracondylar-intracondylar fractures of the femur using the dynamic condylar screw. *J Orthop Trauma* 1989;3:214-222.

46. Bolhofner BR, Carmen B, Clifford P: The results of open reduction and internal fixation of distal femur fractures using a biologic (indirect) reduction technique. *J Orthop Trauma* 1996;10:372-377.

47. Cordeiro EN, Costa RC, Carazzato JG, Silva Jdos S: Periprosthetic fractures in patients with total knee arthroplasties. *Clin Orthop Relat Res* 1990;252:182-189.

48. Davison BL: Varus collapse of comminuted distal femur fractures after open reduction and internal fixation with a lateral condylar buttress plate. *Am J Orthop* 2003;32:27-30.

49. Herrera DA, Kregor PJ, Cole PA, Levy BA, Jönsson A, Zlowodzki M: Treatment of acute distal femur fractures above a TKA: Systematic review of 415 cases (1981-2006). *Acta Orthop* 2008;79:22-27.

50. Cole PA, Zlowodzki M, Kregor PJ: Treatment of proximal tibia fractures using the less invasive stabilization system: Surgical experience and early clinical results in 77 fractures. *J Orthop Trauma* 2004;18:528-535.

51. Haidukewych GJ: Innovations in locking plate technology. *J Am Acad Orthop Surg* 2004;12:205-212.

52. Koval KJ, Hoehl JJ, Kummer FJ, Simon JA: Distal femoral fixation: A biomechanical comparison of the standard condylar buttress plate, a locked buttress plate, and the 95-degree blade plate. *J Orthop Trauma* 1997;11:521-524.

53. Kregor PJ, Hughes JL, Cole PA: Fixation of distal femoral fractures above total knee arthroplasty utilizing the Less Invasive Stabilization System (L.I.S.S.). *Injury* 2001;32:SC64-SC75.

54. Krettek C, Müller M, Miclau T: Evolution of minimally invasive plate osteosynthesis (MIPO) in the femur. *Injury* 2001;32:SC14-SC23.

55. Marti A, Fankhauser C, Frenk A, Cordey J, Gasser B: Biomechanical evaluation of the less invasive stabilization system for the internal fixation of distal femur fractures. *J Orthop Trauma* 2001;15:482-487.

56. Frigg R, Appenzeller A, Christensen R, Frenk A, Gilbert S, Schavan R: The development of the distal femur Less Invasive Stabilization System (LISS). *Injury* 2001;32:SC24-SC31.

57. Zlowodzki M, Williamson S, Zardiackas LD, Kregor PJ: Biomechanical evaluation of the less invasive stabilization system, angled blade plate, and retrograde intramedullary nail for the fixation of distal femur fractures. *J Orthop Trauma* 2004;18:494-502.

58. Farouk O, Krettek C, Miclau T, Schandelmaier P, Guy P, Tscherne H: Minimally invasive plate osteosynthesis: Does percutaneous plating disrupt femoral blood supply less than the traditional technique? *J Orthop Trauma* 1999;13:401-406.

59. Beharrie AW, Nelson CL: Impaction bone-grafting in the treatment of a periprosthetic fracture of the tibia: A case report. *J Bone Joint Surg Am* 2003; 85:703-707.

60. Ortiguera CJ, Berry DJ: Patellar fracture after total knee arthroplasty. *J Bone Joint Surg Am* 2002;84:532-540.

61. Keating EM, Haas G, Meding JB: Patella fracture after post total knee replacements. *Clin Orthop Relat Res* 2003;416:93-97.

62. Parvizi J, Kim KI, Oliashirazi A, Ong A, Sharkey PF: Periprosthetic patellar fractures. *Clin Orthop Relat Res* 2006;446:161-166.

63. Figgie HE III, Goldberg VM, Figgie MP, Inglis AE, Kelly M, Sobel M: The effect of alignment of the implant on fractures of the patella after condylar total knee arthroplasty. *J Bone Joint Surg Am* 1989;71:1031-1039.

64. Reuben JD, McDonald CL, Woodard PL, Hennington LJ: Effect of patella thickness on patella strain following total knee arthroplasty. *J Arthroplasty* 1991;6:251-258.

65. Tria AJ Jr, Harwood DA, Alicea JA, Cody RP: Patellar fractures in posterior stabilized knee arthroplasties. *Clin Orthop Relat Res* 1994;299:131-138.

66. Carpenter JE, Kasman RA, Patel N, Lee ML, Goldstein SA: Biomechanical evaluation of current patella fracture fixation techniques. *J Orthop Trauma* 1997;11:351-356.

67. Berger RA, Crossett LS, Jacobs JJ, Rubash HE: Malrotation causing patellofemoral complications after total knee arthroplasty. *Clin Orthop Relat Res* 1998;356:144-153.

68. Burnett RS, Berger RA, Paprosky WG, Della Valle CJ, Jacobs JJ, Rosenberg AG: Extensor mechanism allograft reconstruction after total knee arthroplasty: A comparison of two techniques. *J Bone Joint Surg Am* 2004;86:2694-2699.

Vancouver Type B3 Periprosthetic Fractures: Evaluation and Treatment

Corey J. Richards, MD, MASc, FRCSC
Donald S. Garbuz, MD, MHSc, FRCSC
Bassam A. Masri, MD, FRCSC
Clive P. Duncan, MD

Abstract

Periprosthetic fracture with preexisting severe loss of bone stock is a challenging condition to treat. Available surgical options can be divided into three categories: complex reconstruction of the deficient proximal femur with secure distal fixation; segmental substitution of the proximal femur with a megaprosthesis or allograft/stem composite; and distally fixed replacement with a modular stem, which acts as a scaffold around which the remaining deficient proximal bone can be assembled, to unite and possibly reconstitute.

Total hip arthroplasty (THA) is an extremely successful procedure, providing excellent pain relief while improving patient function. Complication rates are low but still represent a significant clinical and financial burden to the health care system. Periprosthetic fractures are now the third most common reason for revision THA, after osteolysis (with or without loosening) and recurrent dislocation. The reported prevalence ranges from 0.1% to 2.1%.[1-7] The increasing prevalence of periprosthetic fractures is related to several factors, including an increasing number of patients undergoing THA, an increasing number of elderly patients at risk for falls, and increasing numbers of revision procedures using techniques with distal fixation, resulting in significant stress transfer to the distal tip of the reconstruction and proximal stress shielding.[2,8-10]

The Vancouver classification of postoperative periprosthetic fractures consolidates the three most important factors: location of the fracture, fixation of the femoral stem, and the quality of the surrounding bone stock.[11-13] Type B periprosthetic fractures are those fractures around or just below the femoral stem. These fractures are subdivided depending on the stability of the femoral implant and remaining bone stock: type B1 fractures have a solidly fixed implant; type B2 fractures have a loose implant, but remaining bone stock is good; and type B3 fractures have a loose implant with severe bone stock loss (osteopenia, osteolysis, or comminution; Figure 1). The treatment of type B1 and type B2 fractures is relatively straightforward. Treatment of type B1 fractures is with retention of the component and open or indirect reduction and internal fixation of the fracture. Treatment of type B2 fractures is with component removal and reduction and fixation of the fracture, followed by revision of the femoral component. In contrast, the treatment of type B3 fractures is more complex and depends on various factors, including the age of the patient, the quality of the remaining distal host bone, and the experience and preference of the surgeon.

The surgical management of type B3 periprosthetic fractures can be divided into three broad generic groups, with some overlap: complex reconstruction of the deficient proximal femur with secure distal fixation, using either impaction allografting or strut allografts; segmental substitution of the proximal femur with a megaprosthesis or an allograft/prosthetic composite; and an extensively fixed, modular, fluted, tapered titanium im-

Donald S. Garbuz, MD, MHSc, FRCSC or the department with which he is affiliated has received research or institutional support from Zimmer and is a consultant for or an employee of Zimmer. Clive P. Duncan, MD, FRCSC or the department with which he is affiliated has received research or institutional support from Zimmer and Smith & Nephew, has received miscellaneous nonincome support, commercially derived honoraria, or other nonresearch-related funding and royalties from Zimmer.

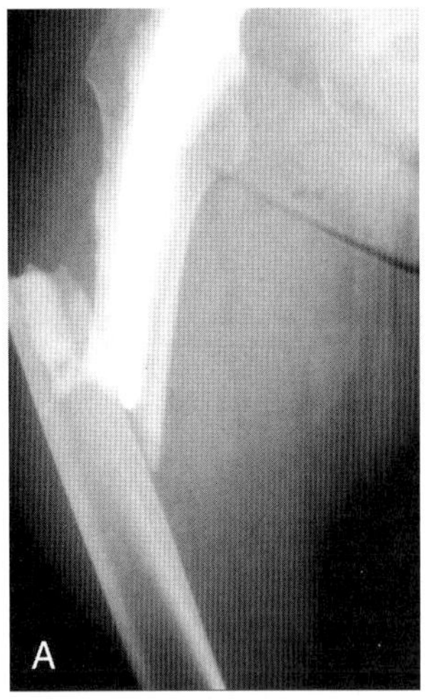

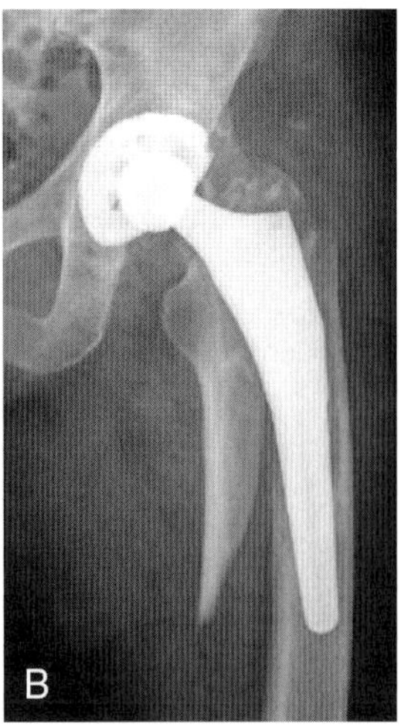

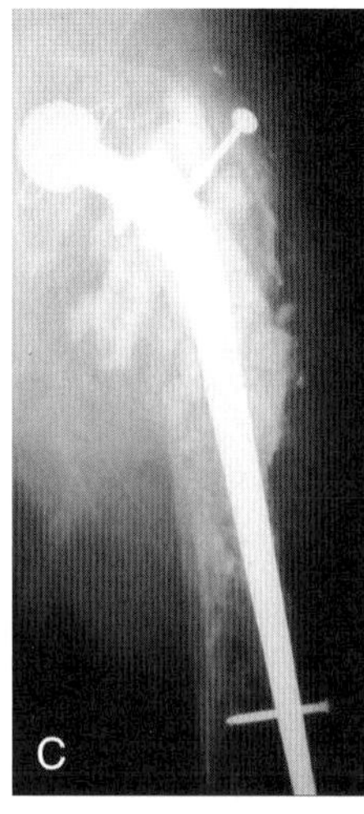

Figure 1 **A,** Vancouver type B1 periprosthetic fracture. **B,** Type B2 periprosthetic fracture. **C,** Type B3 periprosthetic fracture.

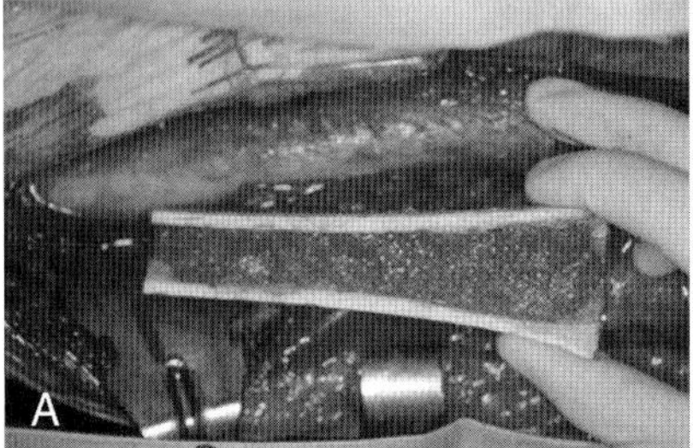

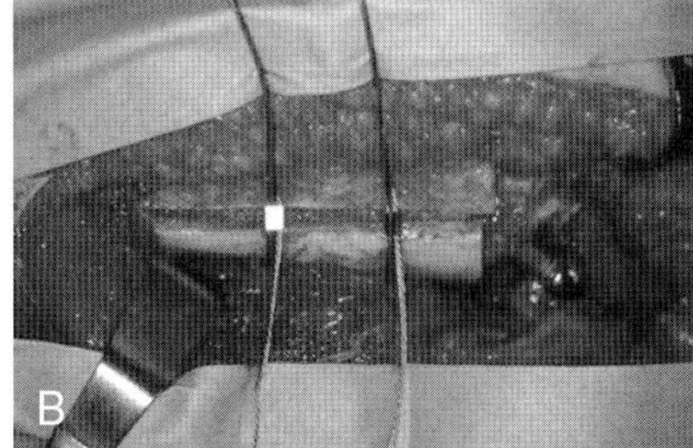

Figure 2 **A** and **B,** Preparation and fixation of strut allograft.

plant replacement, acting as a scaffold around which the remaining proximal bone may be reassembled, with the intention that it will unite and to some extent reconstitute.

Surgical Management of Type B3 Periprosthetic Fractures

Regardless of the specific technique used in the management of a type B3 periprosthetic fracture, the surgeon should be familiar with various extensile approaches to the hip and femur. After removal of the loose implant, the fracture is identified and often can be separated to enhance canal débridement and facilitate femoral reaming. Intraoperative tissue cultures should be obtained and intraoperative prophylactic antibiotics administered. Intraoperative radiographs can be an important adjunct for confirmation of construct integrity before wound closure.

Complex Reconstruction of the Deficient Proximal Femur With Secure Distal Fixation

Strut Allografting With Distally Fixed Stem

Following removal of the prosthesis and cement, the intact distal femur is prepared for a cementless prosthesis. The proximal deficient bone is reduced around the prosthesis and augmented with onlay strut allografts. The use of a whole segmental femoral allograft allows for optimal preparation of the strut graft, if available. The medullary cavity of the allograft femur can be reamed before it is bivalved, to allow good apposition against the host femur. The grafts, 15 cm in length, are secured laterally and anteriorly with at least four multifilament cables and morcellized allograft is spread along the concavity of the strut[14] (Figure 2).

There has been some interest in the reconstruction of femoral defects with cortical strut grafts in the revision setting for aseptic loosening.[15] There are no published reports evaluating their use in the treatment of periprosthetic fractures alone. Emerson and associates[16] have demonstrated that cortical struts unite consistently by 8 months, with a union rate of 96%.

Circumferential Mesh With Impaction Allografting

Following removal of the prosthesis and cement, the fracture is reduced and fixation is achieved or augmented with cerclage wires, cables, plates, or strut allografts. Segmental defects in the femur are reconstructed using wire mesh secured with cerclage wires. A large cement restrictor is inserted. The canal is then packed with allograft bone chips over a central guidewire. The distal canal is impacted until filled to the level of the distal tip of the femoral phantom impactor. The canal is then repeatedly filled and impacted with a femoral phantom impactor until a neomedullary canal is formed. The new canal is then filled with bone cement and pressurized. A polished, collarless, tapered stem is then inserted. Postoperatively, patients are restricted to toe-touch weight bearing for 3 months.[17]

Tsiridis and associates[17] reviewed 89 Vancouver type B2 and B3 fractures treated with impaction allografting and cemented stem fixation. Seventy-four (83%) of the fractures united, with improved re-

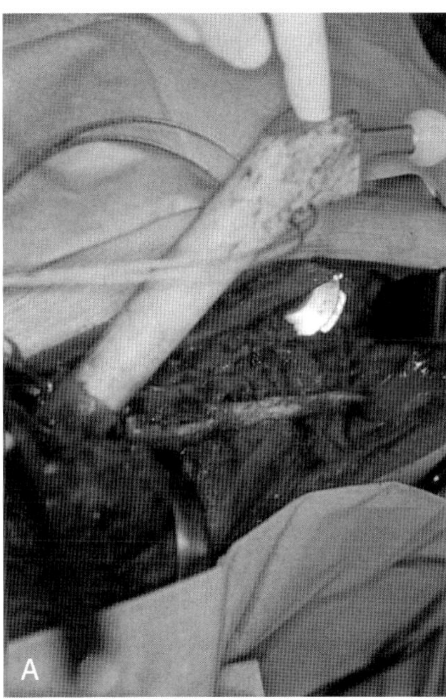

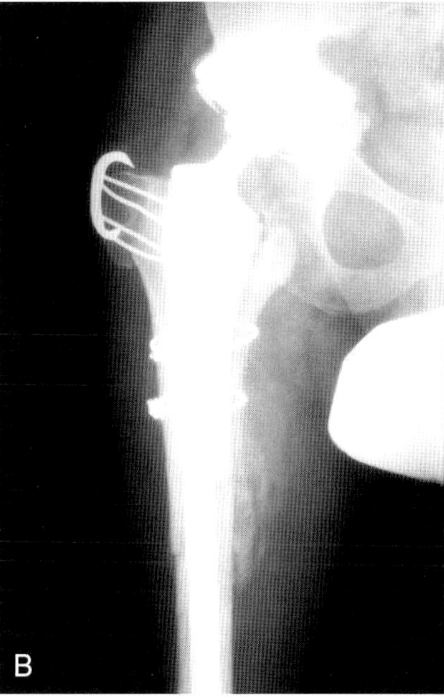

Figure 3 **A,** Insertion of an allograft prosthetic composite. **B,** Postoperative radiograph of the allograft prosthetic composite technique.

sults for patients treated with a long stem prosthesis that bypassed the fracture (66 of 75 fractures [88%]).

Resection of the Proximal Femur With Simple Substitution

Allograft Prosthetic Composite

To ensure adequate fixation of the host greater trochanter to the allograft femur, an extended trochanteric osteotomy or trochanteric slide is favored instead of a classic trochanteric osteotomy. Subsequently, the prosthesis and cement are removed, and a step-cut osteotomy of the host femur at the proximal end of the distal fragment is made. A step-cut is used to maximize stability at the graft-host junction. The structural allograft and femoral stem are selected based on preoperative radiographic templating. The femoral component must bypass the allograft-host bone junction by at least four cortical diameters. The structural allograft should be large enough to ensure a 2-mm cement mantle after the appropriate reaming and broaching. The femoral component is cemented into the allograft on the back table. Once the cement has hardened, the allograft-prosthesis composite is secured to the distal fragment via the step-cut osteotomy. The allograft-host bone junction is secured with Luque wires to ensure rotational stability. If the allograft-host bone junction cannot be adequately secured, a cortical onlay allograft may be used. The remaining osteotomized proximal host bone and autograft reaming from the canal preparation are used to augment the allograft-host bone junction. The host-extended greater trochanteric fragment and remaining host bone are attached to the allograft (Figure 3). Postoperatively, patients are not allowed to bear weight until there is radiographic evidence of allograft-host union, typically after 3 to 6 months.[18]

Maury and associates[19] reported good results in 25 patients with type B3 fractures treated with proximal femoral allograft followed for a minimum of 2 years. Twenty-three of 24 patients were able to walk, and allograft united with host bone in 20 patients. Subsequent union occurred in the four patients requiring repeat allografts. Wong and Gross[20] described using a proximal structural allograft in 15 patients with periprosthetic fracture accompanied by severe host bone loss. Good results were reported in 13 of 15 patients reviewed.

Proximal Femoral Replacement

After removal of the prosthesis and cement, a transverse osteotomy is made at the distal end of the proximal deficient femoral bone for seating of the implant. The distal femur is then prepared in the standard fashion for a proximal femoral replacement prosthesis. When possible, the remaining host bone is attached to the prosthesis with cerclage fixation. Intraoperative hip instability with adequately positioned components is addressed with constrained liners (Figure 4). It is important that the abductors are securely sutured to the implant. The abductors, if still available, promote healing of a soft-tissue envelope to optimize function and stability.

Malkani and associates[21] reported a 64% survivorship at 12 years for 50 patients undergoing proximal femoral replacement for nonneoplastic disorders. Parvizi and associates[22] reported on 43 patients undergoing proximal femoral replacement for nonneoplastic disorders (20 periprosthetic fractures). They found good to excellent results in 22 of 43 patients at a mean follow-up of 36.5 months.

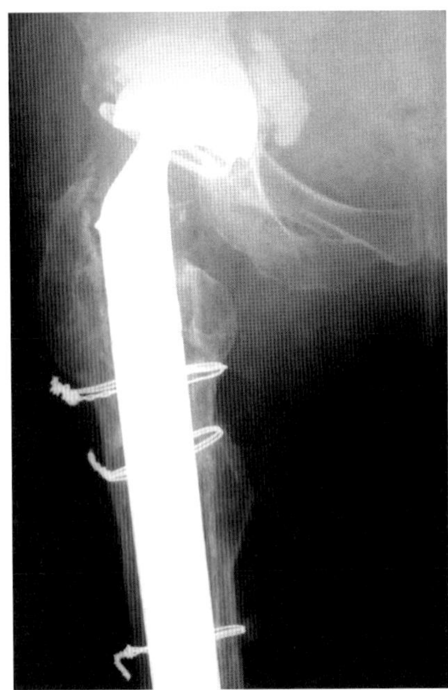

Figure 4 Postoperative radiograph of the proximal femoral replacement technique.

Distally Fixed Replacement That Acts as a Scaffold for the Remaining Proximal Host Bone

Following removal of the prosthesis and cement, a transverse osteotomy is made at the distal end of the deficient femoral bone. The osteotomized proximal portion is split longitudinally, maintaining soft-tissue attachment to the bone fragments. The intact distal femur is then prepared for a cementless modular femoral component, ideally of a tapered and fluted design. The modular body of the stem system is selected next, as well as its length, version, and offset, to achieve satisfactory soft-tissue tension and limb length. Modular body selection is accomplished independent of the native proximal femur that is retracted, with its soft tissues still attached, during this step in the reconstruction.

The remaining fragments of the deficient proximal femur are then wrapped around the proximal part of the stem and secured in place with cerclage fixation, with particular attention paid to the greater trochanter. Joint stability is achieved with attention to soft-tissue tension, leg length, and offset, augmented with large-head components, enhanced offset liners, or a constrained articulation when necessary (Figure 5). Postoperatively, patients are usually managed with limited weight bearing for 12 weeks or until there is clinical and radiographic evidence of union.[23]

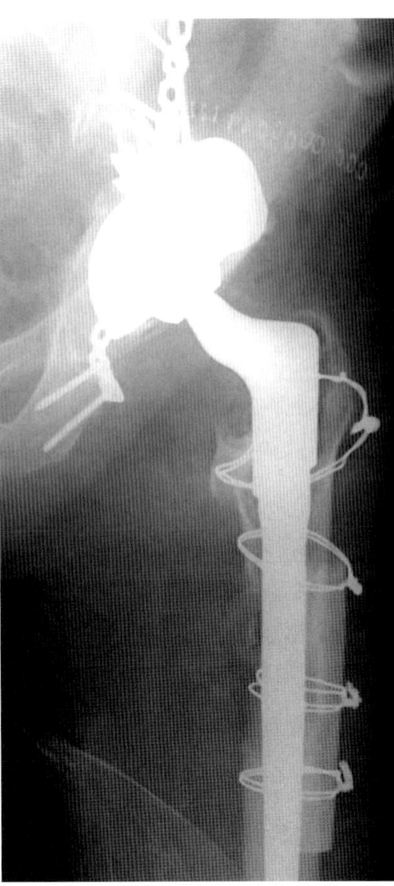

Figure 5 Postoperative radiograph of the scaffold technique with standard unipolar articulation.

Klein and associates[23] reported on a series of 21 patients with type B3 fractures treated with this distally secured, proximal scaffold technique. Twenty of 21 patients were able to ambulate and had minimal to no pain. Berry[24] successfully treated eight patients using a modular, fluted, tapered cementless stem with retention of the proximal femur. At a mean follow-up of 1.5 years, all patients had stable implants, and all acute fractures were healed.

Summary

Periprosthetic femoral fractures with associated severe bone loss remains a difficult treatment challenge. A failure rate of approximately 25% is reported throughout the literature for the various options. The newly introduced scaffold technique has had early promising results (95% success), but additional long-term data are required. The treatment protocol for Vancouver type B3 periprosthetic fractures has evolved over the years. The distally fixed, proximally reassembled scaffold technique is preferable because it is a rapid procedure with reduced blood loss, high versatility, and facilitation of early mobilization.

References

1. Adolphson P, Jonsson U, Kalen R: Fractures of the ipsilateral femur after total hip arthroplasty. *Arch Orthop Trauma Surg* 1987;106:353-357.
2. Berry DJ: Epidemiology: Hip and knee. *Orthop Clin North Am* 1999;30: 183-190.
3. Bethea JS III, DeAndrade JR, Fleming LL, Lindenbaum SD, Welch RB: Proximal femoral fractures following total hip arthroplasty. *Clin Orthop Relat Res* 1982;170:95-106.
4. Fredin H: Late fracture of the femur following perforation during hip arthroplasty: A report of 2 cases. *Acta Orthop Scand* 1988;59:331-332.
5. Garcia-Cimbrelo E, Munuera L, Gil-Garay E: Femoral shaft fractures after cemented total hip arthroplasty. *Int Orthop* 1992;16:97-100.

6. Lowenhielm G, Hansson LI, Karrholm J: Fracture of the lower extremity after total hip replacement. *Arch Orthop Trauma Surg* 1989;108:141-143.

7. Schwartz JT Jr, Mayer JG, Engh CA: Femoral fracture during noncemented total hip arthroplasty. *J Bone Joint Surg Am* 1989;71:1135-1142.

8. Garbuz DS, Masri BA, Duncan CP: Periprosthetic fractures of the femur: Principles of prevention and management. *Instr Course Lect* 1998;47:237-242.

9. Elting JJ, Mikhail WE, Zicat BA, Hubbell JC, Lane LE, House B: Preliminary report of impaction grafting for exchange femoral arthroplasty. *Clin Orthop Relat Res* 1995;319:159-167.

10. Gie GA, Linder L, Ling RS, Simon JP, Slooff TJ, Timperley AJ: Impacted cancellous allografts and cement for revision total hip arthroplasty. *J Bone Joint Surg Br* 1993;75:14-21.

11. Duncan CP, Masri BA: Fractures of the femur after hip replacement. *Instr Course Lect* 1995;44:293-304.

12. Brady OH, Garbuz DS, Masri BA, Duncan CP: Classification of the hip. *Orthop Clin North Am* 1999;30:215-220.

13. Brady OH, Garbuz DS, Masri BA, Duncan CP: The reliability and validity of the Vancouver classification of femoral fractures after hip replacement. *J Arthroplasty* 2000;15:59-62.

14. Siegmeth A, Garbuz DS, Masri BA: Salvage procedures and implant selection for periprosthetic femoral fractures. *Injury* 2007;38:698-703.

15. Head WC, Malinin TI, Mallory TH, Emerson RH Jr: Onlay cortical allografting for the femur. *Orthop Clin North Am* 1998;29:307-312.

16. Emerson RH Jr, Malinin TI, Cuellar AD, Head WC, Peters PC: Cortical strut allografts in the reconstruction of the femur in revision total hip arthroplasty: A basic science and clinical study. *Clin Orthop Relat Res* 1992; 285: 35-44.

17. Tsiridis E, Narvani AA, Haddad FS, Timperley JA, Gie GA: Impaction femoral allografting and cemented revision for periprosthetic femoral fractures. *J Bone Joint Surg Br* 2004;86:1124-1132.

18. Kellett CF, Boscainos PJ, Maury AC, Pressman A, Cayen B, Zalzal P, et al: Proximal femoral allograft treatment of Vancouver type-B3 periprosthetic femoral fractures after total hip arthroplasty: Surgical technique. *J Bone Joint Surg Am* 2007;89(suppl 2 pt 1):68-79.

19. Maury AC, Pressman A, Cayen B, Zalzal P, Backstein D, Gross A: Proximal femoral allograft treatment of Vancouver type-B3 periprosthetic femoral fractures after total hip arthroplasty. *J Bone Joint Surg Am* 2006;88:953-958.

20. Wong P, Gross AE: The use of structural allografts for treating periprosthetic fractures about the hip and knee. *Orthop Clin North Am* 1999;30:259-264.

21. Malkani AL, Settecerri JJ, Sim FH, Chao EY, Wallrichs SL: Long-term results of proximal femoral replacement for non-neoplastic disorders. *J Bone Joint Surg Br* 1995;77:351-356.

22. Parvizi J, Tarity TD, Slenker N, et al: Proximal femoral replacement in patients with non-neoplastic conditions. *J Bone Joint Surg Am* 2007;89:1036-1043.

23. Klein GR, Parvizi J, Rapuri V, et al: Proximal femoral replacement for the treatment of periprosthetic fractures. *J Bone Joint Surg Am* 2005;87:1777-1781.

24. Berry DJ: Treatment of Vancouver B3 periprosthetic femur fractures with a fluted tapered stem. *Clin Orthop Relat Res* 2003;417:224-231.

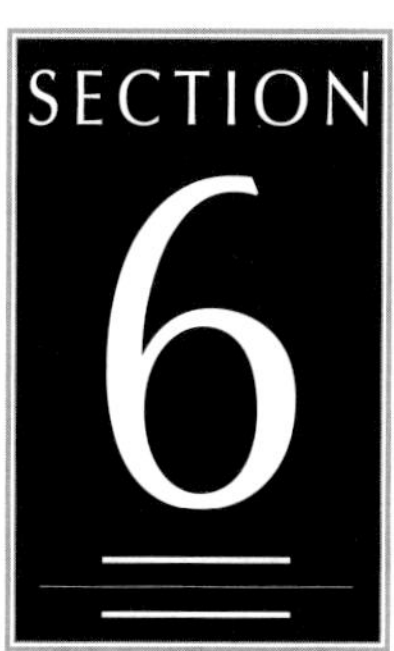

Revision Total Hip Arthroplasty

Revision Total Hip Arthroplasty

Total hip arthroplasty (THA) is among the most successful orthopaedic surgical procedures. As the number of patients requiring THA and the physical demands placed on the hip joints increase, the number of revision surgeries can be expected to increase. Infection, instability, and osteolysis are some of the causes of failure in this generally successful surgical procedure. This section includes six important chapters about revision THA that discuss some of the most challenging and important issues currently faced by orthopaedic surgeons.

In the chapter by Jiranek, the reader is taken through the author's thought process on the best method for choosing an approach for revision THA. Although many articles have described the multiple surgical approaches to revision hip surgery, Jiranek provides perhaps the best overall summary of the various approaches and marries the techniques and intraoperative photographs with tables that succinctly summarize the various techniques, indications, and risks. As the burden of the increasing number of arthroplasty procedures becomes a reality, more surgeons will need to become comfortable with revision arthroplasty if patients are to continue to receive timely care.

Instability remains a common cause for revision hip surgery. Parvizi and associates have done a commendable job of outlining the strategies that can be considered for managing patients with hip instability. The authors present a thorough review of the available surgical techniques for revision THA, include technical tips, and discuss soft-tissue management for instability—a topic that is often glossed over in similar works. Although less experienced surgeons may choose constrained liners as their "knee-jerk" solution for treating hip instability, Parvizi and associates discuss the problems and complications of this seemingly simple approach and provide more durable recommendations. The authors also discuss when constrained liners are best indicated. Modern implants, such as tripolar implants, have added to the armamentarium of treatment modalities for instability and are well described in this chapter.

Managing bone loss remains a major challenge for the arthroplasty surgeon, and multiple THA revisions may present a challenge to even the most experienced orthopaedic surgeons. Infection is one possible etiology of substantial bone loss. Although published data on the incidence of infection after THA vary widely, the average incidence is approximately 1%. Many infections, however, are not diagnosed in a timely manner. If minimally symptomatic and indolent infections are included, the number of infections would likely be higher.

With the improving ability to properly diagnose infection, it appears that a larger number of infected arthroplasties are being seen at tertiary referral centers. Chronic infection can lead to substantial bone loss. In the third chapter in this section, Richards and associates discuss options for managing bone loss on the femoral side. Although modular tapered stems have made femoral reconstruction easier, restoring bone stock remains a complex undertaking because of the wide array of allograft options currently available. The authors discuss the wide range of reconstruction options for these patients and elaborate on the use of a distally fixed stem to act as a template for proximal bone grafting.

The chapter by Richards and associates nicely dovetails with the chapter by Hartman and Garvin, who provide comprehensive summaries on bone loss classification and its subsequent implications on femoral fixation options. Importantly, the authors do an outstanding job of reviewing some key research publications for each of the recommended fixation approaches to give the reader a clear picture of the likely expected outcomes from each technique discussed. The value of modular tapered stems is confirmed, but Hartman and Garvin also comment on the risk of subsidence if these stems are undersized, which I believe is a common mistake for early users of this type of component.

One of the most demanding technical procedures in orthopaedics is acetabular revision, which has its own unique set of surgical challenges. Bone loss about the acetabulum can be severe and is almost always underestimated on preoperative radiographs. The anatomy and orientation of the pelvis, and subsequently the acetabulum, can be variable and complex. An intraoperative understanding of the three-dimensional anatomy of the acetabulum is made exponentially more difficult when large portions of the acetabular bone stock are absent along with the valuable landmarks they provide. Because of the shape and nature of acetabular fixation, creating a stable component is both difficult and imperative.

These technical challenges have been made easier with the advent of highly porous metal augments and acetabular components, but recent decisions from the FDA regarding custom implants have made it somewhat more difficult to treat the most severe cases. Companies are increasingly reluctant to manufacture custom devices, in part because of the way the FDA defines these devices, which seems to have become more restrictive over the years. The compassionate use exemption does not provide a viable alternative pathway for patients who need devices quickly, because it actually takes more time than the pathway for a custom device. Moreover, devices that fall under the compassionate use exemption are labeled experimental, which may create further delays when insurance companies deny coverage. I have personally experienced challenges finding companies willing to create custom implants, as have other orthopaedic surgeons. Such difficulties have led the American Academy of Orthopaedic Surgeons to support regulatory improvements to the FDA Act on medical devices, which strengthen tracking and review of applications for investigational device exemptions and include modifications of the custom device exemption to meet the needs of individual patients.

The last two chapters in this section focus on the acetabulum. The chapter by Sporer presents a well-thought-out and algorithmic approach to acetabular revision. The classification of acetabular bone loss is discussed, along with information to help the surgeon correlate the classification system with the most effective reconstructive options. The chapter includes a helpful table with many tips and technical pearls for each reconstruction plan based on the Paprosky classification system for acetabular defects.

Whereas the Sporer chapter focuses on the most common acetabular revisions, the chapter by Noordin and associates provides an expansive review of the diagnosis and treatment of pelvic dissociation. The authors describe the effective management of this difficult acetabular reconstruction and include some relevant outcomes studies.

All of the chapters in this section discuss the importance of preoperative planning and appropriate pathologic diagnosis. I believe that any surgeon who performs revision surgery will find these chapters extremely valuable. As the complexity of implants continues to increase, orthopaedic surgeons must continue to improve their abilities to manage the complexities of revision surgery. I am confident that this section will help with that responsibility.

David J. Jacofsky, MD
Chairman and Chief Executive Officer
The CORE Institute
Phoenix, Arizona

Dr. Jacofsky or an immediate family member has received royalties from Stryker and Smith & Nephew; serves as a paid consultant to Stryker; has stock or stock options held in Secure Independence; and has received research or institutional support from Biomet, Stryker, Smith & Nephew, and Arthrex.

Approaches for Revision Total Hip Replacement

William Jiranek, MD, FACS

Abstract

Choosing the approach for revision total hip replacement is an essential part of surgical planning and should be done well before the patient enters the operating room. Planning includes selecting patient positioning, the location of the incision, techniques for managing previous incisions, the needed exposure equipment, and the steps needed to extend the exposure. More extensive exposure on both the acetabular and femoral sides is often required in revision surgery.

Considering options for the surgical approach is an essential part of planning for revision total hip replacement. Three basic questions should be asked: (1) Which components are being revised? (2) What defects are present? (3) What approaches were used previously?

In general, it is sensible to honor previous incisions and approaches, with the exception of extensive acetabular work when using the direct lateral approach or extensive femoral work when using the anterior approach. The surgeon also should determine the primary location of the surgery: Is it predominantly acetabular, predominantly femoral, or both?[1]

The chosen approach is influenced by the work that needs to be done. For example, if bulk allografts or buttress augments are required, greater than normal exposure of the ilium will be necessary; posterior plating of a pelvic discontinuity would be difficult to achieve through anterior or anterolateral approaches; and placing a cage or triflange cup is much easier to accomplish through a transtrochanteric approach. For planning purposes, the surgery may use an extensile acetabular exposure, an extensile femoral exposure, or both. An extensile acetabular exposure is needed for managing severe osteolytic lesions, placing bulk allografts, buttress augmentation, posterior column plating for discontinuity, or placing a cage or a triflange cup. An extensile femoral approach is needed for difficult stem or cement extraction, placing a modular stem, managing severe bone loss (type IIIB or IV defects), treating broken femoral stems, or managing a periprosthetic fracture.[2]

Patient Positioning

Because many revision situations require extension of the incision, the surgeon should choose the patient position that provides maximum flexibility. Many surgeons prefer the floppy lateral position because it allows access to both the front and the back of the hip. In this position, the patient is rolled approximately halfway between the supine and lateral decubitus positions, and a beanbag is used to allow some motion forward and backward. The supine position can be used if the surgeon is comfortable with it, but access to posterior structures is difficult. Regardless of the position chosen, there should be clear access to the top of the ilium without impingement by bars or pads that would prevent extension of the incision. Similarly, the positioning should allow a full range of motion of the involved extremity without limitation by the positioning equipment. Numerous positioning guides are available, but the most adjustable may be a beanbag, which allows control of the torso and contralateral limb without restricting the motion of the operated leg.

Dr. Jiranek or an immediate family member has received royalties from DePuy; serves as a paid consultant to DePuy; has received research or institutional support from Stryker; and serves as a board member, owner, officer, or committee member of the American Academy of Orthopaedic Surgeons, the American Association of Hip and Knee Surgeons, and the Knee Society.

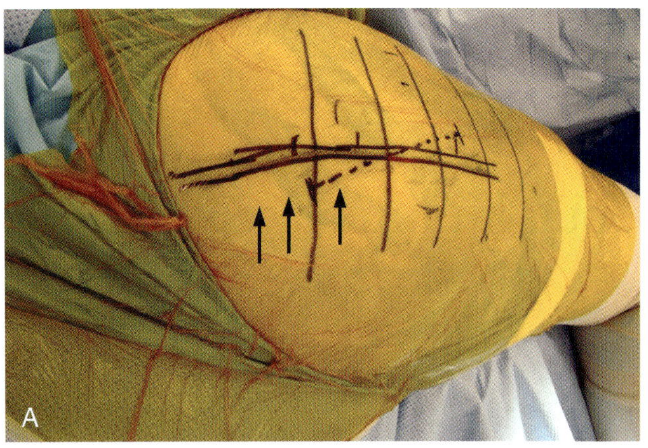

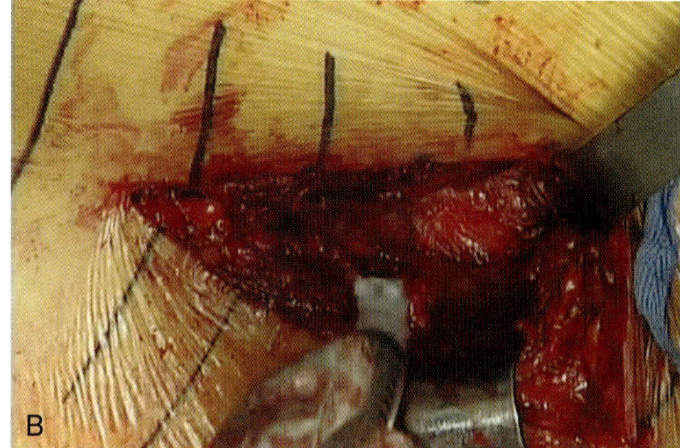

Figure 1 **A,** In managing multiple previous incisions, leaving a small area of potentially devascularized skin (arrows) should be avoided. **B,** Aspirating a hip joint of a failed metal-on-metal total hip replacement before capsulotomy.

Incisions

Rather than making a new incision in a better position, prior incisions should be used wherever possible and extended when necessary. Vascularity in the skin over the hip is considerably better than vascularity in the skin over the knee; however, care must be taken to avoid violating the 1:1 rule of flaps. This rule suggests that in any potential flap created by an old incision and a new incision, the length should be equal to the width (avoiding a strip of potentially devascularized skin) (**Figure 1,** *A*). In the situation where there are multiple prior incisions, the incision that is closest to the planned work should be used, and narrow flaps should be avoided. Attempts should be made to excise the previous incision, rather than merely incising it. This allows the surgeon to excise the dermal scar, which allows better apposition of the flaps on closure and avoids the unsightly appearance of multiple incisions. As with any incision, the surgeon should avoid the creation of large areas of dead space and should mobilize flaps only enough to access the joint and allow adequate closure.

If possible, the deep fascial incision should stay in the interval between the tensor fascia lata and gluteus maximus for both a lateral and a posterior approach. In revision approaches, it is often possible to reflect the posterior pseudocapsule and preserve it for later repair. It can be tagged in much the same manner as is done in a primary arthroplasty. The same is true for a revision performed through an anterolateral approach. Prior to incising the pseudocapsule, the synovial fluid should be aspirated for a cell count, differential, and culture (**Figure 1,** *B*). Findings from the cell count and differential can later help the surgeon differentiate a true positive bacterial culture from a contaminant.[3]

Exposure Equipment

The proper instruments facilitate accomplishing the exposure. Numerous retractors have been developed for revision surgery, including retractors that maintain the greater amounts of exposure required in revision surgery, as well as self-retaining retractors that provide exposure with less assistance. Longer cobra retractors can be used when an osteotomy fragment requires more anterior retraction. High-speed burrs and sharp osteotomes are helpful for creating osteotomies.

Extension of the Exposure

Soft-tissue releases and osteotomies can improve the mobilization of the hip joint. The soft-tissue releases are the anterior capsulectomy (versus capsulotomy), the gluteus maximus tendon release, the rectus strip, and the abductor strip (**Table 1**). Osteotomies include the traditional trochanteric osteotomy, the trochanteric slide, and the extended trochanteric osteotomy (**Table 2**).

Anterior Capsulectomy

The formal anterior capsulectomy is particularly valuable in acetabular revision surgeries performed through a posterior approach in which the femoral component is left in situ. Using this technique, the surgeon can safely differentiate the anterior pseudocapsule from the anterior neurovascular structures. Sufficient anterior capsule can be excised to create a pocket where the femoral trunnion or, in the case of monoblock femoral components, the femoral head can be safely retracted anterior to the anterior rim of the acetabulum. Prior to performing this maneuver, the surgeon should reflect the posterior pseudocapsule in a trapdoor fashion, tagging the capsule for later repair (**Figure 2**). An anterior capsulectomy is facilitated by leaving the prosthetic joint located, which allows the anterior capsule to be placed on tension. This technique is initiated by flexing and externally rotating the affected limb (**Figure 3,** *A*). The anterior border of the gluteus medius muscle belly is delineated, and a Cushing elevator is worked under the gluteus medius and the minimus muscle bellies from anterior to posterior (**Figure 3,** *B*). A long cobra retractor is inserted under the psoas tendon on top of the anterior hip pseudocapsule, with the tip resting over the iliopectineal eminence. The anterior border of the vastus lateralis muscle belly is mobilized, and a rake retractor is used to retract the muscle posteriorly. This provides good exposure of the anterior capsule. The first (superior) triangle is created by releasing the capsule along the vastus lateralis from distal to proximal to the level of the Cushing retractor (**Figure 4**). The release is then turned 90° along the anterior rim of the acetabulum toward the tip of the cobra retractor. The base of the triangle is then excised between these two limbs. The inferior triangle of capsule can be excised under direct vision so that any bleeding can be controlled. Following this excision, the surgeon should be able to place his or her fingers from the front and back of the femur and touch them anteriorly to posteriorly. The hip can then be dislocated, and the femoral head removed if it is modular. The tip of a long cobra retractor can be placed underneath the trunnion of the femoral component and then over the anterior superior rim of the acetabulum. With anterior retraction, the femoral component will slide anteriorly, thus affording wide exposure of the acetabulum.

Gluteus Maximus Tendon Release

The gluteus maximus tendon release aids in anterior mobilization of the femur and will decrease pressure on the sciatic nerve, which can occur with anterior mobilization. Some surgeons will initiate the release by placing a tonsil clamp beneath the tendon to protect the sciatic nerve (**Figure 5**). The tendon can be tagged with suture before release to facilitate later repair. The tendon should be divided with a scalpel or an electrocautery device approximately 1 cm lat-

Table 1 **Soft-Tissue Releases**
Anterior Capsulectomy
Very helpful in acetabular revisions in which femoral component is left in situ and needs to be moved anterior to acetabulum.
Place leg in flexion and external rotation.
Place cobra retractor under iliopsoas and over anterior rim of pelvis.
Place Cushing elevator under abductors.
Remove lateral triangle medial to vastus lateralis and transverse across top of acetabulum.
Remove medial triangle inferior to medial aspect of acetabulum.
Gluteus Maximus Tendon Release
Helpful to mobilize femur anteriorly and takes pressure off sciatic nerve.
Sciatic nerve can be identified beneath gluteus maximus tendon.
Protect nerve by placing a tonsil clamp beneath tendon.
Divide tendon 1 cm lateral to the bony insertion.
Two relatively large vessels run in the deep section of tendon and should be coagulated.
Rectus Strip
Helps mobilize the femur anteriorly.
Place cobra retractor underneath the direct and reflected heads of the rectus femoris at the superomedial corner of the acetabulum.
Release the tendon origin from bone with electrocautery to allow the tendon to slide anteriorly.
Abductor Strip
Helps mobilize scarred abductors.
Identify superior margin of acetabulum.
Use curved 0.75-inch osteotome to slide up the iliac wing.
Avoid diving posteriorly into the sciatic notch.

Table 2 **Osteotomies**
Trochanteric
Use when wide exposure to the ilium is needed and the trochanter needs to be mobilized distally to improve abductor tension.
Trochanteric Slide
Use when wide exposure to the ilium is needed and the trochanter will be repaired in the same position.
Takes advantage of the tenodesis effect of the vastus lateralis attachment to prevent migration.
Place Cushing elevator beneath abductors.
Divide the posterior aspect of vastus lateralis and place Bennett retractor under vastus lateralis and over the femur.
Use oscillating saw to divide trochanter from beneath abductor insertion to beneath vastus tubercle.
Mobilize trochanter anteriorly.
Extended Trochanteric
Use when increased exposure of the femur is needed to remove implants or when femur is remodeled into varus.
Template the needed length to ensure that sufficient distal access is created.
Make posterior limb first; score femur 1 cm anterior to the linea aspera.
Make distal limb transversely; a pencil tip burr can be used to round corners.
Start anterior limb from distal to proximal; make drill holes along the line of the fragment parallel to the posterior limb; try to keep muscle attachments intact to fragment.
Distal to proximally, saw approximately one third the distance of the fragment.
Use an osteotome to complete osteotomy in line with the saw cut.
Make sure the distal corners are complete.
Use the two-osteotomes technique to mobilize the fragment from posterior to anterior.
Use particular care when mobilizing the trochanteric junction with the cortical fragment distal to the vastus tubercle.
The osteotomy weakens the femur approximately 60%, so the femur should be carefully mobilized.
Femoral Univalve
Occasionally indicated when a retained femoral stem for extraction needs to be torsionally mobilized for extraction.

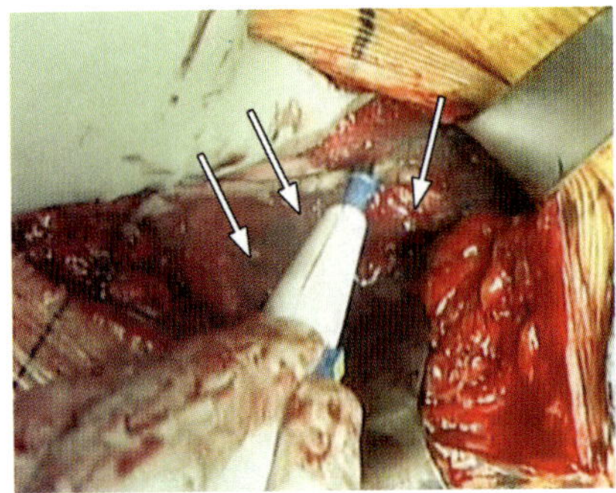

Figure 2 Tagging the posterior pseudocapsule (arrows) facilitates repair and protects the sciatic nerve posteriorly.

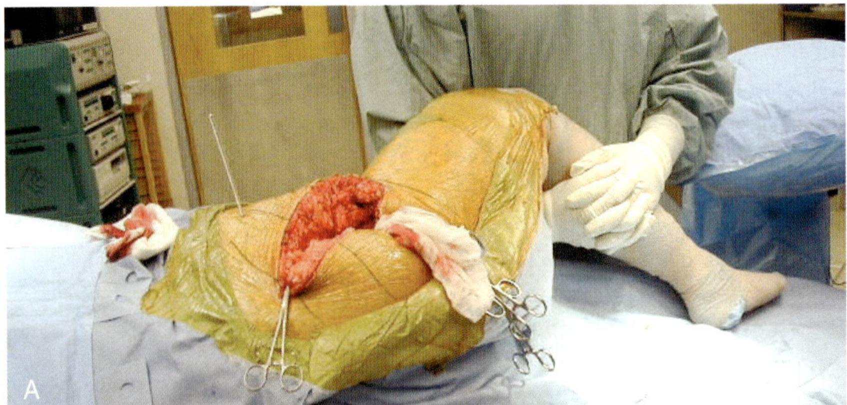

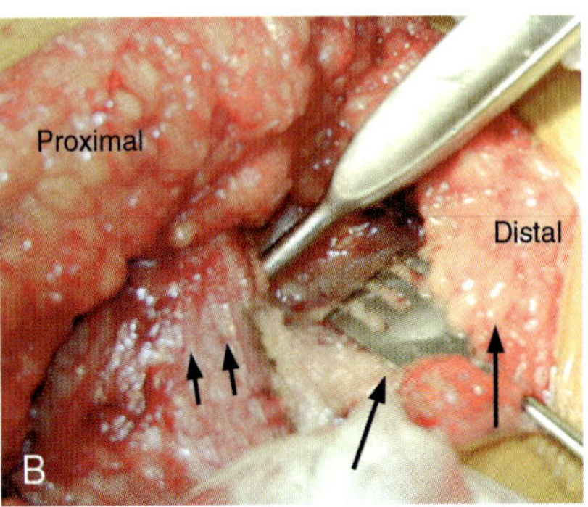

Figure 3 **A,** The capsule is placed on tension by leaving the hip located and flexing and externally rotating the limb. **B,** The anterior capsule is exposed by placing a retractor over the iliopectineal eminence, using a second retractor under the abductor tendons (short arrows), and using a third retractor to pull back the vastus lateralis tendon laterally (long arrows).

eral to the femur. This will facilitate easier repair and also allow control of the two relatively large blood vessels that run in the posterior aspect of the tendon. If exploration of the sciatic nerve is planned proximally, the nerve is located beneath the gluteus tendon.

The Rectus Strip

The rectus strip is used for exposing the superior acetabulum and anterior ilium to facilitate the removal of the acetabular components and the management of anterior bony defects. It allows placement of anterior retractors more medially on the anterior column and protects the anterior rim, which is often weakened and at risk for fracture. It involves releasing the direct head of the rectus femoris in a sliding fashion from anteromedially to posterolaterally. A cobra retractor is placed under the proximal femur and on the ilium superior and anterior to the socket (**Figure 6,** *A*). This placement puts the direct head of the rectus femoris under tension and will allow a window to slide a scalpel or electrocautery under the tendon and release it in a sliding fashion directly off its origin. Once the tendon is released, the surgeon can place the cobra retractor under the tendon in the iliac bone at the superior aspect of the acetabulum.

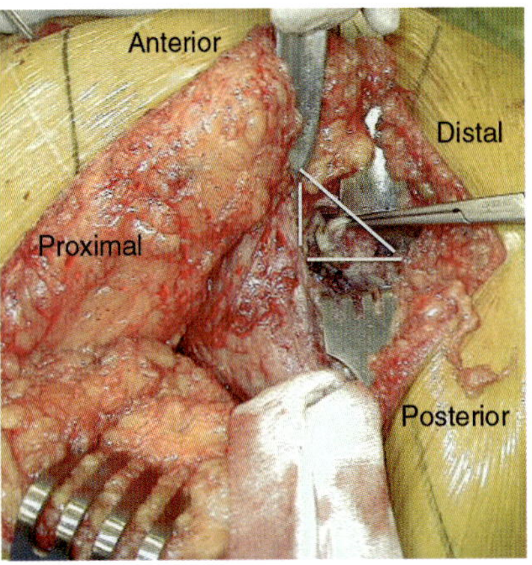

Figure 4 The first triangle of the anterior capsulotomy is excised. The margin of the inferior limb is just anterior to the vastus lateralis muscle belly, and the cephalad limb divides the capsule along the anterior rim of the socket.

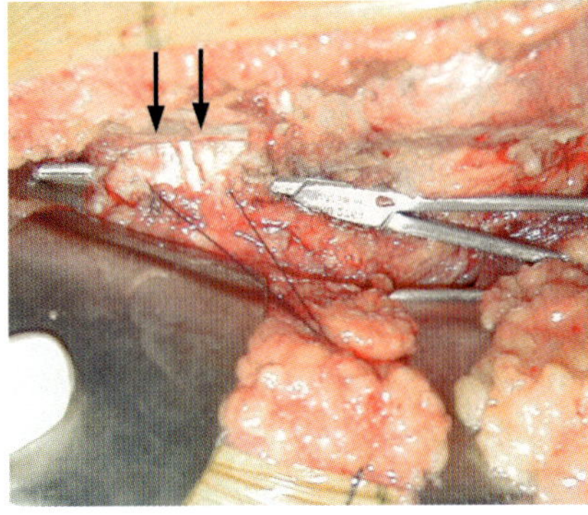

Figure 5 The gluteus maximus tendon (arrows) is isolated by placing a tonsil clamp beneath it; the sciatic nerve is protected inferiorly.

The Abductor Strip

The abductor strip is used to expose the ilium for grafting or hardware placement or mobilize a proximally migrated hip or trochanteric fragment. It releases the muscle belly from its undersurface because the innervation of the muscle belly comes from the other side. The muscle belly may be released all the way to its origin on the iliac crest. The release starts just above the acetabulum, using a 0.75-inch curved osteotome or broad Cobb elevator beneath the muscle, directed in an anterosuperior fashion (**Figure 6,** *B*). Care should be taken to prevent the instrument from sliding into the sciatic

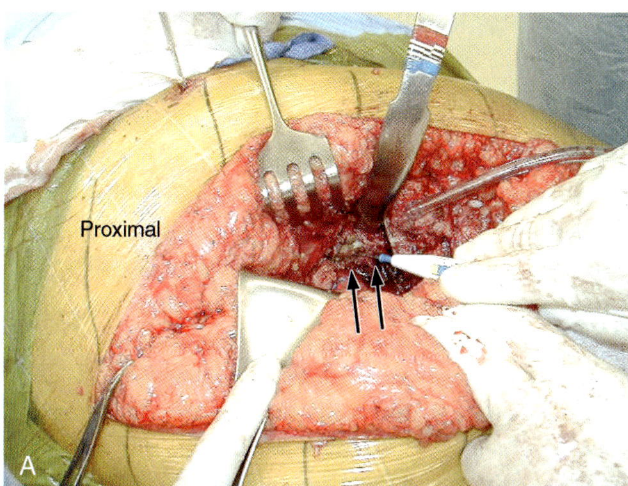

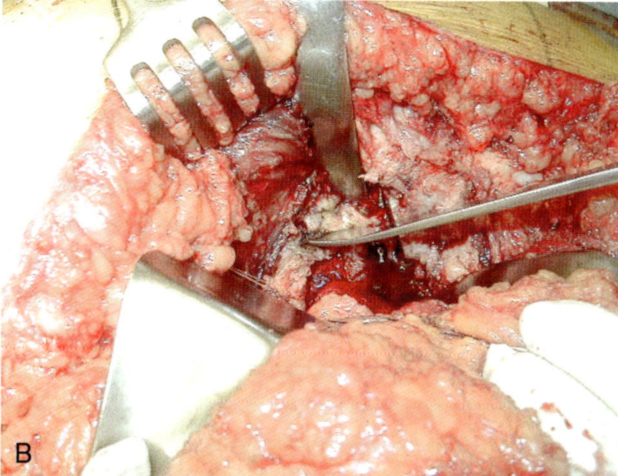

Figure 6 **A,** Sliding a retractor anterior and superior to the socket will place the anterior capsule and the direct head of the rectus femoris under tension (arrows) and allow them to be released in a sliding fashion. **B,** After a space is made between the superior edge of the socket and the rectus tendon, a curved osteotome can slide on bone to the top of the ilium. Caution is needed to prevent the osteotome from sliding posteriorly into the sciatic notch.

notch, which should be palpated before beginning the release. If a trochanteric fragment is present, it can be grasped with a bone-holding clamp, and distal traction can be placed on the fragment to aid in the release. In the case of extreme contracture, if this maneuver does not provide sufficient release, the abductor enthesis may be released from the iliac crest, and the entire muscle belly can be allowed to slide distally.

Osteotomies

A trochanteric osteotomy allows excellent exposure of the hip and femur; however, a trochanteric osteotomy should be used only when it provides clear advantages over soft-tissue releases alone (**Table 3**). The most common osteotomies are the traditional trochanteric osteotomy, the trochanteric slide, and the extended trochanteric osteotomy.[4] Less commonly used but occasionally helpful are the femoral univalve and the femoral window osteotomies.

Traditional Trochanteric

The traditional trochanteric osteotomy detaches the greater trochanter from its distal attachments (the origin of the vastus lateralis muscle belly). It helps provide wide exposure to the acetabulum and also exposes the lateral side of the femoral endosteum to facilitate component exposure. This osteotomy is particularly suited for situations in which the trochanter must be advanced distally. Because of the orientation of the abductor muscles inserting into the proximal greater trochanter, the osteotomized fragment should be reflected proximally and anteriorly. The femur can usually be retracted either anteriorly or posteriorly. The osteotomy is started by templating the obliquity of the cut; a more transverse cut is used if the plan is to advance the trochanter, and a more vertical and superficial cut is used if the fragment is to be placed back onto the bed. The proximal aspect of the trochanter and the inserting abductor tendons should be differentiated from adjacent scar tissue. A Cushing retractor can be placed from anterior to posterior underneath the abductor tendons to delineate the proximal aspect of the osteotomy and protect the tendons from the saw. Distally, the vastus lateralis should be detached from the vastus tubercle. The distal aspect of the osteotomy should come through the tubercle after the muscle is retracted. The osteotomy is repaired by using a four-wire technique (two vertical and two horizontal wires), by horizontal wires or cables, or by using a trochanteric claw device. The healing rate of traditional trochanteric osteotomies in older series was approximately 90% the first time it was repaired, but the rate decreased significantly (to 50% or less) on subsequent attempts at repair.[5]

Table 3
Indications for Osteotomy[a]

Remove solidly ingrown femoral component.
Remove solid cement mantle.
Bypass femoral deformity.
Need to retract abductors for wide exposure to the ilium.
Need to tighten abductor tension.

[a]Because osteotomy adds surgical time and puts the femur at risk for injury, it should be done only for sound indications.

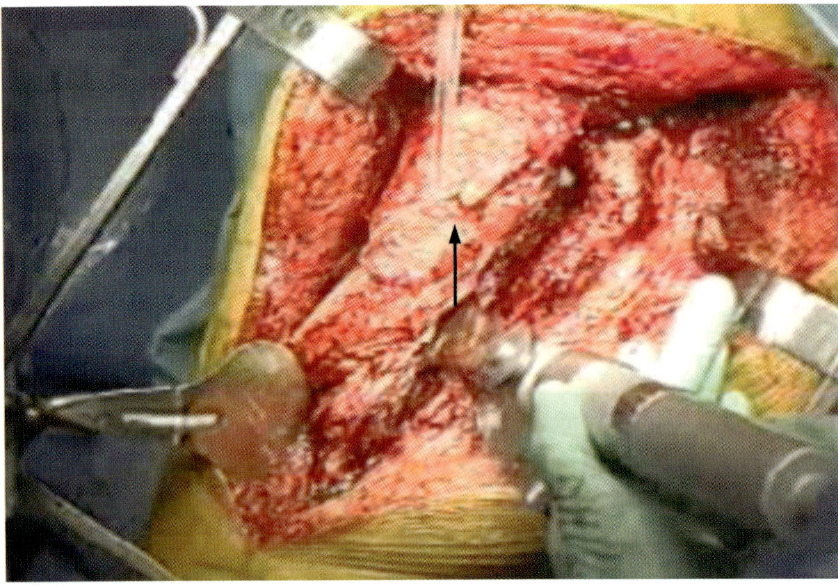

Figure 7 A Bennett retractor is placed beneath the vastus lateralis (arrow) to protect it as the posterior limb of the osteotomy is made through the femur with an oscillating saw. (Courtesy of C. Andrew Engh Jr, MD, Alexandria, VA.)

Trochanteric Slide

The trochanteric slide osteotomy was devised to preserve the distal attachment of the vastus lateralis, which likely improves the blood supply to the fragment and helps function as a tether to prevent proximal migration of the trochanter.[6-8] The only modification from the traditional osteotomy is that the posterior aspect of the vastus lateralis is mobilized just anterior to the intramuscular septum, and a Bennett retractor is used to retract the proximal portion of the muscle anteriorly, which protects the muscle as the osteotomy is made (**Figure 7**). This osteotomy is more appropriate when the trochanter will be repaired in situ and not advanced. Fixation is usually performed with horizontal wires or cables.

Extended Trochanteric

The extended trochanteric osteotomy was popularized by Paprosky in the 1990s to improve access to the femur for removing femoral components and providing more predictable healing of the trochanteric fragment.[9] Because this type of osteotomy weakens the femur to torsional stress by up to 70%, it should be used only with clear indications.[10] The extended trochanteric osteotomy is indicated to allow access to extensively ingrown femoral components or the removal of distal cement, or when varus remodeling of the proximal femur makes placement of a new femoral component very difficult or impossible.

Because the femur is often encased in scar tissue during a revision surgery, the scar tissue should be released and the hip dislocated before starting the osteotomy. If this is not done, there is risk that the remaining femur will fracture as the limb is manipulated to dislocate the hip after the osteotomy. The osteotomy can be planned to include the lateral one third of the femoral circumference or as a more anterior (Wagner type) osteotomy. The Wagner osteotomy is performed 90° more anterior than the traditional extended trochanteric osteotomy and is easier to accomplish when using a Hardinge approach. Because the average femur has a circumference of 6 to 8 cm, an osteotomy width of 2 to 2.5 cm provides sufficient access to the femur without markedly weakening it. The osteotomy can be templated with a 2-mm drill bit. It generally starts just anterior to the posterior intermuscular septum and progresses proximally to the posterior aspect of the greater trochanter and distally to the point that the surgeon determines will provide adequate access to the femoral component for extraction. The osteotomy is then turned 90° anteriorly for a distance of 2 to 2.5 cm and then turned 90° proximal and directed to the anterior aspect of the greater trochanter. Because the fibers of the vastus lateralis originate from this fragment (and presumably carry some of the blood supply), they should be preserved if possible. Consequently, once the anterior limb of the osteotomy has been started for a distance of 4 cm, a straight osteotome can be placed in the osteotomy track underneath the vastus lateralis fibers and impacted toward the anterior aspect of the trochanter (**Figure 8**). After the cortex is divided, the surgeon should ensure that the corners are mobilized. Then, using two wide osteotomes (one proximal and one distal) placed into the posterior limb of the osteotomy, the fragment should be slowly and carefully elevated. If there is extensive bony attachment to the undersurface of the fragment, a curved osteotome is used to gently disrupt the attachment to the underlying cement or prosthesis. The fragment can then be mobilized anteriorly, which provides wide exposure to the acetabulum.

Repair of the osteotomy is usually accomplished with three cables or wires. The proximal wire can be threaded through drill holes in the greater trochanter and passed inferior to the lesser trochanter. The other two wires are evenly spaced between the

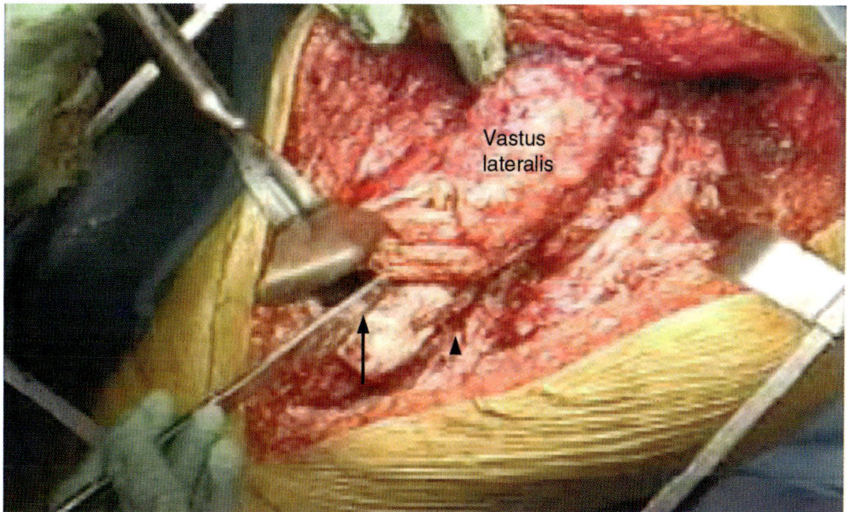

Figure 8 A straight osteotome is placed in the anterior limb (arrow) of the osteotomy from distal to proximal to complete the osteotomy without damaging the overlying muscle fibers. The posterior limb is indicated by the arrowhead. (Courtesy of C. Andrew Engh Jr, MD, Alexandria, VA.)

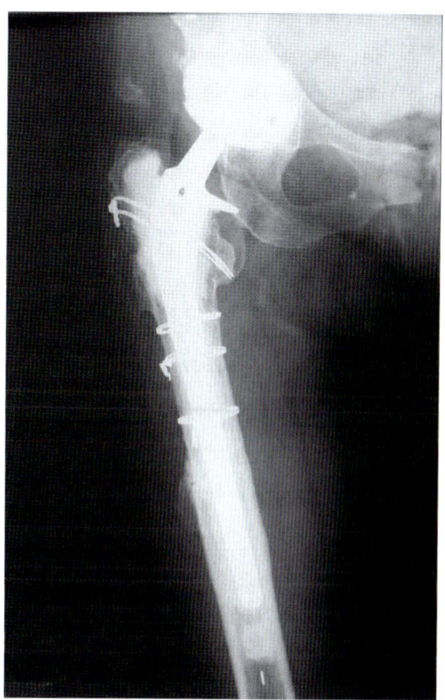

Figure 9 The wire location for repair of the osteotomy is shown. Three or four 18-gauge stainless steel wires or cables are equally spaced. The proximal wire must go under the lesser trochanter and through drill holes in the greater trochanter.

vastus tubercle and the end of the osteotomy fragment (**Figure 9**).

Femoral Univalve

The femoral univalve osteotomy is accomplished by first making the posterior cut of an extended trochanteric osteotomy. If the femoral component is somewhat loose or has fibrous ingrowth, this osteotomy often allows the surgeon to rotate the stem within the canal. The length of the single femoral cut should be close in length to the femoral component that will be removed. The femoral component can then be tapped out in a retrograde fashion. If the univalve is not sufficient to mobilize the femoral component, the remainder of the extended trochanteric osteotomy can be completed.

Femoral Window

The femoral window osteotomy can be an effective procedure for removing a well-fixed cement plug, a distal modular component of a femoral stem, or a broken portion of a femoral component.[11] It also can be helpful in revision surgery to monitor the preparation of the femoral canal. The size of the window should be templated preoperatively; several biomechanical studies have suggested that the anterior third of the femoral cortex causes the least amount of femoral weakening.[11,12]

Summary

Because each revision total hip replacement is unique, the surgeon must consider the previous approaches used, which components require revision, and what defects need to be addressed. Despite the best preparation, unplanned events can occur. The surgeon should be prepared to enhance the surgical exposure with a combination of bony and soft-tissue procedures.

References

1. Masterson EL, Masri BA, Duncan CP: Surgical approaches in revision hip replacement. *J Am Acad Orthop Surg* 1998;6(2):84-92.
2. Taylor JW, Rorabeck CH: Hip revision arthroplasty: Approach to the femoral side. *Clin Orthop Relat Res* 1999;369:208-222.
3. Spangehl MJ, Masri BA, O'Connell JX, Duncan CP: Prospective analysis of preoperative and intraoperative investigations for the diagnosis of infection at the sites of two hundred and two revision total hip arthroplasties. *J Bone Joint Surg Am* 1999;81(5): 672-683.
4. Masri BA, Campbell DG, Garbuz DS, Duncan CP: Seven specialized exposures for revision hip and knee replacement. *Orthop Clin North Am* 1998;29(2):229-240.
5. Glassman AH: Complications of trochanteric osteotomy. *Orthop Clin North Am* 1992;23(2): 321-333.
6. Engh CA Jr, McAuley JP, Engh CS Sr: Surgical approaches for revision total hip replacement surgery: The anterior trochanteric

slide and the extended conventional osteotomy. *Instr Course Lect* 1999;48:3-8.

7. Glassman AH, Engh CA, Bobyn JD: Proximal femoral osteotomy as an adjunct in cementless revision total hip arthroplasty. *J Arthroplasty* 1987;2(1):47-63.
8. Glassman AH, Engh CA, Bobyn JD: A technique of extensile exposure for total hip arthroplasty. *J Arthroplasty* 1987;2(1):11-21.
9. Miner TM, Momberger NG, Chong D, Paprosky WL: The extended trochanteric osteotomy in revision hip arthroplasty: A critical review of 166 cases at mean 3-year, 9-month follow-up. *J Arthroplasty*. 2001;16(8, Suppl 1):188-194.
10. Noble AR, Branham DB, Willis MC, et al: Mechanical effects of the extended trochanteric osteotomy. *J Bone Joint Surg Am* 2005;87(3):521-529.
11. Kerry RM, Masri BA, Garbuz DS, Duncan CP: The vascularized scaphoid window for access to the femoral canal in revision total hip arthroplasty. *Instr Course Lect* 1999;48:9-11.
12. Klein AH, Rubash HE: Femoral windows in revision total hip arthroplasty. *Clin Orthop Relat Res* 1993;291:164-170.

Revision Total Hip Arthroplasty for Instability: Surgical Techniques and Principles

*Javad Parvizi, MD, FRCS
*Elizabeth Picinic, BS
*Peter F. Sharkey, MD

Abstract

Instability is one of the most common complications after total hip arthroplasty. Fortunately, instability usually occurs as a single episode and can successfully be treated nonsurgically in many instances. However, recurrent instability may require surgical treatment. Although many studies related to instability exist, the etiology and the optimal management of recurrent instability are not well known and continue to be investigated. It is important to understand the principles of management and surgical techniques for the treatment of recurrent instability, including the use of constrained liners.

Total hip arthroplasty is one of the most successful orthopaedic procedures and is highly effective in relieving pain and improving function.[1-3] Unfortunately, some patients have complications, with dislocation being one of the most common.[4-8] Dislocation occurs after 0.3% to 10% of primary total hip arthroplasties and after up to 28% of revision total hip arthroplasties.[4-26] The risk of dislocation is influenced by the surgical approach, the underlying diagnosis, the surgical technique, the lifetime of the prosthesis, and the patient's compliance with restrictions.[6,7,25,27-31] An improved understanding of the etiology of dislocation and refinements in surgical techniques have led to a decrease in the rate of dislocation over time.[1,5,6,8,10,19,20,28,32-35] Although most dislocations after total hip arthroplasty are single episodes that can be managed nonsurgically, some patients require surgical intervention to address recurrent dislocation.[7,8,26,28,35]

The choice of surgical technique to manage recurrent dislocation depends on the etiology of the problem.[36] Revision arthroplasty for the treatment of recurrent dislocation is more likely to be successful when a cause for the dislocation has been identified.[26,35] In addition, the timing of the onset of the dislocation influences the decision concerning treatment, especially with regard to surgical intervention.[37,38] Early dislocations—that is, those occurring within a few days to months after the index surgery—are unlikely to recur[26] and are much more likely to respond favorably to nonsurgical measures.[37] Component malpositioning and abductor insufficiency are two of the most important recognized causes of recurrent dislocation.[5,8,19,26,28,39] When malpositioning is the cause, revision of the component is the most effective type of surgical intervention.[6,26,35,39] However, when the etiology of the dislocation is multifactorial or unknown, the best surgical technique for addressing it is often less obvious. The surgical options available for the treatment of recurrent dislocation consist of component revision,[4,16,35,39,40] modular component exchange,[41-44] bipolar arthroplasty,[22,45] use of a larger femoral head,[46-48] soft-tissue reinforcement,[17,30,32,35,49,50] advancement of

Javad Parvizi, MD, FRCS, Elizabeth Picinic, BS, and Peter F. Sharkey, MD or the departments with which they are affiliated have received research or institutional support from Stryker.

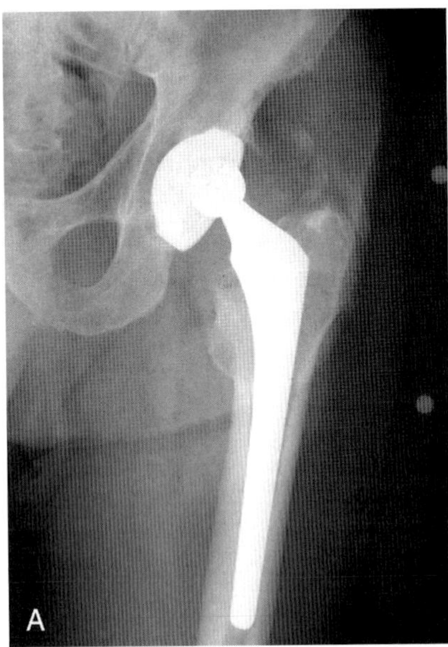

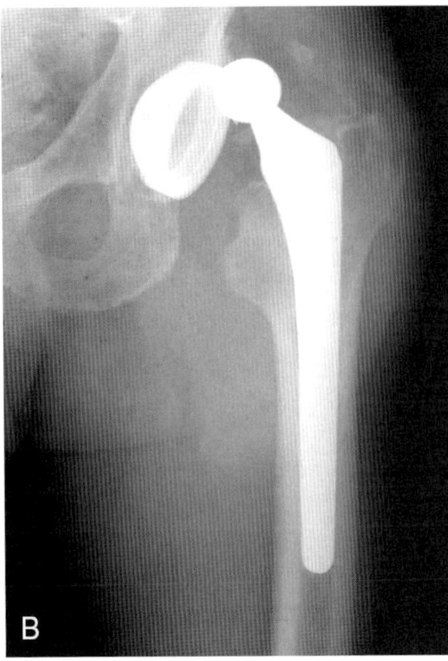

Figure 1 Dislocation following total hip arthroplasty can occur at any time. **A,** AP radiograph made 12 years following a hip arthroplasty. Polyethylene wear is made evident by eccentric seating of the femoral head inside the acetabular liner. **B,** The polyethylene wear was deemed to be responsible for the dislocation in this patient.

the greater trochanter,[11,51] and use of a constrained liner.[9,12,24,33,52-54]

Classification of Dislocation

For treatment purposes, dislocation after total hip arthroplasty can be categorized as early or late on the basis of the timing of the onset.[37,38] Early dislocation usually occurs in the early postoperative period (for example, within 6 months) after the arthroplasty and is often successfully treated with nonsurgical means. In contrast, late dislocation occurs after 5 years and generally requires surgical treatment.[37] Dislocations occurring between 6 months and 5 years may be categorized as intermediate. This temporal classification is useful because it highlights the differences in the etiology of the dislocation in each category, which in turn determine the type of treatment that is selected. Early to intermediate dislocations are usually the result of older age, female gender (muscular laxity), and cognitive or neurologic impairment. In addition, some factors, including a preoperative diagnosis of femoral neck fracture, osteonecrosis of the femoral head, or inflammatory arthritis, may predispose the patient to early dislocation.[6,27,55,56] Late dislocation has a multifactorial etiology that can include polyethylene (bearing surface) wear (Figure 1), deterioration in muscle mass, neurologic impairment, and fractures (such as trochanteric avulsion as a result of wear and osteolysis). Additional predisposing factors for late dislocation include younger age (greater wear), female gender (muscle laxity), unrecognized component malpositioning, and prosthesis-bone impingement as a result of a change in body habitus (weight loss). The incidence of late dislocation may be greater than initially appreciated,[28,37,57,58] and late dislocations account for one third of all dislocations.[37] In addition, their cumulative rate increases with longer follow-up, with reported rates of 1% at 1 month and 1.9% at 1 year, a constant rate of 1% every 5 years, and a 7% rate at 25 years.[27]

Although most dislocations, particularly those in the early to intermediate category, can be treated nonsurgically, the etiology of the dislocation dictates the most appropriate treatment modality.

Surgical Techniques

Surgical options for the treatment of recurrent dislocation include revision of component(s); exchange of modular components such as the acetabular liner and the femoral head; bipolar arthroplasty, which allows motion between the femoral head and the acetabular liner and also between the acetabular liner and the native acetabular cavity; tripolar arthroplasty, which involves placement of a bipolar prosthesis against an acetabular shell; use of a larger femoral head; soft-tissue reinforcement; advancement of the greater trochanter; and use of a constrained liner.

Revision Arthroplasty

As mentioned previously, component malpositioning is one of the primary causes of recurrent dislocation, and component revision can successfully treat this type of dislocation.[3,5,19,26,28,39] Identifying the malpositioned component is not always straightforward. Plain radiographs provide limited information regarding the orientation of the acetabular and femoral components. Hence, CT may be needed to more accurately assess component positioning, especially with regard to version of the acetabulum (Figure 2).[59] Although subtle component malpositioning is difficult to detect on plain radiographs, the radiographs of a dislocated hip should be scrutinized carefully. In addition to showing the direction of the dislocation, these radiographs can convey other important information (Figure 3). Other critical parameters, such as abductor strength and the overall neurologic status of the patient, can be gleaned from clinical examination. Limb-length discrepancy detected on clinical or radiographic examination can be an important finding as it can be associated with component malpositioning[60] because intraoperative instability, which may have been caused by a suboptimally positioned component such as a retroverted socket, may have been addressed by lengthening of the femoral neck to increase the soft-tissue tension (Figure 4). Correction of the malpositioned component can simultaneously correct the limb-length inequality. The ultimate and most accurate information regarding component positioning is obtained from intraoperative inspection of the components during revision surgery. If the component is confirmed to be malpositioned, it should be revised to address the recurrent dislocation. An exception may be made for any frail, elderly, or infirm patient, in whom a slightly malpositioned component may be accepted to prevent prolonged surgery for revision of a well-fixed acetabular or femoral component. In these patients, a constrained liner may be used in an effort to prevent recurrent dislocations.

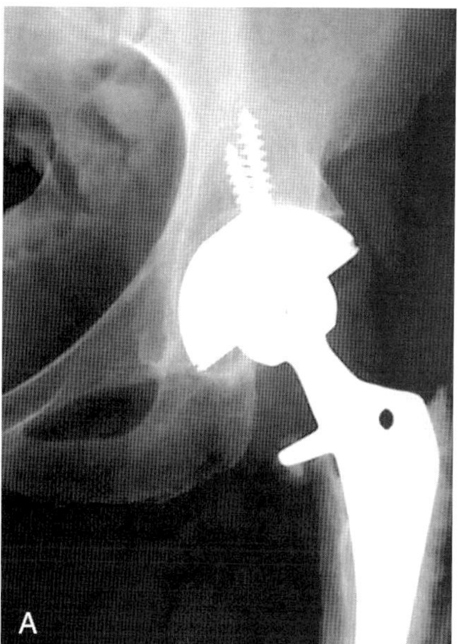

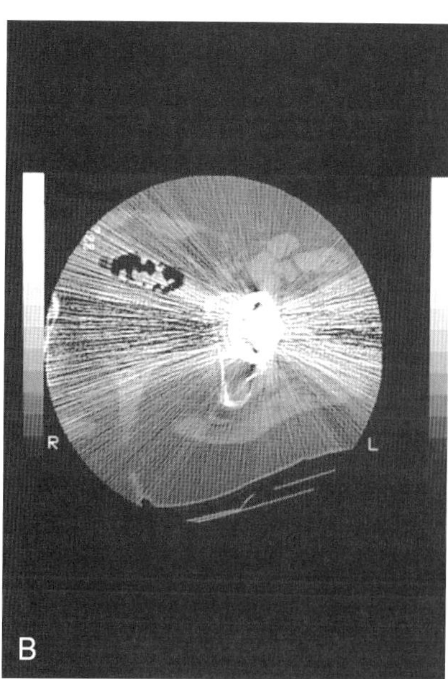

Figure 2 **A,** The components appear to be well positioned on the AP radiograph of the hip of a patient with recurrent dislocation. **B,** CT of the same hip, however, confirms a retroverted acetabular component. Revision of the acetabular component alone in this case was adequate to address the episodes of recurrent dislocation.

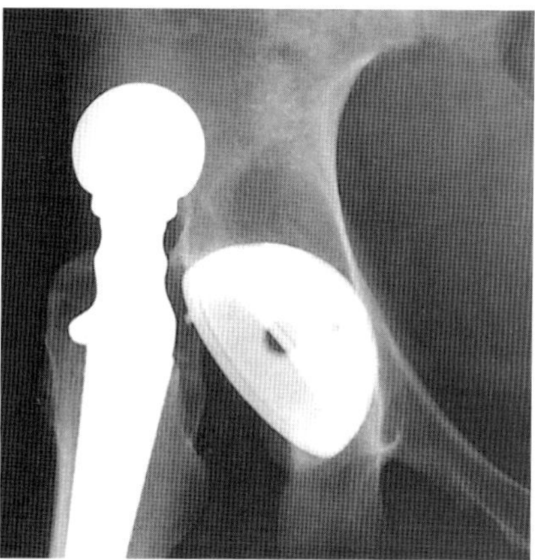

Figure 3 Close scrutiny of the radiographs of a dislocated total hip replacement may be very useful. The retroverted femoral component seen on this radiograph (and confirmed intraoperatively) was the cause of recurrent dislocation in this patient.

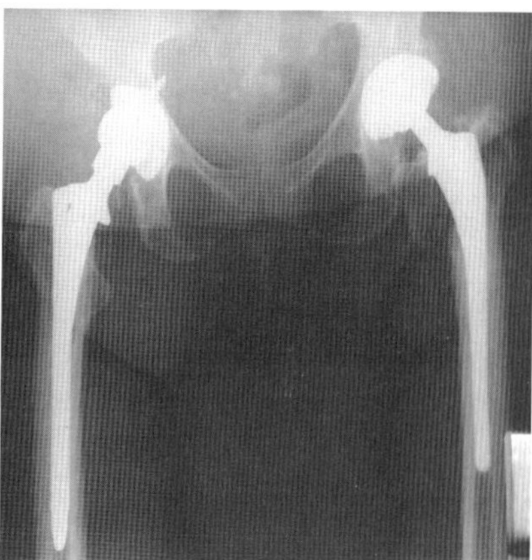

Figure 4 Suboptimal positioning of the components may lead to intraoperative instability, which may be addressed by increasing the soft-tissue tension, resulting in limb-length discrepancy. A vertical and retroverted acetabular component causing intraoperative instability in the right hip of this patient led to the use of a longer femoral neck, resulting in a marked limb-length discrepancy.

Modular Component Exchange

This surgical treatment involves exchanging the acetabular liner and the femoral head, with the main intention being to "upsize" the femoral head and/or use an elevated liner. This treatment can be successful only if the patient has well-positioned and well-fixed acetabular and femoral components. In addition, the acetabular component in place must be sufficiently large to allow an adequate thickness of polyethylene (a minimum of 4 mm) to be used with the larger femoral head. Several studies have demonstrated success with the use of modular component exchange for the correction of recurrent dislocation after total hip arthroplasty.[41-43]

Toomey and associates[41] described a series of 13 patients treated with exchange of the femoral head and/or acetabular liner. One patient was lost to follow-up, and only 1 of the remaining 12 patients had recurrent dislocation at a mean of 5.8 years; thus, this surgical treatment had a success rate of 92%, with less extensive morbidity. However, the authors recommended that modular component exchange be used in only selected cases and that each patient be evaluated thoroughly to identify all factors contributing to the dislocation. Additionally, adequate intraoperative stability must be achieved. Despite the success reported by Toomey and associates, modular components can be problematic. In a report on complications related to 20 hip replacements, Barrack and associates[44] described 15 complications that were related to failure of the modular interface. Complications were attributed to detachment of the femoral head from the trunnion, dislodgment of the polyethylene liner from the shell, and asymmetric rotation of the polyethylene liner. Thus, modular component exchange requires meticulous surgical technique and should be reserved for specific cases.

Bipolar or Tripolar Arthroplasty

Bipolar arthroplasty also has been used as a means of correcting recurrent dislocation.[22,45] The bipolar device is composed of a small femoral head housed inside a polyethylene shell that is covered by a larger femoral head. Theoretically, there is motion at the interface between the smaller femoral head and the polyethylene liner and also between the larger femoral head and the native acetabulum. Placement of the bipolar prosthesis inside an acetabular component with a liner is known as tripolar arthroplasty. The large femoral head and the potential for motion at two interfaces account for the high rate of success of this prosthesis in addressing recurrent instability. Grigoris and associates[46] first described the use of a large bipolar head articulating with a large acetabular shell, also known as tripolar arthroplasty, to treat recurrent dislocation. In their series of eight patients, none had dislocations at a mean of 4.2 years (range, 2.6 to 6.3 years). Ries and Wiedel[22] reported success after using a bipolar prosthesis in three patients who had had recurrent dislocations after failure of multiple surgical procedures to address the problem. Parvizi and Morrey[45] reported the outcomes of bipolar revision total hip arthroplasty for the treatment of recurrent dislocation in a series of 27 patients. Prior to the bipolar hip arthroplasty, all patients had undergone at least two, and a mean of three, stabilizing surgical procedures on the affected hip. At a mean of 5 years after the bipolar arthroplasties, 22 patients (81%) had not had a redislocation. The remaining five patients had had episodes of subluxation or dislocation after the bipolar arthroplasty. Two of the five patients had had only one episode of dislocation, which was treated successfully with immobilization. Two of the remaining three patients required a revision to address continuing dislocation. A constrained liner was used in one patient, and a resection arthroplasty was performed in the second patient. The third patient had continued dislocation episodes but had improved function and pain relief, so a revision was not performed. These studies demonstrate the role of bipolar hip arthroplasty in the salvage management of recurrent dislocation. There are, however, problems associated with the use of bipolar arthroplasty, the most important of which is the potential for medial or superior migration of the prosthesis with time. In addition, groin pain appears to be a frequent problem associated with the use of this prosthesis. Because of these problems, we do not use bipolar arthroplasty as a main-line treatment of recurrent dislocation.

Large Femoral Head

The arc of motion required to dislocate a prosthetic head is directly related to the diameter of the head. Therefore, with larger femoral heads, a greater volume of the head needs to be displaced from the acetabulum for dislocation to occur. Because of this, large femoral heads have been used as a surgical treatment modality to address recurrent dislocation. Beaulé and associates[47] reported on the use of a jumbo femoral head to treat recurrent dislocation in a group of 12 patients who had had an average of four previous operations after an average of seven dislocations. These patients underwent revision total hip arthroplasty with the use of a femoral head with an average diameter of 44 mm (range, 40 to 50 mm). A bipolar head articulating with a fixed socket (a tripolar construct) was used in 10 hips, and a modular head (unipolar) was used in the other two hips. After an average duration of follow-up of 6.5 years (range, 3.2 to 11.8 years), 10 hips had had no additional episodes of dislocation. One hip had dislocated within 1 week after the revision total hip arthroplasty, necessitating revision surgery to reposition the acetabular component. The 12th hip remained stable; however, the patient died 14 months postoperatively of unrelated causes.

Amstutz and associates[48] described the use of a jumbo head in

29 patients with recurrent dislocations. They noted that, in addition to the larger femoral head, reorientation of the bearing surface was required in most patients. Although the early use of jumbo femoral heads has been successful, the downside to the use of a very large femoral head is the necessity to simultaneously insert a thin polyethylene liner. In addition, the longevity of total hip prostheses with a jumbo head has not been determined.

Soft-Tissue Reinforcement and Advancement of the Greater Trochanter

Other, currently less used surgical procedures for addressing recurrent dislocation include reinforcement of the soft tissues—namely, the abductor mechanism—around the hip and trochanteric advancement.[11,51] The main problem associated with these procedures is the variability in outcome.[11,17,30,32,35,49-51] These procedures can also be technically demanding and are likely to fail if used in patients with component malpositioning. Therefore, soft-tissue reinforcement and trochanteric advancement are being used with less frequency and only in cases in which component position has been absolutely determined to be acceptable. Additionally, these procedures should be reserved for patients who are poor candidates for other options such as the use of a constrained liner. For example, soft-tissue enhancement should be considered for a young, high-demand patient or a patient with a well-fixed cemented acetabular component in whom other options cannot be used.

Constrained Liners

The constrained acetabular liner is an invaluable tool in the armamentarium for surgical treatment of recurrent dislocations. Its success has been widely demonstrated.[9,12,24,33,52-54] This device is especially suited for the treatment of recurrent dislocation secondary to soft-tissue (abductor) deficiency. It is also an excellent option for patients with recurrent dislocation of unknown etiology, elderly patients in whom the components are well fixed, and patients with neurologic impairment. In other words, constrained liners are used as a salvage treatment option in the most difficult subset of cases. To our knowledge, Anderson and associates[9] were the first to describe the use of constrained liners in patients with recurrent dislocation. They reported a success rate of 72% in a study of 18 patients followed for a mean of 31 months (range, 24 to 64 months) after the use of this device. Disassembly and disengagement of the Arthropor II constrained component (Joint Medical Products, Stamford, CT) accounted for four of the six failures. The only factor predictive of failure was an increased acetabular abduction angle of the metallic acetabular cup. At the time of follow-up, there was no radiographic or clinical evidence of loosening of the acetabular component.

One of the main advantages of a constrained liner is its ability to provide stability without the need to revise a well-fixed and well-positioned acetabular component. Callaghan and associates[34] reported the clinical and radiographic outcomes of 31 revision total hip arthroplasties in which a constrained liner had been cemented into a well-fixed cementless acetabular shell. At an average of 3.9 years postoperatively, 29 constrained liners (94%) remained securely fixed in the cementless shell, and only 2 liners had failed. One of the failed liners had separated from the cement, and the other had failed as a result of fracture of the capturing mechanism. Each hip was successfully revised with another cemented constrained liner. No acetabular component showed radiographic evidence of progressive loosening or associated osteolysis. The authors drew attention to the importance of proper preparation of the liner, correct sizing of the component, and the use of optimal cementing technique. Their meticulous surgical technique may explain the good results despite the suboptimal outcomes of this technique in other studies.[8,13] This study demonstrated favorable short-term outcomes following cementing of a constrained tripolar liner, but the authors stressed that the shell must be secure and well positioned.

The use of a constrained liner for the treatment of recurrent dislocations can be rewarding when no discrete cause for the dislocations can be identified or when the dislocations are deemed to be caused by soft-tissue deficiency. It is critical that, before using a constrained liner, the surgeon ensure that the components are well positioned and that subtle malpositioning is not the cause of the dislocation. Assessment of component positioning may require preoperative CT and close scrutiny during surgery.

Surgical Technique

There are some important technical details that need to be kept in mind during implantation of a constrained liner to maximize the success of this procedure. The acetabular component needs to be well exposed, and the previous liner must be removed to allow assessment of the positioning of the component. Any previously placed screws also need to be removed to allow testing of the fixa-

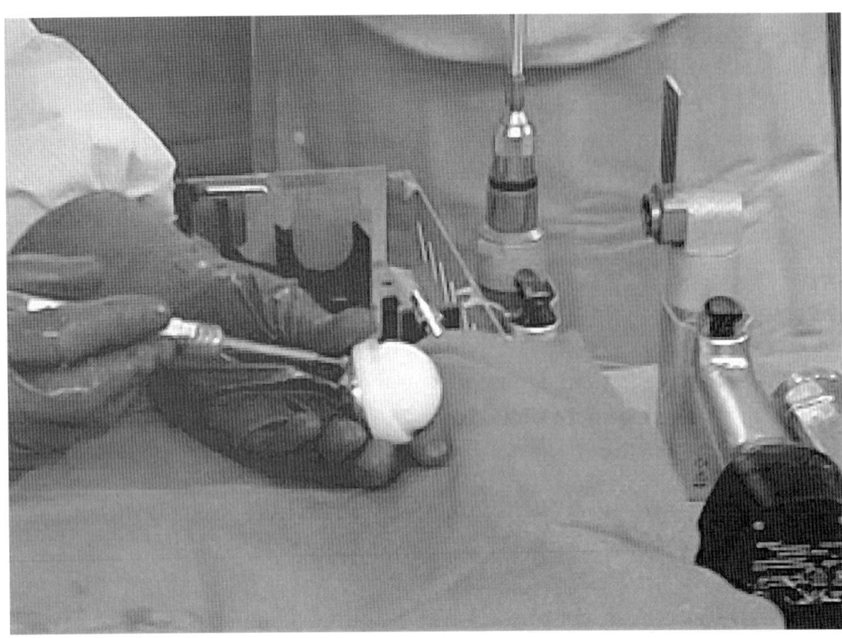

Figure 5 Meticulous attention to detail is pertinent when a constrained liner is being cemented into a well-fixed acetabular liner. Removing the circumferential ring and scoring the back of the constrained liner in a "spider web" manner is being performed here to allow locking of the cement between the liner and the shell.

tion of the acetabular component. If the acetabular liner is well fixed and the locking mechanism is intact, then a matching constrained liner may be snapped into place. When the cup has a suboptimal or nonfunctioning locking mechanism, a constrained liner may be cemented in place. With the introduction of modularity, the latter option is becoming more feasible. It is, however, critical that the retained acetabular component be large enough to allow an adequate cement mantle around the constrained liner. Acetabular shells with polished inner surfaces and no screw holes may be scored in a "spider web" pattern (Figure 5). The cement is pressurized to force it into the screw holes. Then the constrained liner is inserted, with the surgeon making sure that it is seated within the shell while simultaneously trying to prevent it from bottoming out. Usually, 2 mm of cement mantle is optimal. In comparison with revision of the acetabular component, cementation of a constrained liner decreases surgical time, decreases blood loss, and does not compromise acetabular bone stock. Cementation of a constrained liner into a secure cementless shell provides a suitable solution to the problem of recurrent total hip dislocation.

Problems With Acetabular Liners

Although constrained acetabular liners have become popular for treating recurrent dislocation, problems related to premature wear, increased radiolucency, and dislodgment of these liners still remain a major concern.[52] Shrader and associates[52] evaluated the clinical and radiographic outcomes of 110 constrained-liner arthroplasties, 79 of which had been done for the treatment of recurrent dislocation and 31 of which had been performed to address absent or grossly deficient soft-tissue attachments noted at the revision total hip arthroplasty. Ninety-eight percent (108) of these revisions were successful, with no subsequent hip dislocation. Only two patients continued to have sensations of subluxation. Radiographic analysis revealed radiolucent lines around the cup in 15 hips (14%). There were nine revisions: six due to deep infection, two due to loosening of the acetabular component, and one due to periprosthetic fracture of the femur. Over time, the increased stresses on an acetabular cup housing a constrained liner theoretically may cause a high rate of loosening and failure. It was noted that most patients in this study had undergone multiple prior reconstructive procedures, which in some cases had resulted in bone and soft-tissue deficiency. In addition, some of the patients were treated with acetabular bone grafting at the time of the revision operation. Therefore, it is conceivable that the high rate of radiolucency observed in this patient population was due to many factors and was not solely related to the use of the constrained cup.

Cooke and associates[53] identified three types of early failure of a constrained acetabular implant (Figure 6). In their series, 58 patients underwent revision with use of the constrained acetabular implant for various reasons, including recurrent dislocation (46 patients), reimplantation following a Girdlestone resection (8 patients), correction of limb-length discrepancy (3 patients), and periprosthetic fracture (1 patient). Forty-nine of the constrained acetabular components were inserted into a cementless shell, six were cemented into a preexisting cement-

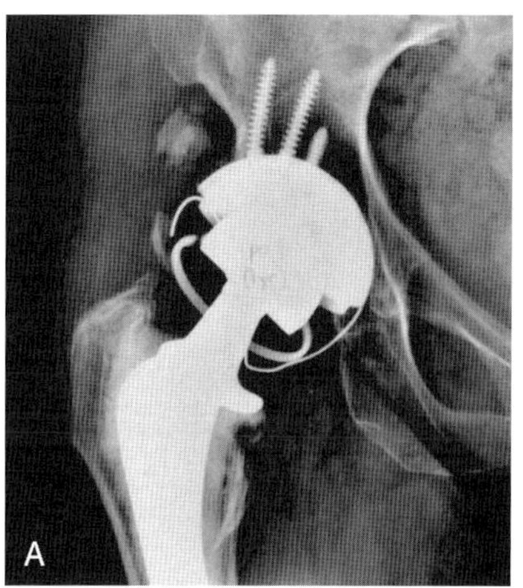

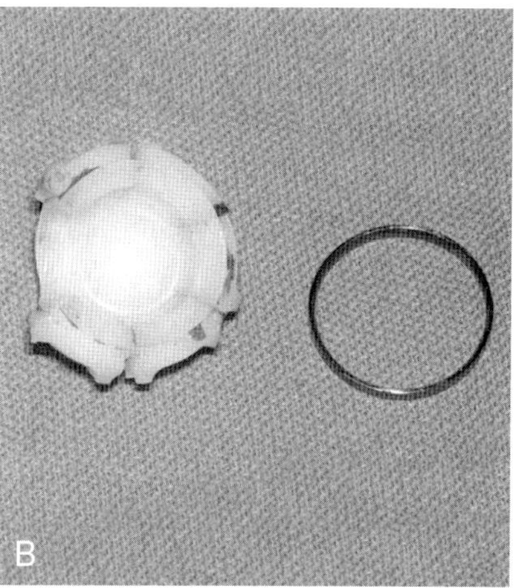

Figure 6 **A,** AP radiograph of the hip demonstrating failure of the constrained liner. **B,** The locking mechanism (ring) of the constrained liner has broken.

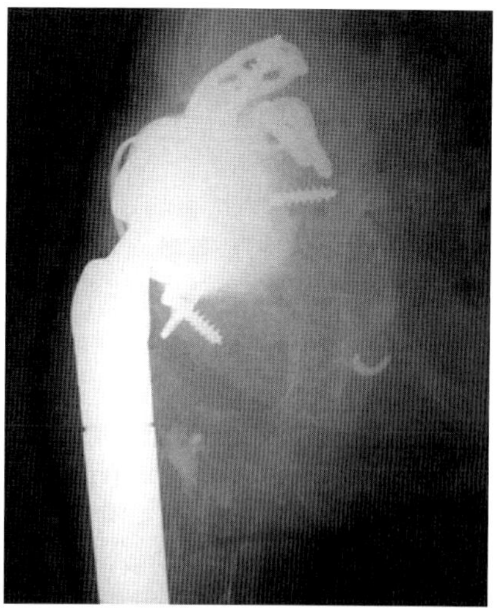

Figure 7 Complete dissociation of the pelvis in a patient in whom the constrained liner had been used in combination with a cage.

less shell, two were cemented into a cage, and one was cemented directly into the acetabular bone. Eight patients (14%) required a revision because of failure of the constrained liner, with seven of them having had recurrent dislocations. Failures were described on the basis of the mechanism of implant failure. There were three type I failures (of the bone-prosthesis interface), two type II failures (of the liner locking mechanism), and one type III failure (of the femoral head locking mechanism). In addition to the failures classified by Cooke and associates, a fourth failure mechanism—complete dissociation of the pelvis (type IV)—has been encountered at our institution when a constrained liner was used in combination with a cage (Figure 7).

Cooke and associates[53] noted that careful attention to surgical technique may decrease failure rates. Type I failures can be avoided by using supplemental screw fixation for the cementless shell before inserting the constrained acetabular component. The risk of type II failures can be minimized when cementing the constrained liner into the cementless shell by seating the liner fully into the shell. Scoring or roughening the polyethylene lightly with a burr enhances the grouting bond of the cement and may minimize debonding of the cement-polyethylene interface. The risk of type III failures can be minimized by ensuring that range of motion does not lead to component-component or component-bone impingement.

In short, hip arthroplasty with a constrained acetabular cup should be considered as an option for the surgical treatment of patients with extensive soft-tissue deficiency, deficiency of the abductor mechanism, dislocation with no discrete or identifiable cause, and/or recurrent dislocation despite prior attempted surgical correction. Patients should be selected carefully for treatment with this technique—that is, only after detailed examination for the cause of the dislocation and after it has been determined that other interventions are unlikely to be successful. Prior to inserting a constrained liner, it is crucial that the positions of the femoral and acetabular components be scrutinized.

Summary

Surgical management of recurrent dislocation following total hip arthroplasty is a challenging problem. Recognition of the etiology is critical for successful treatment. Close scrutiny of component position is a crucial step in the management of these patients. Subtle component malposition should always be suspected. Revision of the malpositioned component is perhaps the most effective type of surgical intervention in the treatment of recurrent dislocation. During revision surgery, it is imperative that the components be carefully inspected to determine if they are optimally positioned. When revision surgery is planned, the necessary equipment should always be available for revision of the malpositioned component. When dislocation is multifactorial or idiopathic, the potential surgical options include modular component exchange, bipolar arthroplasty, use of a large femoral head, and insertion of a constrained acetabular component. Soft-tissue reinforcement and trochanteric advancement have variable and less successful results and should be used in only carefully selected cases.

References

1. Chang RW, Pellisier JM, Hazen GB: A cost-effectiveness analysis of total hip arthroplasty for osteoarthritis of the hip. *JAMA* 1996;275:858-865.
2. Dewal H, Maurer SL, Tsai P, Su E, Hiebert R, Di Cesare PE: Efficacy of abduction bracing in the management of total hip arthroplasty dislocation. *J Arthroplasty* 2004;19:733-738.
3. Jager M, Endres S, Wilke A: Total hip replacement in childhood, adolescence and young patients: A review of the literature. *Z Orthop Ihre Grenzgeb* 2004;142:194-212.
4. Eftekhar NS: Dislocation and instability complicating low friction arthroplasty of the hip joint. *Clin Orthop Relat Res* 1976;121:120-125.
5. Fackler CD, Poss R: Dislocation in total hip arthroplasties. *Clin Orthop Relat Res* 1980;151:169-178.
6. Morrey BF: Instability after total hip arthroplasty. *Orthop Clin North Am* 1992;23:237-248.
7. Rao JP, Bronstein R: Dislocations following arthroplasties of the hip: Incidence, prevention, and treatment. *Orthop Rev* 1991;20:261-264.
8. Ritter MA: Dislocation and subluxation of the total hip replacement. *Clin Orthop Relat Res* 1976;121:92-94.
9. Anderson MJ, Murray WR, Skinner HB: Constrained acetabular components. *J Arthroplasty* 1994;9:17-23.
10. Baldwin KF, Dorr LD: The unstable total hip arthroplasty: The role of postoperative bracing. *Instr Course Lect* 2001;50:289-293.
11. Ekelund A: Trochanteric osteotomy for recurrent dislocation of total hip arthroplasty. *J Arthroplasty* 1993;8: 629-632.
12. Goetz DD, Bremner BRB, Callaghan JJ, Capello WN, Johnston RC: Salvage of a recurrently dislocating total hip prosthesis with use of a constrained acetabular component: A concise follow-up of a previous report. *J Bone Joint Surg Am* 2004;86: 2419-2423.
13. Haft GF, Heiner AD, Dorr LD, Brown TD, Callaghan JJ: A biomechanical analysis of polyethylene liner cementation into a fixed metal acetabular shell. *J Bone Joint Surg Am* 2003;85:1100-1110.
14. Hedlundh U, Ahnfelt L, Hybbinette CH, Wallinder L, Weckstrom J, Fredin H: Dislocations and the femoral head size in primary total hip arthroplasty. *Clin Orthop Relat Res* 1996;333: 226-233.
15. Homesley HD, Minnich JM, Parvizi J, Hozack WJ: Total hip arthroplasty revision: A decade of change. *Am J Orthop* 2004;33:389-392.
16. Krushell RJ, Burke DW, Harris WH: Elevated-rim acetabular components: Effect on range of motion and stability in total hip arthroplasty. *J Arthroplasty* 1991;6(suppl):S53-S58.
17. Lavigne MJ, Sanchez AA, Coutts RD: Recurrent dislocation after total hip arthroplasty: Treatment with an Achilles tendon allograft. *J Arthroplasty* 2001;16(8, suppl 1)13-18.
18. Lee PC, Shih CH, Chen WJ, Tu YK, Tai CL: Early polyethylene wear and osteolysis in cementless total hip arthroplasty: The influence of femoral head size and polyethylene thickness. *J Arthroplasty* 1999;14:976-981.
19. Lewinnek GE, Lewis JL, Tarr R, Compere CL, Zimmerman JR: Dislocations after total hip-replacement arthroplasties. *J Bone Joint Surg Am* 1978;60:217-220.
20. Padgett DE, Warashina H: The unstable total hip replacement. *Clin Orthop Relat Res* 2004;420:72-79.
21. Qassem DM, Smith KB: Effect of elevated-rim acetabular liner and 32-mm femoral head on stability in total hip arthroplasty. *Saudi Med J* 2004;25:88-90.
22. Ries MD, Wiedel JD: Bipolar hip arthroplasty for recurrent dislocation after total hip arthroplasty: A report of three cases. *Clin Orthop Relat Res* 1992; 278:121-127.
23. Schinsky MF, Nercessian OA, Arons RR, Macaulay W: Comparison of complications after transtrochanteric and posterolateral approaches for primary total hip arthroplasty. *J Arthroplasty* 2003;18:430-434.
24. Shapiro GS, Weiland DE, Markel DC, Padgett DE, Sculco TP, Pellicci PM: The use of a constrained acetabular component for recurrent dislocation. *J Arthroplasty* 2003;18:250-258.
25. Williams JF, Gottesman MJ, Mallory TH: Dislocation after total hip arthroplasty: Treatment with an above-knee hip spica cast. *Clin Orthop Relat Res* 1982;171:53-58.
26. Woo RY, Morrey BF: Dislocations after total hip arthroplasty. *J Bone Joint Surg Am* 1982;64:1295-1306.
27. Berry DJ, von Knoch M, Schleck CD, Harmsen WS: The cumulative long-term risk of dislocation after primary Charnley total hip arthroplasty. *J Bone Joint Surg Am* 2004;86:9-14.
28. Dorr LD, Wan Z: Causes of and treatment protocol for instability of total hip replacement. *Clin Orthop Relat Res* 1998;355:144-151.
29. Hedlundh U, Fredin H: Patient characteristics in dislocations after primary total hip arthroplasty: 60 patients compared with a control group. *Acta Orthop Scand* 1995;66:225-228.
30. Hedlundh U, Karlsson M, Ringsberg K, Besjakov J, Fredin H: Muscular and neurologic function in patients with recurrent dislocation after total hip arthroplasty: A matched controlled study of 65 patients using dual-energy X-ray absorptiometry and postural stability tests. *J Arthroplasty* 1999;14:319-325.
31. Soong M, Rubash HE, Macaulay W: Dislocation after total hip arthroplasty. *J Am Acad Orthop Surg* 2004;12: 314-321.
32. Barbosa JK, Khan AM, Andrew JG: Treatment of recurrent dislocation of total hip arthroplasty using a ligament

prosthesis. *J Arthroplasty* 2004;19: 318-321.

33. Bremner BR, Goetz DD, Callaghan JJ, Capello WN, Johnston RC: Use of constrained acetabular components for hip instability: An average 10-year follow-up study. *J Arthroplasty* 2003; 18:131-137.

34. Callaghan JJ, Parvizi J, Novak CC, et al: A constrained liner cemented into a secure cementless acetabular shell. *J Bone Joint Surg Am* 2004;86: 2206-2211.

35. Daly PJ, Morrey BF: Operative correction of an unstable total hip arthroplasty. *J Bone Joint Surg Am* 1992;74: 1334-1343.

36. Bourne RB, Mehin R: The dislocating hip: What to do, what to do. *J Arthroplasty* 2004;19(4, suppl 1)111-114.

37. von Knoch M, Berry DJ, Harmsen WS, Morrey BF: Late dislocation after total hip arthroplasty. *J Bone Joint Surg Am* 2002;84:1949-1953.

38. Paterno SA, Lachiewicz PF, Kelley SS: The influence of patient-related factors and the position of the acetabular component on the rate of dislocation after total hip replacement. *J Bone Joint Surg Am* 1997;79: 1202-1210.

39. Parvizi J, Kim KI, Goldberg G, Mallo G, Hozack WJ: Recurrent instability after total hip arthroplasty: Beware of subtle component malpositioning. *Clin Orthop Relat Res* 2006;447: 60-65.

40. Kavanagh BF, Fitzgerald RH Jr: Multiple revisions for failed total hip arthroplasty not associated with infection. *J Bone Joint Surg Am* 1987;69: 1144-1149.

41. Toomey SD, Hopper RH Jr, McAuley JP, Engh CA: Modular component exchange for treatment of recurrent dislocation of a total hip replacement in selected patients. *J Bone Joint Surg Am* 2001;83: 1529-1533.

42. McGann WA, Welch RB: Treatment of the unstable total hip arthroplasty using modularity, soft tissue, and allograft reconstruction. *J Arthroplasty* 2001;16(8, suppl 1):19-23.

43. Earll MD, Fehring TK, Griffin WL, Mason JB, McCoy T, Odum S: Success rate of modular component exchange for the treatment of an unstable total hip arthroplasty. *J Arthroplasty* 2002;17:864-869.

44. Barrack RL, Burke DW, Cook SD, Skinner HB, Harris WH: Complications related to modularity of total hip components. *J Bone Joint Surg Br* 1993;75:688-692.

45. Parvizi J, Morrey BF: Bipolar hip arthroplasty as a salvage treatment for instability of the hip. *J Bone Joint Surg Am* 2000;82:1132-1139.

46. Grigoris P, Grecula MJ, Amstutz HC: Tripolar hip replacement for recurrent prosthetic dislocation. *Clin Orthop Relat Res* 1994;304:148-155.

47. Beaulé PE, Schmalzried TP, Udomkiat P, Amstutz HC: Jumbo femoral head for the treatment of recurrent dislocation following total hip replacement. *J Bone Joint Surg Am* 2002; 84:256-263.

48. Amstutz HC, Le Duff MJ, Beaulé PE: Prevention and treatment of dislocation after total hip replacement using large diameter balls. *Clin Orthop Relat Res* 2004;429:108-116.

49. Davey JR, Harris WH: Reverse skeletal traction for instability following revision total hip arthroplasty: A report of two cases. *Clin Orthop Relat Res* 1988;234:110-114.

50. Stromsoe K, Eikvar K: Fascia lata plasty in recurrent posterior dislocation after total hip arthroplasty. *Arch Orthop Trauma Surg* 1995;114: 292-294.

51. Kaplan SJ, Thomas WH, Poss R: Trochanteric advancement for recurrent dislocation after total hip arthroplasty. *J Arthroplasty* 1987;2:119-124.

52. Shrader MW, Parvizi J, Lewallen DG: The use of a constrained acetabular component to treat instability after total hip arthroplasty. *J Bone Joint Surg Am* 2003;85:2179-2183.

53. Cooke CC, Hozack W, Lavernia C, Sharkey P, Shastri S, Rothman RH: Early failure mechanisms of constrained tripolar acetabular sockets used in revision total hip arthroplasty. *J Arthroplasty* 2003;18:827-833.

54. Goetz DD, Capello WN, Callaghan JJ, Brown TD, Johnston RC: Salvage of a recurrently dislocating total hip prosthesis with use of a constrained acetabular component: A retrospective analysis of fifty-six cases. *J Bone Joint Surg Am* 1998;80:502-509.

55. Ali Khan MA, Brakenbury PH, Reynolds IS: Dislocation following total hip replacement. *J Bone Joint Surg Br* 1981;63:214-218.

56. Woolson ST, Rahimtoola ZO: Risk factors for dislocation during the first 3 months after primary total hip replacement. *J Arthroplasty* 1999;14: 662-668.

57. Callaghan JJ, Heithoff BE, Goetz DD, Sullivan PM, Pedersen DR, Johnston RC: Prevention of dislocation after hip arthroplasty: Lessons from long-term followup. *Clin Orthop Relat Res* 2001;393:157-162.

58. Coventry MB: Late dislocations in patients with Charnley total hip arthroplasty. *J Bone Joint Surg Am* 1985; 67:832-841.

59. Puri L, Lapinski B, Wixson RL, Lynch J, Hendrix R, Stulberg SD: Computed tomographic follow-up evaluation of operative intervention for periacetabular lysis. *J Arthroplasty* 2006; 21(6, suppl 2):78-82.

60. Parvizi J, Sharkey PF, Bissett GA, Rothman RH, Hozack WJ: Surgical treatment of limb-length discrepancy following total hip arthroplasty. *J Bone Joint Surg Am* 2003;85: 2310-2317.

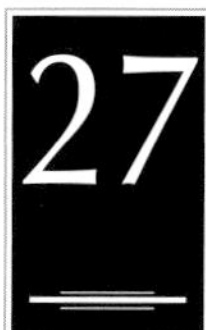

Severe Femoral Bone Loss in Infected Total Hip Arthroplasty: Surgical Management

Corey J. Richards, MD, MASc, FRCSC
*Donald S. Garbuz, MD, MHSc, FRCSC
Bassam A. Masri, MD, FRCSC
*Clive P. Duncan, MD

Abstract

The management of severe bone loss in a patient with a chronically infected total hip arthroplasty is a complex surgical challenge. The surgical alternatives are numerous and include the use of allografts, both structural and morcellized; cemented and cementless femoral components; and segmental replacement megaprostheses.

Infection following a total hip arthroplasty (THA) is a major complication with the potential for devastating long-term sequelae. The risk of infection is generally quoted as being 1%, with reported rates ranging from 0.3% to 2.2%.[1,2] A diagnosis of infection in patients presenting with a painful THA can be challenging, especially for a chronic infection. A delay in diagnosis can result in ongoing host bone destruction, which further hinders the surgeon's ability to perform a successful reconstruction. It is therefore paramount that the work-up of a painful THA includes appropriate measures for investigating infections.

Infected joint arthroplasties are classified based on the timing of presentation, initially described by Coventry:[3] stage I, acute infection within 6 weeks of the index surgery; stage II, delayed presentation with a chronic indolent infection; and stage III, acute presentation of infection secondary to hematogenous spread in a previously well-functioning hip arthroplasty. The management choices available to the treating surgeon include antibiotic suppression alone, débridement with retention of the prosthesis, excision arthroplasty, arthrodesis, amputation, and single- or two-stage revision. The choice of treatment modality will depend on the timing of the presentation, the feasibility of further reconstruction, and the overall health of the patient.

Patients presenting with a clinical scenario consistent with an acute infection (stage I or III) undergo serologic investigations, including erythrocyte sedimentation rate (ESR) and C-reactive protein (CRP), to rule out an infectious process. If these tests are positive, emergent irrigation and débridement with exchange of the modular components of the THA (for example, acetabular liner and femoral head) is performed, followed by 6 weeks of antibiotics directed toward the infecting organism.

If the symptoms are chronic, the diagnosis of an indolent infection (stage II) must be excluded. If the ESR is greater than 30 mm/h, the CRP is greater than 10 mg/L, or the clinical picture is highly suggestive of infection, the patient undergoes a

**Donald S. Garbuz, MD, MHSc, FRCSC or the department with which he is affiliated has received research or institutional support from Zimmer and is a consultant for or an employee of Zimmer. Clive P. Duncan, MD, FRCSC or the department with which he is affiliated has received research or institutional support from Zimmer and Smith & Nephew, has received miscellaneous nonincome support, commercially derived honoraria, or other nonresearch-related funding and royalties from Zimmer.*

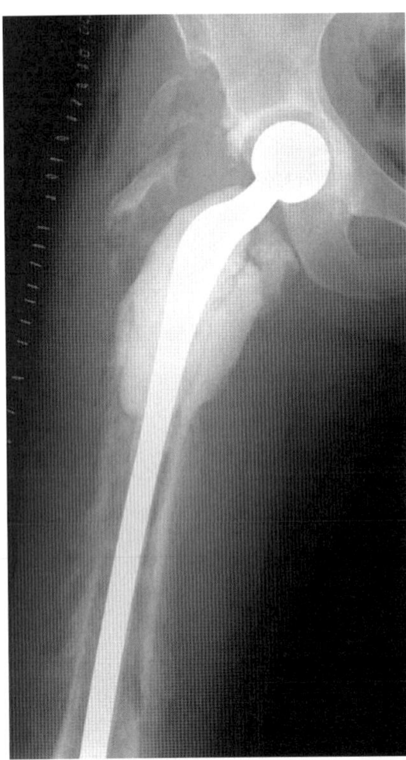

Figure 1 Infected revision THA with segmental bone loss and extensive osteomyelitis, managed first with an antibiotic-loaded, long-stem facsimile of the proximal femur and snap-fit socket (PROSTALAC system).

hip aspiration, with three samples taken under sterile conditions. At least two of three hip aspiration samples must be positive for the diagnosis of infection. For patients in whom a chronic infection is diagnosed, a two-stage revision using an articulated spacer is presently the treatment of choice at most centers in North America and around the world, with reported success rates of 93% to 96%.[4,5]

Management of Bone Loss

An important characteristic of patients with an infected THA is the quality of the remaining femoral host bone. Patients may have severe bone loss secondary either to osteolysis before the onset of the infection or because a delay in the diagnosis of infection resulted in ongoing bone destruction. There are two vital issues to address when planning the surgical management of these patients: how to successfully complete the first-stage procedure to ensure eradication of infection and optimize function while awaiting definitive management; and how to optimally treat the severe bone loss during the second-stage definitive procedure.

Ninety-nine patients who had undergone two-stage revision surgery for infected THA were reviewed in a 10- to 15-year follow-up study.[6] The final recurrence rate of infection was 4%, and a high success rate was also achieved in patients with severe femoral bone loss. These results supported the use of a PROSTALAC (prosthesis of antibiotic-loaded acrylic cement) system (DePuy, Warsaw, IN) for the first stage in these uniquely difficult cases (Figure 1). This has been standard practice at the University of British Columbia since 1986 for maintaining limb length and joint stability, while facilitating early mobilization of the patient as well as the technical details of the second stage.

The surgical options for the management of severe bone loss following the successful eradication of infection are similar to the choices available for the treatment of Vancouver B3 periprosthetic fractures. The surgical alternatives can be divided into three groups: complex reconstruction of the deficient proximal femur with secure distal fixation; segmental substitution of the proximal femur with a megaprosthesis or allograft/prosthesis composite (Figure 2, *A*); and distally fixed replacement with a modular stem that acts as a scaffold around which the remaining deficient proximal bone can be assembled, with or without supplemental bone graft (Figure 2, *B*).

Several of these surgical alternatives require the use of allograft, either morcellized or structural, during the second-stage procedure. Although allograft has been widely used in aseptic revision, there is a theoretical concern that its use following infection may increase the rate of recurrence. Most published articles on the use of allograft in the management of infection have reported excellent success, with recurrence rates ranging from 0 to 7.5%.[7-10] A 2004 report by Ammon and Stockley[11] noted recurrence rates of 14% with the use of allograft at revision for infection. They reviewed 57 patients treated with a two-stage revision for infection with acetabular impaction grafting, femoral impaction grafting, or a combination of these, with 12 requiring a large circumferential allograft. Eight patients had recurrent infections.

The use of a cementless prosthesis at the second stage has been questioned, with early studies reporting rates of reinfection as high as 18% and additional occurrence of loosening.[12] More recent investigations have reported rates of reinfection between 7% and 10%.[13-16] These more promising results demonstrate that modern cementless components can be used at the time of the second-stage revision, with the potential advantage of enhanced survival of the implant. This finding assumes that the infection has been eradicated as a consequence of the first-stage intervention and subsequent antimicrobial management.

The following discussion provides a brief outline of selected articles reporting the results of the various surgical options for the treatment of severe bone loss in infected THAs.

Complex Reconstruction of the Deficient Proximal Femur With Secure Distal Fixation

Circumferential Mesh With Impaction Allografting

English and associates[7] reviewed 53 patients who underwent impaction allografting during the second stage of a two-stage revision for an infected THA. All patients underwent a Girdlestone excision arthroplasty, received local and systemic antibiotics, and subsequently underwent reconstruction using femoral impaction grafting. Four patients (7.5%) had recurrence of their infection.

Bicortical Strut Allografting With Distally Fixed Stem

Although there are no published reports specifically addressing the use of bicortical structural allograft in the setting of infection, Emerson and associates[17] have demonstrated that single cortical struts unite consistently by 8 months with a union rate of 96%.

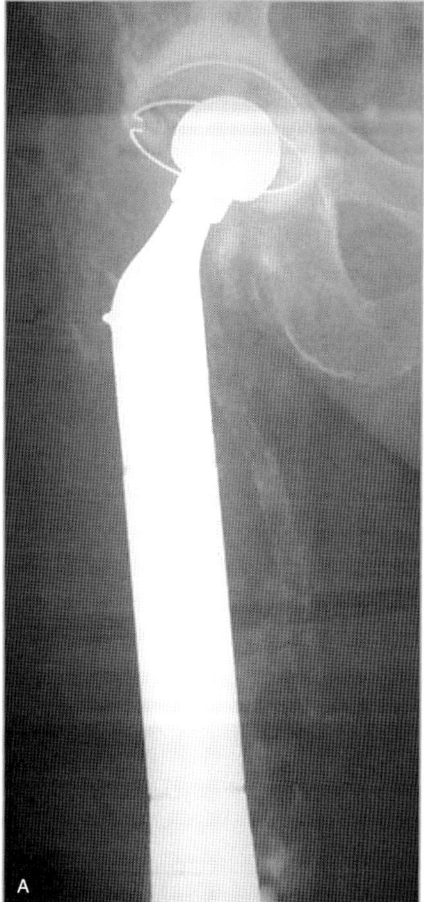
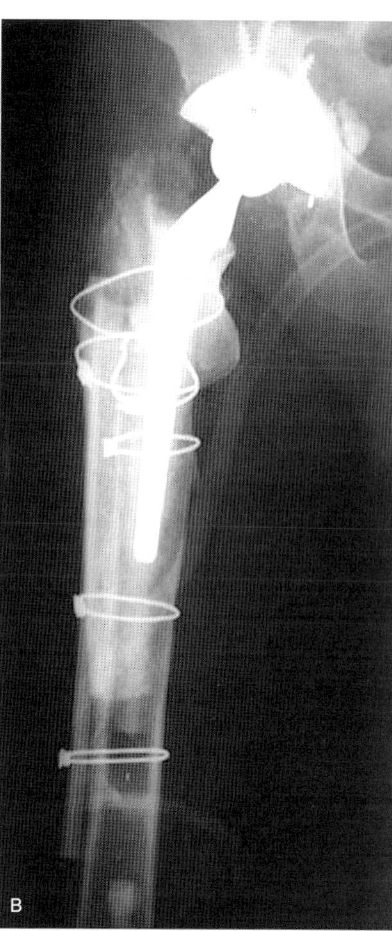

Figure 2 **A,** Postoperative radiograph of a megaprosthesis used for the second-stage revision of a previously infected THA. **B,** Postoperative radiograph of the scaffold technique using a modular tapered titanium femoral component augmented with allograft.

Resection of the Proximal Femur With Segmental Substitution

Allograft-Prosthetic Composite

Alexeeff and associates[8] reviewed 11 patients treated with two-stage revision and structural allograft for infection. There was no recurrence of infection with mean follow-up of 47.8 months (range, 24 to 72 months). Nusem and Morgan[9] reported on the use of structural allografts for bone stock reconstruction in two-stage revision for infected THA in 18 patients. Outcomes were good in 16 of 18 patients followed for 5 to 14 years, with one recurrence of infection. Hsieh and associates[10] reported on the treatment of deep infection of the hip with two-stage revision and structural allograft in 24 patients. There was no recurrence of infection at a mean follow-up of 4.2 years (range, 2 to 7 years).

Proximal Femoral Replacement

Parvizi and associates[18] reported on 43 patients undergoing proximal femoral replacement for nonneoplastic disorders (13 for deep infection). The mean follow-up was 36.5 months, with excellent or good functional outcomes in 22 patients, fair in 10, and poor in 11. Using revision as the end point, the survivorship of the implant was 87% at 1 year and 73% at 5 years. One patient in the series developed a postoperative infection, although it was not stated whether this represented a recurrent infection.

Distally Fixed Replacement That Acts as a Scaffold for the Remaining Proximal Host Bone

This final surgical alternative is a relatively novel technique. The concept is that the deficient proximal femur is wrapped around the proximal part of a distally fixed stem and then secured with cables. Using a modular titanium tapered stem provides a scaffold that encourages healing and possible reconstitution of the proximal femur. This technique requires sufficient proximal host bone support to provide rotational stability of the implant. The adequacy of the remaining host bone is evaluated intraoperatively based on the rotational stability of trial components. Although there are no published reports on the outcome of this technique for the management of infection, early reports of the technique for the management of severe bone loss have been promising.[19]

Summary

The treatment protocol at our institution for a chronic infection with associated severe bone loss remains a two-stage exchange arthroplasty procedure with an antibiotic-loaded facsimile of the joint and proximal femur in the interval between stages. At present, the use of the scaffold technique (distally fixed replacement that acts as a scaffold for the remaining proximal host bone) is recommended during the definitive second stage. Further studies are required to determine the outcome of the scaffold technique for the management of severe bone loss in infections.

References

1. Lidwell OM: Clean air at operation and subsequent sepsis in the joint. *Clin Orthop Relat Res* 1986;211: 91-102.
2. Sculco TP: The economic impact of infected total joint arthroplasty. *Instr Course Lect* 1993;42:349-351.
3. Coventry MB: Treatment of infections occurring in total hip surgery. *Orthop Clin North Am* 1975;6:991-1003.
4. Garvin KL, Fitzgerald RH Jr, Salvati EA, et al: Reconstruction of the infected total hip and knee arthroplasty with gentamicin-impregnated Palacos bone cement. *Instr Course Lect* 1993; 42:293-302.
5. Younger AS, Duncan CP, Masri BA, McGraw RW: The outcome of two-stage arthroplasty using a custom-made interval spacer to treat the infected hip. *J Arthroplasty* 1997;12: 615-623.
6. Kostamo T, Biring GS, Masri BA, Garbuz D, Duncan CP: Two-stage hip revision for infection: A 10-15 year follow-up study in 103 patients. *75th Annual Meeting Proceedings.* Rosemont, IL, American Academy of Orthopaedic Surgeons, 2008, p 391.
7. English H, Timperley AJ, Dunlop D, Gie G: Impaction grafting of the femur in two-stage revision for infected total hip replacement. *J Bone Joint Surg Br* 2002;84:700-705.
8. Alexeeff M, Mahomed N, Morsi E, Garbuz D, Gross A: Structural allograft in two-stage revisions for failed septic hip arthroplasty. *J Bone Joint Surg Br* 1996;78:213-216.
9. Nusem I, Morgan DA: Structural allografts for bone stock reconstruction in two-stage revision for infected total hip arthroplasty: Good outcome in 16 of 18 patients followed for 5-14 years. *Acta Orthop* 2006;77:92-97.
10. Hsieh PH, Shih CH, Chang YH, Lee MS, Yang WE, Shih HN: Treatment of deep infection of the hip associated with massive bone loss: Two-stage revision with an antibiotic-loaded interim cement prosthesis followed by reconstruction with allograft. *J Bone Joint Surg Br* 2005;87:770-775.
11. Ammon P, Stockley I: Allograft bone in two-stage revision of the hip for infection: Is it safe? *J Bone Joint Surg Br* 2004;86:962-965.
12. Nestor BJ, Hanssen AD, Ferrer-Gonzalez R, Fitzgerald RH Jr: The use of porous prostheses in delayed reconstruction of total hip replacements that have failed because of infection. *J Bone Joint Surg Am* 1994;76: 349-359.
13. Haddad FS, Muirhead-Allwood SK, Manktelow AR, Bacarese-Hamilton I: Two-stage uncemented revision hip arthroplasty for infection. *J Bone Joint Surg Br* 2000;82:689-694.
14. Fehring TK, Calton TF, Griffin WL: Cementless fixation in 2-stage reimplantation for periprosthetic sepsis. *J Arthroplasty* 1999;14:175-181.
15. Masri BA, Panagiotopoulos KP, Greidanus NV, Garbuz DS, Duncan CP: Cementless two-stage exchange arthroplasty for infection after total hip arthroplasty. *J Arthroplasty* 2007; 22:72-78.
16. Kraay MJ, Goldberg VM, Fitzgerald SJ, Salata MJ: Cementless two-staged total hip arthroplasty for deep periprosthetic infection. *Clin Orthop Relat Res* 2005;441:243-249.
17. Emerson RH Jr, Malinin TI, Cuellar AD, Head WC, Peters PC: Cortical strut allografts in the reconstruction of the femur in revision total hip arthroplasty: A basic science and clinical study. *Clin Orthop Relat Res* 1992; 285: 35-44.
18. Parvizi J, Tarity TD, Slenker N, et al: Proximal femoral replacement in patients with non-neoplastic conditions. *J Bone Joint Surg Am* 2007;89:1036-1043.
19. Berry DJ: Treatment of Vancouver B3 periprosthetic femur fractures with a fluted tapered stem. *Clin Orthop Relat Res* 2003;417:224-231.

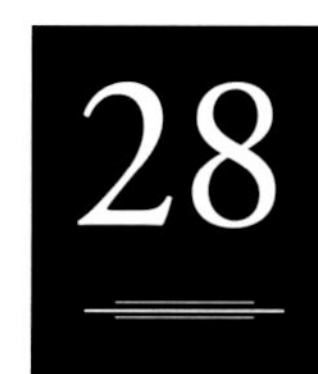

Femoral Fixation in Revision Total Hip Arthroplasty

Curtis W. Hartman, MD
Kevin L. Garvin, MD

Abstract

Management of the femur during revision total hip arthroplasty can be challenging. Strategies for femoral reconstruction are based on understanding the degree of femoral bone loss. Numerous options exist for femoral reconstruction depending on the quantity and quality of the remaining femoral bone stock, including cemented fixation, cementless fixation using proximally porous-coated implants, cylindrical extensively porous-coated implants, modular and nonmodular tapered fluted stems, impaction bone grafting, allograft-prosthetic composites, and proximal femoral replacements (megaprostheses). An understanding of the results of various methods of femoral reconstruction is helpful in guiding the revision surgeon faced with a challenging femoral revision.

Recent data project the number of total hip arthroplasty revisions to grow by 137% between 2005 and 2030.[1] Surgeons who manage the failed total hip replacement will find an ever-increasing workload and must have an understanding of the outcomes and treatment options for the failed femoral implant.

Management strategies for femoral implant revision are based on the femoral defect and the quality and quantity of the remaining femoral bone stock. Numerous options are available for femoral reconstruction, including cemented fixation, cementless fixation with the use of proximally porous-coated implants, cylindrical extensively porous-coated implants, modular and nonmodular tapered fluted stems, impaction bone grafting, allograft-prosthetic composites, and proximal femoral replacements (megaprostheses).

Preoperative Planning

Careful preoperative planning is a necessary step before any revision arthroplasty. An attempt should be made to identify the implants being revised. The implant manufacturer should be contacted for implant removal devices that may be specific to the implant being revised. Even when an isolated femoral revision is planned, it is beneficial to identify the acetabular implant because a modular polyethylene exchange may be possible.

The standard evaluation for preoperative planning includes four radiographic views: an AP view of the pelvis, an AP view of the affected hip, a frog-lateral view, and a shoot-through lateral view of the affected hip.[2] The radiograph should be examined for areas of osteolysis, stress shielding, femoral deformity, a cortical deficiency, and to detect the amount and location of cement. The radiographs provide substantial information as to the difficulty of implant removal and subsequent reconstruction. The degree and pattern of bone loss influence the revision implant choice. The bone stock distal to the implant should be visualized and evaluated because the diaphyseal bone may be essential to obtaining fixation during revision. Additionally, the radiographs should be of sufficient length to determine if a distal implant is present and if it will complicate the proximal reconstruction.

Serial radiographs help to determine whether the femoral stem to be revised is loose or well fixed. Cemented implants that have migrated or subsided, or have a fractured cement

Dr. Hartman or an immediate family member has received research or institutional support from Smith & Nephew. Dr. Garvin or an immediate family member serves as a board member, owner, officer, or committee member of the American Academy of Orthopaedic Surgeons and the American Orthopaedic Association and has received royalties from Biomet.

Table 1
Paprosky Classification System for Femoral Defects

Type	Description
I	Minimal metaphyseal bone loss
II	Extensive metaphyseal bone loss and an intact diaphysis
IIIA	Extensive metadiaphyseal bone loss and a minimum of 4 cm of intact cortical bone in the diaphysis
IIIB	Extensive metadiaphyseal bone loss and < 4 cm of intact cortical bone in the diaphysis
IV	Extensive metadiaphyseal bone loss and a nonsupportive diaphysis

Table 2
AAOS Classification System for Femoral Defects

Type	Description
I	Segmental defect involving loss of cortical osseous support[a]
II	Cavitary defect involving loss of cancellous or endosteal bone with an intact cortical shell
III	Combined segmental and cavitary defects
IV	Femoral malalignment in rotational or angular plane
V	Femoral stenosis with partial or complete occlusion of the intramedullary canal
VI	Femoral discontinuity usually due to fracture nonunion

[a]Type I defects are further specified as level I, indicating bone loss is proximal to the lower edge of the lesser trochanter; level II, loss is within 10 cm of the lower edge of the lesser trochanter; and level III, loss is distal to 10 cm below the lower edge of the lesser trochanter.

Table 3
Mallory Classification System for Femoral Defects

Type	Description
I	Cortex intact with cancellous bone present
II	Cortex intact with cancellous bone absent
IIIA	Cortical deficiency proximal to the lesser trochanter
IIIB	Cortical deficiency between the lesser trochanter and the isthmus
IIIC	Cortical deficiency involving the isthmus and distally

mantle, or implants that have fractured are definitely loose.[3,4] A continuous radiolucent line at the cement-bone interface indicates probable loosening, and a noncircumferential radiolucent line indicates possible loosening.[3,4] Cementless implants that demonstrate progressive subsidence, migration, or divergent radiolucent lines are considered unstable.[5] These femora typically demonstrate a distal pedestal and proximal cortical hypertrophy. An implant with parallel radiolucent lines and without progressive migration is likely to have stable fibrous ingrowth.[5] These femora usually do not have focal proximal cortical hypertrophy. A well-ingrown cementless implant does not have reactive lines or evidence of component migration.[5] These femora typically have proximal stress shielding.

Clear template overlays or digital templates are used to assess the length and the diameter of the proposed revision implant. Templating also helps to determine whether proximal femoral remodeling has occurred. Loose femoral implants are often associated with femoral remodeling into varus alignment and retroversion.[6] If proximal femoral remodeling has occurred, it may be necessary to perform an extended trochanteric osteotomy to reduce the risks of cortical perforation during reaming, fracture during implant insertion, or undersizing the implant because of varus malpositioning.

Classification of Femoral Bone Loss

Multiple authors have proposed systems to characterize femoral bone loss in the setting of revision hip surgery.[7-10] Weeden and Paprosky[10] described a system based on the quantity of metaphyseal and diaphyseal bone stock (**Table 1**). This system uses a simple algorithm for femoral reconstruction based on the severity of the defect. D'Antonio et al[7] reported the classification system developed by the American Academy of Orthopaedic Surgeons (AAOS) (**Table 2**). Although this system is highly descriptive in detailing osseous abnormalities of the femur, it does not provide a guide for reconstructive options based on the femoral defect. Mallory[8] developed a system with three basic categories based on the presence or absence of cancellous bone and the extent of femoral cortical deficiency (**Table 3**). Although this system is simpler and more useful than that of the AAOS for determining the method of femoral reconstruction, as noted by Della Valle and Paprosky,[6] it fails to address several critical determinants of reconstruction. Saleh et al[9,11] also developed a system for classifying femoral bone loss, which is both reliable and valid (**Table 4**).

Paprosky Classification System

The classification system devised by Paprosky is based on the principle that as proximal bone becomes weak and unsupportive, the relatively spared diaphyseal bone can be successfully used to provide reliable, long-term fixation.[10,12-14] The system assigns the femur to one of four categories on the basis of the extent and the location of bone loss (**Figure 1**).

Table 4
Gross Classification System for Femoral Defects

Type	Description
I	No notable loss of bone stock
II	Contained loss of bone stock with cortical thinning
III	Uncontained loss of bone stock involving the calcar and the lesser trochanter
IV	Uncontained circumferential loss of bone stock > 5 cm in length that extends into the diaphysis
V	Periprosthetic fracture with circumferential loss of bone stock proximal to the fracture

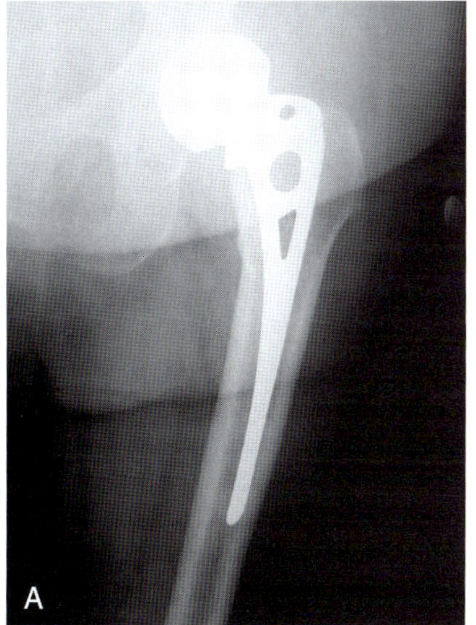
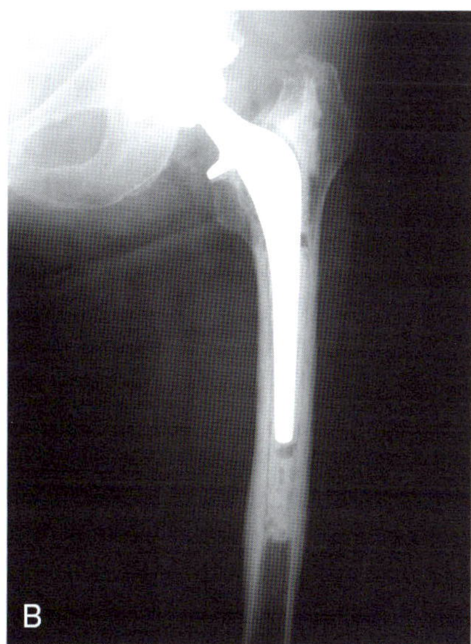
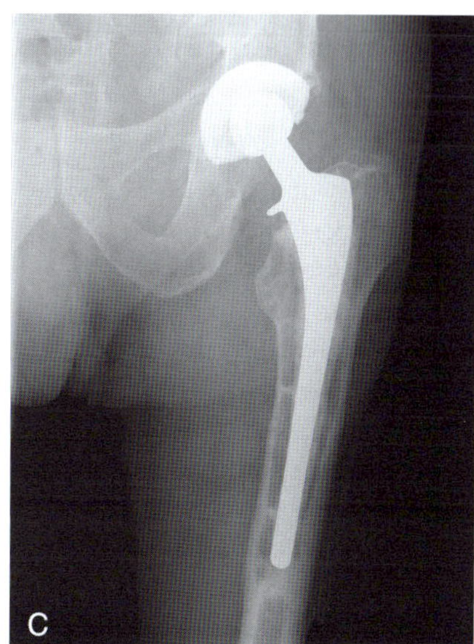
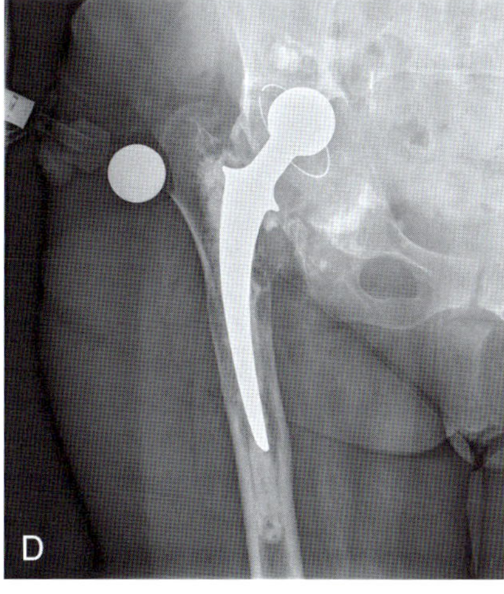
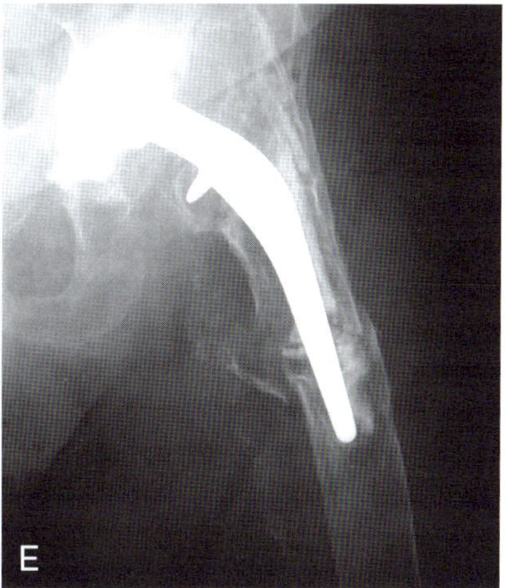

Figure 1 Radiographs showing femoral defects classified according to the Paprosky system. **A,** Type I femoral defect. **B,** Type II femoral defect. **C,** Type IIIA femoral defect. **D,** Type IIIB femoral defect. **E,** Type IV femoral defect. (Panels A, B, and E reprinted with permission from Della Valle CJ, Paprosky WG: Classification and an algorithmic approach to the reconstruction of femoral deficiency in revision total hip arthroplasty. *J Bone Joint Surg Am* 2003;85(Suppl 4):1-6.)

Type I

The femur with a type I defect has minimal loss of metaphyseal cancellous bone and an intact diaphysis (**Figure 1,** *A*).[10] This pattern of bone loss is uncommon in the revision setting and is more common with a failed resurfacing arthroplasty implant or an undersized, non–porous-coated cementless implant.[6]

Type II

The femur with a type II defect has extensive metaphyseal cancellous bone loss and minimal diaphyseal loss (**Figure 1,** *B*).[10] This is a common finding, particularly in the early stages of aseptic loosening.[6]

Types IIIA and IIIB

The femur with a type IIIA defect has extensive metaphyseal bone loss, leaving it unsupportive. The diaphysis is also involved, but a minimum of 4 cm of cortical bone is available at the isthmus to obtain a scratch fit (**Figure 1,** *C*).[10] This is probably the most frequently encountered defect in femoral revision surgery.[10]

The femur with a type IIIB defect has an unsupportive metaphysis secondary to extensive bone loss. Additionally, the diaphysis is more severely damaged, and less than 4 cm of scratch fit can be obtained at the isthmus (**Figure 1,** *D*).[10] This defect seems to be increasing in frequency with improved cementing techniques and the use of longer cementless stems.[6]

Type IV

The femur with a type IV defect has extensive metadiaphyseal bone loss. The femoral canal has expanded, and the isthmic cortical bone cannot provide reliable fixation (**Figure 1,** *E*). Although this pattern of bone loss is rare, its frequency is increasing.[6,10,15]

Results of Reconstruction

Based on the knowledge of this chapter's authors, Iorio et al[16] performed the only randomized, prospective trial of femoral component fixation in revision total hip arthroplasty to date. In that study, femoral component fixation with the use of third-generation cementing techniques was compared with modular metaphyseal cementless fixation in Paprosky type I and type II femora. With a mean follow-up of 8 years, there was no difference in validated outcome measures or 5-year survivorship between the two groups. The relative paucity of comparative trials in revision arthroplasty makes interpretation of the results of revision arthroplasty difficult. Because of these shortcomings, it is most beneficial to evaluate the outcomes of different techniques on an individual basis.[17]

Cemented Fixation

The early results of cemented femoral implant revision had high failure rates. Pellicci et al[18] followed 99 hips for a mean 8.1 years after revision total hip arthroplasty and reported a 19% rate of rerevision and a 29% rate of femoral loosening. Similarly, Kavanagh et al[19] followed 166 hips for a mean 4.5 years and reported a 6% rate of rerevision but a 44% rate of radiographic femoral loosening.

These dismal results were credited to early cementing techniques, and revisions performed with more modern techniques (distal plug, medullary lavage, retrograde cement delivery, and pressurization) have higher rates of success. Callaghan et al[20] reported a 4.3% rate of rerevision in a cohort of 139 hips followed for a mean 3.6 years, with 16% showing definite mechanical loosening and 29% showing progressive radiolucencies. Rubash and Harris,[21] in a study of 43 hips followed for a mean 6.2 years after revision hip arthroplasty with cement, reported a 2% failure rate caused by aseptic loosening, whereas 11% demonstrated radiographic evidence of femoral component loosening. Estok and Harris[22] described the long-term results for this cohort, which included 38 hips that were available for review at a mean follow-up of 11.7 years. They noted a 10.5% rerevision rate for aseptic failure and an additional 10.5% with radiographic evidence of loosening. In a third review of this cohort, Mulroy and Harris[23] reported a 26% rate of femoral component loosening at a mean follow-up of 15.1 years.

The so-called third-generation cementing technique that used pressurized, vacuum-mixed cement did little to improve the results of previous studies. Eisler et al[24] followed 83 consecutive hips after the first revision of the total hip replacement for 1.5 to 6.3 years. At a median follow-up of 3.6 years, the femoral failure rate was 39%.

These generally disappointing failure rates have led to further study in the laboratory in an attempt to understand the failure mechanisms more fully. Biomechanical tests evaluating the shear strength of the cement-bone interface found that a simulated revision setting reduces the interface shear strength to 20.6% of primary strength, and a second revision reduces the shear strength to 6.8% of primary strength.[25]

Impaction Grafting

Femoral impaction grafting was first reported by Simon et al[26] as a technique for femoral revision. The technique is relatively straightforward in concept but is time consuming and technically demanding.[27,28] The premise is that a damaged and ectatic femoral canal can be packed with cancellous allograft, creating a neomedullary canal. A highly polished, collarless, double-tapered stem is cemented into the graft bed with the use of contemporary cementing techniques. The graft is then vascularized and gradually incorporated with subsequent reconstitution of the deficient femoral bone stock (**Figure 2**). Full-thickness cortical defects can be reconstructed with mesh or cortical strut allografts to contain the morcellized cancellous graft.

Although some authors have reported worrisome results with impaction grafting,[29-33] numerous authors have reported short- and long-term success with this technique.[34-38] Meding et al[32] evaluated the results of 34 hips followed for a mean 30 months after femoral impaction grafting. The authors reported a 38% subsidence rate, with a mean subsidence of 10.1 mm and a 12% intraoperative femoral fracture rate. Similarly, Eldridge et al[29] reported massive subsidence (> 10 mm) in 11% of 79 hips followed for a mean 12.6 months. Ornstein et al[27] reported 39 femoral fractures within the first year after 108 femoral component revisions. Sierra et al[39] reviewed a subgroup of femoral revisions with use of stems of 220 mm or more in length, with the hypothesis that the longer stems would decrease the incidence of postoperative femoral fractures. The authors found 6 of the 42 hips reviewed required a reoperation. Survival analysis revealed a survival rate of 90% at 5 and 10 years with revision of the stem as the end point. However, with any femoral reoperation as the end point, the survival rate was 82% at both 5 and 10 years.

Similar to other procedures with a steep learning curve, the results of impaction grafting have improved as surgeons have become more comfortable with the procedure. Ornstein et al[34] reported the long-term results of a large cohort of femoral revisions in Sweden. They followed 1,305 femoral revisions for 5 to 18 years, identifying 70 repeat revisions. Survivorship for all causes of failure was 94% for women and 94.7% for men at 15 years. Survivorship at 15 years was 99.1% with aseptic loosening as the end point, 98.6% with infection as the end point, 99.0% with subsidence as the end point, and 98.7% with fracture as the end point. Wraighte and Howard[38] reported the results for 75 consecutive hips that had revision total hip replacement with a mean follow-up of 10.5 years. Survivorship with any further femoral operation as the end point was 92% at 10.5 years. They also found that subsidence correlated with the preoperative Endo-Klinik bone loss score, and the degree of subsidence at 1 year had a strong association with long-term subsidence. Halliday et al[36] reported that the survival of 226 hip replacements at 10 to 11 years was 90.5%, with any femoral operation as the end point. Mahoney et al[37] reviewed the results of 44 hips followed for a mean 4.7 years. With reoperation as the end point, the survivorship was 97%. These data support the use of impaction femoral bone grafting in select patients with substantial proximal femoral bone loss.

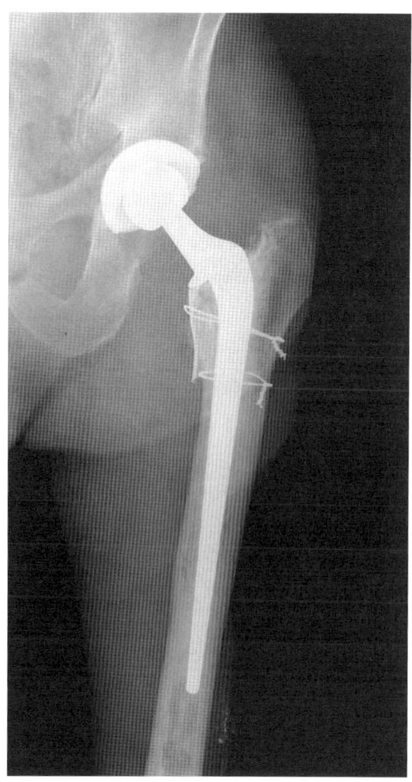

Figure 2 Radiograph of the femur after treatment of extensive osteolysis with impaction bone grafting. The patient had a cemented femoral stem and required revision because of extensive osteolysis. See Figure 1C for a radiograph of the femur before revision.

Cementless Fixation

The initial poor outcomes for cemented stems in revision arthroplasty led some to question their utility and search for other options. As a result, the use of cementless stems gained popularity. Multiple design philosophies have been used in cementless femoral fixation and have had important effects on the durability of the revision.

Proximally Porous-Coated Stems

The results of femoral implant revision with proximally porous-coated stems have been inferior compared with more modern techniques.[8,40-43] The primary reason for failure is the inability to obtain stable fixation of the stem in the deficient metaphysis. The results of proximally porous-coated stems in revision surgery can be summarized by the work of Berry et al.[44] The authors reviewed a series of 375 total hip arthroplasty revisions performed without cement and with the use of at least six different proximally porous-coated femoral components. A survivorship analysis at 8 years found that the survival rate, with revision for aseptic femoral failure as the end point, was 58%. The survival rate with aseptic femoral loosening (revision for aseptic loosening or radiographic loosening) as the end point was only 20%. In this series, greater preoperative bone loss correlated with worse survivorship. The authors concluded that the damaged and weakened proximal part of the femur does not provide an optimal

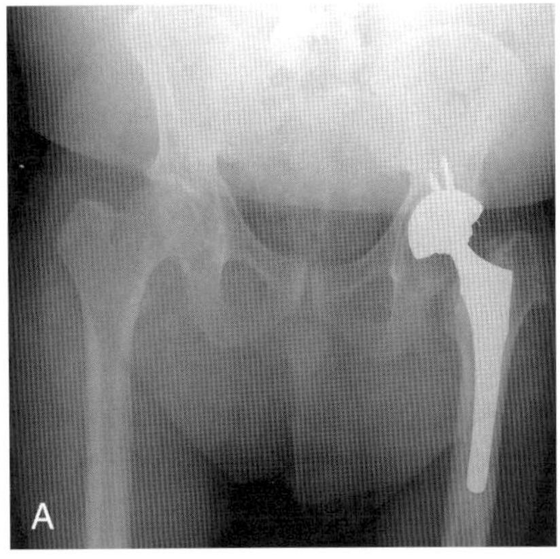

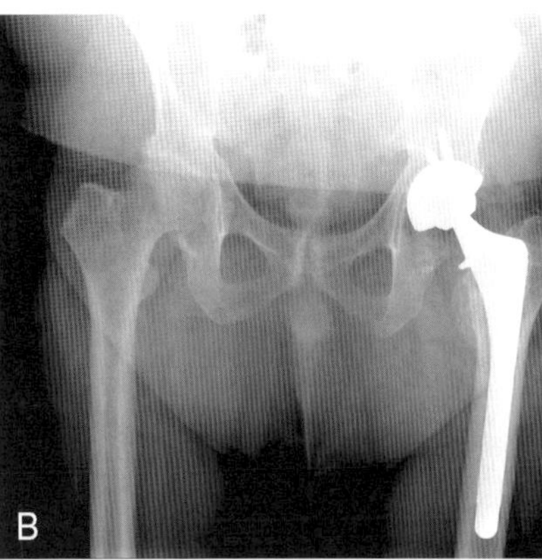

Figure 3 **A,** Radiograph of a hip with a loose, proximally porous-coated femoral stem before revision. **B,** Radiograph of the hip made after revision with an extensively porous-coated femoral stem.

environment for initial or long-term biologic fixation.

Fracture of the proximal part of the femur is a frequent complication in revisions with the use of proximally porous-coated implants. Berry et al[44] reported a 26% rate of intraoperative fracture. Malkani et al[45] reported a 45.9% incidence of intraoperative femoral fracture. The authors reported an overall 5-year survivorship free of moderate pain or revision of 82%; however, the fracture subgroup had survivorship of only 58% at 4 years. The difference in the survivorship between the groups was significant. Mulliken et al[46] reported a 40% intraoperative fracture rate. The authors did not report the failure rates in the fracture group but did find that the deficient proximal part of the femur was more likely to fracture, and most of the failures were in femora with severe proximal bone loss.

Proximally Porous-Coated Modular Stems

Proximally porous-coated modular femoral stems have appeal for cementless femoral revision because of their ability to obtain independent metaphyseal sizing and fixation relative to the diaphyseal portion of the implant. The goal of this technique is to reduce stress shielding by attaining stable implant fixation in the proximal part of the femur.[47] This stem type has performed well for revisions with minimal bone loss (Paprosky types I and II);[47-49] however, for more difficult cases with more extensive bone loss, the results have been inferior. For example, McCarthy and Lee,[50] in a retrospective review of the results of revision hip replacement in 67 hips with a mean follow-up of 14 years, reported that 78% of the femora had Paprosky type III or IV defects. With revision as the end point, 14-year survival was 60%. All aseptic failures were in Paprosky type IIIB or IV femora. There were no long-term failures in femora classified as Paprosky type II or IIIA. Bolognesi et al[51] performed a randomized, prospective trial comparing hydroxyapatite-coated metaphyseal sleeves and porous-coated metaphyseal sleeves with use of the S-ROM prosthesis (DePuy, Warsaw, IN) in 53 patients followed for a mean of 4 years. The authors found that, with Paprosky type III defects, the hydroxyapatite-coated sleeve was 2.6 times more likely to achieve osseous ingrowth than the porous-coated sleeve. The authors also reported that regardless of which sleeve was used, the Harris hip scores were significantly worse with worsening bone loss. For the entire cohort, the probability of femoral stem survival, with revision as the end point, was 95% at 3.9 years.

Cylindrical, Extensively Porous-Coated Stems

The use of extensively porous-coated femoral stems in revision arthroplasty is based on the principle that bypassing the damaged proximal part of the femur and engaging the diaphysis can reliably provide an ingrown and stable reconstruction (**Figure 3**). Despite concerns over proximal stress shielding, this technique is popular among surgeons who perform revisions because of the high rate of success and relative ease of technique. The results of revision with cylindrical, extensively porous-coated stems have been excellent[10,12,52-55] and are summarized in **Table 5**.

Several authors have reported the difficulty of using cylindrical, extensively porous-coated implants for femoral revision in the face of extensive bone loss.[10,52,56,57] Weeden and Paprosky[10] found that patients with type II or IIIA defects had a 5% failure rate, whereas patients with type IIIB defects had a 21% failure rate. Engh et al[57] identified 26 hips with bone loss extending 10 cm or more distal to the lesser trochanter that were followed for a mean of 13.3 years. The authors reported a 15% rate of mechanical loosening and a 10-year survivorship of 89%, with femoral revision as the end point. In another study by Engh et al,[52] the survival of femoral stems was significantly less if the preoperative bone loss extended more than 10 cm distal to the lesser trochanter. Sporer and Paprosky[56] investigated the failure rates of 51 patients with Paprosky type IIIA, IIIB, or IV femoral defects and reported no failures in 17 patients with type IIIA de-

Table 5
Results of Revision With Extensively Porous-Coated Femoral Stems

Study (Year)	Number of Hips	Implant Type[a]	Mean Patient Age (Years)	Mean (Range) of Follow-up (Years)	Results
Engh et al[52] (2004)	777	AML and Solution	NA	20[b]	Survival with revision for any reason as end point: 97.7% at 5 years, 95.8% at 10 years, and 95.8% at 15 years
Weeden and Paprosky[10] (2002)	170	AML and Solution	61.2	14.2	4.1% mechanical failure rate
Moreland and Moreno[55] (2001)	137	AML and Solution	63.0	9.3 (5-16)	4% revision rate for aseptic femoral loosening
Krishnamurthy el al[12] (1997)	297	AML	59.6	8.3 (5-14)	2.4% mechanical failure rate
Moreland and Bernstein[54] (1995)	175	AML and Solution	62.4	5 (2-10)	4% mechanical failure rate
Lawrence et al[53] (1994)	81	AML and Solution	57.0	9 (5-13)	11% mechanical failure rate

[a]AML = Anatomic Medullary Locking total hip replacement (DePuy, Warsaw, IN); Solution System (DePuy). [b]Twenty-year experience. NA = not available.

fects. They also found no failures in 15 patients with type IIIB femora if the endosteal canal was less than 19 mm; however, in the 11 patients with type IIIB femora and an endosteal canal diameter greater than 19 mm, the mechanical failure rate was 18%. Three of the eight patients with type IV femoral defects had mechanical failure. The authors noted that an additional 13 patients with type IV femora were treated with either impaction bone grafting or modular tapered fluted stems; patients treated with these techniques had no failures at the time of publication.

Tapered Fluted Stems

The concerns over proximal stress shielding and the difficulty of reconstructing femora with advanced bone loss with use of the cylindrical, extensively porous-coated stems have led to the development of other designs. Several authors have reported a generally favorable experience using the Wagner SL Revision stem (Zimmer, Warsaw, IN).[58-60] Although fixation with the Wagner SL Revision stem was reasonably good, most authors have also reported a relatively high rate of subsidence,[59,61] leading to the development of modular, fluted, tapered stems[62] (**Figure 4**). The results with modular, fluted, tapered stems have been excellent, with midterm survival rates of greater than 95% in several series.[63-70] The results of revision with modular, fluted, tapered stems are summarized in **Table 6**.

Richards et al[15] compared outcomes of femoral revisions with the use of either a tapered, fluted, modular titanium stem (ZMR Hip System; Zimmer) or a cylindrical, nonmodular cobalt-chromium implant (Solution System; DePuy). Despite the fact that patients in the tapered stem group had substantially worse osseous defects (65% had Paprosky type IIIB and IV defects), the cohort had better Western Ontario and McMaster Universities Osteoarthritis Index, Oxford-12, and

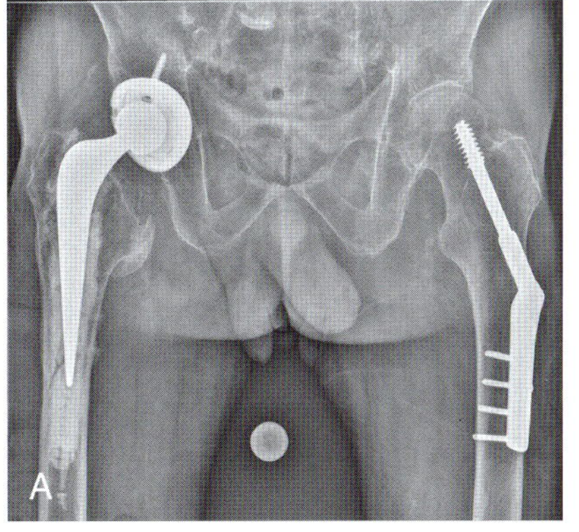

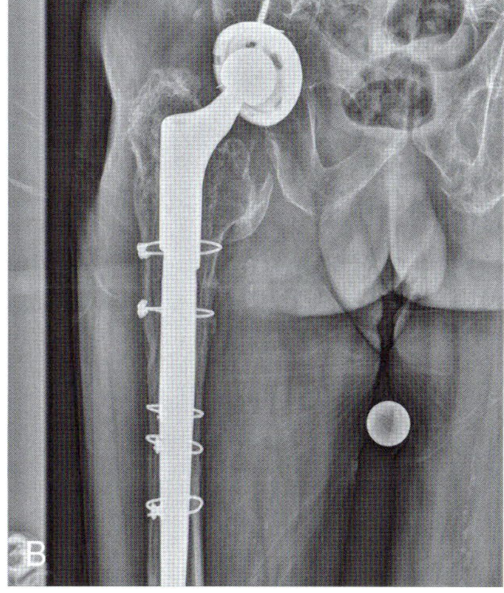

Figure 4 **A,** Radiograph of a hip with a periprosthetic femoral fracture and a loose cemented femoral stem before revision. **B,** Radiograph of the hip made after revision with a modular tapered fluted stem.

Table 6
Results of Revision With Tapered Fluted Stems

Study (Year)	Number of Hips	Implant Type[a]	Mean Duration of Follow-up (Months)	Stem Rerevision (%)	Any Rerevision (%)	Intraoperative Fractures (%)	Subsidence[c] (mm)
Wirtz et al[70] (2000)	142	MRP-Titan	28	1.4	4.9	NR	6 stems with > 5
Kwong et al[63] (2003)	143	Link MP	40	2.8	NR	2.1	2.1 (0-11.3)
Schuh et al[67] (2004)	79	MRP-Titan	48	3.8	NR	5.1	1 stem with > 2
Murphy and Rodriguez[65] (2004)	54	Link MP	42.6	2.9	16.3	NR	0
McInnis et al[64] (2006)	70	PFM	47	2.9	8.6	18.6	10 (0-52)
Park et al[66] (2007)	62	Lima-Lto	50	1.6	4.8	12.9	1 (0-25)
Rodriguez et al[87] (2009)	97	Link MP	39	5	NR	NR	5 stems with ≤ 2
Ovesen et al[69] (2010)	125	ZMR	50	3.2	6.4	3.2	2 (0-20)
Weiss et al[68] (2011)	90	Link MP	50[b]	2.0	10.0	1.0	2.7 (0-30)

[a]MRP-Titan (Peter Brehm Chirurgie Mechanik, Weisendorf, Germany); Link MP (Waldemar Link, Hamburg, Germany); PFM (Sulzer Orthopaedics, Baar, Switzerland); Lima-Lto (Lima Corporate, Udine, Italy); ZMR prosthesis (Zimmer, Warsaw, IN). [b]Median follow-up. [c]The values are given as the mean, with the range in parentheses, unless otherwise indicated. NR = not reported.

satisfaction scores. The authors also found that patients with a tapered stem had fewer fractures and more proximal osseous restoration.

Several authors have reported femoral stem fractures distal to the proximal modular junction.[15,69] Richards et al[15] reported four stem fractures in a cohort of 105 patients but noted that all the fractures occurred at the modular junction of an older design that is no longer in use. Although Berry[62] warned of the engineering challenges, given the location of this modular junction in a high-stress area, Postak and Greenwald[71] found the structural characteristics of the Link MP hip stem (Waldemar Link, Hamburg, Germany) are such that it offers the prospect of in vivo longevity.

Allograft-Prosthetic Composites

Proximal femoral allograft replacement has been used successfully for the reconstruction of massive proximal femoral bone loss in the setting of multiple revision arthroplasties or oncologic resection. The obvious advantages to proximal femoral allograft are the ability to restore bone stock, particularly in younger patients, the provision of a biologic anchor for the abductor complex, and the ability to precisely adjust limb length.[72] The risks associated with proximal femoral allografts are the risk of disease transmission, graft resorption, and nonunion. Several authors have reported encouraging results of this technique with variable lengths of follow-up. Safir et al[73] reviewed the cases of 50 patients with a mean follow-up of 16.2 years who had been managed with a proximal femoral allograft. Survival at 15 years was 82.2%, with revision femoral surgery as the end point. Five patients required bone grafting and plate fixation for symptomatic nonunion of the graft-host junction. The authors reported minor resorption of the graft in 58% of the patients, but only one patient in whom resorption led to failure of the construct. Graham and Stockley[74] reviewed the results of 25 allografts in 24 patients with a mean follow-up of 53 months. Two allografts required revision: one for aseptic failure and one for late infection. Another patient required augmentation of the graft-host junction for symptomatic nonunion. Babis et al[75] reported the results for 56 patients managed with an allograft-prosthetic composite. Survivorship of the reconstruction was 69% at 10 years with 26 hips remaining at risk. The authors reported the causes of failure were aseptic loosening in four, allograft resorption in three, allograft nonunion in two, allograft fracture in four, fracture of the femoral stem in one, and deep infection in five.

The authors also evaluated survival on the basis of the femoral defect and the number of previous revisions. Survival of the reconstructions was significantly worse for hips with Paprosky type IV defects than for those with type IIIB defects, and three or more previous femoral revisions significantly affected survival compared with one previous revision.

These results suggest that the use of proximal femoral allografts for massive segmental bone loss in revision total hip arthroplasty can provide durable long-term results, although the survival seems to be adversely affected by the amount of bone loss and the number of previous revisions.

Proximal Femoral Replacement

Proximal femoral replacements have been used extensively in the management of proximal femoral bone loss secondary to neoplastic disease.[76-82] There are few reports regarding the use of these prostheses in nonneoplastic conditions.[83-86] Parvizi and Sim[84] cautioned that these prostheses should be reserved for elderly or sedentary patients with massive proximal bone loss that cannot be reconstructed by other means.

Sim and Chao[83] reported encouraging results in a cohort of 21 patients who had been followed for 25 to 92 months after proximal femoral replacement. Two femoral components were revised: one because of recurrent instability and one because of acetabular loosening with substantial bone loss; the patient elected to have the well-fixed prosthesis removed. The authors cautioned that the results were preliminary, and longer term follow-up might change the results. In a follow-up report, Malkani et al[86] reviewed the 11.1-year results of 50 proximal femoral replacements. They reported that four femoral and seven acetabular components had been revised because of aseptic loosening. With any revision as the end point, survivorship was predicted to be 64% at 12 years following proximal femoral replacement. They also found that 11 of 50 hips had dislocated. Parvizi et al[85] reviewed the cases of 43 patients who had a proximal femoral replacement for a nonneoplastic condition at a mean of 36.5 months. With revision used as the end point, 37 of 43 implants had survived at 1 year and 31 of 43 implants at 5 years. Eight patients had hip instability, and six required revision for recurrent dislocation. Although the use of proximal femoral replacements can provide functional long-term results, the prostheses should be reserved for salvage situations in which massive proximal femoral bone loss cannot be reconstructed with other techniques.

Summary

Revision of a femoral implant is a challenging endeavor when there is substantial proximal bone loss. Numerous reconstructive options have been studied, and surgeons considering revision of a failed femoral prosthesis should be familiar with them. Careful preoperative planning is central to a successful outcome. Part of the preoperative plan will include a critical review of the radiographs in an effort to assess the degree of anticipated bone loss. Although several authors have proposed classification schemes for femoral bone loss, the Paprosky classification system provides a useful guide to femoral reconstruction based on the degree of bone loss. The rare type I defects can be treated with essentially any implant used in primary arthroplasty. The type II and IIIA defects can be reliably reconstructed with a cylindrical, extensively porous-coated implant. The type IIIB defect can usually be treated with a tapered, fluted, modular stem. The complex type IV defect has been treated successfully with impaction grafting, modular tapered stems, allograft-prosthetic composites, and proximal femoral replacements. As technology and techniques have evolved, the success of femoral reconstruction in the face of extensive bone loss has improved. Continued follow-up and further evolution in technique and technology will continue to guide the management of femoral revision.

References

1. Kurtz S, Ong K, Lau E, Mowat F, Halpern M: Projections of primary and revision hip and knee arthroplasty in the United States from 2005 to 2030. *J Bone Joint Surg Am* 2007;89(4):780-785.
2. Agarwal S, Freiberg AA, Rubash HE: Preoperative planning for revision hip arthroplasty, in Callaghan JJ, Rosenberg AG, Rubash HE, eds: *The Adult Hip*, ed 2. Philadelphia, PA, Lippincott Williams & Wilkins, 2007, p 1313.
3. Harris WH, McCarthy JC Jr, O'Neill DA: Femoral component loosening using contemporary techniques of femoral cement fixation. *J Bone Joint Surg Am* 1982;64(7):1063-1067.
4. O'Neill DA, Harris WH: Failed total hip replacement: Assessment by plain radiographs, arthrograms, and aspiration of the hip joint. *J Bone Joint Surg Am* 1984;66(4):540-546.
5. Engh CA, Bobyn JD, Glassman AH: Porous-coated hip replacement: The factors governing bone ingrowth, stress shielding, and clinical results. *J Bone Joint Surg Br* 1987;69(1):45-55.
6. Della Valle CJ, Paprosky WG: The femur in revision total hip arthroplasty evaluation and classification. *Clin Orthop Relat Res* 2004;420:55-62.

7. D'Antonio J, McCarthy JC, Bargar WL, et al: Classification of femoral abnormalities in total hip arthroplasty. *Clin Orthop Relat Res* 1993;296:133-139.

8. Mallory TH: Preparation of the proximal femur in cementless total hip revision. *Clin Orthop Relat Res* 1988;235:47-60.

9. Saleh KJ, Holtzman J, Gafni A, et al: Reliability and intraoperative validity of preoperative assessment of standardized plain radiographs in predicting bone loss at revision hip surgery. *J Bone Joint Surg Am* 2001;83-A(7):1040-1046.

10. Weeden SH, Paprosky WG: Minimal 11-year follow-up of extensively porous-coated stems in femoral revision total hip arthroplasty. *J Arthroplasty* 2002;17(4, Suppl 1):134-137.

11. Saleh KJ, Holtzman J, Gafni A, et al: Development, test reliability and validation of a classification for revision hip arthroplasty. *J Orthop Res* 2001;19(1): 50-56.

12. Krishnamurthy AB, MacDonald SJ, Paprosky WG: 5- to 13-year follow-up study on cementless femoral components in revision surgery. *J Arthroplasty* 1997;12(8): 839-847.

13. Lawrence JM, Engh CA, Macalino GE: Revision total hip arthroplasty: Long-term results without cement. *Orthop Clin North Am* 1993;24(4):635-644.

14. Della Valle CJ, Paprosky WG: Classification and an algorithmic approach to the reconstruction of femoral deficiency in revision total hip arthroplasty. *J Bone Joint Surg Am* 2003;85-A(Suppl 4):1-6.

15. Richards CJ, Duncan CP, Masri BA, Garbuz DS: Femoral revision hip arthroplasty: A comparison of two stem designs. *Clin Orthop Relat Res* 2010;468(2):491-496.

16. Iorio R, Healy WL, Presutti AH: A prospective outcomes analysis of femoral component fixation in revision total hip arthroplasty. *J Arthroplasty* 2008;23(5): 662-669.

17. Barrack RL, Folgueras AJ: Revision total hip arthroplasty: The femoral component. *J Am Acad Orthop Surg* 1995;3(2):79-85.

18. Pellicci PM, Wilson PD Jr, Sledge CB, et al: Long-term results of revision total hip replacement: A follow-up report. *J Bone Joint Surg Am* 1985;67(4):513-516.

19. Kavanagh BF, Ilstrup DM, Fitzgerald RH Jr: Revision total hip arthroplasty. *J Bone Joint Surg Am* 1985;67(4):517-526.

20. Callaghan JJ, Salvati EA, Pellicci PM, Wilson PD Jr, Ranawat CS: Results of revision for mechanical failure after cemented total hip replacement, 1979 to 1982: A two to five-year follow-up. *J Bone Joint Surg Am* 1985;67(7):1074-1085.

21. Rubash HE, Harris WH: Revision of nonseptic, loose, cemented femoral components using modern cementing techniques. *J Arthroplasty* 1988;3(3):241-248.

22. Estok DM II, Harris WH: Long-term results of cemented femoral revision surgery using second-generation techniques: An average 11.7-year follow-up evaluation. *Clin Orthop Relat Res* 1994;299: 190-202.

23. Mulroy WF, Harris WH: Revision total hip arthroplasty with use of so-called second-generation cementing techniques for aseptic loosening of the femoral component: A fifteen-year-average follow-up study. *J Bone Joint Surg Am* 1996;78(3):325-330.

24. Eisler T, Svensson O, Iyer V, et al: Revision total hip arthroplasty using third-generation cementing technique. *J Arthroplasty* 2000; 15(8):974-981.

25. Dohmae Y, Bechtold JE, Sherman RE, Puno RM, Gustilo RB: Reduction in cement-bone interface shear strength between primary and revision arthroplasty. *Clin Orthop Relat Res* 1988;236: 214-220.

26. Simon JP, Fowler JL, Gie GA, Ling RS, Timperley AJ: Impaction cancellous grafting of the femur in cemented total hip revision arthroplasty. *J Bone Joint Surg Br* 1991;73(Suppl 1):73.

27. Ornstein E, Atroshi I, Franzén H, Johnsson R, Sandquist P, Sundberg M: Early complications after one hundred and forty-four consecutive hip revisions with impacted morselized allograft bone and cement. *J Bone Joint Surg Am* 2002;84-A(8):1323-1328.

28. Oakes DA, Cabanela ME: Impaction bone grafting for revision hip arthroplasty: Biology and clinical applications. *J Am Acad Orthop Surg* 2006;14(11):620-628.

29. Eldridge JD, Smith EJ, Hubble MJ, Whitehouse SL, Learmonth ID: Massive early subsidence following femoral impaction grafting. *J Arthroplasty* 1997;12(5): 535-540.

30. Jazrawi LM, Della Valle CJ, Kummer FJ, Adler EM, Di Cesare PE: Catastrophic failure of a cemented, collarless, polished, tapered cobalt-chromium femoral stem used with impaction bone-grafting: A report of two cases. *J Bone Joint Surg Am* 1999;81(6): 844-847.

31. Masterson EL, Masri BA, Duncan CP: The cement mantle in the Exeter impaction allografting technique: A cause for concern. *J Arthroplasty* 1997;12(7): 759-764.

32. Meding JB, Ritter MA, Keating EM, Faris PM: Impaction bone-grafting before insertion of a femoral stem with cement in revision total hip arthroplasty: A minimum two-year follow-up study. *J Bone Joint Surg Am* 1997; 79(12):1834-1841.

33. Pekkarinen J, Alho A, Lepistö J, Ylikoski M, Ylinen P, Paavilainen T: Impaction bone grafting in

revision hip surgery: A high incidence of complications. *J Bone Joint Surg Br* 2000;82(1): 103-107.

34. Ornstein E, Linder L, Ranstam J, Lewold S, Eisler T, Torper M: Femoral impaction bone grafting with the Exeter stem: The Swedish experience. Survivorship analysis of 1305 revisions performed between 1989 and 2002. *J Bone Joint Surg Br* 2009;91(4): 441-446.

35. Edwards SA, Pandit HG, Grover ML, Clarke HJ: Impaction bone grafting in revision hip surgery. *J Arthroplasty* 2003;18(7): 852-859.

36. Halliday BR, English HW, Timperley AJ, Gie GA, Ling RS: Femoral impaction grafting with cement in revision total hip replacement: Evolution of the technique and results. *J Bone Joint Surg Br* 2003;85(6):809-817.

37. Mahoney CR, Fehringer EV, Kopjar B, Garvin KL: Femoral revision with impaction grafting and a collarless, polished, tapered stem. *Clin Orthop Relat Res* 2005; 432:181-187.

38. Wraighte PJ, Howard PW: Femoral impaction bone allografting with an Exeter cemented collarless, polished, tapered stem in revision hip replacement: A mean follow-up of 10.5 years. *J Bone Joint Surg Br* 2008;90(8):1000-1004.

39. Sierra RJ, Charity J, Tsiridis E, Timperley JA, Gie GA: The use of long cemented stems for femoral impaction grafting in revision total hip arthroplasty. *J Bone Joint Surg Am* 2008;90(6):1330-1336.

40. Gustilo RB, Pasternak HS: Revision total hip arthroplasty with titanium ingrowth prosthesis and bone grafting for failed cemented femoral component loosening. *Clin Orthop Relat Res* 1988;235: 111-119.

41. Harris WH, Krushell RJ, Galante JO: Results of cementless revisions of total hip arthroplasties using the Harris-Galante prosthesis. *Clin Orthop Relat Res* 1988;235: 120-126.

42. Hedley AK, Gruen TA, Ruoff DP: Revision of failed total hip arthroplasties with uncemented porous-coated anatomic components. *Clin Orthop Relat Res* 1988;235: 75-90.

43. Woolson ST, Delaney TJ: Failure of a proximally porous-coated femoral prosthesis in revision total hip arthroplasty. *J Arthroplasty* 1995;10(Suppl):S22-S28.

44. Berry DJ, Harmsen WS, Ilstrup D, Lewallen DG, Cabanela ME: Survivorship of uncemented proximally porous-coated femoral components. *Clin Orthop Relat Res* 1995;319:168-177.

45. Malkani AL, Lewallen DG, Cabanela ME, Wallrichs SL: Femoral component revision using an uncemented, proximally coated, long-stem prosthesis. *J Arthroplasty* 1996;11(4):411-418.

46. Mulliken BD, Rorabeck CH, Bourne RB: Uncemented revision total hip arthroplasty: A 4-to-6-year review. *Clin Orthop Relat Res* 1996;325:156-162.

47. Christie MJ, DeBoer DK, Tingstad EM, Capps M, Brinson MF, Trick LW: Clinical experience with a modular noncemented femoral component in revision total hip arthroplasty: 4- to 7-year results. *J Arthroplasty* 2000;15(7): 840-848.

48. Cameron HU: The long-term success of modular proximal fixation stems in revision total hip arthroplasty. *J Arthroplasty* 2002; 17(4, Suppl 1):138-141.

49. Smith JA, Dunn HK, Manaster BJ: Cementless femoral revision arthroplasty: 2- to 5-year results with a modular titanium alloy stem. *J Arthroplasty* 1997;12(2): 194-201.

50. McCarthy JC, Lee JA: Complex revision total hip arthroplasty with modular stems at a mean of 14 years. *Clin Orthop Relat Res* 2007;465:166-169.

51. Bolognesi MP, Pietrobon R, Clifford PE, Vail TP: Comparison of a hydroxyapatite-coated sleeve and a porous-coated sleeve with a modular revision hip stem: A prospective, randomized study. *J Bone Joint Surg Am* 2004;86-A(12): 2720-2725.

52. Engh CA Jr, Hopper RH Jr, Engh CA Sr: Distal ingrowth components. *Clin Orthop Relat Res* 2004; 420:135-141.

53. Lawrence JM, Engh CA, Macalino GE, Lauro GR: Outcome of revision hip arthroplasty done without cement. *J Bone Joint Surg Am* 1994;76(7):965-973.

54. Moreland JR, Bernstein ML: Femoral revision hip arthroplasty with uncemented, porous-coated stems. *Clin Orthop Relat Res* 1995; 319:141-150.

55. Moreland JR, Moreno MA: Cementless femoral revision arthroplasty of the hip: minimum 5 years followup. *Clin Orthop Relat Res* 2001;393:194-201.

56. Sporer SM, Paprosky WG: Revision total hip arthroplasty: The limits of fully coated stems. *Clin Orthop Relat Res* 2003;417: 203-209.

57. Engh CA Jr, Ellis TJ, Koralewicz LM, McAuley JP, Engh CA Sr: Extensively porous-coated femoral revision for severe femoral bone loss: Minimum 10-year follow-up. *J Arthroplasty* 2002;17(8): 955-960.

58. Böhm P, Bischel O: Femoral revision with the Wagner SL revision stem: Evaluation of one hundred and twenty-nine revisions followed for a mean of 4.8 years. *J Bone Joint Surg Am* 2001; 83-A(7):1023-1031.

59. Kolstad K, Adalberth G, Mallmin H, Milbrink J, Sahlstedt B: The

Wagner revision stem for severe osteolysis: 31 hips followed for 1.5-5 years. *Acta Orthop Scand* 1996;67(6):541-544.

60. Suominen S, Santavirta S: Revision total hip arthroplasty in deficient proximal femur using a distal load-bearing prosthesis. *Ann Chir Gynaecol* 1996;85(3): 253-262.

61. Grünig R, Morscher E, Ochsner PE: Three- to 7-year results with the uncemented SL femoral revision prosthesis. *Arch Orthop Trauma Surg* 1997;116(4): 187-197.

62. Berry DJ: Femoral revision: Distal fixation with fluted, tapered grit-blasted stems. *J Arthroplasty* 2002; 17(4, Suppl 1):142-146.

63. Kwong LM, Miller AJ, Lubinus P: A modular distal fixation option for proximal bone loss in revision total hip arthroplasty: A 2- to 6-year follow-up study. *J Arthroplasty* 2003;18(3, Suppl 1):94-97.

64. McInnis DP, Horne G, Devane PA: Femoral revision with a fluted, tapered, modular stem seventy patients followed for a mean of 3.9 years. *J Arthroplasty* 2006;21(3):372-380.

65. Murphy SB, Rodriguez J: Revision total hip arthroplasty with proximal bone loss. *J Arthroplasty* 2004;19(4, Suppl 1):115-119.

66. Park YS, Moon YW, Lim SJ: Revision total hip arthroplasty using a fluted and tapered modular distal fixation stem with and without extended trochanteric osteotomy. *J Arthroplasty* 2007;22(7): 993-999.

67. Schuh A, Werber S, Holzwarth U, Zeiler G: Cementless modular hip revision arthroplasty using the MRP Titan Revision Stem: Outcome of 79 hips after an average of 4 years' follow-up. *Arch Orthop Trauma Surg* 2004;124(5): 306-309.

68. Weiss RJ, Beckman MO, Enocson A, Schmalholz A, Stark A: Minimum 5-year follow-up of a cementless, modular, tapered stem in hip revision arthroplasty. *J Arthroplasty* 2011;26(1):16-23.

69. Ovesen O, Emmeluth C, Hofbauer C, Overgaard S: Revision total hip arthroplasty using a modular tapered stem with distal fixation: Good short-term results in 125 revisions. *J Arthroplasty* 2010;25(3):348-354.

70. Wirtz DC, Heller KD, Holzwarth U, et al: A modular femoral implant for uncemented stem revision in THR. *Int Orthop* 2000; 24(3):134-138.

71. Postak PD, Greenwald AS: *The Influence of Modularity on the Endurance Performance of the LINK MP Hip Stem.* Cleveland, OH, Orthopaedic Research Laboratories, 2001.

72. Lee SH, Ahn YJ, Chung SJ, Kim BK, Hwang JH: The use of allograft prosthesis composite for extensive proximal femoral bone deficiencies: A 2- to 9.8-year follow-up study. *J Arthroplasty* 2009;24(8):1241-1248.

73. Safir O, Kellett CF, Flint M, Backstein D, Gross AE: Revision of the deficient proximal femur with a proximal femoral allograft. *Clin Orthop Relat Res* 2009; 467(1):206-212.

74. Graham NM, Stockley I: The use of structural proximal femoral allografts in complex revision hip arthroplasty. *J Bone Joint Surg Br* 2004;86(3):337-343.

75. Babis GC, Sakellariou VI, O'Connor MI, Hanssen AD, Sim FH: Proximal femoral allograft-prosthesis composites in revision hip replacement: A 12-year follow-up study. *J Bone Joint Surg Br* 2010;92(3):349-355.

76. Bosquet M, Burssens A, Mulier JC: Long term follow-up results of a femoral megaprosthesis: A review of thirteen patients. *Arch Orthop Trauma Surg* 1980;97(4): 299-304.

77. Donati D, Zavatta M, Gozzi E, Giacomini S, Campanacci L, Mercuri M: Modular prosthetic replacement of the proximal femur after resection of a bone tumour a long-term follow-up. *J Bone Joint Surg Br* 2001;83(8): 1156-1160.

78. Kawai A, Backus SI, Otis JC, Inoue H, Healey JH: Gait characteristics of patients after proximal femoral replacement for malignant bone tumour. *J Bone Joint Surg Br* 2000;82(5):666-669.

79. Johnsson R, Carlsson A, Kisch K, Moritz U, Zetterström R, Persson BM: Function following mega total hip arthroplasty compared with conventional total hip arthroplasty and healthy matched controls. *Clin Orthop Relat Res* 1985;192:159-167.

80. Morris HG, Capanna R, Del Ben M, Campanacci D: Prosthetic reconstruction of the proximal femur after resection for bone tumors. *J Arthroplasty* 1995;10(3): 293-299.

81. Ogilvie CM, Wunder JS, Ferguson PC, Griffin AM, Bell RS: Functional outcome of endoprosthetic proximal femoral replacement. *Clin Orthop Relat Res* 2004; 426:44-48.

82. Zehr RJ, Enneking WF, Scarborough MT: Allograft-prosthesis composite versus megaprosthesis in proximal femoral reconstruction. *Clin Orthop Relat Res* 1996; 322:207-223.

83. Sim FH, Chao EY: Hip salvage by proximal femoral replacement. *J Bone Joint Surg Am* 1981;63(8): 1228-1239.

84. Parvizi J, Sim FH: Proximal femoral replacements with megaprostheses. *Clin Orthop Relat Res* 2004;420:169-175.

85. Parvizi J, Tarity TD, Slenker N, et al: Proximal femoral replacement in patients with non-neoplastic conditions. *J Bone Joint Surg Am* 2007;89(5):1036-1043.

86. Malkani AL, Settecerri JJ, Sim FH, Chao EY, Wallrichs SL: Long-term results of proximal femoral replacement for non-neoplastic disorders. *J Bone Joint Surg Br* 1995;77(3):351-356.

87. Rodriguez JA, Fada R, Murphy SB, Rasquinha VJ, Ranawat CS: Two-year to five-year follow-up of femoral defects in femoral revision treated with the link MP modular stem. *J Arthroplasty* 2009;24(5): 751-758.

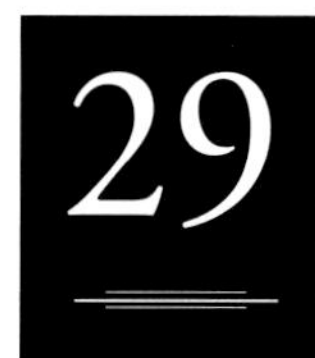

How to Do a Revision Total Hip Arthroplasty: Revision of the Acetabulum

Scott M. Sporer, MD

Abstract

The need for revision total hip arthroplasty continues to increase as the indications for total hip replacement broaden and the average life expectancy of patients and their demands for activity increase. To achieve a successful long-term outcome after revision acetabular surgery, the surgical reconstruction must provide a mechanically stable construct that will minimize micromotion, allow bone ingrowth, and restore appropriate hip biomechanics. Achieving these goals during revision acetabular surgery can be challenging because of periacetabular bone loss and a compromised biologic environment. Acetabular classifications can help to preoperatively predict areas of bone loss to guide treatment options. Most acetabular defects can be managed with a hemispheric or elliptic porous acetabular component; however, large areas of segmental or cavitary bone loss may require alternative treatments such as custom implants, metal/allograft augmentation, or an acetabular cage reconstruction.

The most common indications for acetabular revision include instability, infection, polyethylene wear, and aseptic loosening.[1] The prevalence of these conditions remains essentially unchanged despite improved prosthetic component designs and enhanced surgical techniques. A successful acetabular revision must provide intimate contact between the acetabular implant and the host bone, a stable mechanical construct minimizing micromotion to allow bone ingrowth into a cementless acetabular component, and a mechanical construct that distributes the physiologic stresses to the surrounding acetabular bone. Additionally, the acetabular reconstruction must allow appropriate component orientation to minimize the risk of dislocation and reestablish the anatomic hip center to improve the overall joint kinematics. Biologic methods of acetabular reconstruction are advised except in cases of severe bone loss or prior radiation treatment in the hip region because nonbiologic revisions eventually fail.[2] Periacetabular bone loss can compromise component fixation, resulting in early loosening of the revised acetabulum. The amount of bone loss undoubtedly influences the ability to obtain initial optimal fixation. The location of remaining supportive bone, however, has a more important role in providing durable fixation than does the quantity of bone loss.

Defect Classification Systems

Acetabular defect classification systems can be used to predict the extent of bone loss seen intraoperatively and guide subsequent reconstructive options. The three most common classification systems for acetabular defects are the American Academy of Orthopaedic Surgeons (AAOS) classification system described by D'Antonio et al[3] (**Table 1**), the Gross classification system described by Saleh et al[4] (**Table 2**), and the Paprosky classification system[5] (**Table 3**). The AAOS classification system identifies the pattern of acetabular bone loss but does not quantify the size or location of the defect. Despite being the most commonly cited system, the AAOS defect classification system does not guide the

Dr. Sporer or an immediate family member serves as a paid consultant to Smith & Nephew and Zimmer and has received research or institutional support from Coolsystems.

identification of reconstructive options. The system described by Saleh et al[4] is based on the degree of bone loss seen on preoperative standard AP and lateral radiographs of the hip. A bone defect is considered uncontained if morcellized bone graft cannot be used to fill the defect. The Paprosky classification system is based on four radiographic criteria from an AP pelvic radiograph: (1) superior migration of the hip center, (2) ischial osteolysis, (3) acetabular teardrop osteolysis, and (4) position of the implant relative to the Kohler line[5] (**Figure 1**). Superior migration of the hip center represents bone loss of the acetabular dome involving the anterior and posterior columns. Ischial osteolysis indicates bone loss from the posterior column including the posterior wall, whereas teardrop osteolysis and migration beyond the Kohler line represent medial acetabular bone loss. Type III defects require structural support from bulk allograft, metallic augmentation, an acetabular cage, or a custom acetabular component. The Paprosky classification system is often used clinically, because it not only predicts bone loss encountered intraoperatively but also assists in determining reconstructive options.

Table 1
AAOS Classification System for Acetabular Defects

Type	Description
I	Segmental defect
II	Cavitary defect
III	Combined segmental and cavitary defect
IV	Pelvic discontinuity
IVa	Discontinuity with mild segmental or cavitary bone loss
IVb	Discontinuity with moderate to severe segmental or cavitary bone loss
IVc	Discontinuity with prior pelvic irradiation
V	Hip arthrodesis

AAOS = American Academy of Orthopaedic Surgeons

Table 2
Gross Classification System for Acetabular Defects

Type	Description
I	No substantial loss of bone stock
II	Contained loss of bone stock (columns and/or rim intact)
III	Uncontained loss of bone stock (< 50% acetabulum)
IV	Uncontained loss of bone stock (> 50% acetabulum)
V	Contained loss of bone stock with pelvic discontinuity

Component Removal

Successful acetabular reconstruction begins with a meticulous surgical technique to remove a well-fixed acetabular component. The use of acetabular "explant osteotomes" (**Figure 2**) facilitates the safe removal of well-fixed components. An osteotome blade, which is the outer diameter of the acetabular component, is used with a so-called femoral head that matches the diameter of the bearing surface. The osteotome is rotated around the periphery of the socket, disrupting the interface between the implant and the host bone. Areas of the pelvis that are crucial for subsequent reconstruction are the anterosuperior and posteroinferior aspects of the acetabulum. Monoblock

Table 3
Paprosky Classification System for Acetabular Defects

	Description			
Type	Femoral Head Center Migration	Ischial Osteolysis	Kohler Line	Teardrop
I	Minimal (< 3 cm)	None	Intact	Intact
IIA	Mild (< 3 cm)	Mild	Intact	Intact
IIB	Moderate (< 3 cm)	Mild	Intact	Intact
IIC	Mild (< 3 cm)	Mild	Disrupted	Moderate lysis
IIIA	Severe (> 3 cm)	Moderate	Intact	Moderate lysis
IIIB	Severe (> 3 cm)	Severe	Disrupted	Severe lysis

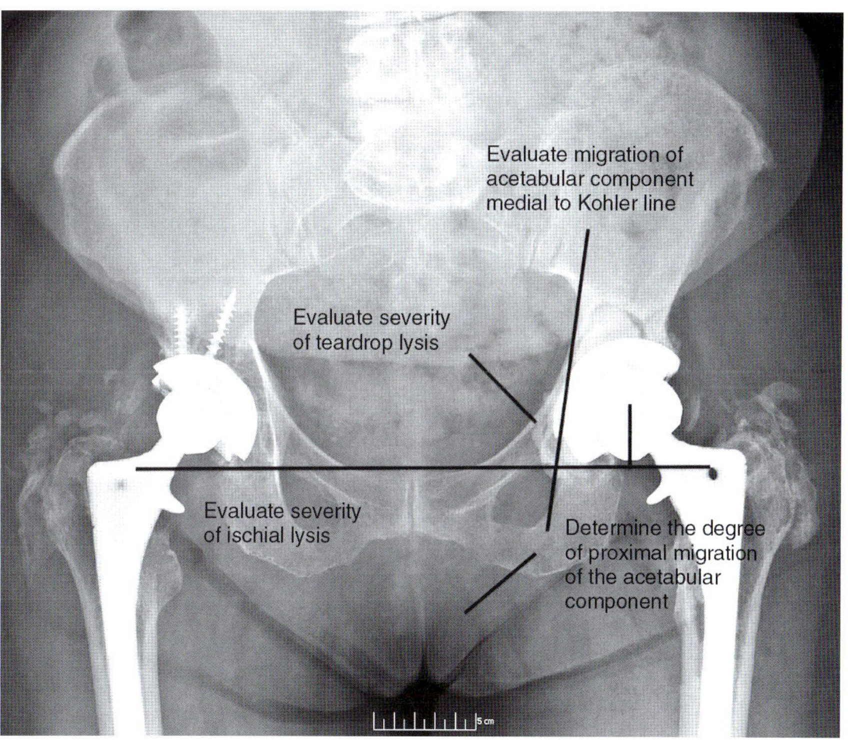

Figure 1 Components of the radiographic criteria in the Paprosky classification system for acetabular defects.

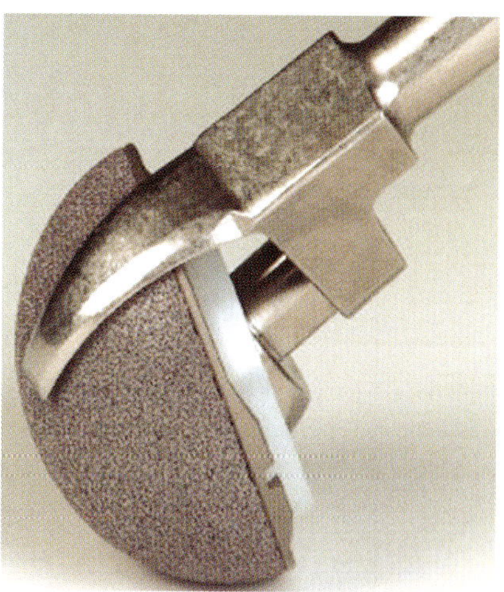

Figure 2 Acetabular component extraction tool. A bipolar femoral head may be used to remove a monoblock cobalt-chromium acetabular component. (Reproduced with permission from Taylor PR, Stoffel KK, Dunlop DG, Yates PJ. Removal of the well-fixed hip resurfacing acetabular component: A simple, bone preserving technique. *J Arthroplasty* 2009;24:484-486.)

acetabular components are removed with the use of a so-called bipolar articulation with a curved osteotome blade matching the outer diameter of the acetabular component. Alternatively, manual instruments such as curved chisels and motorized burrs can be used to disrupt the prosthesis-bone interface or section the cup. Forceful manipulation of the component during removal should be avoided because severe bone loss and associated pelvic discontinuity may occur. A preoperative angiogram and/or vascular surgery consultation should be obtained if the acetabular component has migrated medially past the Kohler line (**Figure 3**).

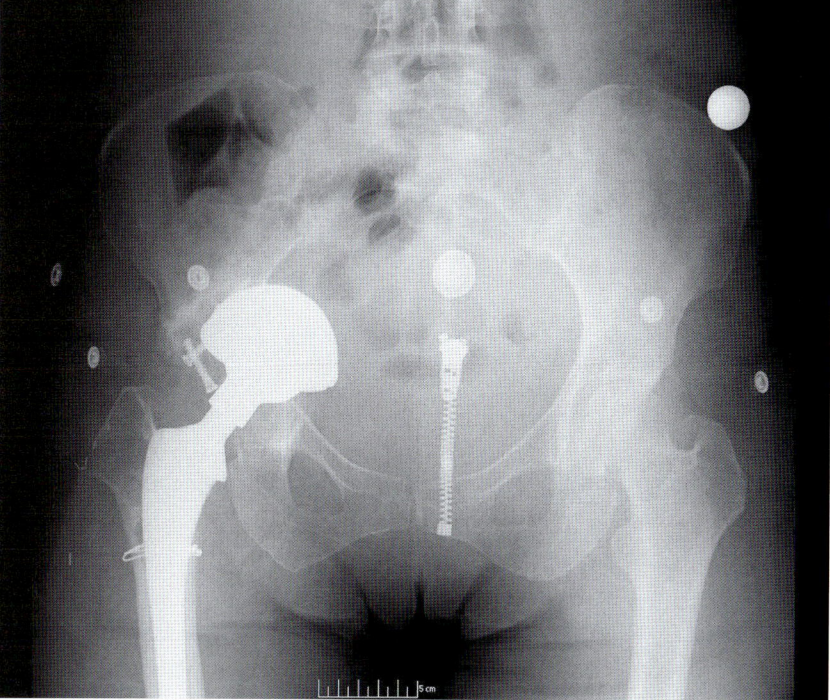

Figure 3 Intrapelvic migration of the acetabular component, a Paprosky type IIIB defect. A preoperative angiogram or vascular surgery consultation should be considered to minimize the risk of injury to the iliac vessel during revision arthroplasty.

Treatment Algorithm

The treatment of acetabular defects depends on the degree and location of bone loss in addition to the potential for biologic fixation. Prior irradiation of the pelvis can result in periacetabu-

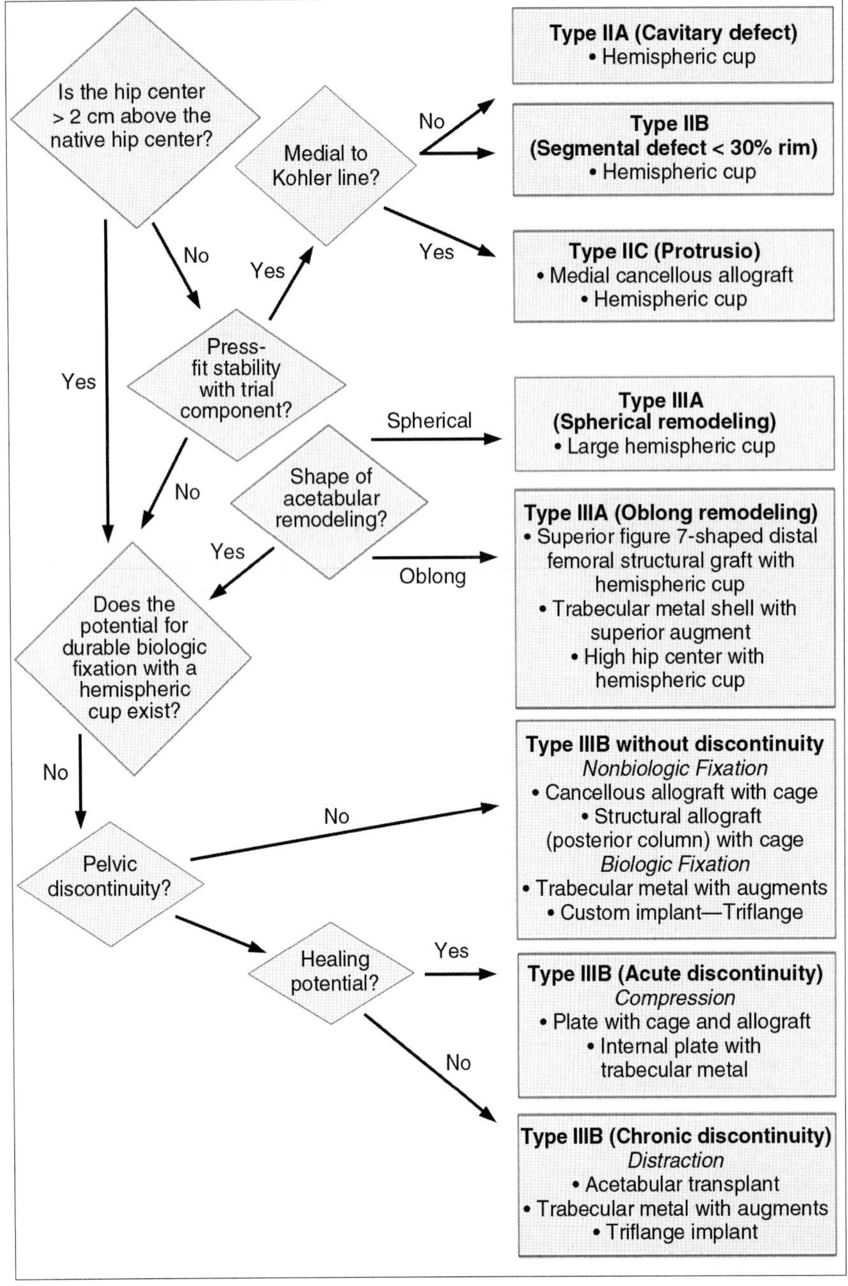

Figure 4 Treatment algorithm for acetabular revision surgery. (Reproduced from Sporer SM, Paprosky WG, O'Rourke MR: Managing bone loss in acetabular revision. *Instr Course Lect* 2006;55:287-298.)

lar osteonecrosis with limited ingrowth potential.[2] In these situations, nonbiologic fixation options, such as acetabular cages, custom implants, and fixed-angle devices, which offload the host bone, should be considered. Fortunately, most acetabular revisions can be managed successfully with a hemispheric component alone.[6-9] The goals of revision surgery are to obtain stable fixation on the remaining host bone and restore the hip center with the acetabular component near the Kohler line and the inferomedial aspect of the acetabular component near the inferior portion of the acetabular teardrop. An algorithmic approach to acetabular defects helps preoperative planning as well as surgical decision making (**Figure 4**).

Acetabular Reconstruction

Hemispheric or Elliptic Component

An acetabular component with a hemispheric or elliptic design can be used in patients when the hip center of rotation has not migrated more than 3 cm proximally (Paprosky types I, IIA, IIB, and IIC).[10,11] After acetabular component removal, the remaining host bone should be exposed, and all granulation tissue should be thoroughly débrided. Pelvic discontinuity is assessed by looking for motion between the superior and the inferior hemipelvis when applying a caudal stress to the ischium with a Cobb elevator.

A retractor is placed in the obturator foramen to determine the level of the true acetabulum, which is the level of the inferior border of the acetabulum. Sequentially larger hemispheric acetabular reamers are used to determine the size of the acetabulum until the anterior and posterior columns are engaged by the reamer. To minimize the likelihood of creating pelvic discontinuity while reaming, in general, anterior acetabular bone should be sacrificed before posterior column bone. Trial acetabular components are used to assess the stability of the acetabular socket along with the degree of component coverage. Most acetabular defects have 5% to 20% of the acetabular component uncovered posterosuperiorly if the trial cup is placed in 40° of vertical inclination and 15° of anteversion. The temptation to place the component more vertically to improve coverage should be avoided because this can increase the risk of dislocation and wear. Cavitary bone defects are packed with either local autograft or allograft with the use of a reamer 2 mm smaller

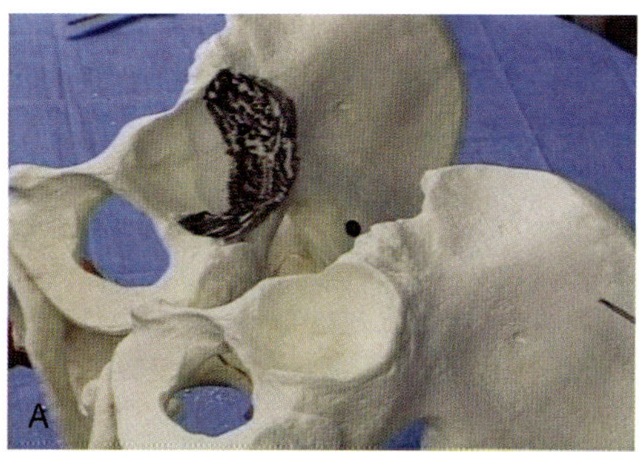

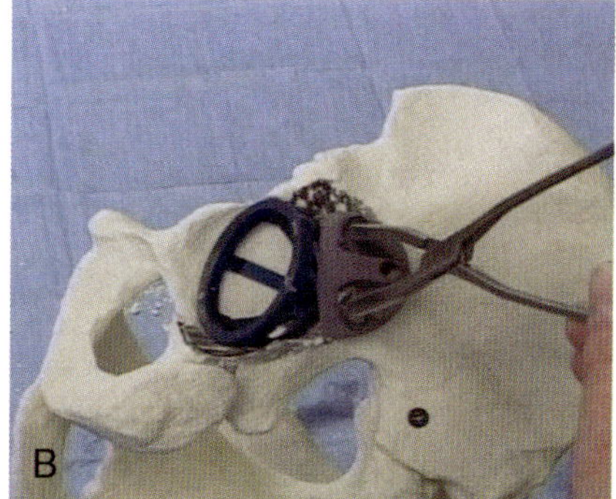

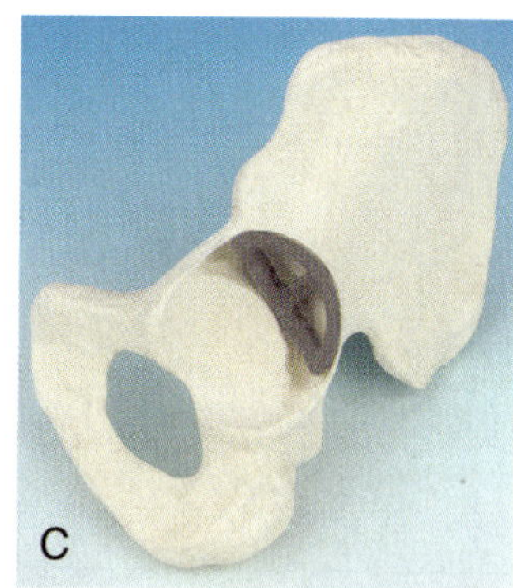

Figure 5 **A,** Type IIIA acetabular defect with superior and posterior bone loss. **B,** Acetabular augment used as a buttress to provide additional superior coverage. **C,** Augment used as a cavitary graft to fill cavitary bone defect and lower hip center.

than the last reaming in reverse. An acetabular component that is 2 mm larger at the periphery than the last reamer is used in most patients to obtain a so-called press-fit and initial fixation. Supplemental fixation with multiple screws is advised in all revisions to minimize micromotion and promote bone ingrowth. Screws should be placed not only posterosuperiorly into the dome of the acetabulum but also inferiorly into the ischium.

Surgical Treatment of Type IIIA Defects

Proximal and lateral migration of the acetabular component of more than 3 cm results in an acetabular dome deficiency that does not provide enough stability for a hemispheric acetabular component alone. Treatment options for patients with superior segmental bone loss include the use of structural bulk allograft, dual-geometry monoblock components, hemispheric components with metallic superior augmentation, or the placement of an implant with a high hip center. A high hip center places the hip abductor muscles at a mechanical disadvantage and necessitates the use of a small acetabular component. It can be challenging to obtain stable fixation and appropriate component orientation with use of a monoblock dual-geometry acetabular component.[12,13] This chapter's author prefers to use a hemispheric acetabular component placed at the level of the true acetabulum and to create superior cup coverage with the use of metallic augmentation.

Hemispheric Component With Metallic Augmentation

The surgical treatment of a superior segmental bone defect with a hemispheric shell and augment begins by identifying the location of the true acetabulum with a retractor placed into the obturator foramen. Hemispheric reamers are then used to ream in the anatomic position until the anterior and posterior columns are engaged, which results in partial stability of a trial acetabular component. A superior augment is used either as a buttress in patients with primarily segmental bone loss or as a superior graft in patients with primarily oblong cavitary bone loss (**Figure 5**). It is crucial that the position of the augment not influence the ultimate position of the acetabular component. With the trial component in place, the augment is secured to the host bone with screws. The augment is then packed with bone graft, leaving the portion facing the cup exposed. Polymethyl methacrylate cement is placed directly on the porous revision cup only in the areas mating with the augment. The acetabular component is firmly impacted to achieve a press-fit against the host bone. In severe bone loss, the polyethylene liner can be cemented into the acetabular shell to place screws at a fixed angle. Multiple screws are used in different planes to maximize stability and minimize the likelihood of component loosening.[14]

Hemispheric Component With Distal Femoral Allograft

The use of bulk allograft has been largely abandoned except in young patients because of the increased surgical time, the need for more soft-tissue exposure, and the concern for graft resorption.[15] Similar to metallic augmentation, the first step in the acetabular reconstruction with bulk allograft is to identify the location of the desired hip center and use acetabular reamers to size and shape the anteroposterior dimensions of the acetabulum to accept a hemispheric cementless implant. The distal femoral allograft is prepared to accommodate the segmental dome defect once it has been determined that there is inadequate coverage of a hemispheric component. The cortex of the distal femoral allograft shaft in the coronal plane relative to the condyles is removed.

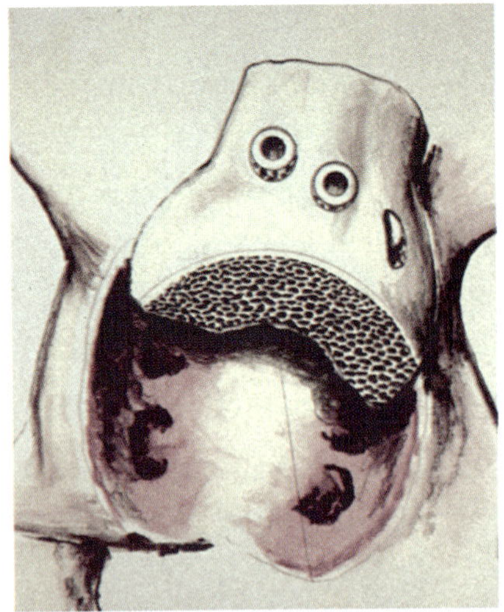

Figure 6 Distal femoral structural allograft used to reconstruct the superior dome of the acetabulum. (Reproduced with permission from Sporer SM, O'Rourke M, Chong P, Paprosky WG: The use of structural distal femoral allografts for acetabular reconstruction: Average ten-year follow-up. *J Bone Joint Surg Am* 2005;87:760-765.)

The posterior aspect of the condyles is then shaped to correspond with the superior acetabular defect with the use of a female reamer measuring 2 mm larger than the last reamer used to size the defect. The anterior to posterior aspect of the distal femoral allograft should correspond to the medial to lateral depth of the defect. The superior cortical limb of the graft should be approximately 4 to 5 cm to allow adequate fixation to the lateral aspect of the ilium. The contoured graft is impacted into the superior defect, obtaining a press-fit. The allograft is secured with three or four parallel 6.5-mm cancellous screws with washers. The screws are oriented obliquely into the ilium in the direction of loading to provide compression of the graft against the remaining ilium. The acetabular cavity is reamed to contour the portion of the graft that will contact the hemispheric component[16] (**Figure 6**).

Surgical Treatment of Type IIIB Defects

Proximal and medial migration of the acetabular component of more than 3 cm results in an acetabular dome deficiency as well as a medial wall deficiency that does not provide enough intrinsic stability for a hemispheric acetabular component alone. Treatment options for patients with superomedial segmental bone loss include structural bulk allograft, custom implants spanning the iliac wing to the ischium, hemispheric components with multiple metal augments, or an acetabular cage. Pelvic discontinuity frequently occurs in patients with severe proximal medial migration of the acetabular component.

Acetabular Transplant With Cage

Acetabular reamers are used to size the acetabular cavity and identify the location of remaining bone along the superior aspect of the ilium that will abut the allograft. The acetabulum of the hemipelvic allograft is reamed on the back table to accept the cage. A curvilinear osteotomy is made in the allograft from the greater sciatic notch to the anterior-superior iliac spine. The pubic and ischial portions of the allograft are removed distal to the confluence of the acetabulum with enough length to accommodate any inferior defects. Leaving excessive inferior bone on the allograft that may prevent optimal medialization of the graft should be avoided because this leads to subsequent vertical cup placement and lateralization of the hip center. A female reamer, 1 to 2 mm larger than the acetabular reamer used to size the acetabulum, should be used to mark and shape the medial aspect of the graft to fit the defect. A groove is made in the superior aspect of the ilium of the allograft to correspond to the ledge of bone along the superior aspect of the native acetabulum. This tongue-and-groove junction provides a stable buttress between the host and the allograft. A burr is used to debulk the inner table of the allograft ilium, while a shelf that will fill the defect of the acetabulum is maintained distally. The graft is secured with Steinmann pins provisionally until four 6.5-mm partially threaded screws are placed obliquely into the ilium from both the intra-articular and lateral aspects of the ilium of the graft. A pelvic reconstruction plate contoured to the posterior column with three screws in the native ilium and ischium is used for fixation. A cage is recommended to protect all transplants, and, if possible, the inferior flange of a cage is inserted into a slot in the ischium for fixation. A metal shell or a polyethylene liner is cemented into the cage-allograft composite, with care taken to avoid the tendency to place the acetabular component in a vertical and retroverted position.

Type IIIB Defect: Modular Metal Augmentation

The acetabulum is reamed in the anatomic location and direction (anterior to posterior, anterior-inferior to posterior-inferior, or posterior-superior to anterior-inferior) for the eventual reconstruction until two points of fixation are achieved, because this determines the size of the acetabular defect. Acetabular augments are used to decrease the acetabular volume and restore a rim to support a revision cup. The location and orientation of augments depends on the pattern of bone loss. Augments are frequently placed along the medial aspect of the ilium or are stacked together to reconstruct the superomedial defect. It is more common to use augments with the wide base placed laterally and the apex medially, which is the opposite of how the augments are often used in

Table 4
Tips and Pearls for Acetabular Revision

Paprosky Classification of Defect	Tips and Pearls
Type IIB	Ream until the anterior and posterior columns are engaged to allow intrinsic stability of the trial component Ream slightly superiorly to improve coverage. Avoid attempts to provide coverage of the superior dome; the superior portion of the acetabular component may remain uncovered. Reverse ream with a reamer that is 1 to 2 mm undersized to pack cavitary defects. Use a cup with multiple holes. Avoid a spiked cup.
Type IIC	Ream until the anterior and posterior columns are engaged to allow intrinsic stability of trial cup along the acetabular rim. Medial bone graft is added until the reverse reamer, which is 1 to 2 mm undersized, disengages from the drive shaft. Use an acetabular component that is 2 mm larger than the last reamer to achieve press-fit fixation. Use a cup with multiple holes.
Type IIIA—distal femoral allograft	Verify that the surgical site is free of infection before opening the distal femoral allograft. Culture the femoral allograft. Avoid the use of femoral head allograft. Elevate abductor musculature with use of a Taylor retractor to allow adequate visualization of the iliac wing. Cut a figure 7-shaped portion of allograft at slightly less than 90° to allow intrinsic stability. Use 6.5-mm cancellous screws and always use with a washer. Tap screws in the allograft to avoid fracture. Avoid the tendency to place the component in excessive abduction and retroversion (the cup may remain uncovered). Place screws through cup-allograft-host bone if possible.
Type IIIA—hemispheric component with metal augment	Progressively ream in the anatomic position to engage the anterior and posterior columns to allow intrinsic stability to the acetabular trial component. Place the superior augment with the trial component in place (with appropriate version and abduction); the augment can be placed in any position or orientation to allow improved initial stability; leave 1 to 2 mm between the cup and the augment for the placement of cement. Use a motorized burr along the superior dome to fit the host bone to the augment to improve intrinsic stability and maximize bone contact. Pack the augment with bone graft, leaving the metal of the augment that faces the cup exposed. Place cement directly onto the porous revision cup only in areas mating with the augment. Insert the cup with cement in the doughy phase to improve interdigitation between the cup and the augment Consider the use of cement with antibiotics. Before the cement hardens, attempt to place a screw in the revision cup to eliminate motion during the final seating of the screws. Place bone wax in the end of the screws to facilitate cup removal.
Type IIIB—hemispheric component with metal augment and no discontinuity	Use augments to reconstruct the pelvis with nonbiologic material. Expose all margins of the acetabular defect. Progressively ream (anterior-posterior, anterior-inferior, and posterior-inferior) until two points of fixation are achieved. Loss of inferior bone stock (ischium) is often involved. Intrinsic stability will not be obtained with the trial component. Use augments to decrease acetabular volume and facilitate press-fit between the cup and the augment (attempt to place the augment in direct contact with the revision cup). Secure the augment first. Reverse ream with the augment in place to pack the bone graft. Clear bone graft from the exposed host bone (maximize the contact area between the host bone and the revision porous cup). Attempt to place screws inferiorly into the ischium to avoid cup pullout.
Type IIIB—pelvic discontinuity distraction	Use a porous acetabular component to reconstruct the pelvis with biologic material as an internal fixation device. Expose all margins of the acetabular defect and discontinuity thoroughly. Progressively ream (anterior to posterior, anterior-inferior to posterior-inferior, or posterior-superior to anterior-inferior) until two points of fixation are achieved. Intrinsic stability will not be obtained. Use augments to decrease acetabular volume and facilitate press-fit between the cup and the augment (attempt to place the augment in direct contact with the revision cup). Bridge the discontinuity with the augment and place screws cephalad and caudal to the discontinuity. Remove fibrous tissue in the discontinuity and place the bone graft. Reverse ream with the augment in place to pack the bone graft. Clear bone graft from exposed host bone (maximize contact area between the host bone and the revision cup).

the type IIIA defect. The revision acetabular cup directly contacts the augments, and the augments are necessary to achieve a press-fit of the acetabular component. Similar to the treatment of a type IIIA defect, augments for a type IIIB defect are initially secured to the host bone with the use of multiple screws. Portions of the augments are removed with a burr or a reamer as needed to optimize the surface area contact between the revision shell and the augments. Particulate bone graft is placed into any remaining cavities before the hemispheric revision shell is impacted in place. Similar to the treatment of a type IIIA defect, the interface between the revision shell and the augment is cemented to minimize micromotion and subsequent fretting. Multiple screws into both the ilium and ischium are used for fixation.

Pelvic Discontinuity

A hemispheric acetabular component alone does not provide adequate implant stability in patients with a pelvic discontinuity. Treatment options for a pelvic discontinuity include compression plating of the posterior column with use of a hemispheric component, placement of an acetabular cage, use of a custom implant that spans the discontinuity, or use of metal acetabular augments to "distract" across the pelvic discontinuity.[17] In patients with a chronic pelvic discontinuity, the amount of bone loss along the posterior column is often too severe to provide direct bone apposition during compression plating.

Modular Metal Augmentation With Distraction for Pelvic Discontinuity

The goal of the distraction technique for a pelvic discontinuity is to use ligamentotaxis secondary to the lengthening across the discontinuity to provide initial component stability. The location and severity of bone loss determine the type and position of the acetabular augments used to enhance initial component stability. Acetabular augments are frequently used to reconstruct portions of the anterosuperior aspect of the acetabulum as well as the posteroinferior aspect of the acetabulum to provide two secure points of fixation for the acetabular component both cephalad and caudal to the discontinuity. A porous acetabular component, which is 6 to 8 mm larger than the hemispheric reamer that engaged the anterior and posterior columns, is used to distract the superior hemipelvis from the inferior hemipelvis. Multiple screws are placed into the remaining ilium and ischium through the acetabular shell, and the augments are secured to the cup with polymethyl methacrylate. A polyethylene liner is cemented into the acetabular component, allowing screws to be placed at a fixed angle. A successful reconstruction of a pelvic discontinuity requires ingrowth of the host bone into both the superior and inferior portions of the acetabular component to bridge the discontinuity. Consequently, as much contact as possible should be obtained between the host bone and the porous augments and acetabular component.

Tips and Pearls for Acetabular Revision

Tips and pearls for the acetabular revision of various types of Paprosky defects are listed in **Table 4**.

References

1. Bozic KJ, Kurtz SM, Lau E, Ong K, Vail TP, Berry DJ: The epidemiology of revision total hip arthroplasty in the United States. *J Bone Joint Surg Am* 2009;91(1):128-133.
2. Jacobs JJ, Kull LR, Frey GA, et al: Early failure of acetabular components inserted without cement after previous pelvic irradiation. *J Bone Joint Surg Am* 1995;77(12):1829-1835.
3. D'Antonio JA, Capello WN, Borden LS, et al: Classification and management of acetabular abnormalities in total hip arthroplasty. *Clin Orthop Relat Res* 1989;243:126-137.
4. Saleh KJ, Holtzman J, Gafni ASaleh L, et al: Development, test reliability and validation of a classification for revision hip arthroplasty. *J Orthop Res* 2001;19(1):50-56.
5. Paprosky WG, Perona PG, Lawrence JM: Acetabular defect classification and surgical reconstruction in revision arthroplasty: A 6-year follow-up evaluation. *J Arthroplasty* 1994;9(1):33-44.
6. Della Valle CJ, Berger RA, Rosenberg AG, Galante JO: Cementless acetabular reconstruction in revision total hip arthroplasty. *Clin Orthop Relat Res* 2004;420:96-100.
7. Gaffey JL, Callaghan JJ, Pedersen DR, Goetz DD, Sullivan PM, Johnston RC: Cementless acetabular fixation at fifteen years: A comparison with the same surgeon's results following acetabular fixation with cement. *J Bone Joint Surg Am* 2004;86-A(2):257-261.
8. Hallstrom BR, Golladay GJ, Vittetoe DA, Harris WH: Cementless acetabular revision with the Harris-Galante porous prosthesis: Results after a minimum of ten years of follow-up. *J Bone Joint Surg Am* 2004;86-A(5):1007-1011.
9. Templeton JE, Callaghan JJ, Goetz DD, Sullivan PM, Johnston RC: Revision of a cemented acetabular component to a cementless acetabular component: A ten to fourteen-year follow-up study. *J Bone Joint Surg Am* 2001;83-A(11):1706-1711.

10. Leopold SS, Rosenberg AG, Bhatt RD, Sheinkop MB, Quigley LR, Galante JO: Cementless acetabular revision: Evaluation at an average of 10.5 years. *Clin Orthop Relat Res* 1999;369:179-186.

11. Silverton CD, Rosenberg AG, Sheinkop MB, Kull LR, Galante JO: Revision total hip arthroplasty using a cementless acetabular component: Technique and results. *Clin Orthop Relat Res* 1995; 319:201-208.

12. Chen WM, Engh CA Jr, Hopper RH Jr, McAuley JP, Engh CA: Acetabular revision with use of a bilobed component inserted without cement in patients who have acetabular bone-stock deficiency. *J Bone Joint Surg Am* 2000;82(2): 197-206.

13. Schutzer SF, Harris WH: High placement of porous-coated acetabular components in complex total hip arthroplasty. *J Arthroplasty* 1994;9(4):359-367.

14. Sporer SM, Paprosky WG: The use of a trabecular metal acetabular component and trabecular metal augment for severe acetabular defects. *J Arthroplasty* 2006; 21(6, Suppl 2):83-86.

15. Sporer SM, O'Rourke M, Chong P, Paprosky WG: The use of structural distal femoral allografts for acetabular reconstruction: Average ten-year follow-up. *J Bone Joint Surg Am* 2005;87(4): 760-765.

16. Sporer SM, O'Rourke M, Chong P, Paprosky WG: The use of structural distal femoral allografts for acetabular reconstruction: Surgical technique. *J Bone Joint Surg Am* 2006;88(Suppl 1 Pt 1): 92-99.

17. Paprosky WG, O'Rourke M, Sporer SM: The treatment of acetabular bone defects with an associated pelvic discontinuity. *Clin Orthop Relat Res* 2005;441: 216-220.

Pelvic Dissociation in Revision Total Hip Arthroplasty: Diagnosis and Treatment

Shahryar Noordin, MBBS, FCPS
Clive P. Duncan, MD, MSc, FRCSC
Bassam A. Masri, MD, FRCSC
Donald S. Garbuz, MD, MHSc, FRCSC

Abstract

Pelvic dissociation is a distinct but uncommon condition, which occurs in association with total hip arthroplasty, in which the superior aspect of the pelvis is separated from the inferior aspect by fracture. Because radiodense implants and cement can obscure pelvic discontinuity on plain radiographs, not all dissociations can be diagnosed preoperatively; therefore, a high index of suspicion for this condition should be maintained. In selected patients, CT angiography may be indicated. Successful treatment requires achieving initial stability of the socket, establishing conditions for long-term stability of the socket, stabilizing the pelvic dissociation, and producing conditions favorable for healing. Applying a posterior pelvic reconstruction plate to the ilium and ischium will achieve stabilization of the dissociation in most patients if sufficient posterior wall and column are present. Occasionally, if there is adequate space, a second plate may be applied. In selected patients, it may be feasible to place anterior column fixation screws using image guidance, which is the preferred technique of the authors rather than the alternate option of using anterior column plating through an anterior exposure. Residual bone loss is then reevaluated and possible options such as a hemispherical socket, a jumbo cup, or a highly porous metal component and augment can be considered. If there is not enough room for a posterior pelvic reconstruction plate, a cup-cage construct with or without an allograft can be used as a reconstruction option.

Dr. Duncan or an immediate family member is a member of a speakers' bureau or has made paid presentations on behalf of Zimmer; and has received research or institutional support from DePuy, Stryker, and Zimmer. Dr. Masri or an immediate family member serves as a board member, owner, officer, or committee member of the Canadian Orthopaedic Association; and has received research or institutional support from Stryker. Dr. Garbuz or an immediate family member has received research or institutional support from Zimmer. Neither Dr. Noordin nor an immediate family member has received anything of value from or owns stock in a commercial company or institution related directly or indirectly to the subject of this chapter.

Pelvic dissociation is a distinct but uncommon condition that occurs in association with total hip arthroplasty (THA). In pelvic dissociation the superior aspect of the pelvis is separated from the inferior aspect by fracture.[1] Pelvic dissociation may be a result of massive bone loss caused by osteolysis, infection, mechanical abrasion, or fracture. In this setting, revision hip arthroplasty is challenging because of the need to achieve fracture stabilization, to replenish bone stock, to accomplish immediate stabilization of the new socket, and to produce an environment that will permit fracture union, bone regeneration, and long-term implant fixation.

Pelvic osteolysis is a common and well-recognized complication associated with THA.[2-4] It affects cemented and uncemented sockets and has been attributed to the biologic reaction to particulate wear debris, particularly polyethylene debris.[2,5] In instances of massive osteolysis and structural failure, the acetabular rim, quadrilateral plate, and associated columns become

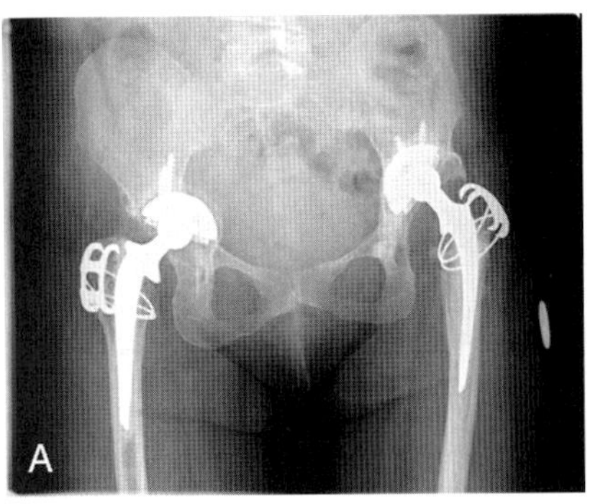

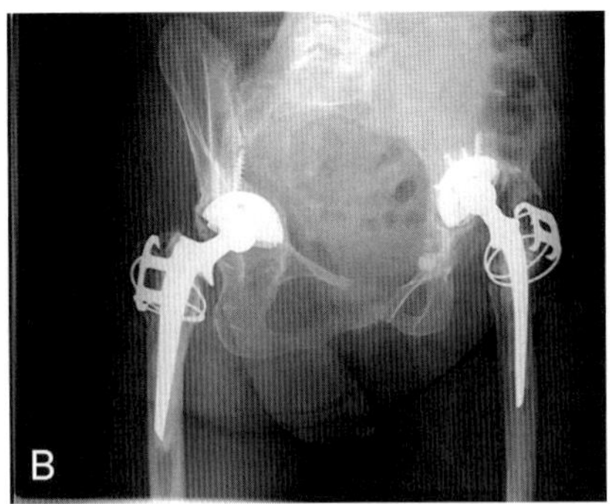

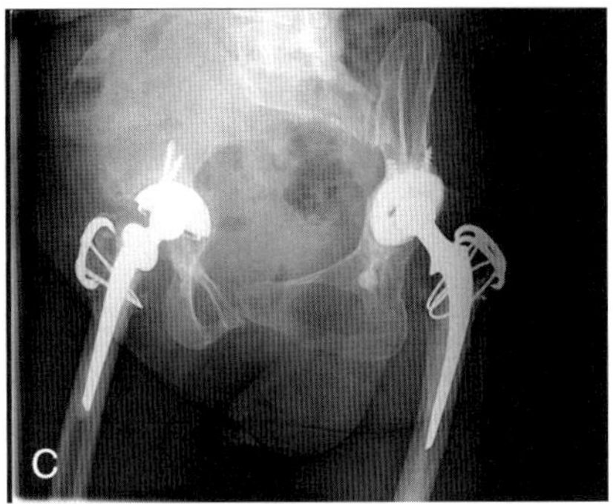

Figure 1 AP **(A)**, obturator oblique **(B)**, and iliac oblique **(C)** views of the pelvis showing pelvic dissociation of the right hip.

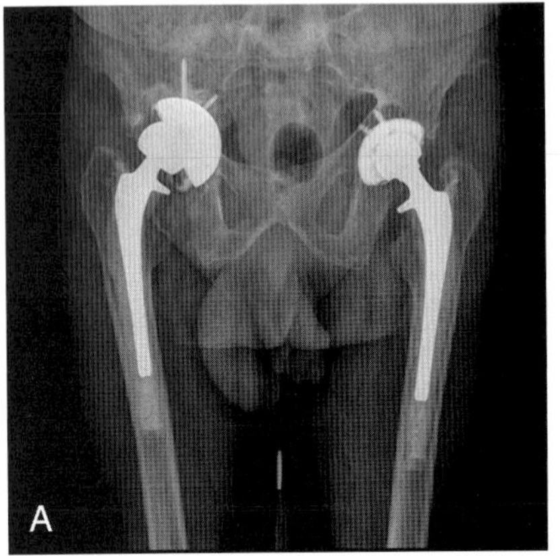

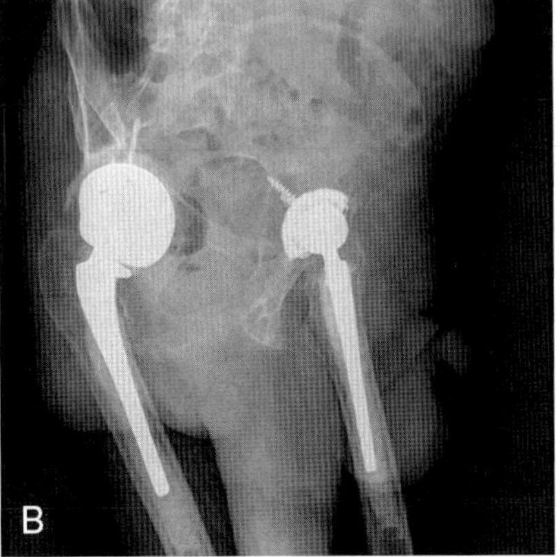

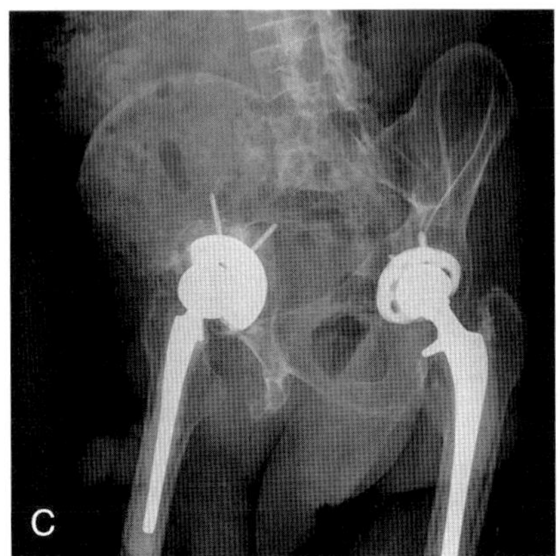

Figure 2 AP **(A)**, obturator oblique **(B)**, and iliac oblique **(C)** views of the pelvis of a patient with pelvic dissociation.

nonsupportive and deficient. In the worst-case scenario, this deficiency occurs in conjunction with pelvic dissociation in which the connection between the ilium and the ischium is disrupted.[6] The incidence of such acetabular destruction is low and most of the literature consists of case reports or small studies. Berry and associates[1] identified this condition in 31 of 3,505 consecutive acetabular revisions. Identified risk factors for pelvic dissociation are female gender, massive pelvic bone loss, and rheumatoid arthritis.

Diagnosis and Radiologic Investigations

Plain Radiographs and Special Views

Because pelvic dissociation is often associated with osteolysis, any investigation for pelvic discontinuity also should have a high predictive value for pelvic osteolysis. In 1999, using computer simulations and cadaver studies, Southwell and associates[7] reported that three radiographic views—the AP view, 45° iliac oblique view, and 60° obturator oblique view—were optimal for accurately assessing pelvic osteolysis. With the AP view alone, linear osteolysis (3 mm or more deep) would be obscured in more than 83% of the cup surface. With two views, 30% to 50% of the cup surface would be obscured. However, with three views, only 7% of the cup surface would be obscured. This assumes that the cup is not severely displaced in a medial direction, which could potentially obscure the posterior column regardless of the radiographic view. Once the degree and location of osteolysis has been determined, signs of pelvic dissociation should be evaluated. These include (1) a visible transverse acetabular fracture on AP, Judet obturator oblique, or iliac oblique pelvic radiographs (Figure 1); (2) medial offset of the inferior pelvis relative to the superior pelvis as seen by a break in the Köhler line (Figure 2); and (3) rotation of the inferior versus superior hemipelvis seen as asymmetry of the obturator rings on a true AP pelvic radiograph.[1] Because radiodense implants and cement can obscure pelvic dissociation on radiographs, not all cases can be diagnosed preoperatively with radiographs, and a high index of suspicion should remain so that such missed cases can be diagnosed intraoperatively. CT scanning is another imaging option to aid in the diagnosis.

CT Scans

The difficulty with observing and underestimating the presence of osteolytic lesions with plain radiographs have led some physicians to advocate CT to evaluate these lesions.[4,8,9] With advances in technology and the development of helical multidetector CT scanners, image quality has greatly improved. The helical CT scanner obtains images in a continuous fashion and has a shorter image acquisition time. Sequential images of the osteolytic lesions can provide volumetric measurements and the shorter scan time decreases the motion artifact. This provides precise information about the lesions located in the ilium, acetabular roof, medial wall, anterior column, posterior column, ischium, or pubic ramus. In patients with significant protrusio, preoperative CT angiography may be required to show the anatomic position of the iliac vessels and other important structures within the pelvis.

Classification and Decision Making

In its classification of acetabular bone loss, the American Academy of Orthopaedic Surgeons (AAOS) defined pelvic dissociation as a type IV deficiency[10] (Table 1). Berry and associates[1] subclassified the degree of bone loss associated with pelvic dissociation as type IVa if the dissociation is associated with cavitary (type II) or mild segmental (type I) bone loss, type IVb if the dissociation is associated with a large segmental (type I) or a combined (type III) defect, and type IVc if the pelvis had been previously irradiated regardless of the presence of cavitary or segmental bone loss.

The treatment of pelvic dissociation requires a full understanding of not only the presence of the fracture but also the degree of bone loss. Preoperatively, the Paprosky classification of bone loss can be used to better plan the equipment and implants required for surgery.[11] This system is based on the severity of bone loss and the ability to support cementless fixation. It is important to assess four radiographic criteria: (1) superior migration of the hip center, (2) ischial osteolysis, (3) teardrop osteolysis, and (4) the position of the implant relative to the Köhler line. Type I and II defects indicate mild to moderate bone loss, and reconstruction is generally straightforward.

With a type IIIa defect, adequate host bone is available and in contact with the ingrowth surface to obtain durable biologic fixation. Preoperative radiographs will show superior and lateral migration of the component more than 3 cm above the obturator line. Ischial lysis will be mild to moderate, extending less than 15 mm inferior to the obturator line. The teardrop will be partially destroyed; however, the medial limb of the teardrop will generally be present. The component will be at or lateral to the Köhler line, and the ilioischial and iliopubic lines will be intact. Pelvic dissociation rarely occurs in type IIIa defects.

In a type IIIb defect, there is less than 40% host bone remaining in contact with the ingrowth surface. The rim defect is greater than 50% of the circumference, usually from the 9 o'clock to 5 o'clock positions. Preoperative radiographs show more extensive ischial osteolysis (> 15 mm below the superior obturator line), complete destruction of the teardrop, migration medial to the Köhler line, and more than 3 cm of superior migration to the obturator line. The failed component migrates superiorly and medially in the type IIIb defect compared with the type IIIa defect in which the migration is superior and lateral. Patients with type IIIb defects are at high risk for occult pelvic dissociation.[11] This condition may be associated with scarring of vital structures, such as the femoral vessels, femoral nerve, ureter, and bowel.

Table 1
Classification of Acetabular Deficiencies

Type I	Segmental deficiencies Peripheral Superior Anterior Posterior Central (medial wall absent)
Type II	Cavitary deficiencies Peripheral Superior Anterior Posterior Central (medial wall intact)
Type III	Combined deficiencies
Type IV	Pelvic discontinuity
Type V	Arthrodesis

(Reproduced with permission from D'Antonio JA, Capello WN, Borden LS, et al: Classification and management of acetabular abnormalities in total hip arthroplasty. *Clin Orthop Relat Res* 1989;243:123-137.)

Intraoperatively, once the acetabulum is fully exposed, the anterior and posterior columns are compressed with a Cobb elevator and motion between the superior and inferior hemipelvis is assessed. Important intraoperative findings include the amount of host bone present, the location of structural defects, and the location of the dissociation.

Surgical Treatment

Goals

Surgical goals include pain relief and restoration of ambulatory status in patients who are suitable candidates for surgery. Successful treatment achieves initial stability of the socket, establishes conditions for long-term stability of the socket, stabilizes the pelvic dissociation, and produces conditions favorable for healing.[1]

Treatment Algorithm

If a trial component has partial inherent stability, there is generally enough contact with host bone to support ingrowth and the defect is type IIIa.[12] Options for reconstruction include a structural distal femoral graft with a cementless hemispherical cup, a modular highly porous metal component (such as the Trabecular Metal cup [Zimmer, Warsaw, IN]) augment with a hemispherical cup, or a high hip center hemispherical cup. When there is no inherent stability of the hemispherical trial component, the defect is type IIIb. Treatment options for these defects include augments and pelvic reconstruction plates (posterior and/or anterior). If there is not enough room for a posterior reconstruction plate, a cup-cage construct with or without an allograft can be used.

Principles of Treatment

Guiding principles for the treatment of pelvic dissociation include identifying the condition, stabilizing or effectively bypassing the dissociation, bone grafting at the site of the discontinuity, treating any associated bone loss, and placing a stable acetabular implant.[1] Once pelvic dissociation is detected, the posterior column and wall should be evaluated first. If there is sufficient wall and column, a posterior pelvic reconstruction plate into the ilium and ischium will stabilize the dissociation in most patients. Occasionally, if there is adequate space, a second plate may be applied. In selected cases, under image guidance, the use of an anterior column fixation screw may be feasible. Alternatively, plating of the anterior column can be used. The residual bone loss is then reevaluated; possible treatment options include a hemispherical socket or highly porous metal socket and augment. If there is not enough room for a posterior pelvic reconstruction plate, then a cup-cage construct with or without an allograft can be used as a reconstruction option.[13] Osseointegration of the implant provides secondary stability to the pelvic dissociation and effectively eliminates the instability, protecting the hardware from fracture. To achieve stability of the dissociated fragments, it may be necessary to intentionally distract them, placing the highly porous metal socket to act as a biointegrative bridge.

Results

Cementless Sockets

Reliable and durable fixation of cementless acetabular components requires an environment with adequate biologic potential and mechanical stability to allow bone ingrowth.[12] Sporer and Paprosky[12] reported on a 6-year follow-up study of 13 patients (13 hips) with type IIIb acetabular defects and an associated pelvic dissociation. A highly porous metal socket acetabular component with or without an augment was used to obtain fixation proximal and distal to the dissociation. At a mean follow-up of 2.6 years, two patients required the use of a walker, two required the use of a cane, and nine walked without support for more than six blocks. Eleven patients had no pain or mild pain, whereas two had moderate pain. Clinically, the modified Postel-Merle d'Aubigné score improved from 6.1 preoperatively to 10.3 postoperatively ($P < 0.05$). Radiographically, one patient had possible acetabular loosening secondary to screw breakage, despite being clinically asymptomatic. None of the remaining patients required any repeat surgery.

Acetabular Cages and Ring

When bone loss and instability preclude the use of a hemispherical cementless socket, another approach involves the use of reconstruction metal cages that distribute forces to a larger area to bypass areas of bone loss into which a cup is cemented (Figure 3).

Paprosky and associates[14] reported on 15 patients with 16 acetabular cage reconstructions at a mean follow-up of 5 years (range, 2 to 8 years). The presence of pelvic dissociation was based on intraoperative findings after removing any pseudomembrane and exposing the remaining host bone. There were two Paprosky type IIc defects, six type IIIa defects, and eight type IIIb defects. Posterior column plate fixation was used in 11 of 16 patients and structural allograft was used in 7 patients. Revision or resection occurred in 5 of 16 hips (31%) at intermediate-term follow-up. Four hips were revised for aseptic loosening including three fractured cages. The cage type did not correlate with the revision. More type IIIb defects (3 of 8) were associated with rerevision compared with type IIIa defects (1 of 6). Use of a plate and the type of allograft used did not seem to affect rerevision rates. Complications included one infection, four nerve palsies, and one dislocation. Study limitations included missing data, heterogeneity of the underlying diagnoses, the heterogeneity of the implants and/or allografts used, and the small number of patients studied. Despite these limitations, with a 31% revision rate and 44% rate of overall loosening, the authors concluded that acetabular cages in the setting of pelvic dissociation did not provide encouraging results at intermediate term follow-up.

Eggli and associates[15] reported the clinical outcome of seven patients with pelvic dissociation following revision THA after a mean follow-up of 96 months. Surgical treatment consisted of three consecutive steps beginning with mechanical stabilization of the two acetabular columns, followed by bony acetabular reconstruction (filling the osteolytic defect with allograft chips covered with autologous bone to achieve a contained defect after healing of the autograft), and anchorage of the cup using an acetabular reinforcement ring (five with a hook and two without a hook). A high complication rate was reported, including a partial ischial nerve lesion, one intraoperative femoral shaft fracture, and one recurrent dislocation. One patient had revision surgery after 12 months because of aseptic loosening; another patient required removal of two prominent screws.

Goodman and associates[13] reported the results of 61 acetabular revisions with ilioischial cages at 1 to 7 years showing an overall successful result in 76%; however, in patients with pelvic dissociation only 5 of 10 revisions (50%) were considered successful and 8 of 10 (80%) had complications.

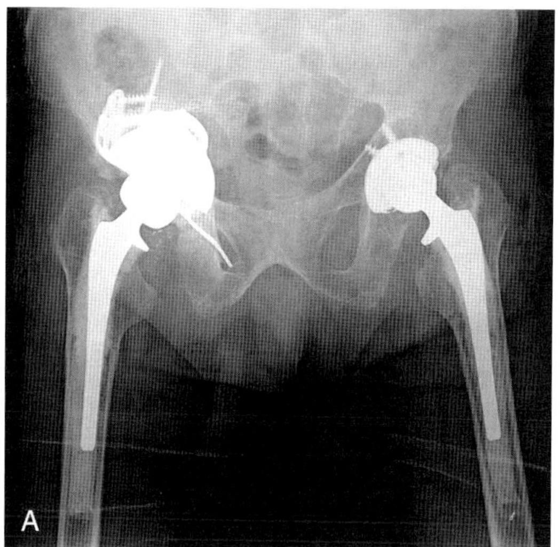

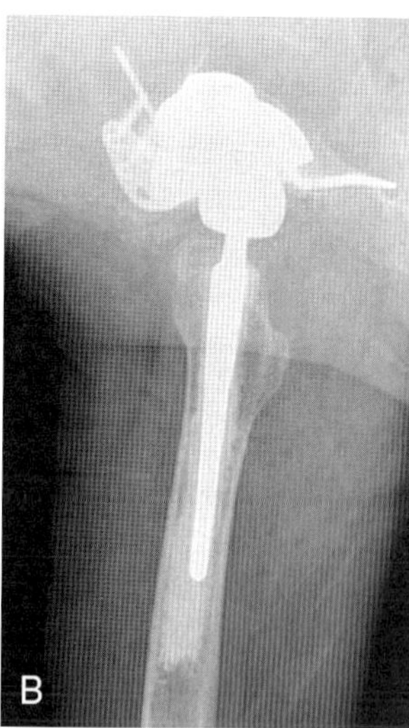

Figure 3 AP (**A**) and lateral (**B**) views showing 1-year postoperative radiographs of a pelvic dissociation treated with a cup-cage construct.

Custom Triflange Acetabular Prosthesis

A triflange cup provides another option for difficult acetabular reconstruction in a patient with pelvic dissociation and massive bone loss. It achieves stable implant fixation on host bone, reapproximates anatomic load bearing, and provides the potential for biologic fixation. DeBoer and associates[16] reported the results of 28 patients (30 hips) with failed THA and pelvic dissociation (most were type IVb). The prosthesis was custom manufactured on the basis of a three-dimensional model of the hemipelvis created with CT. The locations of the three flanges were identified by the surgeon on the ilium, ischium, and pubis; the center of rotation of the femoral head and orientation of the cup were then determined. Initial stability of the implant was provided with screw fixation, which was first placed in the ischial flange. The iliac flange was then fixed with screws that pulled the flange into intimate contact with bone, often reduced the dissociation, and rotated the caudad half of the hemipelvis into correct orientation relative to the cephalad aspect of the hemipelvis. Twenty hips in 18 patients were followed for a mean of 10 years (range, 7.4 to 13 years). Definite healing of the pelvic dissociation was indicated by the presence of bridging callus in 18 of the 20 hips. There were no broken screws and no implant migration, even when the discontinuity persisted. Small nonprogressive radiolucent lines were observed in six hips. Complications included one partial sciatic nerve palsy that resolved completely and one instance of loose ischial screws in a radiographically stable implant in the same patient. Five patients had one or more dislocations postoperatively. The mean Harris hip score improved from 41 points preoperatively to 80 points at the time of the latest follow-up (range, 7.4 to 13 years). Eleven patients required ambulatory aids postoperatively. No component was revised.

Structural Allografts

Bulk acetabular bone grafting has been used with bulk femoral heads with limited screw fixation as well as with whole acetabular allografts. Acetabular reamers are used to size the acetabular cavity and identify the location of the remaining bone to support the allograft. A pelvic recon-

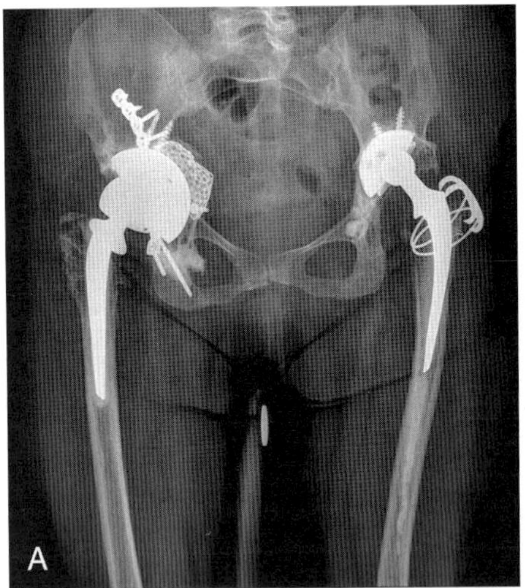

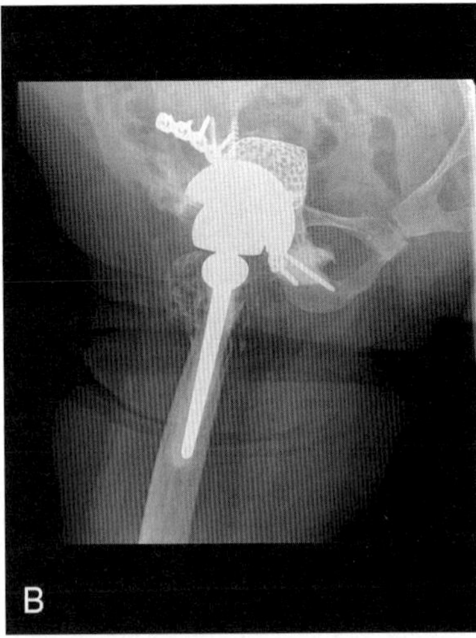

Figure 4 Two-year postoperative AP **(A)** and lateral **(B)** radiographs of a pelvic dissociation reconstructed with porous tantalum implant and posterior plating.

struction plate may be required to stabilize the posterior column as previously mentioned. A cage is recommended to protect allografts. Cage-host bone screws and cage-allograft bone screws achieve fixation. The inferior flange of the cage should be inserted into a slot in the ischium for fixation. Some cages have an inferior flange designed for screw fixation into ischium; however, because of complications associated with screws in the ischium, this technique is not preferred. A metal shell or a polyethylene liner is then cemented into the cage or allograft composite, avoiding the tendency to place the component in a vertical and retroverted position.

Type IIIb acetabular defects treated with an acetabular allograft and a cemented acetabular component have shown poor clinical results. Sporer and associates[11] reported on 16 patients at a minimum 8-year follow-up (mean follow-up, 10 years). Six hips were functioning without loosening, six were revised for aseptic loosening at an average of 2.9 years, and four hips showed radiographic loosening.

Stiehl and associates[6] reported on 17 patients with massive acetabular bone loss. Ten of these patients had a type IV pelvic dissociation, with nine having a type IVb deficiency and one having a type IVc deficiency. Bulk structural allograft was used in combination with posterior and/or anterior column plates. At follow-up (mean, 7 years postoperatively), 6 of 10 patients (60%) required rerevision surgery. Cementless cups that rested on a bulk allograft had high failure rates.

Highly Porous Metal Modular Implants With or Without Plating

Porous coated acetabular components provide effective long-term stability in the revision setting through biologic fixation to the host bone in addition to plating (Figure 4). Porous tantalum, with a high volumetric porosity (ranging from 70% to 80%) and low modulus of elasticity, has a propensity for bony ingrowth and biologic fixation.[17,18]

The acetabular defect is sized with acetabular reamers in the desired location to find the dimension of the cavity until two points of fixation are achieved (anterior to posterior, anteroinferior to posteroinferior, posterosuperior to anteroinferior). Augments are used to decrease acetabular volume and restore a rim to support a revision cup. The location and orientation of the augments are highly variable depending on the bone-loss pattern. Augments are often placed on the medial aspect of the ilium, or they may be stacked. It is more common to use the augments with the wide base placed laterally and the apex medially. The augments are initially secured to the host bone with the use of multiple screws. Portions of the augments may need to be removed with a burr to optimize the surface area contact between the revision shell and the augments. Multiple screw fixation is then used through the revision shell.[11]

Potential Complications

In addition to the risk of mechanical and biologic failure of the construct, serious complications related to these large-scale, difficult reconstructions include intraoperative fractures, recurrent dislocations, deep infections, injuries to the sciatic nerve, nonunions, and fixation failures. Delayed sciatic neuropathy following complex acetabular reconstruction for pelvic dissociation has been reported by Stiehl and Stewart.[19] Sciatic nerve exploration at 12 months postoperatively showed dense scar tissue directly over the plate as the nerve crossed the ischium. One pelvic plate screw had worked out approximately 3 mm and was directly pressing on the nerve. Substantial improvement in clinical symptoms resulted from screw removal and nerve release. Palmer and associates[20] reported a hip-vagina fistula in a 46-year-old woman who had multiple revision procedures complicated by infection after a primary THA that failed because of recurrent dislocation. The patient presented with a hip-vagina fistula 18 months after reconstruction of pelvic dissociation using an antiprotrusio cage. Radiographs showed a fracture of the cage with superomedial migration into the pelvis. The fistula was possibly formed by pressure necrosis from the failed acetabular cage against the intrapelvic vaginal wall. The patient was treated with a salvage procedure that included primary closure of the fistula with rotational muscle flaps, the use of an oversized bipolar acetabular component to avoid Girdlestone resection, and chronic bacterial suppression with antibiotics.

Summary

Pelvic dissociation following THA is a challenging condition requiring complex reconstructive procedures. Despite the technical feasibility of such revisions and the good clinical results, the main goal should be early recognition of acetabular loosening to minimize osteolytic loss of bone stock. Modular highly porous metal component revision systems have not been used long enough to provide definitive recommendations; however, early results from various centers are encouraging. For large defects in patients with pelvic dissociation, highly porous metal cups should be supported with either augments or a cage, when indicated, to improve initial mechanical stability and long-term biologic fixation.

References

1. Berry DJ, Lewallen DG, Hanssen AD, Cabanela ME: Pelvic discontinuity in revision total hip arthroplasty. *J Bone Joint Surg Am* 1999;81:1692-1702.
2. Harris WH: Wear and periprosthetic osteolysis: The problem. *Clin Orthop Relat Res* 2001;393:66-70.
3. Hozack WJ, Mesa JJ, Carey C, Rothman RH: Relationship between polyethylene wear, pelvic osteolysis, and clinical symptomatology in patients with cementless acetabular components: A framework for decision making. *J Arthroplasty* 1996;11:769-772.
4. Chiang PP, Burke DW, Freiberg AA, Rubash HE: Osteolysis of the pelvis: Evaluation and treatment. *Clin Orthop Relat Res* 2003;417:164-174.
5. Jacobs JJ, Roebuck KA, Archibeck M, Hallab NJ, Glant TT: Osteolysis: Basic science. *Clin Orthop Relat Res* 2001;393:71-77.
6. Stiehl JB, Saluja R, Diener T: Reconstruction of major column defects and pelvic discontinuity in revision total hip arthroplasty. *J Arthroplasty* 2000;15:849-857.
7. Southwell DG, Bechtold JE, Lew WD, Schmidt AH: Improving the detection of acetabular osteolysis using oblique radiographs. *J Bone Joint Surg Br* 1999;81:289-295.
8. Puri L, Wixson RL, Stern SH, Kohli J, Hendrix RW, Stulberg SD: Use of helical computed tomography for the assessment of acetabular osteolysis after total hip arthroplasty. *J Bone Joint Surg Am* 2002;84:609-614.
9. Stulberg SD, Wixson RL, Adams AD, Hendrix RW, Bernfield JB: Monitoring pelvic osteolysis following total hip replacement surgery: An algorithm for surveillance. *J Bone Joint Surg Am* 2002;84:116-122.
10. D'Antonio JA, Capello WN, Borden LS, et al: Classification and management of acetabular abnormalities in total hip arthroplasty. *Clin Orthop Relat Res* 1989;243 :126-137.
11. Sporer SM, O'Rourke M, Paprosky WG: The treatment of pelvic discontinuity during acetabular revision. *J Arthroplasty* 2005;20:79-84.
12. Sporer SM, Paprosky WG: Acetabular revision using a trabecular metal acetabular component for severe acetabular bone loss associated with a pelvic discontinuity. *J Arthroplasty* 2006;21:87-90.
13. Goodman S, Saastamoinen H, Shasha N, Gross A: Complications of ilioischial reconstruction rings in revision total hip arthroplasty. *J Arthroplasty* 2004;19:436-446.
14. Paprosky W, Sporer S, O'Rourke MR: The treatment of pelvic discontinuity with acetabular cages. *Clin Orthop Relat Res* 2006;453:183-187.
15. Eggli S, Müller C, Ganz R: Revision surgery in pelvic discontinuity: An analysis of seven patients. *Clin Orthop Relat Res* 2002;398:136-145.
16. DeBoer DK, Christie MJ, Brinson MF, Morrison JC: Revision total hip arthroplasty for pelvic discontinuity. *J Bone Joint Surg Am* 2007;89:835-840.
17. Levine B, Della Valle CJ, Jacobs JJ: Applications of porous tantalum in total hip arthroplasty. *J Am Acad Orthop Surg* 2006;14:646-655.
18. Weeden SH, Schmidt RH: The use of tantalum porous metal implants for Paprosky 3A and 3B defects. *J Arthroplasty* 2007;22:151-155.
19. Stiehl JB, Stewart WA: Late sciatic nerve entrapment following pelvic plate reconstruction in total hip arthroplasty. *J Arthroplasty* 1998;13:586-588.
20. Palmer SW, Luu HH, Finn HA: Hip-vagina fistula after acetabular revision. *J Arthroplasty* 2003;18:533-536.

Index

D

E

F

N

O

P

R

S

T

U

V

W

X

Z